Medicine and Social Justice

Medicine and Social Justice

Essays on the Distribution

of Health Care

Edited by

ROSAMOND RHODES

MARGARET P. BATTIN

ANITA SILVERS

OXFORD

UNIVERSITY PRESS

2002

OXFORD
UNIVERSITY PRESS

Oxford   New York
Auckland   Bangkok   Buenos Aires   Cape Town   Chennai
Dar es Salaam   Delhi   Hong Kong   Istanbul   Karachi   Kolkata
Kuala Lumpur   Madrid   Melbourne   Mexico City   Mumbai   Nairobi
São Paulo   Shanghai   Singapore   Taipei   Tokyo   Toronto

and an associated company in Berlin

Published by Oxford University Press, Inc.
198 Madison Avenue, New York, New York 10016
http://www.oup-usa.org

Library of Congress Cataloging-in-Publication Data

Medicine and social justice :
essays on the distribution of health care /
edited by Rosamond Rhodes,
Margaret P. Battin, Anita Silvers.
p. cm.
Includes bibliographical references and index.
ISBN 0-19-514354-X
1. Medical care—Social aspects.
2. Right to health care.
3. Social justice.
4. Medical ethics.
5. Medical economics—Moral and ethical aspects.
I. Rhodes, Rosamond.
II. Battin, M. Pabst.
III. Silvers, Anita.
RA445.M385 2002
362.1'042—dc21
2002022910

2 4 6 8 9 7 5 3 2 1

Printed in the United States of America
on acid-free paper

Preface

This ample and challenging set of essays—by philosophers, doctors, lawyers, bioethicists, political scientists, and economists—seeks to deepen our understanding of issues in social justice through a detailed examination of both theory and practice in health care. It asks big, difficult questions: What is justice? What is it for a health-care system to be just? Are some national health-care systems more just than others? What conditions of social justice—or injustice—in the background society affect issues of justice in health care, and how does this vary from one country to another? What choices and trade-offs made within health-care systems are just, and which ones are not? What requests from patients, seeking access to specific forms of health care, does justice require be answered—does their history matter, their prognosis, or the anguish of their desperation? What exactly is social justice, and what would it be for health care to be justly distributed across a society as a whole?

This volume serves two immediate purposes: It both explores a wide range of different approaches to the issues of justice in health care, and it also probes the connections between theoretical accounts of justice and observations of justice (and injustice) in practice. It does not impose a single way of looking at justice; rather, readers will be introduced to the repleteness of theory and the many ways that different approaches to theory frame the problems at hand, and they will be invited to observe how theory is used in practice and is itself changed as the conditions of practice demand.

The theoretical discussion of justice, in a sense, begins with Aristotle. Still definitive in this point, Aristotle defines "justice" as treating like cases alike, different cases differently. This is known as the "formal principle of justice," and it still holds in all of the specific forms of justice: *distributive* justice (how, in a situation of scarcity, things are parceled out among the parties who claim them), *retributive* justice (how those harmed respond to the party who caused the offense), *compensatory* justice (how to repair harms done to a party), *restorative* justice (how to return someone who has harmed another to the moral community), and so on. Although other spheres of justice play a role as well, distributive justice issues are central in a discussion of health-care justice because health systems virtually always operate under conditions of scarcity: How should providers parcel out care among patients who need or want it when there are not enough resources to satisfy everyone's needs and desires?

The term "social justice" refers to relationships between a society and the groups and individuals that comprise it. Social justice sets out what the society owes to its members and what individuals owe to the whole. Social justice can be opposed to the individual conception of justice, which explains what individuals owe to one another (e.g., a doctor to a patient, a parent to a child, neighbors to each other). Although the term "social justice" is used by various authors in widely different ways, it incorporates the various specific senses of justice, with particular emphasis on distributive justice in light of the immensely complex relationships within a society involving rights, opportunities, access to services, past deprivations, economic relationships, prejudice, and many other factors that create obligations within a society as a whole. Social justice is the ultimate goal of the various specific forms of justice as they might be practiced interactively, in concert, within a society as a whole.

Many discussions of health care and social justice are framed in terms of health and disease. "Health" is often defined as a condition that approximates normal species function. Basing decisions about the allocation of health-care resources on the concept of health makes allocation decisions turn on whether or not to classify some condition as an illness or a disease: Resources are provided only for cure or amelioration of disease. Despite the prominence of this line of argument, health may not be the single appropriate standard for designing a health-care system because, as others argue, it is hard to make sense of the notion of "a right to health" and because the illusive ideal of health may not be the best standard for assessing the justice of a system. Also, the skills and knowledge of medicine are typically called upon to address conditions that are not directly related to disease (e.g., abortion service, genetic counseling, plastic surgery). In that sense, the domain of medicine goes beyond health. Moreover, the concept of "health care" goes still further by including services such as immunization, ambulette transportation, and care for caregivers. Chapters in this volume employ all of these concepts and debate whether to funnel the dialogue through one concept rather than the other.

Four groupings of chapters address these issues. Those in Part I address underlying theoretical issues about the nature and requirements of justice. Some of these chapters draw on John Rawls's influential theory of justice, a theory that, particularly in the application by Norman Daniels, has shaped much of contemporary thinking about justice in health care. In Chapter 1, Daniels emphasizes the importance of health in equalizing people's abilities to pursue opportunities in the world; he also develops the "life span" approach to justice in health care, according to which the young, the middle-aged, and the old are not seen as groups in competition for scarce health resources, but persons at different stages of their lives. Other chapters in this section falling within the Rawlsian framework focus on different ways in which health care can contribute to justice. Still other chapters are non-Rawlsian in their conception of justice and their views of justice in health care. The chapters in Part I, sometimes in agreement and sometimes in tension with one another, explore and expand the deepest roots of the issues.

Part II deals with a variety of issues concerning whether specific national health systems are just, examining those of the United States, the United Kingdom, Australia, Italy, the Scandinavian countries, and the relationship of economically developed nations to the developing world. Many of these chapters point to dilemmas and inadequacies in the systems they examine, and to failures to reach or even to approximate justice in the distribution of health-care resources; others identify policies and practices that do approach a condition of genuine justice in health care. It is this section that begins to show the realities of putting into practice the theoretical considerations explored in Part I, as well as the magnitude of the obstacles—economic, political, and ideological—to the accomplishment of justice in actual health-care situations and systems.

The chapters in Part III pose some of the hardest challenges concerning justice in health care; they consider the claims and needs of disadvantaged groups, including racial minorities, people with disabilities, women, children, the elderly, the poor, and other groups that are typically defined by social criteria—this often means prejudice—and not by health-care needs alone. This is where troubling practical questions arise: What do theories, and national health-care systems, say about these claims of people who are politically powerless or socially disadvantaged? Do the systems even recognize or appreciate their special needs? Do health-care systems deal with inequities of influence, do they acknowledge them with hollow rhetoric, do they address long histories of unfairness and maldistribution? Many of the chapters in Part III deal with social problems that can be traced to painful group experiences of denial and deprivation and to frustration with the limitations of health-care systems. The issues they raise are shaped by a profound sense of human need in matters of health care and by recognition of the difficulty of responding to social differences in a way that is just to all parties concerned.

Finally, Part IV explores serious challenges in assessment and priority-setting for health-care policy design. Those who actually make the hard choices involved in preferring one set of claims to another when there is not enough care to go around have to address the details that can be ignored on the theoretical level. They have to make decisions on the allocation of medical resources between individuals (e.g., who gets the liver?) and on which treatments and procedures to support or deny (e.g., drugs for schizophrenia or acupuncture). The chapters in Part IV address the range of bias that can infect policy decisions. They also deal with the fundamental issue of whether a just system should focus on efficiency by trying to make the greatest difference with limited resources or on equality of outcomes by prioritizing health care for those who are worse off than others. Furthermore, health-care systems have to take a position on the legitimacy of weighing individual needs against desires—should only health needs be considered in allocation or should issues that are profoundly important to many people (e.g., assisted reproduction, care for seriously compromised newborns) be funded even when health per se is not involved? Many of the chapters in Part IV involve practical explorations of the theoretical issues already addressed in Part I; the chapters in this fourth and culminating section of the text exhibit the challenging dilemmas that remain in designing a just health-care system.

Whereas the following chapters have been organized into these four parts, many of them are complex and deal with multiple issues; some could have been appropriately placed within more than one section of the text. Similarly, the disciplinary concerns of the contributors overlap considerably: Some contributors are involved in policy consultations, some in bedside treatment decisions, some in academic discussion, and some in legal proceedings, but many of them are involved in all of these domains. The introduction to each section of the text provides a more detailed guide to the chapters within it, but all are concerned with a range of deeply troubling and profoundly important issues—the issues of justice in health care—in contemporary societies. All are also concerned with sharpening and refining our conception of justice. Taken together, the chapters in this volume enrich our understanding of the concept of justice and what a just health-care system should be.

R. R.
M. P. B.
A. S.

Contents

Contributors, xiii

I THEORETICAL FOUNDATIONS

1. Justice, Health, and Health Care, 6
   Norman Daniels
2. Justice and the Basic Structure of Health-Care Systems, 24
   Paul T. Menzel
3. Multiculturalism and Just Health Care: Taking Pluralism Seriously, 38
   Jeffrey Blustein
4. Utilitarian Approaches to Justice in Health Care, 53
   Matti Häyry
5. Aggregation and the Moral Relevance of Context in
   Health-Care Decision Making, 65
   David Wasserman
6. Why There Is No Right to Health Care, 78
   Bernard H. Baumrin
7. Specifying the Content of the Human Right to Health Care, 84
   Kristen Hessler and Allen Buchanan

II RATIONING AND ACCESS IN TODAY'S WORLD

8. Unequal by Design: Health Care, Distributive Justice, and the American
   Political Process, 102
   Bruce C. Vladeck and Eliot Fishman

9. Health-Care Justice and Agency, 121
   Patricia S. Mann

10. Treatment According to Need: Justice and the British
    National Health Service, 134
    Roger Crisp

11. Rationing Decisions: Integrating Cost-Effectiveness with Other Values, 144
    Tony Hope, John Reynolds, and Siân Griffiths

12. Resources and Rights: Court Decisions in the United Kingdom, 156
    Richard H.S. Tur

13. Justice and the Social Reality of Health: The Case of Australia, 169
    Mark Sheehan and Peter Sheehan

14. Justice for All? The Scandinavian Approach, 183
    Tuija Takala

15. Ethics, Politics, and Priorities in the Italian Health-Care System, 191
    Giovanna Ruberto

16. Philosophical Reflections on Clinical Trials in Developing Countries, 197
    Baruch A. Brody

III SPECIAL NEEDS OF SOCIAL GROUPS

17. Racial Groups, Distrust, and the Distribution of Health Care, 212
    Howard McGary

18. Gender Justice in the Health-Care System: Past Experiences, Present
    Realities, and Future Hopes, 224
    Rosemarie Tong and Nancy Williams

19. Bedside Justice and Disability: Personalizing Judgment,
    Preserving Impartiality, 235
    Anita Silvers

20. The Medical, the Mental, and the Dental: Vicissitudes of
    Stigma and Compassion, 248
    Michael Teitleman

21. Children's Right to Health Care: A Modest Proposal, 259
    Loretta M. Kopelman

22. Age Rationing Under Conditions of Injustice, 270
    Leslie Pickering Francis

23. Just Expectations: Family Caregivers, Practical Identities, and Social Justice
    in the Provision of Health Care, 278
    James Lindemann Nelson

24. Caring for the Vulnerable by Caring for the Caregiver: The Case of
    Mental Retardation, 290
    Eva Feder Kittay

25. Justice, Health, and the Price of Poverty, 301
    Patricia Smith

IV DILEMMAS FOR MEDICINE AND HEALTH-CARE SYSTEMS: ASSESSMENT AND PRIORITIES

26. Alternative Health Care: Limits of Science and Boundaries of Access, 319
    E. Haavi Morreim

27. Justice in Transplant Organ Allocation, 345
    Rosamond Rhodes

28. Priority to the Worse Off in Health-Care Resource Prioritization, 362
    Dan W. Brock

29. Whether to Discontinue *Non*futile Use of a Scarce Resource, 373
    F.M. Kamm

30. Disability, Justice, and Health-Systems Performance Assessment, 390
    Jerome E. Bickenbach

31. Responsibility for Health Status, 405
    Lance K. Stell

32. Does Distributive Justice Require Universal Access to Assisted Reproduction? 426
    Mary Anne Warren

33. Premature and Compromised Neonates, 438
    Ian R. Holzman

34. Just Caring: Do Future Possible Children Have a Just Claim to a Sufficiently Healthy Genome? 446
    Leonard M. Fleck

Index, 459

Contributors

MARGARET P. BATTIN, PH.D.
Department of Philosophy and Division of Medical Ethics
University of Utah
Salt Lake City, Utah

BERNARD H. BAUMRIN, PH.D., J.D.
Department of Philosophy
Graduate Center and Lehman College
City University of New York
New York, New York

JEROME E. BICKENBACH, PH.D., LL.B.
Department of Philosophy
Queen's University
Kingston, Ontario
Canada

JEFFREY BLUSTEIN, PH.D.
Department of Epidemiology and Social Medicine
Division of Bioethics
Albert Einstein College of Medicine/Montefiore Medical Center
Bronx, New York

DAN W. BROCK, PH.D.
Department of Philosophy and Medical School
Brown University
Providence, Rhode Island

BARUCH A. BRODY, PH.D.
Center for Medical Ethics and Health Policy
Baylor College of Medicine
Houston, Texas

ALLEN BUCHANAN, PH.D.
Department of Philosophy
University of Arizona
Tucson, Arizona

ROGER CRISP, B.PHIL., M.A., D.PHIL.
St Anne's College, Oxford
Oxford, England
United Kingdom

NORMAN DANIELS, PH.D.
Department of Philosophy
Tufts University
Medford, Massachusetts

ELIOT FISHMAN, PH.D.
Institute for Medicare Practice
Mount Sinai School of Medicine
New York, New York

LEONARD M. FLECK, PH.D.
Department of Philosophy and Center for Ethics and Humanities in the Life Sciences
Michigan State University
East Lansing, Michigan

LESLIE PICKERING FRANCIS, PH.D., J.D.
Department of Philosophy, School of Law, and Division of Medical Ethics
University of Utah
Salt Lake City, Utah

SIÂN GRIFFITHS
Directorate of Public Health and Health Policy Oxfordshire Health Authority
Oxford, England
United Kingdom

MATTI HÄYRY, B.A., M.A., M.SC, LIC.SC., D.SC.
Centre for Professional Ethics and Department of Philosophy
University of Central Lancashire
Preston, England
United Kingdom

KRISTEN HESSLER, PH.D.
Department of Philosophy
Iowa State University
Ames, Iowa

IAN R. HOLZMAN, M.D.
Department of Pediatrics
Division of Newborn Medicine

Mount Sinai School of Medicine
New York, New York

TONY HOPE, M.A., PH.D., MB., BCH., FRCPSYCH
Professor of Medical Ethics and Director of Ethox Institute of Health Sciences
University of Oxford
Oxford, England
United Kingdom

F.M. KAMM, PH.D.
Department of Philosophy
New York University
New York, New York

EVA FEDER KITTAY, PH.D.
Department of Philosophy
State University of New York at Stony Brook
Stony Brook, New York

LORETTA M. KOPELMAN, PH.D.
Department of Medical Humanities
Brody School of Medicine at East Carolina University
Greenville, North Carolina

PATRICIA S. MANN, PH.D.
Department of Philosophy
Temple University
Philadelphia, Pennsylvania

HOWARD McGARY, PH.D
Department of Philosophy
Rutgers, The State University of New Jersey
New Brunswick, New Jersey

PAUL T. MENZEL, PH.D.
Department of Philosophy
Pacific Lutheran University
Tacoma, Washington

E. HAAVI MORREIM, PH.D.
College of Medicine
University of Tennessee
Memphis, Tennessee

JAMES LINDEMANN NELSON, PH.D.
Department of Philosophy and Center for Ethics and Humanities in the Life Sciences
Michigan State University
East Lansing, Michigan

JOHN REYNOLDS
Department of Clinical Pharmacology
John Radcliffe Hospital
Oxford, England
United Kingdom

ROSAMOND RHODES, PH.D.
Department of Medical Education
Mount Sinai School of Medicine
New York, New York

GIOVANNA RUBERTO, M.D.
Immunology and Bioethics
Dipartimento di Medicina Interna ed Oncologia
Università di Pavia
Pavia, Italy

MARK SHEEHAN
Department of Philosophy
Keele University
Straffordshire, England
United Kingdom

PETER SHEEHAN, PH.D.
Centre for Strategic Economic Studies
Victoria University
Melbourne, Australia

ANITA SILVERS, PH.D.
Philosophy Department
San Francisco State University
San Francisco, California

PATRICIA SMITH, PH.D.
Department of Philosophy
Graduate Center and Bernard Baruch College
City University of New York
New York, New York

LANCE K. STELL, PH.D., FACFE
Department of Philosophy and Program in Medical Humanities
Davidson College
Davidson, North Carolina

TUIJA TAKALA, PH.D.
Research Fellow
Department of Practical Philosophy
University of Helsinki
Helsinki, Finland

MICHAEL TEITLEMAN, PH.D., M.D.
New York, New York

ROSEMARIE TONG, PH.D.
Center for Professional and Applied Ethics
University of North Carolina
Charlotte, North Carolina

RICHARD H.S. TUR, M.A., LL.B.
Benn Fellow and Senior Law Tutor
Oriel College, Oxford

Oxford, England
United Kingdom

BRUCE VLADECK, PH.D.
Institute for Medicare Practice
Mount Sinai School of Medicine
New York, New York

MARY ANNE WARREN, PH.D.
Philosophy Department
San Francisco State University
San Francisco, California

DAVID WASSERMAN, J.D.
Department of Philosophy
University of Maryland, College Park
College Park, Maryland

NANCY WILLIAMS
Department of Philosophy
University of Georgia
Atlanta, Georgia

I
THEORETICAL FOUNDATIONS

Justice, said Aristotle, involves treating like cases alike and different cases differently. This formal principle of justice would be easy to satisfy if it were possible to tell which cases are alike and which cases are different, and if, when distributive questions arose, enough resources were available in every situation so that everyone who needs or wants something could have it. But it is not so, and the real challenges of theories of distributive justice involve showing how the merely formal demands of the Aristotelian principle are to be met in cases of scarcity—whether that scarcity is real or the result of various policy constraints.

What counts as justice in medicine, or in health care more generally? Are "like cases alike" when two people have the same illness? Or have the same prognosis? Or when they are the same age, or are in the same social situation, or have suffered the same past deprivation, or have made the same social contributions, or are the same in other specific respects? The chapters in this section seek not only to resolve the basic issues in theories of justice as they apply to health care but also to examine the appropriateness of various sorts of conceptual machinery for applying these theories to practical dilemmas.

In "Justice, Health, and Health Care," the first of the theoretical selections in Part I, Norman Daniels provides a succinct but comprehensive statement of his well-known theory of justice in health care, now expanded to examine three basic questions: First, is health care special, different from other goods? Second, when are inequalities in health—not simply health care, but health itself—unjust? And third, can there be a fair process for making rationing decisions? Daniels's theory of justice in health care is developed as an application of John Rawls's theory of justice to the special circumstances of health care, an issue Rawls did not address. Daniels's theory holds that health—and hence health care—is important because it affects the range of opportunities in life that are open to a person—

offices, employments, relationships, aesthetic capabilities, political roles, even the capacity to think. Thus, health care can affect virtually every area of human experience and activity: If poorer health care means poorer health, it may also mean poorer experience in every aspect of human existence. Hence, health care is not just one among many things that are good, but something of central, crucial importance.

Recent empirical work shows, however, that people's level of health is correlated not only with the level of health care they receive, but strongly associated with the characteristics of their social environment. Does this mean that health care is unimportant, or that concerns of justice in health care are no longer pressing? To answer this challenge, Daniels expands upon his celebrated theory and shows how justice is good for health and also how health is good for justice.

Paul Menzel, in "Justice and the Basic Structure of Health-Care Systems," explores what have been assumed to be basic, irreconcilable conflicts between different types of health-care systems—specifically, between the basic liberties of individual choice and responsibility on the one hand, and the basic goals of cost-efficiency and equity on the other. What would make one form of health-care system more just than another? More freedom to choose? More equality in care or outcome? Or what? Menzel tries to reconcile what is commonly believed to be a basic conflict between egalitarian social-welfare systems, which tax richer persons to pay for the health care of poorer persons and impose some restrictions, like cost constraints, on the liberty of all, versus, in contrast, free-market systems in which health care is treated much more like other consumer goods: Those who can pay can get excellent health care, and those who cannot pay go without or rely on minimally funded public or charity care. This tension between egalitarian and free-market values, Menzel believes, can be reduced. He shows how to do so by taking careful account of five considerations: what a free-rider would actually choose if forced to make choices; what is involved when a patient's prior consent is accurately presumed; what is at stake in personal integrity and whether a person ought to be held to the later implications of personal choices he or she has made at an earlier time; equal opportunity for welfare; and a secondary principle of a just sharing of financial burdens between well and ill individuals.

Jeffrey Blustein raises another question about reconciling diverse values to further justice in health care. In Chapter 3 he examines the views of Tristram Engelhardt, Norman Daniels, and Ezekiel Emanuel on the issue of what conception of justice is appropriate for a pluralistic or multicultural society. Blustein's objective is a political conception of justice that can secure allegiance from diverse people with different ideas of the good, of disease and disability, and of the moral importance of health care.

Matti Häyry's account of "Utilitarian Approaches to Justice in Health Care" examines the assumption that the goal of a just health-care system ought to be the "greatest good for the greatest number," the utilitarian ideal. The challenge of achieving the greatest good for the greatest number is particularly great under conditions of scarcity, as all actual systems are. Häyry acknowledges that, in many respects, actual health-care systems are utilitarian in character, weighing benefits to some people against benefits to others and trying to achieve the fairest balance between them, but he seeks to explore a broad range of issues this situation presents. To do so, he examines the use of *quality-adjusted life-years,* or QALYs, as a measurement model intended to approximate the utilitarian paradigm. To show the problems thus raised, Häyry considers various paradoxes, like John Harris's utilitarian paradox: If a number of people need various transplant organs and will die without them, why not find a single person who would be a perfect match as a donor for all, and simply kill him to harvest his

organs? After all, one person would die, but many other people would be saved. Häyry concludes that standard utilitarianism cannot yield an adequate theory of justice in health care, but—insisting that the greatest happiness of the greatest number is still a laudable ideal—defends a skeptical utilitarian approach.

Part I continues with a discussion that addresses both utilitarian and non-utilitarian, non-consequentialist approaches to justice in health care. In Chapter 5, "Aggregation and the Moral Relevance of Context in Health-Care Decision Making," David Wasserman focuses on dilemmas of "tragic choices," namely whom to save when one cannot save all. These dilemmas have often been framed as distributive choices among individuals in situations of scarcity—for example, choosing between two patients in an emergency room, both of whom will die without a respirator, when only one respirator is available—but Wasserman expands the discussion to focus on "tragic choices" made by institutions and governments about allocating health-care resources among different groups of prospective patients. He observes that different distributional rules are thought to apply in "macro" contexts and in the standard "micro" contexts of bioethics, particularly in rules concerning trade-offs between a small number of great harms, such as the loss of life, and a larger number of lesser harms, such as the loss of a limb. Yet the differences between the two contexts are poorly defined and the justification for different rules is rarely articulated. Wasserman examines three possible differences among these contexts—the imminence of the harm, the social or institutional role of the decision maker, and the identifiability of the claimants—and offers several explanations of their moral relevance. Although he does not claim to have resolved the issue, Wasserman's exploration presents serious challenges to any account of justice in health care.

The final two chapters in Part I consider whether there is a right to health care. In

Chapter 6, "Why There Is No Right to Health Care," Bernard Baumrin applies the conceptually important distinction between negative and positive rights in an analysis of the purported right. Negative rights, also called "liberty rights," are rights not to be interfered with in doing something you want to do or impeded in acquiring something you want to possess: the right to do or to have something if you can do it or obtain it yourself, or if you have found someone willing to assist you or to provide it to you. Positive rights, in contrast—also called "claim rights"—are rights to be provided with something. Baumrin considers whether health care is a right in either of these senses, and if so whether it could be the product of contract, oath, legislation, or simple expectation. He also considers what a right to health care, if there were such, might cover. Here, he constructs three lists of services, one covering minimal emergency and acute care and control of epidemic disease, a second also including chronic and reconstructive care, and a third including all of those plus well care, dental care, and nutrition. Baumrin argues that there is no general right to health care, despite broad expectations, and that this issue will be "the main social battlefield of the 21st century."

The final chapter of Part I, which explores the question of whether there is a right to health care, takes a somewhat different view. In "Specifying the Content of the Human Right to Health Care," Kristen Hessler and Allen Buchanan address this question by identifying two distinct trends in the discussion of this issue—one of which, they argue, is on the mark, the other misguided. The one they find praiseworthy is the increasingly broad approach to the issue of justice in health care, discussed by Norman Daniels earlier in this section, in which the social determinants of health are included. What they find misguided is a range of attempts to analyze the precise content of the alleged "right to health" by specifying what levels and sorts of health care a person is entitled to. Thus, any attempt to specify a "decent minimum" of components of reproductive-health care or mental-health care, for example (much the sort of list the preceding chapter by Baumrin had constructed)—the specific sorts of services a person should expect to receive— is, they believe, defective. They point out that a "right to health" as distinct from a "right to health care" would be impossibly expensive and ultimately unattainable (after all, all patients eventually die, and so cannot have been guaranteed an open-ended right to health). Hessler and Buchanan's argument reviews several accounts of rights to health care in the recent literature; all of them are found wanting. Instead, they suggest that we should think of "rights" to health care not as a foundation of justice in health care, but as established— that is, created—by the political process, especially by the procedures of a democratic state. We should thus look to the realities of human experience and political decision making, rather than to ideals of moral principle, to ascertain "rights" to health care.

1

Justice, Health, and Health Care

Norman Daniels

THREE QUESTIONS OF JUSTICE

A theory of justice for health and health care should help us answer three central questions. First, is health care special? Is it morally important in ways that justify (and explain) the fact that many societies distribute health care more equally than many other social goods? Second, when are health inequalities unjust? After all, many socially controllable factors besides access to health care affect the levels of population health and the degree of health inequalities in a population. Third, how can we meet competing health-care needs fairly under reasonable resource constraints? General principles of justice that answer the first two questions do not, I argue, answer some important questions about rationing fairly. Is there instead a fair process for making rationing decisions?

About 20 years ago I answered the first question by claiming health care was special because of its impact on opportunity (Daniels, 1981, 1985). Specifically, the cen-

tral function of health care is to maintain normal functioning. Disease and disability, by impairing normal functioning, restrict the range of opportunities open to individuals. Health care thus makes a distinct but limited contribution to the protection of equality of opportunity. Though I construed health care broadly to include public health as well as individual preventive, acute, and chronic care, I ignored other factors that have a profound effect on population health. Unfortunately, focusing on just health care adds to the popular misconception that our vastly improved health in the last century is primarily the result of health care.

During the last 20 years a major literature has emerged exploring the social determinants of health. We have long known that, the richer that people are, the longer and healthier their lives. The powerful findings of the last several decades, however, have deepened our understanding of the factors at work producing these effects on population health and the distribution of health within populations. It is less tenable to believe that it is simply poverty and true deprivation that diminishes the health of some people, for there is growing evidence that the effects of race and class operate across a broad range of inequalities. Because social policies—not laws of human nature or economic development—are responsible for the social and economic inequalities that produce these health effects, we are forced to look upstream from the point of medical delivery and ask about the fairness of the distributions of these goods. John Rawls's theory of justice as fairness, quite serendipitously, contains principles that give a plausible account of the fair distribution of those determinants, thus providing an answer to the second question (Daniels et al., 1999, 2000).

During the 1980s, I became aware that my account of a just health-care system, like other general theories, failed to give specific guidance, or gave implausible answers, to certain questions about rationing (Daniels, 1993). Though philosophers may work out middle-level principles that can supplement general accounts of distributive justice and solve these unsolved rationing problems, it is unlikely that there will be consensus on them in the foreseeable future. Distributive issues remain highly contested.

In the absence of consensus on distributive principles, we need a fair process to establish legitimacy for critical resource allocation decisions. My account of fair process for addressing these distributive issues is called "accountability for reasonableness" (Daniels and Sabin, 1997, 1998a, 2002). It is an attempt to connect views about deliberative democracy to decision making at various institutional levels, whether public or private, in our complex health systems.

My goal in this chapter is to sketch the central ideas behind my approach to all three questions and to suggest how they all fit together. Detailed arguments can be found in the references. By pushing a theory of justice toward providing answers to all three questions, and not simply the first,

I hope to give a fuller demonstration that justice is good for our health.

WHAT IS THE SPECIAL MORAL IMPORTANCE OF HEALTH CARE?

For purposes of justice, the central moral importance of preventing and treating disease and disability with effective health-care services (construed broadly to include public health and environmental measures, as well as personal medical services) derives from the way in which protecting normal functioning contributes to protecting opportunity.[1] Specifically, by keeping people close to normal functioning, health care preserves for people the ability to participate in the political, social, and economic life of their society. It sustains them as fully participating citizens—normal collaborators and competitors—in all spheres of social life.

By maintaining normal functioning, health care protects an individual's fair share of the normal range of opportunities (or plans of life) that reasonable people would choose in a given society. This normal opportunity range is societally relative, depending on various facts about its level of technological development and social organization. Individuals' fair shares of that societal normal opportunity range are the plans of life it would be reasonable for them to choose were they not ill or disabled and were their talents and skills suitably protected against misdevelopment or underdevelopment as a result of unfair social practices and the consequences of socioeconomic inequalities. Individuals generally choose to develop only some of their talents and skills, effectively narrowing their range of opportunities. Maintaining normal functioning preserves, however, their broader, fair share of the normal opportunity range, giving them the chance to revise their plans of life over time.

This relationship between health care and the protection of opportunity suggests that the appropriate principle of distributive justice for regulating the design of a health-care system is a principle protecting equality of opportunity. Any theory of justice that supports a principle assuring equal opportunity (or giving priority to improving the opportunities of those who have the least opportunity) could thus be extended to health care. At the time I proposed this approach, the best defense of such a general principle was to be found in John Rawls's theory of justice as fairness (Rawls, 1971). One of the principles that Rawls's social contractors would choose is a principle assuring them *fair equality of opportunity* in access to jobs and offices. This principle not only prohibits discriminatory barriers to access, but requires positive social measures that correct for the negative effects on opportunity, including the underdevelopment of skills and talents, that derive from unfair social practices (e.g., a legacy of gender or race bias) or socioeconomic inequalities. Such positive measures would include among other things the provision of public education and other opportunity improving early childhood interventions.

Rawls, however, had deliberately simplified the formulation of his general theory of justice by assuming that people are fully functional over a normal life span. His social contractors thus represented people who suffered no disease or disability or premature death. By subsuming the protection of normal functioning under (a suitably adjusted version of) Rawls's principle assuring fair equality of opportunity, I showed how to drop that idealization and apply his theory to the real world (Rawls, 1993, supports this approach). In the last two decades, however, other work on egalitarianism has suggested alternative ways to connect health care to opportunity or to positive liberty or capabilities, and I shall comment on them shortly. First, I want to highlight some key elements of my approach.

The fair equality of opportunity account does not use the impact of disease or disability on welfare (desire satisfaction or happiness) or utility as a basis for thinking about distributive justice. One might have thought, for example, that what was special about health care was that good health was important for happiness. But illness and disability may not lead to unhappiness, even if they restrict the range of opportunities open to an individual. Intuitively, then, there is something attractive about locating the moral importance of meeting health-care needs in the more objective impact on opportunity than in the more subjective impact on happiness.

This analysis fits well with and extends Rawls's (1971) non-welfarist account of primary social goods. For purposes of justice, Rawls argued, we should not seek to determine what we owe each other by measuring our satisfaction or welfare, but we should measure our levels of well-being by publicly accessible measures. For Rawls this means an index of primary social goods that includes rights and liberties, powers and opportunity, income and wealth, and the social bases of self-respect. My account includes the protection of normal functioning within the scope of the primary good of opportunity. Drawing on insights from Scanlon's (1975) discussion of the "urgency" of meeting some "preferences" to relieve decrements in well-being but not others, my account explains why we believe we have obligations to assist others in meeting health-care needs but not necessarily to provide them with other things they say they need to make them happier.

Consider an actual issue where the contrast is important. People with long-standing disabilities will often rank their welfare higher than would other people who are merely imagining life with such disabilities. Perhaps people with disabilities accommodate by adjusting their goals and expectations. Even if they are more satisfied with their lives than people without disabilities might expect, there is an objective loss in their range of capabilities and opportunities, and that loss is captured by the appeal to a fair share of an opportunity range. The fair equality of opportunity account thus avoids a troubling feature that haunts cost-utility analysis and its treatment of such disabilities.[2]

Health care is of special moral importance because it helps to preserve our status as fully functioning citizens. By itself, however, this does not distinguish health care from food, shelter, and rest, which also meet the basic needs of citizens by preserving normal functioning. Because medical needs are more unequally distributed than these other needs and can be catastrophically expensive, they are appropriately seen as the object of private or social insurance schemes. It might be argued that we can finesse the problem of talking about the medical needs we owe it to each other to meet if we assure people fair income shares from which they can purchase such insurance. We cannot, however, define a minimal but fair income share unless it is capable of meeting such needs (Daniels, 1985).

Some economists and philosophers may object that giving special status to health insurance will be "paternalistic" and inefficient as some people prefer to trade income for things other than health care.[3] Our social obligation, however, is to provide institutions (such as social insurance or subsidies to buy private insurance) that protect opportunity, not to maximize aggregate welfare or achieve efficiency above all else. The principles of justice defended here thus depart from utilitarian goals.

The account sketched here has several implications for the design of our health-care institutions and for issues of resource allocation. Perhaps most important, the account supports the provision of universal access to appropriate health care—including traditional public health and preventive measures—through public or mixed public and private insurance schemes. Health care aimed at protecting fair equality of opportunity should not be distributed according to ability to pay, and the burden of payment should not fall disproportionately on those who are ill (Daniels, 1985, 1995; Daniels et al., 1996).

Properly designed universal coverage health systems will be constrained by reasonable budgets, for health care is not the only important good. Reasonable resource constraints will then require judgments about which medical needs are more important to meet than others. Both rationing and setting priorities are requirements of justice; this is because meeting health-care needs should not and need not be a bottomless pit.

The elderly might object that an opportunity-based account of a just system of health care will leave them out in the cold, for their opportunities might seem to be in the past. We can avoid this by not biasing our allocations in favor of one stage of life and instead considering the age-relative opportunity range. Still, treating people differently at different stages of life—for example, saving resources from one stage of life for use at another—does not produce inequalities across individuals in the way that differential treatment by race or gender does. We all age—though we do not change gender or race. Fairness among age groups in designing a health-care system is appropriately modeled by the idea of prudent allocation over a life span (Daniels, 1988). Under some conditions of scarcity, this implies that "pure" rationing by age (where age is not a proxy for other traits) is permissible.[4]

Some universal coverage health care systems permit a supplementary tier that is then purchased by those who are best off in society. For example, the British private insurance sector allows about 10% of the population to have quicker access to services that others must wait longer for in the British National Health Sevice. Other countries, such as Norway, prohibit a supplementary tier, fearing it will undermine the political solidarity needed to sustain their generous health-care system. The fair equality of opportunity account constrains, but does not rule out, all tiering (Daniels et al., 1996; Daniels, 1998a).

One controversial implication of my approach provides a way to contrast the fair equality of opportunity view with some alternative egalitarian accounts. In aiming at normal functioning, my approach views the prevention and treatment of disease and disability as the primary rationale for what we owe each other by way of assistance in cooperative health-care schemes (Buchanan et al., 2000). Enhancing otherwise normal conditions—even when they put us at a disadvantage compared to others through no fault of our own—is then viewed as "not medically necessary." For example, there is support in my view for the common insurance practice of covering treatment for very short children who have growth-hormone deficiencies but not covering it for equally short children who are otherwise normal.

The objection to my view is that this coverage policy seems to place too much weight on the presence of disease and disability and too little on what really should matter to an account aiming at protecting opportunity—namely, reducing the disadvantage that extreme shortness brings. This objection might be pressed by those who defend "equal opportunity for welfare or advantage" (Arneson, 1988; G.A. Cohen, 1989). Their view rests on claiming that anyone who suffers bad "brute luck"—a deficit in welfare or advantage that is no fault of their own—has a claim on others for assistance or compensation. In contrast, bad "option luck," the result of the choices we make or are responsible for making, does not give rise to claims on others. A disadvantage in talents or skills or even height that is not our fault thus provides a basis for claims on others for compensation or possibly enhancement. I argue (Daniels, 1990, 2000a) that this view gives too much centrality to choice or responsibility, a centrality we do not and should recognize when we want to protect our capilities as citizens in a democratic society; there are good policy objections to it as well (Sabin and Daniels, 1994).

A similar objection might be raised from a perspective grounded in the importance of positive liberty or freedom, thought of as our capability to do or be what we choose (Sen, 1980, 1992, 1999). The claim is that we should not necessarily be focused on a concept such as disease or disability but rather on whether individuals have the appropriate set of capabilities to do or be what they choose. Perhaps the very short child who is otherwise normal still lacks a key trait or capability that we should address.

If we consider more carefully, however, when differences in capabilities give rise to claims on others, support for treating the short but normal child may disappear. Sen (1992) himself notes that many differences in capabilities will be "incommensurable" as there will be no consensus about whether a person is worse off than others. The short but normal child, for example, may have an excellent temperament or wonderful social or cognitive skills. The cases where there is likely to be agreement that someone is clearly worse off in capabilities are likely to be captured by the categories of (serious) disease and disability. In practice, then, this view converges much more with the view I defend than it appears at first.[5]

These alternative views obviously deserve more careful discussion than I can offer here. Still, my answer to the original question, that the special moral importance of health care derives from the protection of our opportunities, remains a defensible member of a family of views connecting health care to our opportunities and capabilities. Moreover, its practical implications converge more with those of its cousins than is apparent from the family quarrels among them.

WHICH HEALTH INEQUALITIES ARE UNJUST?

Universal access to appropriate health care—health care that is just—does not break the link between social status and health that I noted earlier, a point driven home in studies of the effects on health inequality of the British National Health Service (Black et al., 1988; Acheson et al., 1998; Marmot et al., 1998) and confirmed by work in other countries as well (Kawachi et al., 1999). Our health is affected not simply by the ease with which we can see a doctor—though that surely matters—but also by our social position and the underlying inequality of our society. We cannot, of course, infer causation from these correlations between social inequality and health inequality (though later I explore some ideas about how the one might lead the other). Suffice to say that, although the exact processes are not fully understood, the evidence suggests that social determinants of health exist (Marmot, 1999).

If social factors play a large role in determining our health, then efforts to ensure greater justice in health outcomes should not focus simply on the traditional health sector. Health is produced not merely by having access to medical prevention and treatment, but also, to a measurably greater extent, by the cumulative experience of social conditions over the course of one's life. By the time a 60-year-old heart attack victim arrives at the emergency room, bodily insults have accumulated over a lifetime. For such a person, medical care is, figuratively speaking, "the ambulance waiting at the bottom of the cliff." Much contemporary discussion about reducing health inequalities by increasing access to medical care misses this point. Of course, we still want that ambulance there, but we should also be looking to improve social conditions that help to determine the health of societies.

As I noted earlier, Rawls's theory of justice as fairness was not designed to address issues of health care. Rawls assumed a completely healthy population, and he argued that a just society must assure people equal basic liberties, guarantee that the right of political participation has roughly equal value for all, provide a robust form of equal opportunity, and limit inequalities to those that benefit the least advantaged. When these requirements of justice are met, Rawls argued, we can have reasonable confidence that others are showing us the respect that is essential to our sense of self-worth. The fair terms of cooperation specified by these principles promote our social and political well-being.

The conjecture I explore is that by establishing equal liberties, robustly equal opportunity, a fair distribution of resources, and support for our self-respect—the basics of Rawlsian justice—we would go a long way in eliminating the most important injustices in health outcomes. To be sure, social justice is valuable for reasons other than its effects on health (or Rawls could not have set aside issues of health when arguing for justice as fairness). And social reform in the direction of greater justice would not eliminate the need to think hard about fair allocation of resources within the health-care system. Still, acting to promote social justice is a crucial step toward improving our health because there is this surprising convergence between what is needed for our social and political well being and for our mental and physical health.

To see the basis for this conjecture about Rawlsian principles, let us review very briefly some of the central findings in the recent literature on the social determinants of health. If we look at cross-national studies, we see that a country's prosperity is related to its health, as measured, for example, by life expectancy: In richer countries, people tend to live longer. But the relationship between per capita gross domestic product (GDPpc) and life expectancy levels off at about $8,000 to $10,000; beyond this threshold, further economic advance buys virtually no further gains in life expectancy. This leveling effect is most apparent among the advanced industrial economies. Nevertheless, even within this relationship, telling variations exist. Though Cuba and Iraq are equally poor (each has a GDPpc of about $3,100), life expectancy in Cuba exceeds that in Iraq by 17.2 years. The poor state of Kerala in India, which invested heavily in education, especially female literacy, has health outcomes far superior to the rest of India and more comparable to those in much wealthier countries. The difference between the GDPpc for Costa Rica and the United States is enormous (about $21,000), yet Costa Rica's life expectancy exceeds that of the United States (76.6 to 76.4 years).

Taken together, these observations show that the health of nations depends, in part, on factors other than wealth. Culture, social organization, and government policies also help determine population health. Variations in these factors—not fixed laws of economic development—may explain many of the differences in health outcomes among nations.

One especially important factor in explaining the health of a society is the distribution of income: The health of a population depends not just on the size of the economic pie, but on how the pie is shared. Differences in health outcomes among developed nations cannot be explained simply by the absolute deprivation associated with low economic development—lack of access to the basic material conditions necessary for health such as clean water, adequate nutrition and housing, and general sanitary living conditions. The degree of relative deprivation within a society also matters.

Numerous studies support this *relative-income hypothesis*, which states, more precisely, that inequality is strongly associated with population mortality and life expectancy across nations (Wilkinson, 1992, 1994, 1996). Rich countries vary in life expectancy, and that variation dovetails with income distribution. In particular, wealthier countries with more equal income distributions, such as Sweden and Japan, have higher life expectancies than does the United States, despite their having lower per capita GDP. Likewise, countries with low GDPpc but remarkably high life expectancy, such as Costa Rica, tend to have a more equitable distribution of income.

We find a similar pattern when we compare states within the United States. If we control for differences in state wealth, income inequality accounts for about 25% of the between-state variation in age-adjusted mortality rates (Kennedy et al., 1996, 1998b). Furthermore, a recent study across U.S. metropolitan areas found that regions with high income inequality had an excess of death compared to regions with low inequality—a very large excess, equivalent in magnitude to all deaths due to heart disease (Lynch et al., 1998). Longitudinal studies, which look at a single place over time and examine widening income differentials, support similar conclusions.

At the individual level, we also find that inequality is important. Numerous studies have documented what has come to be known as the "socioeconomic gradient": At each step along the economic ladder we see improved health outcomes over the rung below (including in societies with universal health insurance). Differences in health outcomes are not confined to the extremes of rich and poor; they are observed across all levels of socioeconomic status.

The slope of the socioeconomic gradient varies substantially across societies. Some societies show a relatively shallow gradient in mortality rates: Being better off confers a health advantage, but not so large an advantage as elsewhere. Others, with comparable or even higher levels of economic development, show much steeper gradients. The slope of the gradient appears to be fixed by the level of income inequality in a society: The more unequal a society is in economic terms, the more unequal it is in health terms. Moreover, middle-income groups in a country with high income inequality typically do worse in terms of health than comparable or even poorer groups in a society with less income inequality. We find the same pattern within the United States when we examine state and metropolitan area variations in inequality and health outcomes (Kennedy at al., 1998a; Lynch et al., 1998).

Earlier, I cautioned that correlations between inequality and health do not necessarily imply causation. Still, there are plausible and identifiable pathways through which social inequalities appear to produce

health inequalities to make a reasonable case for causation. In the United States, the states with the most unequal income distributions invest less in public education, have larger uninsured populations, and spend less on social safety nets (Kaplan et al., 1996; Kawachi and Kennedy, 1997). Studies of educational spending and educational outcomes are especially striking: Controlling for median income, income inequality explains about 40% of the variation between states in the percentage of children in the fourth grade who are below the basic reading level. Similarly strong associations are seen for high school dropout rates. It is evident from these data that educational opportunities for children in high income-inequality states are quite different from those in states with more egalitarian distributions. These effects on education have an immediate impact on health, increasing the likelihood of premature death during childhood and adolescence (as evidenced by the much higher death rates for infants and children in the high-inequality states). Later in life, they appear in the socioeconomic gradient in health.

When we compare countries, we also find that differential investment in human capital—in particular, education—is a strong predictor of health. Indeed, one of the strongest predictors of life expectancy among developing countries is adult literacy, particularly the disparity between male and female adult literacy, which explains much of the variation in health achievement among these countries after accounting for GDPpc. For example, among the 125 developing nations with a per capita GDP of less than $10,000, the difference between male and female literacy accounts for 40% of the variation in life expectancy (after factoring out the effect of GDPpc). In the United States, differences between the states in women's status—measured in terms of their economic autonomy and political participation—are strongly correlated with higher female mortality rates.

These societal mechanisms—for example, income inequality leading to educa-

tional inequality leading to health inequality—are tightly linked to the political processes that influence government policy. For instance, income inequality appears to affect health by undermining civil society. Income inequality erodes social cohesion, as measured by higher levels of social mistrust and reduced participation in civic organizations. Lack of social cohesion leads to lower participation in political activity (such as voting, serving in local government, volunteering for political campaigns). And lower participation, in turn, undermines the responsiveness of government institutions in addressing the needs of the worst-off. States with the highest income inequality, and thus lowest levels of social capital and political participation, are less likely to invest in human capital and provide far less generous social safety nets (Kawachi and Kennedy, 1999).

Rawls's principles of justice thus turn out to regulate the key social determinants of health. One principle assures equal basic liberties, and specifically provides for guaranteeing *effective* rights of political participation. The fair equality of opportunity principle assures access to high-quality public education, early childhood interventions, including day care, aimed at eliminating class or race disadvantages, and universal coverage for appropriate health care. Rawls's "Difference Principle" permits inequalities in income only if the inequalities work (e.g., through incentives) to make those who are worst-off as well-off as possible. This is not a simple "trickle down" principle that tolerates any inequality as long as there is some benefit that flows down the socioeconomic ladder; it requires a maximal flow downward. It would therefore flatten socioeconomic inequalities in a robust way, assuring far more than a "decent minimum" (J. Cohen, 1989). In addition, the assurances of the value of political participation and fair equality of opportunity would further constrain allowable income inequalities.

The conjecture is that a society complying with these principles of justice would

probably flatten the socioeconomic gradient even more than we see in the most egalitarian welfare states of northern Europe. The implication is that we should view health inequalities that derive from social determinants as unjust unless the determinants are distributed in conformity with these robust principles. Because of the detailed attention Rawls's theory pays to the interaction of these terms of fair cooperation, it provides us—through the findings of social science—with an account of the just distribution of health.

The inequalities in the social determinants that are still permitted by this theory may still produce a socioeconomic gradient, albeit a much flatter one than we see today. Should we view these residual health inequalities as unjust and demand further redistribution of the social determinants?

I believe the theory I have described does not give a clear answer. If the Rawlsian theory insists that protecting opportunity takes priority over other matters and cannot be traded for other gains (and Rawls generally adopts this view), then residual health inequalities may be unjust. If health can be traded for other goods—and all of us make such trades when we take chances with our health to pursue other goals—then the account may be more flexible (Daniels et al., 1999, 2002). Still, Rawls's principles provide more specific guidance in thinking about the distribution of the social determinants than is provided by the fair equality of opportunity account of a just health-care system alone.

I noted earlier that considerable convergence exists between the opportunity-based view I defend and Sen's (1992) appeal to a capabilities-based account (or freedom-based account) of the target of justice. The convergence is even more pronounced when Sen (1999) discusses the ways in which health in developing countries is affected by different development stategies and when Sen emphasizes the importance of education and the growth of democratic culture and institutions. Rawls's focus on the "capabilities of free and equal citizens"

suggests the convergence works in both directions (Daniels, 2000a). Both approaches allow us talk informatively about justice and the distribution of health.

WHEN ARE LIMITS TO HEALTH CARE FAIR?

Justice requires that all societies meet health-care needs fairly under reasonable resource constraints. Even a wealthy, egalitarian country with a highly efficient health-care system will have to set limits to the health care it guarantees everyone (whether or not it allows supplementary tiers for those who can afford them). Poorer countries have to make even harder choices about priorities and limits. However important, health care is not the only important social good. All societies must decide which needs should be given priority and when resources are better spent elsewhere.

How should fair decisions about such limits be made? Under what conditions should we view such decisions as a legitimate exercise of moral authority?

Answering these questions would be much simpler if people could agree on principles of distributive justice that would determine how to set fair limits to health care. If societies agreed on such principles, people could simply check social decisions and practices against the principles to determine whether they conform with them. Where decisions, practices, and institutions fail to conform, they would be unjust and people should then change them. Disagreements about the fairness of actual distributions would then be either disagreements about the interpretation of the principles or about the facts of the situation. Many societies have well-established and reliable, if imperfect, legal procedures for resolving such disputes about facts and interpretations.

Unfortunately, there is no consensus on such distributive principles for health care. Reasonable people, who have diverse moral and religious views about many mat-

ters, disagree morally about what constitutes a fair allocation of resources to meet
competing health-care needs—even when
they agree on other aspects of the justice of
health care-systems, such as the importance
of universal access to whatever services are
provided. We should expect, and respect,
such diversity in views about rationing
health care. Nevertheless, we must arrive at
acceptable social policies despite our disagreements. This moral controversy raises
a distinctive problem of legitimacy: Under
what conditions should we accept as legitimate the moral authority of those making
rationing decisions?

I shall develop the following argument:
(1) We have no consensus on principled solutions to a cluster of morally controversial
rationing problems, and general principles
of justice for health and health care fail to
provide specific guidance about them (Daniels, 1993). (2) In the absence of such a
consensus, we should rely on a fair process
for arriving at solutions to these problems
and for establishing the legitimacy of such
decisions (Rawls, 1971). (3) A fair process
that addresses issues of legitimacy will have
to meet several constraints that I shall refer
to as "accountability for reasonableness"
(Daniels and Sabin, 1998a, 2002); these
constraints tie the process to deliberative
democratic procedures (Daniels and Sabin,
1997). This issue of legitimacy and fair
process arises in both public and mixed
public–private health-care systems, and it
must be addressed in countries at all levels
of development.

To support the first step of the argument,
consider a problem that has been labeled
the "priorities problem" (Daniels, 1993;
Kamm, 1993): How much priority should
we give to treating the sickest or most disabled patients? To start with, imagine two
extreme positions. The Maximin position
("maximize the minimum") says that we
should give complete priority to treating
the worst-off patients. One might think
that Maximin is implied by the fair equality of opportunity account (though I believe my account is only committed to giv-

ing *some* priority to the worst off, placing
it in a broad family of views that leave the
degree of priority unspecified). The Maximize position says that we should give priority to whatever treatment produces the
greatest net health benefit (or greatest net
health benefit per dollar spent) regardless
of which patients we treat.

Suppose comparable resources could be
invested in Technology A or in B, but the
resources are "lumpy" (we cannot introduce some A and some B) and we can only
afford one of A or B in our health-care
budget. The Maximin position would settle
the matter by determining whether patients
treated by A are worse off before treatment
than patients treated by B. If so, we introduce A; if patients treated by B are worse
off, we introduce B. If the two sets of patients are equally bad off, we can break the
tie by considering whom we can provide
the most benefit. The Maximize position
chooses between A and B solely by reference to which produces greatest net
benefit.[6]

In practice, most people are likely to reject both extreme positions (Nord, 1995,
1999). If the benefits that A and B produce
are nearly equal, but patients needing A
start off much worse than patients needing
B, most people seem to believe we should
introduce A. They prefer to provide A even
if they know we could produce somewhat
more net health benefit by introducing B.
But if the net benefit produced by A is very
small, or if B produces significantly more
net benefit, then most people will overcome
their concern to give priority to the worst
off and will prefer to introduce B to A.
Some people who would give priority to
patients needing A temper their preference
if those patients end up faring much better
than patients needing B. Disagreement persists: A definite but very small minority are
inclined to be *maximizers* and a definite
but very small minority are inclined to be
maximiners. Most people fall in between,
and they vary considerably in how much
benefit they are willing to sacrifice to give
priority to worse off patients.

Two other types of rationing problems also suggest we are not straight maximizers or maximiners, though we lack principled characterizations of acceptable middle-course solutions (Daniels, 1993). The Fair Chances Best Outcomes Problem asks, Should we give all who might benefit some chance at a resource or should we give the resource to those who get the best outcome? The Aggregation Problem asks, When do lesser benefits to many outweigh greater benefits to a few?

Two strategies have been pursued to address these kinds of rationing problems, one philosophical, one empirical. The philosophical approach, brilliantly exemplified in Kamm's (1993) work, examines subtly varied hypothetical cases, seeking to reveal agreement on a complex set of underlying principles that can account for the judgments the philosophical inquirer makes about these cases. This strategy may well help us arrive at middle-level principles for addressing these rationing problems, and it should be pursued by others. Nevertheless, given the subtlety of the method and the likelihood that some disagreements about cases will reflect broader moral disagreements about other matters, I do not believe this method will produce consensus on such principles in the foreseeable future. The insights from this approach are important inputs into a fair, deliberative process of decision making, but they are not a substitute for such a fair process.

The empirical approach has been ingeniously developed by the economist Erik Nord (1999), who also explores hypothetical cases by asking groups of people "person–trade-off" questions. These questions are a variation on a standard economic approach seeking "indifference" points or curves reflecting when an individual finds two benefits or outcomes equivalent. For example, if we can invest only in treatments *A* and *B*, and treatment *A* is used for people more seriously ill than treatment *B*, we might ask how many treatments with *B* would someone trade for some number of

treatments with *A*. Nord hopes this approach can uncover the structure of moral concerns in a population of people. A key risk of the method is that it disguises moral disagreement by talking about a "range" of responses. For this, and other reasons I discuss elsewhere (Daniels, 1998c, 2002b), the results of Nord's work can help inform fair, deliberative decision processes but cannot substitute for them.

If we have persistent disagreement about principles for resolving rationing problems, then we must retreat to a process all can agree is a fair way to resolve disputes about them. The "retreat to procedural justice" as a way of determining what is fair when we lack prior agreement on principles is a central feature of Rawls's account (thus "justice as [procedural] fairness"). Rather than argue for this familiar approach (the second step of my argument above), I shall move directly to characterizing the features of such a fair process.

We would take a giant step toward solving the problems of legitimacy and fairness that face public agencies and private health plans making limit-setting decisions if the following four conditions were satisfied (Daniels and Sabin, 1997):

- *Publicity condition:* Decisions regarding coverage for new technologies (and other limit-setting decisions) and their rationales must be publicly accessible.
- *Relevance condition:* The rationales for coverage decisions should aim to provide a *reasonable* construal of how the organization (or society) should provide "value for money" in meeting the varied health needs of a defined population under reasonable resource constraints. Specifically, a construal will be "reasonable" if it appeals to reasons and principles that are accepted as relevant by people who are disposed to finding terms of cooperation that are mutually justifiable.
- *Appeals condition:* There is a mechanism for challenge and dispute resolution regarding limit-setting decisions, including

the opportunity for revising decisions in light of further evidence or arguments.

• *Enforcement condition:* There is either voluntary or public regulation of the process to ensure that the first three conditions are met.

The guiding idea behind the four conditions is to convert private health plan or public agency decisions into part of a larger public deliberation about how to use limited resources to protect fairly the health of a population with varied needs.[7] The broader public deliberation envisioned here is not necessarily an organized democratic procedure, though it could include the deliberation underlying public regulation of the health-care system. Rather, it may take place in various forms in an array of institutions, spilling over into legislative politics only under some circumstances. Meeting these conditions also serves an educative function: The public is made familiar with the need for limits and appropriate ways to reason about them.

The first condition (Publicity condition) requires that rationales for decisions be publicly accessible to everyone affected by them. One American health plan, for example, decided to cover growth-hormone treatment but only for children who are growth hormone deficient or who have Turner syndrome. It deliberated carefully and clearly about the reasons for its decision. These included the lack of evidence of efficacy or good risk benefit ratios for other groups of patients, and a commitment to restrict coverage to the treatment of disease and disability (as opposed to enhancements). It did not, however, state these reasons in its medical director's letter to clinicians or in support materials used in "shared decision making" with patients and families about the procedure. Its reasons were defensible ones aimed at a public good that all people can understand and see as relevant, the provision of effective and safe treatment to a defined population under resource constraints. The restriction

to treatment rather than enhancement requires a moral argument, however, and remains a point about which reasonable people can disagree, as we saw earlier.

One important effect of making public the reasons for coverage decisions is that, over time, the pattern of such decisions will resemble a type of "case law." A body of case law establishes the presumption that if some individuals have been treated one way because they fall under a reasonable interpretation of the relevant principles, then similar individuals should be treated the same way in subsequent cases. In effect, the institution generating the case law is saying, "We deliberate carefully about hard cases and have good reasons for doing what we have done, and we continue to stand by our reasons in our commitment to act consistently with past practices." To rebut this presumption requires showing either that the new case differs in relevant and important ways from the earlier one, justifying different treatment, or that there are good grounds for rejecting the reasons or principles embodied in the earlier case. Case law does not imply past infallibility, but it does imply giving careful consideration to why earlier decision makers made the choices they did. It involves a form of institutional reflective equilibrium, a commitment to both transparency and coherence in the giving of reasons.

The benefits of publicity in the form of case law are both internal and external to the decision-making institution. The quality of decision making improves if reasons must be articulated. Fairness improves over time, both formally, because like cases are treated similarly, and substantively, because there is systematic evaluation of reasons. To the extent that we are then better able to discover flaws in our moral reasoning, we are more likely to arrive at fair decisions. Over time, people will understand better the moral commitments of the institutions making these decisions.

The Relevance condition imposes two important constraints on the rationales that are made publicly accessible. Specifically, the rationales for coverage decisions should aim to provide (a) a *reasonable* construal of (b) how the organization (or society) should provide "value for money" in meeting the varied health needs of a defined population under reasonable resource constraints. Both constraints need explanation.

We may think of the goal of meeting the varied needs of the population of patients under reasonable resource constraints as a characterization of the *common* or *public good* pursued by all engaged in the enterprise of delivering and receiving this care. Reasoning about that goal must also meet certain conditions. Specifically, a construal of the goal will be "reasonable" only if it appeals to reasons (evidence, values, and principles) that are accepted as relevant by "fair-minded" people. By "fair-minded" I mean people who seek mutually justifiable terms of cooperation. The notion is not mysterious; we encounter it all the time in sports. Fair-minded people are those who want to play by agreed-upon rules in a sport and prefer rules that are designed to bring out the best in that game. Here we are concerned with the game of delivering health care that meets population needs in a fair way.

Recall the restriction on the use of growth-hormone treatment to those with growth-hormone deficiency. As I noted earlier, some individuals object that a theory that emphasizes protecting equal opportunity, as mine does, should also use medical interventions to eliminate extreme but normal shortness if it is disadvantaging to the person. Still, proponents on both sides of this dispute can recognize that reasonable people might disagree about the specific requirements of a principle protecting opportunity. Both sides of the dispute about the scope of the goals of medicine nevertheless must recognize the relevance and appropriateness of the kind of reason offered by the other, even if they disagree with the interpretation of the principle or the applications to which it is put.

Consider further the implications of the Relevance condition. "Including this treatment benefits me (and other patients like me)," just like "excluding this treatment disadvantages me (or other patients like me)," is not the kind of reason that meets the constraints on reasons. Because comparative coverage decisions always advantage some and disadvantage others, mere advantage or disadvantage is not a relevant reason in debates about coverage. If, however, a coverage decision disadvantages me compared to other patients similar to me in all relevant ways, then this is a reason based on disadvantage that all must think is relevant. Also, if a coverage decision disadvantages someone (and others like him) more than anyone need be disadvantaged under alternatives available, then this too is a reason that all must consider relevant.

How should we view the claim that a treatment "costs too much"? First, suppose this is a claim about relative cost-effectiveness or worthiness. People who share in the goal of meeting the varied medical needs of a population covered by limited resources would consider relevant the claim that a particular technology falls below some defensible threshold of cost-effectiveness or relative cost-worthiness. Suppose, however, the claim that something "costs too much" refers to its effects on profits or competitiveness. Supporting this claim often requires providing information that private health plans will not reveal (for good business reasons); it often turns on economic and strategic judgments requiring special experience and training, and it ultimately depends on a much more fundamental claim about the design of the system—namely, that a system involving competition in this sort of market will produce efficiencies that work to the advantage of all who have medical needs. My point is not that these reasons fail to meet the Relevance condition, but that providing support for them requires information that is often not available, that is hard to understand when it is available, and that ultimately depends on fundamental moral and political judgments about the feasibility of quite different alternative systems for delivering health care. Nevertheless, if for-profit health plans are to comply with the Relevance condition, they must either be willing to provide information they would ordinarily not make public, or make their decisions on the basis of reasons that they can defend to other relevant stakeholders.

The constraints here imposed on reasons have a bearing on a philosophical debate about the legitimacy of democratic procedures. An aggregative or proceduralist conception of democratic voting sees it as a way of aggregating preferences. Where, however, we are concerned with fundamental differences in values, not mere preferences, an aggregative view seems inadequate. It seems insensitive to how we ideally would like to resolve moral disputes, namely through argument and deliberation. An alternative "deliberative" view imposes constraints on the kinds of reasons that can play a role in deliberation. Not just any preferences will do. Reasons must reflect the fact that all parties to a decision are viewed as seeking terms of fair cooperation that they accept as reasonable. Even if we have to rely on a majority vote to settle a disagreement where there are serious moral issues involved, if the reasons are constrained to those all must view as relevant, then the minority can at least assure itself that the preference of the majority rests on the kind of reason that even the minority must acknowledge appropriately plays a role in deliberation. The majority does not exercise brute power of preference but is instead constrained by having to seek reasons for its view that are justifiable to all who seek mutually justifiable terms of cooperation.

The Appeals and Enforcement conditions involve mechanisms that go beyond the publicity requirements of the first two conditions. When patients or clinicians use these procedures to challenge a decision, and the results of the challenge lead effectively to reconsideration of the decision on its merits, the decision-making process is made iterative in a way that broadens the input of information and argument. Parties that were excluded from the decision-making process, and whose views may not have been clearly heard or understood, find a voice, even if after the original fact. The dispute resolution mechanisms do not empower enrollees or clinicians to play a direct, participatory role in the actual decision-making bodies, but that does not happen in many public democratic processes as well. Still, it does empower them to play a more effective role in the larger social deliberation about the issues, including deliberation within those public institutions that can play a role in regulating private health plans or otherwise constraining their acts. The mechanisms we describe thus play a role in assuring broader accountability of private organizations to those who are affected by limit-setting decisions. The arrangements required by the four conditions provide connective tissue to, not a replacement for, broader democratic processes that ultimately have authority and responsibility for guaranteeing the fairness of limit-setting decisions.

Together these conditions hold institutions—public or private—and decision makers in them "accountable for the reasonableness" of the limits they set. All must engage in a process of establishing their credentials for fair decision making about such fundamental matters every time they make such a decision. Whether in public or mixed systems, establishing the accountability of decision makers to those affected by their decisions is the only way to show, over time, that arguably fair decisions are being made and that those making them have established a procedure we should view as legitimate This is not to say that public participation is an essential ingredient of the process in either public or mixed systems, but the accountability to the public in both cases is necessary to facilitate broader democratic processes that regulate the system.

In many public systems the reasoning that lies behind decisions that affect the length of queues—a rationing device—are inscrutable to the public. They are made in a "black box" of budgetary decisions. Queues may then be adjusted if the public complains too much—there is this kind of accountability to the squeaky wheel. But there is in general too little accountability of the sort demanded by the four conditions I describe (Ham and Pickard, 1998; Coulter and Ham, 2000). Only through such accountability and the way in which it facilitates or enables a broader social deliberation will there be a wider perception that rationing decisions are fair and are made through an exercise of legitimate authority.

One issue facing this "process" approach to rationing seems to be more problematic in public systems than it does in mixed ones. In a mixed system, two different insurers or health plans might arrive at different judgments about what limits to set. I have suggested both might be "right" if their decisions are the results of fair procedures (Daniels and Sabin, 1998b). The anomaly is that some patients will then have access to services that others will not have, and this might seem to violate a formal constraint on fairness— that society treat like cases similarly. In a mixed system, we might see this variation as a price we pay for whatever virtues (if any) the mixed system brings (the variation might ultimately lead us to better decisions over time). In a public system, however, such variation (e.g., between districts) might seem more objectionable if all are governed by the same public legislation and funding. Still, despite such anomalies, fair process may be the best we can do wherever we have no prior consensus on fair outcomes.

CONCLUDING REMARKS

A comprehensive approach to justice, health, and health care must address all three questions I have discussed. My extension of Rawls's theory of justice to health and health care provides a way to link answers to the first and second questions. There are also three ways in which Rawls's theory also provides support for my approach to the third question. First, I propose that we use a fair process to arrive at what is fair in rationing; this is because we lack prior consensus on the relevant distributive principles. This "retreat to procedural justice" is at the heart of Rawls's own invocation of his version of a social contract. Second, Rawls places great emphasis on the importance of publicity as a constraint on theories of justice: Principles of justice and the grounds for them must be publicly acknowledged. This constrain is central to the conditions that establish accountability for reasonableness. Finally, Rawls develops the view that "public reason" must constrain the content of public deliberation and decision about fundamental matters of justice, avoiding special considerations that might be elements of the comprehensive moral views that people hold (Rawls, 1993). Accountability for reasonableness pushes decision makers toward finding reasons all can agree are relevant to the goals of cooperative health-delivery schemes. In this way, accountability for reasonableness promotes the democratic deliberation that Rawls also advocates.

In pointing out these connections, I am not suggesting that this is the only approach to developing a theory of justice that applies to all aspects of health and health care. Indeed, I have pointed to other theories that converge in practice and to some extent in theory with the approach adopted here. I am proposing that concerns about justice and fairness in health policy should look to political philosophy for guidance and that some specific guidance is forthcoming. At the very same time, seeing how we have to modify and refine work in political philosophy if it is to apply to real issues in the world suggests that we should abandon the unidirectional implications of the term "applied ethics" or "applied political philosophy" (Daniels, 1996, 1996b).

Acknowledgments

Bruce Kennedy and Ichiro Kawachi collaborated with me to write the material on which I draw for the section "Which Health Inequalities Are Unjust?" James Sabin collaborated on the research and writing on which I draw for the section "When Are Limits to Health Care Fair?" Research for this chapter was supported by a Robert Wood Johnson Investigator Award and Tufts Sabbatical Leave. I have benefited from discussions with Richard Arneson, Allen Buchanan, Dan Brock, G.A. Cohen, Joshua Cohen, John Rawls, and Dan Wikler about the relationship between my approach and that of other recent work on egalitarianism.

NOTES

1. Disease and disability, both physical and mental, are construed as adverse departures from or impairments of species-typical normal functional organization, or "normal functioning," for short. The line between disease and disability and normal functioning is drawn in the relatively objective and non-evaluative context provided by the biomedical sciences, broadly construed (though glaring misclassifications have also occurred). I ignore the considerable controversy in the philosophy of biology about how to analyze the concept of function (Daniels, 1985).

2. Daniels (1996a) discusses the relationship between the equal opportunity account and the rationale for "reasonable accommodation" required of employers under the Americans with Disabilities Act; see also Brock, 1995. Brock (1998) discusses the implication of disabilities for cost-effectiveness analysis.

3. Economists view an arrangement as efficient or "pareto optimal" if no one can be made better off without making someone else worse off. If some people would trade their access to health care through socially provided insurance for other goods, they are not in a pareto optimal situation.

4. The age rationing implied by this account is different in rationale from that advocated by Callahan (1987), who believes the elderly have a duty to step aside in favor of the young: It is also different from those who argue for a version of the "fair innings" view, which gives priority to the young on the grounds that the old have already had their opportunity to acquire years lived (cf. Brock, 1989; Williams, 1997); it is also different in rationale from Kamm (1993), who argues that the young would be worse off than the old and in that sense "need" years more than the old. The considerable disagreement about what justice permits, even among those who accept some forms of age rationing, argues for the importance of the type of fair process described later in this chapter.

5. See Daniels, 2000a; also Rawls, 1993. The convergence is clearer still when Sen (1999) addresses the ways in which we should focus on our capabilities as citizens—see Anderson, 1999.

6. Kamm insists on exploring hypothetical cases or "thought experiments," rather than real ones, attempting to isolate more clearly in these cases the relevant features that motivate our judgments. Kamm believes that her method will uncover an "internal program" or underlying moral structure to our beliefs; crucial to this approach is the claim that people will agree on a central range of cases—that is, that others will have the same responses that Kamm has to them. For doubts about the method, see Daniels, 1998b.

7. The conditions described were developed independently but fit reasonably well with the framework of principles for democratic deliberation developed by Gutmann and Thompson, 1996. For some reservations about their approach, see Daniels, 1999.

REFERENCES

Acheson, D. (1998). *Report of the Independent Inquiry into Inequalities in Health*. London: Stationery Office.

Anderson, E. (1999). What is the point of equality? *Ethics* 109, 287–337.

Arneson, R.J. (1988). Equality and equal opportunity for welfare. *Philosophical Studies*. 54, 79–95.

Black, D., Morris, J.N., Smith, C., Townsend, P., and Whitehead, M. (1988). *Inequalities in Health: The Black Report: The Health Divide*. London: Penguin Group.

Brock, D. (1989). Justice, health care, and the elderly. *Philosophy and Public Affairs* 18, 297–312.

Brock, D. (1995). Justice and the ADA: Does prioritizing and rationing health care discriminate against the disabled? *Social Philosophy and Policy* 12, 159–184.

Brock, D. (1998). Ethical issues in the development of summary measures of health status. In Institute of Medicine, *Summarizing Population Health: Directions for the Development and Application of Population Metrics*. Washington, DC: National Academy Press, pp. 73–86.

Buchanan, A., Brock, D., Daniels, N., and Wikler, D. (2000). *From Chance to Choice: Genetics and the Just Society*. New York: Cambridge University Press.

Callahan, D. (1987). *Setting Limits: Medical Goals in an Aging Society*. New York: Simon & Schuster.

Cohen, G.A. (1989). On the currency of egalitarian justice. *Ethics* 99, 906–44.

Cohen, J. (1989). Democratic equality. *Ethics* 99, 727–51.

Coulter, A. and Ham, C. (2000). *The Global Challenge of Health Care Rationing*. Philadelphia: Open University Press.

Daniels, N. (1981). Health-care needs and distributive justice. *Philosophy and Public Affairs* 10, 146–79.

Daniels, N. (1985). *Just Health Care*. New York: Cambridge University Press.

Daniels, N. (1988). *Am I My Parents' Keeper? An Essay on Justice Between the Old and the Young*. New York: Oxford University Press.

Daniels, N. (1990). Equality of what: Welfare, resources, or capabilities? *Philosophy and Phenomenological Research* 50 (Suppl), 273–96.

Daniels, N. (1993). Rationing fairly: programmatic considerations. *Bioethics* 7 (2/3), 224–33. (Reprinted in Daniels, 1996b, pp. 317–26).

Daniels, N. (1995). *Seeking Fair Treatment: From the AIDS Epidemic to National Health Care Reform*. New York: Oxford University Press.

Daniels, N. (1996a). Mental disabilities, equal opportunity and the ADA. In R.J. Bonnie and J. Monahan (eds.), *Mental Disorder, Work Disability, and the Law*. Chicago: University of Chicago Press, pp. 282–97.

Daniels, N. (1996b). *Justice and Justification: Reflective Equilibrium in Theory and Practice*. New York: Cambridge University Press.

Daniels, N. (1998a). Rationing medical care: A philosopher's perspective on outcomes and process. *Economics and Philosophy* 14, 27–50.

Daniels, N. (1998b). Kamm's moral methods. *Philosophy and Phenomenological Research*. 58(4), 947–54.

Daniels, N. (1998c). Distributive justice and the use of summary measures of population health status. In Institute of Medicine, *Summarizing Population Health: Directions for the Development and Application of Population Metrics*. National Academy Press, pp. 58–71.

Daniels, N. (1999). Enabling democratic deliberation: How managed care organizations ought to make decisions about coverage for new technologies. In S. Macedo (ed.), *Deliberative Politics: Essays on Democracy and Disagreement*. New York: Oxford University Press, pp. 198–210.

Daniels, N. (2002a). Democratic equality: Rawls's complex egalitarianism. In S. Freeman (ed.), *Cambridge Companion to Rawls*. Cambridge: Cambridge University Press.

Daniels, N. (2002b). Legitimacy, fair process, and limits to health care. World Health Organization Project on Fairness and Goodness (in press).

Daniels, N., Kennedy, B., and Kawachi, I. (1999). Why justice is good for our health: Social determinants of health inequalities. *Daedalus* 128(4), 215–51.

Daniels, N., Kennedy, B., and Kawachi, I. (2000). Justice is good for our health: How greater economic equality would promote public health. *Boston Review* 25, 4–9, 18–19.

Daniels, N., Light, D., and Caplan, R. (1996). *Benchmarks of Fairness for Health Care Reform*. New York: Oxford University Press.

Daniels, N. and Sabin, J.E. (1997). Limits to health care: Fair procedures, democratic deliberation, and the legitimacy problem for insurers. *Philosophy and Public Affairs* 26, 303–50.

Daniels, N. and Sabin, J. (1998a). The ethics of accountability and the reform of managed-care organizations. *Health Affairs* 17(5), 50–69.

Daniels, N. and Sabin, J. (1998b). Last-chance therapies and managed care: Pluralism, fair procedures, and legitimacy. *Hastings Center Report* 28(2), 27–41.

Daniels, N. and Sabin, J. (2002). *Setting Limits Fairly: Can We Learn to Share Medical Resources?* New York: Oxford University Press.

Gutmann, A. and Thompson, D. (1996). *Democracy and Disagreement*. Cambridge, MA: Harvard University Press.

Ham, C. and Pickard, S. (1998). *Tragic Choices in Health Care: The Story of Child B*. London: Kings Fund.

Kamm, F.M. (1993). *Morality, Modality. Vol. 1: Death and Whom to Save from It*. Oxford: Oxford University Press.

Kaplan, G.A., Pamuk, E.R., Lynch, J.W., Cohen, R.D., and Balfour, J.L. (1996). Inequality in income and mortality in the United States: Analysis of mortality and potential pathways. *British Medical Journal* 312, 999–1003.

Kawachi, I. and Kennedy, B.P. (1997). Health and social cohesion: Why care about income inequality? *British Medical Journal* 314, 1037–40.

Kawachi, I. and Kennedy, B.P. (1999). Income inequality and health: Pathways and mechanisms. *Health Services Research* 34, 215–27.

Kawachi, I., Kennedy, B.P., and Wilkinson, R. (1999). *Income Inequality and Health: A Reader.* New York: The New Press.

Kennedy, B.P., Kawachi, I., and Prothrow-Stith, D. (1996). Income distribution and mortality: Test of the Robin Hood Index in the United States. *British Medical Journal* 312, 1004–8. Published erratum appears in *British Medical Journal* 312, 1194.

Kennedy, B.P., Kawachi, I., Glass, R., and Prothrow-Stith, D. (1998a). Income distribution, socioeconomic status, and self-rated health: A US multi-level analysis. *British Medical Journal* 317, 917–21.

Kennedy, B., Kawachi, I., Glass, R., and Prothrow-Stith, D. (1998b). Social capital, income inequality and mortality. *American Journal of Public Health* 87, 1491–98.

Kennedy, B., Kawachi, I., Prothrow-Stith, D., and Gupta, V. (1998c). Income inequality, social capital and firearm-related violent crime. *Social Science and Medicine* 47, 7–17.

Lynch, J.W., Kaplan, G.A., Pamuk, E.R., Cohen, R.D., Balfour, J.L., and Yen, I.H. (1998). Income inequality and mortality in metropolitan areas of the United States. *American Journal of Public Health* 88, 1074–80.

Marmot, M.G. (1999). *Social Causes of Social Inequalities in Health.* Harvard Center for Population and Development Studies, Working Paper Series 99.01, January 1999.

Marmot, M.G., Fuhrer, R., Ettner, S.L., Marks, N.F., Bumpass, L.L., and Ryff, C.D., (1998). Contribution of psychosocial factors to socioeconomic differences in health. *Milbank Quarterly* 76(3), 403–48.

Nord, E. (1995). The person-tradeoff approach to valuing health care programs. *Medical Decision Making* 15, 201–8.

Nord, E. (1999). *Cost-Value Analysis in Health Care: Making Sense Out of QALYs.* Cambridge: Cambridge University Press.

Rawls, J. (1971). *A Theory of Justice.* Cambridge, MA: Harvard University Press.

Rawls, J. (1993). *Political Liberalism.* New York: Columbia University Press.

Sabin, J. and Daniels, N. (1994). Determining medical necessity in mental health practice: A study of clinical reasoning and a proposal for insurance policy. *Hasting Center Report* 24(6), 5–13.

Scanlon, T.M. (1975). Preference and urgency. *Journal of Philosophy* 77(19), 655–69.

Sen, A.K. (1980). Equality of what? In S. McMurrin (ed.), *Tanner Lectures on Human Values, Vol. 1.* Cambridge: Cambridge University Press.

Sen, A.K. (1992). *Inequality Reexamined.* Cambridge, MA: Harvard University Press.

Sen, A.K. (1999). *Development as Freedom.* New York: Alfred A. Knopf.

Wilkinson, R.G. (1992). Income distribution and life expectancy. *British Medical Journal* 304, 165–68.

Wilkinson, R.G. (1994). The epidemiological transition: From material scarcity to social disadvantage? *Daedalus* 123, 61–77.

Wilkinson, R.G. (1996). *Unhealthy Societies: The Afflictions of Inequality.* London: Routledge.

Williams, A. (1997). Intergenerational equity: An exploration of the "fair innings" argument. *Health Economics* 6, 117–32.

2

Justice and the Basic Structure of Health-Care Systems

Paul T. Menzel

Health-care systems are sometimes thought to fall on a spectrum, from those that are characterized by great equity but employ considerable collective coercion to those that achieve little equity but encroach less on individual liberty[1] (Culyer et al., 1981). Usually, systems lying in the equity-emphasizing and arguably liberty-diminishing direction are also surmised to be more efficient (cost-effective). More centralized, they seem better able to control costly provider behavior and insurance-distorted patient demand. Their structural paradigm is a unitary public system, either single-payer insurance or national health service. The structural paradigm on the other, decentralized end of the spectrum is a pluralistic system of market competition that does not achieve universal access to even a basic minimum of services.

The stereotypical conflicts of liberty with equity or with cost-effectiveness are admittedly understood to have their limits. Unitary public systems can fully respect an individual's right of informed refusal of care, and pluralistic systems that utilize competitive private markets can achieve virtually universal access through publicly subsidized vouchers (Pauly et al., 1992). Nonetheless, the trade-offs and conflicts are still commonly thought to be significant enough that health policy tends to remain an ideological battleground between the political left willing to compromise liberty to achieve both greater equity and aggregate efficiency and the political right willing to sacrifice equity and universal access to avoid any encroachment on liberty.

These allegedly deep conflicts of individual liberty with collective equity and efficiency, however, cannot be straightforwardly translated into conflict between justice and pluralistic market system. For one thing, senses of justice vary widely across the political spectrum. To be sure, utilitarian views of justice are likely to focus on a system's cost-worthiness; then, given some common empirical assumptions, a more unitary system is usually favored. And egalitarian views of justice would insist from the start on both universal access to a robust basic minimum of care and financially equitable burdens of financing (for example, community-rated premiums); because both appear to be difficult to achieve in a pluralistic market system, justice is then viewed as simply requiring a more unitary public system. There are more libertarian senses of justice, however, in which it is claimed that a pluralistic market not only respects liberty but also constitutes a more just arrangement for health care (Engelhardt, 1996).

This chapter articulates my own view of why at least some of the apparently fundamental conflicts between the values of individual liberty and responsibility on the one hand, and those of both equity and cost-efficiency on the other, are fewer and less intractable than is usually assumed. The result will be to break the rigid and stereotypical association of senses of justice with the two paradigms of basic organizational structure for a health-care system: libertarian-leaning senses of justice with pluralistic market systems that employ little central coercion, and egalitarian senses with unitary public systems.[2] Understanding better the ingredients of liberty, equity, and justice as well as the complexity of how they actually intersect in a health-care system opens up possibilities for their significant reconciliation.

I will, in fact, defend such a partial reconciliation. I will conclude, among other things, that even non-egalitarian views of distributive justice should strongly embrace compulsory, universal coverage of health care for some significant level of care, and that egalitarian views ought not to regard different levels of coverage for people of different income levels as necessarily unjust. To begin, I will need to clarify at length an important *Anti-Free-Riding Principle* (AFRP). Later I will invoke four other substantive principles: *Presumed Prior Consent*, which contends that under certain restricted conditions we are allowed to presume individuals' consent to restrictions on their care; *Personal Integrity*, which ex-

pands the time-frame of the health-related events in people's lives to which consent pertains and allows us to see how liberty can be reconciled with significant rationing of health care for cost-efficiency; *Equal Opportunity for Welfare* (EOW), an understanding of distributive justice that harbors considerable potential for reducing the tension of liberty with equity; and *Just Sharing*, a secondary principle that follows from EOW and directly speaks to the matter of community-rated as opposed to experience-rated premiums.

THE ANTI-FREE-RIDING PRINCIPLE

We might first look at more general arguments for state power for suggestions about whether a society may restrict the liberty of providers, insurers, subscribers, and patients for the sake of equity or efficiency. One argument in particular, the argument from "public goods," has often been thought by classical liberals to justify a state's limited coercive power: Because the most essential benefits of the state accrue to everyone—the goods are "public" and "nonexclusive"[3]—the state may extract from all people their individual fair share of taxes as well as obedience. From a liberty-emphasizing perspective, the powerful element in this argument for state coercion is that behind coercion lies individual preference for a collective enterprise.

One way to see this is to flesh out the argument in terms of a more fundamental Anti-Free-Riding Principle (AFRP), also sometimes known as the "principle of fairness." The AFRP speaks to two situations, one where people actively impose costs on others and the other where they receive benefits without paying their share of expense.

The Anti-Free-Riding Principle (AFRP): A person should pay for any costs she imposes on others through voluntary action that she initiates without their informed consent, and a person should be required to pay her share of a collective enterprise that produces benefits from which she cannot be excluded unless she would actually prefer to lose all of the benefits of the enterprise rather than pay her fair share of its cost.[4]

I have argued elsewhere (Menzel, 1990, pp. 29–31) that the correct limiting condition in the second part of AFRP is precisely the hypothetical preference and consent of the person receiving the benefits that is conveyed in the principle as I have stated it here. It is not the weaker condition of a person's mere acceptance of the benefits, and unless consulting her for her actual consent is feasible and not prohibitively costly, it is not the stronger condition of her actual consent. If, in fact, were push actually to come to shove, she would agree to pay her share rather than forgo the benefits, and if it is very difficult if not impossible to exclude noncontributors from receiving the (public) good at issue, then it is entirely respectful of people as free individuals to hold them responsible for contributing their share, and even to coercively require them to contribute.[5]

For example, suppose that individual residents cannot feasibly be excluded from receiving many of the benefits of a park in their neighborhood, and suppose that they would agree to pay their share of its expense were that necessary for them to receive those benefits. Then, even if we can hardly any longer feasibly ask their consent (by putting the matter to a vote, say, for the park already exists), we may compel them to pay their share of expense. At the same time, their mere "acceptance" of the park's benefits (say, by not moving away, or by a slightly active participation on their part, like watching the park's birds from their porch across the street) would not so clearly justify taxing them for the park's collective expense.

If this, then, is the right version of the AFRP, any argument that a person must pay her fair share is of course only as good as the descriptive accuracy of the claim that in fact she would have agreed to pay that share if she had had to in order to receive the benefits. It is often difficult to be confident in such a claim. For one thing, we have trouble putting people to a true test of whether they will consent to contribute their share so as to avoid losing all benefits; if they cannot realistically be excluded from the benefits, any consent we might attribute to them remains forever hypothetical.

Furthermore, even if we could technically exclude people in order to give a sense of reality to the test, they might still be tempted to "hold out," hoping both that others will come forth to get the collective enterprise off the ground and that subsequently it will be too expensive or bothersome for others to exclude them from the benefits. We end up in a situation where we must depend on fallible judgments about hypothetical consent unless we are just going to turn a blind eye to free-riding.

Even if we embrace hypothetical consent as a conceptual ingredient in any AFRP used in the real social world, though, we still need to confront a major difficulty in using such a principle to justify coercion: There will virtually always still be "honest holdouts," people for whom the likely benefits received from the enterprise are less than their share of the costs. Coercion laudably catches free-riders, but it also catches people who honestly prefer not to pay their share of the enterprise's required costs in order to obtain its benefits (Schmidtz, 1991, p. 84). Why, then, should *they* have to fund what is essentially other people's project? The point cannot be dismissed simply by claiming that the gain in catching free-riders outweighs the loss to liberty in coercing honest holdouts, for if aggregate social value could just straightforwardly trump individual liberty, we will have begged the question against all conceptions of liberty that were not fundamentally utilitarian. Perhaps, then, all we have is an AFRP that proclaims free-riding to be regrettable. We will not yet have shown that free-riding is objectionable enough to justify the *coercive* extraction of contribution.

However, AFRP is powerful enough to justify coercion despite commitment to individualistic values once the following points are recognized.

1. Honest holdouts and free-riders are not necessarily different people. If the good that the collective enterprise produces is virtually universal, then even if one is an honest holdout because one judges the benefit in one's own case to be insufficient to outweigh one's fair-share cost, the matter may be a close call. Even if a person's status as an honest holdout should prevent requiring participation, the fact remains that if the enterprise proceeds and one is not required to help pay for its costs, one is still getting a free ride.

2. Free-riding is certainly objectionable enough to justify coercion when persons have actually agreed to set up the collective enterprise. Yet as noted earlier, trying to procure people's *actual* consent is often not realistic given the nonexclusive character of benefits and the existence of a residuum of strategic holdout psychology. Short of actual consent, however, I would argue that coercion can still be selectively justified. The strength of the case for coercing a person's contribution will vary with the degree to which we are justifiably confident that she *would* have consented to the arrangement if she had to in order to receive its benefits (Menzel, 1990, pp. 29–34).

Whether coercion is finally justified will also depend on other contextual factors. For example, how close do alternative arrangements of private contract come to achieving the same benefits? One has to see the full context of a situation before a considered judgment can be rendered about whether coercion is justified to prevent free-riding.

3. The AFRP is itself fundamentally a pro-individualist principle compatible with libertarian senses of justice. In holding people responsible not just for the effects of their voluntary actions on others but also for the costs of the collective enterprises from which they benefit, the AFRP keeps collective solutions to human needs in tow, tying them tightly to people's ability and willingness to pay their costs. Thus, AFRP provides a strong connection between social arrangements and individual preference. Although AFRP is a powerful principle in justifying social coercion of membership and contribution, properly understood it is also a principle that fits squarely within a social philosophy that highly values individual liberty.

To summarize: Society may coercively extract contributions to a collective enterprise whose benefits are nonexclusive whenever the individual members would actually, if put to the test, prefer paying their share of costs rather than entirely forgoing those benefits. Ideally, to be sure, honest holdouts should not be forced to contribute, but several factors must be considered before rejecting coercion in an actual context: the degree to which potential[6] honest holdouts still benefit considerably from the arrangement, and how close the alternate, noncoercive contractual arrangements come to producing equivalent benefits.

FREE-RIDING AND COMPULSORY UNIVERSAL INSURANCE

An important question in shaping the basic structure of a health-care system concerns compulsory coverage: Must everyone in the society be insured, or should people be at liberty to go uninsured?

From a liberty-focused perspective, health care is good only insofar as it contributes to people's ultimately preference-based welfare or to their opportunity for that; thus, it might seem that people should be at liberty to have not only as much but as little insurance as they desire (even none). The matter, though, is significantly more complex, largely because of free-riding.

To understand why, let us clear away from our discussion two cases: (1) the person who could definitely (perhaps even easily) pay "out of pocket" for any care from which he might later significantly benefit, and (2) the person who will not subscribe to even the leanest plan because she simply does not have the necessary resources after paying for more immediate needs (food, minimal shelter, clothing, etc.). (The person in the second case, let us assume, is either provided basic insurance itself or the means to make it realistically affordable.) Then the question becomes: Should people who cannot afford to pay for their care out-of-pocket be required to insure? Let us designate as "rejecters" the subset of such persons who would not subscribe, were the decision left entirely up to them.

Suppose that most people of roughly the same economic status as a given set of rejecters do, by contrast, subscribe. Their behavior benefits the rejecters in a variety of ways. Because of them, rejecters seldom see friends and relatives die or suffer from disease and disability for lack of insurance, and thus they seldom find themselves pulled by powerful moral and emotional attachments into bailing out people who need crisis care. They also find themselves living in a more buoyant and healthy society owing to the preventive care that people would not get without insurance. Suppose, furthermore, that when put to the test, rejecters would be willing to pay a certain amount of their own resources if they simply had to in order to obtain these benefits from other people's insurance. To the extent of these benefits, then, rejecters are free-riding on the payments of others for insurance.

A converse point concerns costs that rejecters impose on others. If a person does not insure, others will be faced with torturous decisions about whether to bail her out if she becomes ill beyond her means. To the extent that the moral and emotional pull on their heartstrings is a peculiar function of their individual values, it might be said that they, not she, bear responsibility for the cost and inconvenience that they carry. To the extent, however, that their anguish and willingness to take on such cost and inconvenience are the eminently reasonable reactions that people are expected to have (and that perhaps even the individ-

ual rejecter, too, would have) then she—not they—is responsible.

Whether, then, in terms of the costs that they impose on others or in terms of the benefits from collective activities whose costs they do not fairly share, rejecters are free-riding on other people's insurance. To be sure, this does not tell us whether requiring them to join the collective insurance scheme would be an at least break-even deal for them. It does tell us, however, that whether the benefits to a potential rejecter of a virtually universal practice of insurance exceed a fair share of its individual costs *cannot* be accurately gauged by her unfettered choice about whether to subscribe. Thus, the door is opened to requiring insurance universally.

Such free-rider considerations may, in fact, explain a great deal of the predominant attitude toward insurance in Germany and the Netherlands (Kirkman-Liff, 1991; Heubel, 2000). All non-indigent, low- and middle-income citizens there are expected to insure themselves. Concomitantly, insurers are considered obligated to operate at lowest possible cost. In those countries, much more so than in the United States, a person who needed care but who had not insured would be socially and morally disgraced. This may reflect not so much paternalistic disdain for people who fail to care for themselves as it is condemnation of those who neglect their social responsibilities and free-ride on others.

Some may believe that this moral aversion to free-riding is powerful only in societies more oriented toward collective solidarity than in the United States today, but such an observation would fail to recognize the strongly individualistic foundation of AFRP. Such an observation would also fail to account for the fact that even in the United States, the provision of basic emergency care for those who have not subscribed to insurance is mandated by the Emergency Medical Treatment and Active Labor Act (EMTALA, 1998). Moreover, such a belief would ignore the vicious circle of even a small initial element of free-riding. As a few of the healthier members of a society go uninsured, premiums rise for those who remain in the pool. That rise in premiums leads more of those on the healthier side to go without insurance, which leads to even higher premiums for those who stay in. But then, of course, the phenomenon of people opting out of insurance escalates, and eventually enough people are deliberately uninsured or underinsured so as to create great dislocation. That may lead people to conclude that, even strictly from self-interest, it would be best to press for some coercive arrangement to reduce the ranks of the uninsured. One commentator surmises that this instability of private insurance will eventually cause the United States to require a basic level of universal coverage (Banja, 2000).

This may be too rosy a predictive picture to paint for the future of universal health insurance in the United States. Nonetheless, one can say that the AFRP and honest recognition of the full costs of the vicious circle of an increasing percentage of people opting not to procure insurance create a strong moral argument for compulsory insurance from the perspective of even libertarian theories of justice. Mandatory insurance is one element of the basic structure of a health-care system that is justified from the perspective of all major social philosophies.

COST-EFFICIENCY, FAIRNESS, AND THE PRINCIPLE OF PERSONAL INTEGRITY

What is the relationship between liberty and the achievement of cost-efficiency[7] in health care? It might initially be thought that only social philosophies residing on the collectivist end of the philosophical spectrum—utilitarian and egalitarian views—would endorse coercive rationing to achieve cost-efficiency. I will argue that even significantly libertarian views of justice, however, can endorse a structure for health-care systems that allows a great deal of rationing. Furthermore, in the right empirical circumstances this structure might even include significantly unitary and public health-care systems. The argument is based on three claims:

1. *The integrity of free persons and the morally objectionable nature of free-riding require that health care be limited beyond the extent to which any set of currently ill patients will consent.*

Given the insurance-centered structure of many modern health-care economies, controlling the use of even very high-cost-per-benefit care is extremely difficult. Once patients are insured, whether in private or in public arrangements, both they and providers have strong incentives to use care even when its statistical benefits approach zero and its cost is enormous. To respond to this problem and regain some control over insurance-supported medicine's otherwise virtually endless draw on resources, patients and subscribers must see resource use from a longer temporal vantage point than simply that of the patient. Admittedly, it should not be the perspective of an earlier subscriber who does not imagine realistically what it is to be ill, but it should also not be the perspective of someone who now thinks only as a more temporally limited "patient." Knowing what incentives are created by insurance, the problem of controlling the use of care has to be addressed at an early point in the process—insuring—where the essential trouble starts. Patients and subscribers of integrity will not shrink from this challenge. A stated principle of "personal integrity" may add clarity at this point:

The Principle of Personal Integrity: People ought to be held to the implications of their beliefs, values, and preferences as they confront both later events and other dimensions of their current lives.

People of integrity have this mark of serious consistency: They wrestle with what one belief, value, or preference that they are inclined to hold, means for others, and they wrestle with how to live out their beliefs and values over time, not just change or ignore them when the going gets rough. This has direct application to the rationing of their health care. In their later situation as insured ill patients, their capacity to control the resources of their larger lives is sharply diminished. Whether in communities or as individuals, people of integrity will retrieve that control by referring to what, at an earlier point in time, they would have thoughtfully consented to by way of rationing.

The argument for rationing is also linked to free-riding. If better alternate use of resources is the good that persons in a private or public insurance pool receive by constraining the use of high-cost/low-benefit care, any person desiring to receive that benefit must pay his or her fair share to produce it. This share is simply abiding by limitations on care when they are applied to one's own later case as a patient. Not to abide by those restrictions when others largely do abide would simply be free-riding, namely receiving the benefit of more efficiently directed premiums without paying one's own share of the denial of marginally beneficial services.

2. *If patient–subscribers very likely would have consented to rationing out certain non-cost-worthy care, even though they have not actually consented, then as long as consulting them explicitly beforehand is virtually impossible or prohibitively costly, they still should be denied such care.*

Ideally, of course, subscribers or their representatives should be involved in shaping the major priorities and guidelines for rationing services to improve efficiency. For one thing, people see intrinsic value in making their own explicit choices. But this is not the sole value of consent (Menzel, 1990, pp. 30–31). Bringing decisions in line with a person's values and beliefs is also a major factor in consent's moral importance. To test this out, just imagine examples where the only consent possible is hypothetical and presumed. If you are comatose, should we simply say that, because there is obviously no intrinsic value any longer in your explicit participation, we are going to make the decision about whether to keep you alive solely on the basis of *our* values? I doubt it. (On this larger point about the scope of the concept of liberty, see Sen, 1983.) A formal principle about presumed prior consent can then be stated.

Principle of Presumed Prior Consent: A person's prior consent to welfare-limiting or liberty-restricting policies or actions may be presumed by others both to the extent that it is impossible, not feasible, or prohibitively costly to have solicited the person's actual consent, and to the extent that others can reasonably accurately judge what the person's prior preferences would have been (Menzel, 1990, pp. 22–36)

This statement of the principle makes clear that the moral legitimacy of presuming the hypothetical consent of actual persons is bolstered or weakened by various circumstantial factors. The more clearly and explicitly, for example, the entire context of health care and its coverage consist of lean delivery of services and acknowledgment of concern for efficiency, the more ethical room we have for presuming a person's consent to health-care rationing.

Conversely, the more an insurer or provider publicly proclaims that cost is never any consideration in covering care and that proclamation is relied on by people making insurance decisions, the less plausible it probably is for others to claim that a particular patient would previously have consented to restrictions. Increasingly in the environment of managed care in the United States, however, insurers are cautious in making such claims that cost is never any consideration, and acknowledgment of concern for efficiency has become increasingly widespread. In that context, claims of presumed prior consent to rationing become increasingly legitimate.[8]

3. *Whether the overriding of honest con-*

trary preferences of particular individuals by a larger group's rationing decisions offends against individual liberty depends on numerous larger circumstantial factors in a health-care system, including "translation barriers" to consent-based efficiency.

The clearest case of ethical rationing for cost-efficiency will occur when subscribers voluntarily bind themselves to a plan either by freely joining it when its rationing policies have been publicly disclosed or by cooperatively helping to construct its policies once they join. That clear case of ethical rationing is plainly dependent on a plurality of competing insurers and pre-paid providers.

Nevertheless, more unitary systems cannot be condemned as necessarily violating individual liberty and libertarian senses of justice. First, limiting care in accordance with people's considered desires about the use of resources is not just compatible with moral respect for the dignity of individual patients; it is morally required by that respect. In the case where care is rationed for a large group of subscribers or a whole society of citizens, it is admittedly unfortunate, and a diminution of their liberty, that dissenters do not have their choices reflected in the final shape of their care. Yet *equally*, if care is *not* rationed, individuals who would prefer not to pay for coverage of some of the care that is then provided also have their choices rebuffed. Whereas in the former case dissenters are left without care they would prefer to have covered even with its higher cost, in the latter case dissenters have their resources taken from them without reference to their preferences.

Unitary systems have both an advantage and disadvantage on this score. They can simply globally cap the aggregate resources used and thereby force providers to limit the use of care; not every agent in the system can keep passing the buck of responsibility for rationing up or down in the system, with the result that *no one* acts to restrain the consumption of resources. Unitary systems achieve this, however, at the

cost of not accommodating well the desires of honest dissenters who would rather endure later possible denial of care to gain the benefit of lower taxes or premiums, or pay the price of higher taxes or premiums to gain the benefits of more robust coverage.

Just where this balance finally comes out in our moral calculus may depend in large part on how difficult it is to translate potential patient desire to conserve resources into actual restraints on care—difficulties I call "translation barriers." Market system and mixed-system providers, for example, may strongly resist denying their patients dubiously cost-worthy care. In contrast, if private providers in a mixed system are readily willing to create lean plans and adopt distinctly cost-restraining practice styles, there would be much less to gain in adopting a more unitary, budget-capped system.[9]

In seriously considering support for unitary, budget-capped systems because of the extra bite they give preference-based rationing, however, people with libertarian-leaning views of justice must still ask whether autonomy will be diluted by shifting the place in which values generate rationing trade-offs from an individual context of market choice to a communal context of politically hammering out policies with fellow citizens. Worries here should not automatically lead libertarians to reject unitary systems. Autonomous, responsible resource decisions might be enhanced rather than diminished by the "legislative" conceptual framework in which citizens would begin to confront the hard trade-off issues. Perhaps the best way to get people to think about allocating resources over their extended lives is to place them in the shoes of legislators responsible for an entire health-care system. (For the more general claim here about political discussions, see Sunstein, 1991.)

I would thus conclude: The libertarian sense of justice and the autonomy-respecting ideal that cost-efficiency in health care should ultimately reflect the preferences of individual subscribers do not dictate the choice of health-care system structure in abstraction from a host of particular economic and political facts about the society (Menzel, 1992a).

JUSTICE, EQUAL OPPORTUNITY FOR WELFARE, AND MEDICAL EGALITARIANISM

If people are left to their own choices, some will insure for much less health care than others. Those who insure little are likely to be either healthier or poorer (or less realistic, like the young, for instance) than those who insure more completely. Respecting the choices of subscribers will apparently allow the likely well not to share at all equally in the cost of care for others who through no fault of their own are more likely to need health services; and those who are well-off financially will insure for much more complete care than the relatively poor. To achieve greater equity both between well and ill people and between rich and poor, it seems that a considerable amount of individual subscriber liberty must be sacrificed.

In response to this view that liberty and equity collide with each other in choosing a pluralistic market versus unitary public structure for a health-care system, I want to endorse a more "liberty-friendly" conception of justice generally and work out some claims about the equitable distribution of health care in particular that blunt the conflict between liberty and equity.

A strong case can be made for the claim that egalitarian distributive justice is best captured by the principle of "equal opportunity for welfare" (Arneson, 1989, 1990):

Principle of Equal Opportunity for Welfare (EOW): People should not be worse off than others through no fault or voluntary choice of their own. Situations where people are much worse off than others because of their own sufficiently blameworthy actions or choices may be tolerated, as painful or distasteful as those situations may be.

The equality at which justice should aim, says EOW, obtains among people "when all of them face equivalent decision trees—[when] the expected value of each person's ...most prudent...choice of options, second-best [choice], ...nth-best is the same." Such equal opportunity for welfare differs not only from equality of resources but from equality of welfare per se, although in EOW the opportunities still get ranked by the prospects for welfare they afford (Arneson, 1989, 1990).

Emphasis on equality of opportunity for welfare preserves the possibility of a far greater role for individual choice than is seen in other egalitarian accounts of distributive justice. Furthermore, the focus of EOW on equality of opportunity for welfare, instead of on either equal opportunity unspecified or equal opportunity for some other conceptual item, is more compatible with the liberty to make widely varying financial investments in health care than are many other accounts of distributive justice. The more restrictive ideal of equality of health, for example, even if it legitimately rests on some special contribution that health makes to opportunity, limits freely chosen trade-offs between health and other goods in a way that EOW does not.

The EOW vision of distributive justice allows us to see that the tension between egalitarian and more libertarian accounts of justice in health care is overdrawn. Also, EOW does not involve us in the liberty-denying claims of "medical egalitarianism," the view that care for persons of equal medical needs ought to be equal regardless of a patient's income. That is a view, of course, that pushes distinctly away from pluralistic market systems, but it is dubious.

Take the argument by Daniels for a modified version of some such special equality for health care (Daniels, 1985a, 1985b). Because illness and disability are major, unequal barriers to equal opportunity, health care ought to be distributed straightforwardly according to medical need. Daniels defines illness and disease as deviations from "the natural functional organization of a typical member of a species." A person has a health-care need when care is necessary to achieve or maintain that "species-typical normal functioning." Maintaining or regaining health is not important simply because it is necessary for satisfying people's desires. The role of health care is something further: preserving or restoring the "normal opportunity range."

To see how problematic this argument is, note that the concept of opportunity involves three sorts of references: some goal or set of goals toward which we are striving, a particular obstacle or set of obstacles to that goal from which we are free, and the absence of all insurmountable obstacles to that goal. Equal opportunity in particular then refers to people's mutual freedom from the same set of particular obstacles to the same set of goals (Westen, 1985). The argument for the special equality of health care based on equal opportunity omits one of these elements: a set of goals to which illnesses are impediments.

The argument is then caught on the horns of an impossible dilemma (Menzel, 1990, pp. 124–25). If its point is merely that the opportunity to pursue *any* set of goals is set back by disease and disability, then, though that may in fact be largely true, it would certainly seem appropriate for a rational poor person to adjust her level of medical care downward from what the middle class selects in order to balance out her health-care needs with other important goals. The set of all goals, after all, is the point of the project.

In contrast, if the implicit goals of the opportunities that health care helps to equalize exclude or downgrade the competing goals which might lead a rational poor person to adjust his preferred level of health care downward, we get locked in an argument about why the ultimate goals of health care are more important. The concept of "opportunity" performs no magic here at all in abstraction from the real lives

of preferring individuals. And once we get to those real lives, we see different, plausible opinions about what resources to invest in health care in order to maximize opportunity; EOW allows that.

Thus, EOW helps us to see that the notion of an equitable distribution of care between rich and poor is much less rigid a notion than commonly thought, and certainly not captured by "medical egalitarianism" (a one-tier system). The attraction we have to the proposition that a decent minimum of health care for the poor is roughly equal to the care that others who are not at all poor receive reflects at best only practical considerations, not moral principle (Menzel, 1992a). Perhaps, for example, providers just inevitably fall into the routine of using a uniform conception of "good" and "basic" care, so there is no way other than complete exclusion of specific services to distinguish a decent minimum from the common care for the middle class.

Moreover, in particular historical circumstances, lumping the poor in with the middle class under a unitary standard of required care may seem to be the only politically feasible way of getting additional resources to the poor. In a sense, then, the public is justified in giving resources to poor people in the form of medical care even when the poor would benefit more from devoting some of those resources to other things. But note: Those attitudes that politically restrict government to that form of provision may themselves be the problem. They are public attitudes, for which the public is still on the hook (Menzel, 1983, pp. 92–93; Menzel, 1990, pp. 126–28).

If these considerations make a pluralistic and multitiered system not at all necessarily inequitable for lower-income citizens, so, conversely, other factors may make a unitary system less objectionable to higher-income citizens. Problems of preference translation, monopoly, and administrative efficiency might push free individuals of widely varying incomes toward a unified single-payer system (with buyouts, though not necessarily extra-billing, permitted). Honest holdouts against a more unitary system may be fewer than we think once the operation of a health-care economy is more carefully considered.

JUST SHARING BETWEEN WELL AND ILL

To assess the prospect that pluralistic market systems, in their best form, might be potentially as compatible with justice as so far I have painted them to be, a remaining question must be addressed: Must the premiums that relatively well persons pay be virtually the same as the premiums paid by more likely ill people of similar income?

We might think that placing a high value on liberty requires us to permit a wide range of bargain-seeking behavior by subscribers and insurers, but more careful consideration gives us pause. Suppose that something close to EOW's moderate and relatively liberty-accommodating conception of equity is the considered view of distributive justice held by a great majority of citizens. Applied to the distribution of costs between ill and well, EOW generates a secondary principle:

The Principle of Just Sharing: The financial burdens of medical misfortunes ought to be shared equally by well and ill alike unless individuals can be reasonably expected to control those misfortunes by their own choices.

Note, first, that this "Principle of Just Sharing" is not a strong principle of general redress for natural misfortune that would call on us to equalize the entire life chances of the well and ill, perhaps a futile and significantly wasteful effort. The principle's goal is more modest: equalizing the financial costs of illness. Second, whereas the principle makes a stronger claim than merely that such a distribution is a supererogatory ideal (that is, it may indeed speak to something stronger, like moral obligation), it does not by itself justify the use of coercion to achieve an equitable distribution.

I suspect that EOW and the Principle of Just Sharing are very close to the values held by most Americans. To be sure, there are opponents of even such moderate notions of equity. Arch-libertarians, for example, may argue that short of contract, actual individuals have no obligations of justice to others; obligations never arise out of fate alone. Their position has some intuitive attraction: If through no act or oversight or inaction of yours, I am struck, say, by lightning, why should you be obligated to help me? I am not worse off because of you; you are not better off because of me.

Even in the United States, however, few people think about the overall burdens of health care along such strictly "separatist" lines. Most, I suspect, hold a conception of equitable distribution that simply flips the whole initial burden of proof: If there is no relevant difference between people (for example, if one person is no more deserving than another, or made no shrewder choices), why should one not be obligated to share in another's most unfortunate, life-agenda-setting burdens? After all, the very business of being alive at all is a gratuitous fortune for each of us, so on what basis might a person legitimately complain if truly undeserved burdens are pooled in order to help equalize the life chances and overall opportunities for welfare of well and ill alike? Obligations of justice are simply not grounded only in contract by actual individuals.

If people do indeed widely share some such view similar to EOW and the Principle of Just Sharing, then a public-goods, anti-free-rider argument comes into play. Residing in a society that lives by the Principle of Just Sharing will then be a benefit, not just to the more likely ill, but to all who morally agree with that principle. One's fair share of costs will then be the equal premium or tax assessment necessary to implement the principle.

Although we must still acknowledge an "honest holdout" problem for those who do not share the Principle of Just Sharing, the mere existence of honest holdouts does not by itself block the use of coercion to implement AFRP. Ideally, we should use coercion only on those who share the Principle of Just Sharing, but in practice there may be no way to confine our use of coercion to that group. We have to ask which is worse: Out of respect for truly honest holdouts, do we put up with the free-riding behavior of many of the likely well who do share the principle, or do we regrettably coerce contributions from a few honest holdouts to eliminate the unfairness of a greater number of likely well free-riders paying lower premiums? Because the larger set of individualistic values includes not only various liberties but something like the AFRP, and because the principle of EOW from which the Just Sharing principle is derived is already a significantly liberty-incorporating principle, the use of coercion cannot be ruled out a priori. Where the argument finally comes out on the question of coercion in a context where the AFRP is highly relevant may depend on empirical facts about how widely held the Just Sharing principle is in a particular society.

CONCLUSION

Neither justice nor cost-efficiency in a health-care system requires a fundamentally communalist, non-individualist social ethic. As long as an individualist social philosophy takes careful account of free-riding, presumed prior consent, personal integrity, justice as equal opportunity for welfare, and a principle of just sharing, such philosophies can accommodate both cost-efficiency and the equitable distribution of health care.

Egalitarian social philosophies can also tolerate a wider range of structural type of health-care system than is commonly thought. Equal medical care for persons with similar medical needs regardless of their level of income is not required by principles of equity and egalitarian justice.

Also, a basic minimum of insurance coverage for all citizens is mandatory even if a pluralistic market system is chosen. The only plausible exception would be for those individuals who are able to purchase insurance and do not, and who wish neither to receive care if they end up needing care that they then cannot afford nor to live in a society that rescues those who find themselves in medical emergencies without insurance. And even in a pluralistic market system, premiums for the likely ill and likely well should be roughly equivalent unless the insurance is for conditions widely known to be caused by the person's voluntary choice.

Moreover, a final choice between more pluralistic as opposed to more unitary health-care systems cannot be made solely on the basis of any theory of justice. Such choice will ultimately depend on many details of empirical social fact about a particular culture. This means, for one thing, that a relatively unitary public system can be selected for reasons highly respectful of the value of liberty, just as an appropriately bridled pluralistic market system may be chosen for reasons highly sensitive to equity.

NOTES

1. At least not on "negative liberty" (the liberty not to be interfered with).

2. And utilitarian senses of justice, perhaps, most paradigmatically with mixed private/public systems.

3. Public safety, national defense, or the education of the population to support a modern economy, for example. Once a certain mass of contributors is in place, it is difficult if not impossible to exclude from the benefits of these enterprises an individual who chooses not to contribute to them.

4. This second component of the larger AFRP is widely known in the philosophical literature as the "Principle of Fairness" or the "Duty of Fair Play." See Hart (1955, p. 185), Nozick (1974, pp. 93–95), Simmons (1979), Arneson (1982), Klosko (1987), and the excellent survey of the philosophical literature by Morelli (1985). Note that the "fair share" and "willing to pay" elements in my statement of

the principle already include the exemption that would often be claimed for people unable to pay. In their case, either the fair share of payment is virtually nothing, or, with their meager resources they would not have been willing to pay to get the benefits; they thus have no duty to pay just because we cannot now exclude them from the benefits. On the general point about not obligating people unable to pay, see Schmidtz (1991, p. 146).

5. I will not here attempt anything like a justification of AFRP, no matter which version. It is possible that though AFRP is one of a larger coherent set of principles, there are no more fundamental reasons that it itself that can be used to justify it. Indeed, AFRP might even be needed to explain why any moral principles bind people: Morality as a whole is the collective enterprise, and a reasonable degree of obedience is the fair share everyone is obligated to pay to gain the nonexcludable benefits of morality as a social institution.

6. I say "potential" only because it is notoriously difficult to know who the honest holdouts are if the benefits are actually nonexclusive.

7. My preferred term here would be "costworthiness" (Menzel, 1983, pp. 2–4, 17), but I suspect that to most people it conveys less of the bite of comprehensive economic frugality than "cost-efficiency." "Cost-effectiveness" is well-defined in health economics, but it is technically too narrow to capture the issue discussed here. In this section I will address not only whether the liberty of patients and providers may be restricted when another course of action is likely to produce greater health, or equal health more cheaply, but whether that liberty might be restricted because a particular investment in health at all is not worth its cost. Perhaps we should devote the resources to something other than health care entirely.

8. See here the extensive work by Mark Hall (1997). For a complex and interesting case for applying the Principle of Presumed Prior Consent, one might look at the 1991 Minnesota case of Helga Wanglie. I have argued elsewhere that even in this complex situation, a patient may be legitimately denied care on the assumption that she would not have been willing to pay the added insurance costs of covering life-support for certifiedly persistent vegetative-state patients (Menzel, 1992b).

9. Translation problems in the U.S. current mixed system may stem primarily not from provider resistance but from the peculiar historical fact of an inadequate incentive framework for patients and subscribers: the large and politically well entrenched tax break that the IRS gives for health care purchased through insurance obtained through employer-paid premiums. Perhaps only without that subsidy, a subsidy that the American public seems incapable of repealing, will subscribers realistically confront decisions about what portion of their lifetime available resources they believe should be devoted to medicine. Translation barriers like this may tip the balance of argument back away from pluralistic, mixed systems toward more unitary, budget-capped ones.

REFERENCES

Arneson, R. (1982). The principle of fairness and free-rider problems. *Ethics* 92, 616–33.

Arneson, R. (1989). Equality and equal opportunity for welfare. *Philosophical Studies* 56, 77–93.

Arneson, R. (1990). Liberalism, distributive subjectivism, and equal opportunity for welfare. *Philosophy and Public Affairs* 19 (2), 158–93.

Banja, J.D. (2000). The improbable future of employment-based insurance. *Hastings Center Report* 30 (3), 17–25.

Culyer, A.J., Maynard, A. and Williams, A. (1981). Alternative systems of health care provision: An essay on motes and beams. In M. Olson (ed.), *A New Approach to the Economics of Health Care*. Washington, DC: American Enterprise Institute, pp. 131–50.

Daniels, N. (1985a). *Just Health Care*. Cambridge: Cambridge University Press.

Daniels, N. (1985b). Fair equality of opportunity and decent minimums: A reply to Buchanan. *Philosophy and Public Affairs* 14, 106–10.

Daniels, N. (1990). Equality of what: Welfare, resources, or capabilities? *Philosophy and Phenomenological Research* 50 (Suppl.), 273–96.

EMTALA (The Emergency Medical Treatment and Active Labor Act). (1998). Publ. Law 99–272, 100 Stat. 164 (codified as amended at 42 U.S.C. 1395dd).

Engelhardt, H.T. (1996). *The Foundations of Bioethics*, 2nd ed. New York: Oxford University Press.

Hall, M.A. (1997). *Making Medical Spending Decisions: The Law, Ethics, and Economics of Rationing Mechanisms*. New York: Oxford University Press.

Hart, H.L.A. (1955). Are there any natural rights? *Philosophical Review* 64, 175–91.

Heubel, F. (2000). Patients or customers: Ethical limits of market economy in health care. *Journal of Medicine and Philosophy* 25, 240–53.

Kirkman-Liff, B. (1991). Health insurance values and implementation in the Netherlands and the Federal Republic of Germany. *JAMA* 265, 2496–2502.

Klosko, G. (1987). Presumptive benefit, fairness, and political obligation. *Philosophy and Public Affairs* 16, 241–59.

Menzel, P.T. (1983). *Medical Costs, Moral Choices: A Philosophy of Health Care Economics in America*. New Haven, CT: Yale University Press.

Menzel, P.T. (1990). *Strong Medicine: The Ethical Rationing of Health Care*. New York: Oxford University Press.

Menzel, P.T. (1992a). Equality, autonomy, and efficiency: What health care system should we have? *Journal of Medicine and Philosophy* 17, 33–58.

Menzel, P.T. (1992b). Some ethical costs of rationing. *Law, Medicine and Health Care* 20 (1–2), 57–66. Reprinted in J. Arras and B. Steinbock (eds.), *Ethical Issues in Modern Medicine*, 5th ed. 1999, pp. 715–24. Moun-

tain View, CA: Mayfield Publishing Company.

Morelli, J. (1985). The fairness principle. *Philosophy and Law Newsletter* (American Philosophical Association), Spring 2–4.

Nozick, R. (1974). *Anarchy, State, and Utopia.* New York: Basic Books.

Pauly, M.V., Danzon, P., Feldstein, P.J., and Hoff, J. (1992). *Responsible National Health Insurance*. Washington, DC: American Enterprise Institute Press.

Schmidtz, D. (1991). *The Limits of Government: An Essay on the Public Goods Argument.* Boulder, CO: Westview Press.

Sen, A. (1983). Liberty and social choice. *Journal of Philosophy* 80, 5–28.

Simmons, A.J. (1979). The principle of fair play. *Philosophy and Public Affairs* 8, 307–37.

Sunstein, C.R. (1991). Preferences and politics. *Philosophy and Public Affairs* 20(1), 3–34.

Westen, P. (1985). The concept of equal opportunity. *Ethics* 95, 837–50.

3

Multiculturalism and Just Health Care: Taking Pluralism Seriously

Jeffrey Blustein

Ours is a culturally diverse society. A major source of this diversity is the influx of foreign-born populations fleeing economic hardship and social deprivation and hoping for a better life and greater opportunities in the United States. Immigration to the United States is not a recent phenomenon, of course. The arrival of ethnic and minority populations from various Asian and Hispanic countries is only the latest in a long history of immigration to America. In past years mainstream American society expected the new arrivals to quickly discard their distinctive beliefs, customs, and traditions and join the great "melting pot"; today this assimilationist expectation is increasingly being branded as "culturally insensitive." Not only do we now understand that, as a matter of sociological fact, ethnic and minority groups retain parts of their cultural belief systems while incorporating elements of the broader society, but there is also a growing appreciation of the *moral* claims of cultural pluralism. The call for assimilation has been replaced or supple-

mented by a new emphasis on respect for cultural diversity,[1] grounded in the recognition that it is insulting to the members of these cultural groups to neglect or belittle the importance of their cultural identities.

MULTICULTURALISM, PLURALISM, AND JUSTICE

Multiculturalism, as I understand it, is an amalgam of descriptive, pragmatic, and ethical claims.[2] The descriptive claim is that there are diverse culturally based and conditioned belief systems that help to shape the ways in which individuals view themselves, their relations with others, and their world. Pragmatically, multiculturalism advises us that efforts to communicate, to establish trust, and possibly to bring about change in the behavior of members of cultural groups are unlikely to be successful if those who interact with them are unfamiliar with the ways in which language is used in different cultures, with their particular cultural belief systems, and with the cultural context of their practices. The ethical claims are of two sorts. First, multiculturalism admonishes us to be humble. It is presumptuous of us to suppose that our moral values, rules, and practices are the best ones for human beings and that we have nothing to gain in terms of moral wisdom from communication with so-called inferior cultures. Our moral understanding of complex issues is furthered by respectful discussion with people with whom we disagree, especially when these people have cultural identities different from our own.[3] Second, multiculturalism espouses an egalitarian ethos. As Charles Taylor puts it, "Just as all must have equal civil rights, and equal voting rights, regardless of race and culture, so all should enjoy the presumption that their traditional culture has value" (Taylor, 1993, p. 68). The political implication of this presumption is that a state's institutions and policies should create a political framework that does not discriminate against individuals with different cultural belief systems merely because their conceptions of the good life are not shared by the majority culture.

As we shall see, a central question in debates about the proper scope of government action in general, and the role of government in the provision of health care in particular, is whether it is legitimate for the state to promote a particular conception of the good life. Because the term "conception of the good or the good life" has various meanings in these debates and is often not very clearly defined, it is necessary to indicate how I use the term in this chapter. Roughly, I understand it to refer to a way of life—that is, to a person's pattern of living—which embodies a particular ranking of goods or values that constitute or contribute to the good life for a person and a particular way of realizing them.[4] Multiculturalism is or should be a concern of theories of legitimate state action because a person's conception of the good, understood in this way, is partly constituted and shaped by aspects of his or her culture.

Cultural diversity is part of the expla-nation of the diverse conceptions of the good life among members of a pluralistic society such as ours, but not all the members of a particular cultural group necessarily share the same conception of the good life and not all differences in conceptions of the good life can be traced to distinctive cultural traditions and values. Indeed, as John Rawls and others have pointed out, modern constitutional democracies are characterized by an irreversible pluralism, that is, by often conflicting and incommensurable fundamental value systems, and this pluralism is only partly explained by culture and cultural diversity. Even in democratic societies that are much more culturally homogeneous than ours—certain European democracies, for example—pluralism "is the normal result of the exercise of human reason within the framework of the free institutions of a constitutional democratic regime" (Rawls, 1996, p. xviii).

The very pluralism that democratic regimes foster, however, creates the following serious problem for these societies: When people disagree so fundamentally about the good life, where are the grounds of social unity to be found? This is a quite general problem for liberal political theory, but in this chapter I want to focus on a related but narrower set of issues having to do with what justice requires with respect to the provision of health care in modern democratic societies. Rawls himself has not taken up this question, but a number of other philosophers, including Tristram Engelhardt (Engelhardt, 1991, 1999), Ezekiel Emanuel (Emanuel, 1991), and Norman Daniels in recent work (Daniels, 1990, 1996, 2000) have written on pluralism and its implications for a theory of just health care.

What these authors say about health-care justice, and their sensitivity to the problem of irresolvable pluralism, permit us to understand their proposals as varying responses to the problem posed by John Rawls in his later writing on political liberalism. Briefly put, the Rawlsian question is this: When full agreement on fundamental value conceptions cannot be reached among the members of society, conceived as free and equal persons who are concerned to live with one another on fair terms, can there be a societal consensus—what Rawls calls an "overlapping consensus"[5]—on the basic political arrangements for their society? The object of this consensus is, in Rawls's terminology, a *political conception* of justice. In the case of health care, the question is whether there can be general agreement among such persons on what they owe each other by way of medical assistance or health-care protection, that is, on a political conception of health-care justice. The oppressive use of state power to overcome pluralism might be able to impose uniformity, but, as in Rawls, this is ruled out by a normative commitment to noncoercion and to the achievement of free and willing agreement among citizens. Again as in Rawls, it is not sufficient that the consensus be a mere "modus vivendi," that is, the result of a political accommodation that is advantageous for parties with conflicting individual and group interests.

In contrast to an overlapping consensus, a modus vivendi is inherently unstable, for it is contingent on the balance of power remaining favorable to a political compromise, and it is affirmed on prudential, not principled, grounds. A theory of just health care of the right sort is a political conception of justice that can secure the voluntary and principled allegiance of persons who are divided by diverse conceptions of the good life, including, among other things, diverse understandings of disease and disability and the contributions different medical and health-related services make to the good life.

Pluralism is a general fact of political sociology that any political conception of justice in health care must accept and, in liberal societies with relatively permissive immigration policies, multiculturalism contributes significantly to that pluralism. But both the possibility of an overlapping consensus on a political conception and the content of that conception depend on how deep and extensive the pluralism is. Or rather, because not every conception of the good is compatible with basic tenets of a society of free institutions, the context within which these questions about an overlapping consensus are to be asked is a pluralism of what Rawls calls "reasonable" conceptions.[6] Engelhardt, for example, believes the pluralism of reasonable doctrines is so thoroughgoing that public agreement on a "content-full" or fully substantive political conception of justice for health care cannot be achieved except through state coercive measures.

Daniels, in contrast, is much more sanguine about the possibility, within a democratic society, of an overlapping consensus on a substantive criterion by which to determine the just distribution of health care resources. Emanuel, in contrast to Daniels, argues from the fact of pluralism against a substantive principle that determines an overarching set of medical services that citizens should be guaranteed by the polity as a matter of social justice. In contrast to Engelhardt, he argues for a conception of liberalism according to which society is entitled to differentially support and encourage those conceptions of the good life that embody certain substantive ideals, including political autonomy and individual self-development.[7]

The citizens of a democratic regime, in the free exercise of their reason, may come to espouse diverse theories of just health care that reflect their particular moral or religious or philosophical beliefs. But the justification of a theory of just health care for a democratic society of free institutions cannot rest on such doctrines as they are bound to be highly controversial. It must be independent of them, yet at the same time the theory must be one that citizens who affirm reasonable though opposing conceptions of the good have reason to endorse. Hence, it must not conflict too sharply with such reasonable conceptions. The three authors whose arguments I examine in this chapter have different views of the content of a theory of just health care that accommodates reasonable pluralism and multiculturalism insofar as cultural diversity contributes to reasonable pluralism. But they pose a similar question for themselves—namely, is there a theory of just health care for a democratic society that can win widespread support, where the basic fact of political life that constitutes the context of inquiry is a reasonable pluralism of conceptions of the human good, and if so, what does this theory require?

The two sections that follow deal with Engelhardt and Emanuel. Though as we shall see, there are some commonalities between them, their views on health care justice can be thought of as falling to the political right and the political left of liberalism, respectively. In expounding on their views, I have not dwelt at length on the conception of liberalism they reject, but have chosen instead to let the conception they are attacking emerge from their criticisms of it. In a later section, I turn to liberalism. After discussing recent developments in Rawlsian liberalism and fleshing out the Rawlsian problematic, I consider arguments for a liberal conception of just health care as the proper response to the political challenge Rawls poses.

A LIBERTARIAN RESPONSE TO PLURALISM

Great diversity in beliefs about philosophical, religious, and moral matters is especially likely in a liberal democratic society characterized by freedom of thought and expression, but the conditions that Tristram Engelhardt emphasizes as giving rise to value pluralism are quite general features of what he calls our "postmodern age." The contemporary world, he claims, is marked by two contrasting forces. There is a loss of faith in the power of human reason "to provide for morality and political theory what we long took for granted: a rationally justified content-full moral vision" (Engelhardt, 1991, p. xi). At the same

time, "there remains a plurality of faith and moral commitments" that give rise to passionate conflicts among proponents of "irreconcilable competing moral visions" (1991, p. 9). Not only are there disagreements about such controversial matters as "contraception, abortion, third-party-assisted reproduction, and physician-assisted suicide," but in addition, "there are as many secular accounts of equality, justice, and fairness as there are religious groups, sects, and cults" (Engelhardt, 1999, p. 642). But if there are such deep disagreements about the requirements of justice itself, we have to wonder whether it is possible for diverse moral and religious communities to converge on a common conception of justice and just health care that can span differences among them, and whether such a conception can be justified to them, given fundamental disagreements among them. Engelhardt believes that convergence on a common moral framework for deliberating about health care can be secured, despite the moral fragmentation characteristic of the postmodern age, and it is important to understand how he arrives at this conclusion.

As I interpret Engelhardt's argument, it draws a boundary between two domains with very different justificatory practices, the private and the public. Diverse conceptions of equality, justice, and fairness exist in the individual normative outlooks of members of a pluralistic society, conceptions that are grounded in and justified by (or taken to be justified by) particular religious, philosophical, and moral beliefs. Because these conceptions are justified by irreconcilable conceptions of the good, no theory of justice can possibly fit with all the particular beliefs that support these diverse conceptions. If the goal is convergence on a conception of justice that is *fully* justified to all reasonable members of a pluralistic society, plainly the goal can never be achieved. However, some kind of justification may still be possible, but this depends on putting aside particular moral, religious, and philosophical beliefs, as matters of *pri-*

vate or group conviction, and recasting the problem of justifying a theory of justice as a problem of political justification in the *public* domain. Perhaps there is a basis for common agreement that forms a bridge across diverse communities with differing normative commitments, a conception of justice to regulate public life in a pluralistic society on which there can be an overlapping consensus. These are not exactly the terms in which Engelhardt articulates and defends his view, but I believe he could accept them as a faithful reconstruction.

Given the fact of pluralism, the only conception of justice that Engelhardt believes will be generally acceptable to reasonable people—that is, to people who are concerned to live with others on fair terms of association and who respect one another as free and equal persons—is a libertarian one:

The necessary condition for participating in that world [i.e., a common moral world with moral strangers] is mutual respect, the non-use of others without their consent. This side-constraint is not grounded in a value given to autonomy, liberty, or to persons. . . . Mutual respect is accepted because it is the one way to ground a common moral world for strangers without arbitrarily endorsing a particular ranking of values. (Engelhardt, 1991, p. 119)

There can be an overlapping consensus on a political conception of justice in a pluralistic society, but the conception is a limited and negative one. Coercion and deception are prohibited, but any more robust notion of what we owe to others as a matter of justice is ruled out as involving substantive moral intuitions about which individuals are deeply divided.

Engelhardt bases his libertarian response to pluralism on the claim that our postmodern age is defined in part by widespread rejection of the assumption that serious moral disagreements are in principle amenable to rational resolution. This skeptical thesis about the resolution of moral disagreements is controversial and libertarians are not committed to it. In any case, we might ask whether Engelhardt's politi-

cal solution is sustainable if, as he claims, we live in a world characterized by a loss of faith in the power of reason to establish a common moral framework.[8] Perhaps such a loss of faith undercuts Engelhardt's own solution and dashes hopes for uncoerced general agreement on a content-less, as well as a content-full, political conception. But I will set aside questions about the foundation and coherence of Engelhardt's account and focus instead on the implications of his libertarianism for the delivery and conduct of health care.

The mechanism for the distribution of health care that, in Engelhardt's view, best exemplifies the only defensible political conception for a pluralistic society is the free market. He explains the connection between the conception and the free market this way:

By requiring only peaceable, non-coerced, non-fraudulent exchanges, the market can allow strangers to transfer goods for services without endorsement of a particular morality. . . . Because a free market in health care requires. . . . only the consent of the participants, the market will always have an intellectual advantage over egalitarian health care systems that depend on a particular content-full vision of proper health care distributions. (1991, pp. 134–35)

In a just society, individuals would be able to join with like-minded others to form health-care systems or health-care delivery networks that are congenial to their normative outlooks. Their members would collectively decide how they will use common funds to insure themselves against various eventualities—in other words, what their health care entitlements will be—and because different systems would presumably reach different conclusions based on their particular vision of health care, there would be no universally mandated set of entitlements to health care. In addition, if some people wished to use their private resources to purchase more health care than that provided by common funds, they would be able to do so.

One question this proposal raises has to do with how the common funds are to be collected. If common funds are to be pooled from the private resources of the participants in each health-care delivery network, and if incomes are not fair, affluent networks would have an unfair advantage over poor ones in their ability to provide coverage for a more comprehensive set of benefits. In later writing, perhaps partly in recognition of this problem, Engelhardt added new details to his proposal by advocating the establishment of a system of vouchers or health-care purchase accounts. Two interrelated features of this proposal are worth underscoring. First, Engelhardt's voucher system is intended to attach to a free market system. Vouchers are introduced into this system for use by the poor to purchase health care from the delivery network of their choice. The vouchers function as specially dedicated money to be used by individuals to buy protection against health-care needs as defined by them. Second, the government's role with respect to the distribution of health care is confined to protecting the operation of the free market, and "a limited welfare right to health care"—involving government provision of vouchers—is defended on this basis. Under Engelhardt's proposal, there are no positive rights to health care that government should guarantee to all citizens as a matter of justice, for this "would involve the secular equivalent of establishing a particular religious morality" (1999, p. 650).

A further question about Engelhardt's libertarian solution to the lack of common agreement on a set of basic health-care entitlements concerns the extent to which reasonable people with diverse conceptions of the good life actually disagree about what is and is not a disease. If for the most part there is little controversy among reasonable people about this, then we might be able to mount an argument, at least with respect to the more important diseases, that society is obligated to provide people with medical services to treat them, resources permitting. At least Engelhardt could not object that recognition of a positive right to be given treatments for these conditions would in-

volve the illicit imposition of a single "content-full" morality on a morally diverse society, *if* the way in which reasonable people draw the line between disease and its absence is largely independent of the fact of pluralism.

Engelhardt, however, believes that pluralism plays an important role here, and he takes this to provide further support for a libertarian solution: "The identification of a state of disease or health involves appeal to . . . particular rankings of human goals," and understandings of disease will therefore necessarily be "culture-influenced and relative" (1991, p. 113). It is relevant here to consider what the large body of cross-cultural and multicultural research on the interplay between culture and disease has shown us about the cultural relativity of disease.[9] We know from this literature that cultures vary in their understandings of how the human body works and how to fix it when it stops working properly. We also know that different cultures will use different terms to describe the diseases their members suffer from and that significant variations exist in how people from different cultures explain the causes of disease. None of this shows that there are significant differences across cultures with respect to what members count as a disease state. Indeed, Engelhardt himself is willing to concede that many diseases "(e.g., cancer of the lung or coronary artery disease) are identified as such because they tend to impede whatever goals humans might have" and that they will appear as diseases across cultures (1991, p. 113). Apparently more telling are those historical examples in which certain behaviors or conditions were once classified as diseases, (e.g., masturbation and the running-away disease of slaves) (Engelhardt, 1974). But merely mentioning these cases does not establish that they were properly so classified or that no reasonable consensus on particular substantive health-care issues can be achieved. Reasonable people recognize that the classification was erroneous and in doing so implicitly reject the view that, as Engelhardt puts its, disease categories are just "human cultural constructs" or "human social fabrications" (1991, p. 114).[10]

A LIBERAL COMMUNITARIAN RESPONSE TO PLURALISM

A central tenet of many contemporary liberalisms—collectively referred to as "neutralist liberalism"—is that government may legitimately exercise a range of coercive powers, including the power of taxation, only if it uses these powers neutrally. Exactly what this *neutrality constraint* on government action involves has been a matter of considerable debate among liberals, but I shall understand the claim to be that government actions and policies should not intend to favor some conceptions of the good and some particular ways of life over others. State neutrality is appealing on two counts. The first is that neutrality is a moderately uncoercive means of securing the consent of persons who are concerned with living in a pluralistic society of free and equal citizens. Persons so conceived recognize that the government may not act on their behalf to coercively impose their particular way of life on others, but at the same time they reasonably want assurance that their own way of life will not be seriously threatened, and they are more likely to be confident of this when state coercive power is used on them neutrally than when it is used non-neutrally. The second source of the appeal is the requirement to treat people with equal respect and to protect their autonomy. When government uses coercive power on some citizens for reasons they morally reject, it is argued, they may reasonably feel that the government is failing to respect them as persons.[11]

Despite what many liberals regard as the powerful moral appeal of the notion of neutrality, Ezekiel Emanuel argues that it blocks solutions to crucial ethical questions about termination of medical care for incompetent individuals and rationing of scarce medical resources. We cannot solve these problems without appealing to some robust conception of the good, and liberalism, with its commitment to neutrality about what counts as the good life, cannot allow this. Only communities of individuals organized around shared visions of the good have the moral resources to make progress on these problems without violating the terms of their cooperative arrangement. But we live in a pluralistic society and so we must tolerate—indeed, as Emanuel sees it, more than just tolerate—a plurality of incompatible solutions, each driven by commitment to a particular conception of the good life. There are some similarities here with Engelhardt, but one significant difference between them is that Emanuel argues for a pluralistic system of health care on the ground that a commitment to neutrality precludes the solution of pressing questions in medical ethics, whereas Engelhardt bases it on the implausibility of supposing that serious moral disagreements, in medicine and elsewhere, can in principle be rationally resolved. In one case, neutrality is the problem, in the other, rationality.

"Liberalism accepts pluralism as a fact and permits individual diversity," Emanuel admits. But the neutrality condition, while it may yield a principle of toleration of diversity, provides no basis for positive encouragement of it. Emanuel's political vision, embracing elements of both liberalism and communitarianism, goes further in giving a more prominent place to pluralism: It "affirms pluralism as a positive value enhancing the realization of human potentialities and seeks not only to permit it but to foster it through political diversity" (Emanuel, 1991, p. 175).

Emanuel's conception of pluralism is communal and dynamic. From his perspective, conceptions of the good provide the framework for communal processes of deliberation among individuals who share the same basic normative commitments. They are not just held as matters of private conviction by those who may or may not participate with like-minded others in deliberations about their meaning and implications. Pluralism, for Emanuel, is decidedly not just a pluralism of conceptions of the good that guide people in the conduct of their private lives. It is also, and chiefly, a pluralism of *communities* with shared traditions, ideals, and practices, and liberalism, in his view, is ill-equipped to give the latter any special status. What is called for instead, he argues, is a political philosophy that, although liberal insofar as it recognizes the claim of pluralism and protects individual rights, is also communitarian in that it espouses a "pluralism of affirmation" whose realization "requires recognizing a plurality of communities of deliberation" (1991, p. 161).

Liberal communitarianism also has important implications for how we are to understand the liberal commitment to respect cultural diversity, because respect for cultural diversity occupies an important place in liberal political thought as a way of acknowledging the claim of pluralism. On the liberal communitarian view, it is not enough to tolerate reasonable cultural diversity. Respect requires more—namely, conditions that support and promote ongoing collective deliberations within diverse cultural groups about fundamental elements of their communal life.

As with Engelhardt, we can think of Emanuel as engaged in the task of articulating a political conception of justice for a democratic pluralistic society (and perhaps a multicultural society as well). More specifically, both authors offer a political conception of justice in health care that is suitable for a society characterized by a reasonable pluralism of conceptions of the good. Further, both hold that, because there are deep disagreements regarding appropriate moral understandings of health care, there will be no general agreement on how to rank the value of different medical services, no consensus on which basic medical services society should guarantee to citizens as a matter of justice. A just society is not one that establishes some uniform set of equal basic health-care entitlements for all citizens. Rather, it is a society in which individuals are free to join and receive benefits from the health-care network of their choice (Engelhardt) or, with an important qualification to be mentioned below, a community health program of like-minded individuals, each group espousing and pursuing its own particular conception of the good insofar as it bears on health care (Emanuel).[12] Both writers therefore embrace a political conception of just health care that includes a universal right of citizens to participate in health care organizations they find congenial to their moral, religious, and cultural outlooks, and a corresponding obligation on the part of government to protect this right.

Unlike Engelhardt, however, Emanuel's political conception incorporates a substantive conception of the good, a communitarian conception. Communitarianism, as Emanuel conceives of it, makes a number of claims about the good of persons and how this is achieved:

Informing this ideal [of liberal communitarianism] is a vision of a person who is (*1*) autonomous, (*2*) with fully developed capacities, including those capacities that can only be fully developed through participation in democratic deliberations, and (*3*) who has transcended his contingent existence through participation in the shaping and sustaining of his community. (Emanuel, 1991, p. 157)

Emanuel presumably believes that there can be a consensus among reasonable people on a political conception of justice that includes these liberal communitarian beliefs, and as his political conception includes them, he argues that government, acting on behalf of its citizens, may give extra support and encouragement to those community health programs with a philosophy and mode of operation that are congenial to the liberal communitarian vision. In doing so, of course, the neutrality constraint on government action is violated; but it is the commitment to neutrality, after all, that Emanuel regards as the principal problem with liberalism.

Emanuel is at pains to show that his vision of a health-care system organized along liberal communitarian lines is not just an exercise in utopian thinking, and he provides numerous details to flesh out his proposal. In his plan, several thousand individuals would devise their own community health program, possibly organized around preexisting neighborhood health centers, unions, community hospitals, or health maintenance organizations (HMOs), and based on a shared notion of the good. The programs would be funded by federal vouchers that are given to each person or family in the program and pooled in some sort of health-care trust fund supervised by a federal oversight board. What some may find particularly troubling are the significant exclusionary powers that community health programs have. In Emanuel's (1991) scheme, the right of individuals to participate in this pluralistic health-care system does not entail that a particular community health program is obligated to accept them, even if they agree to live by its policies. A program may exclude them if this is "necessary to sustain a community's commitment to a particular conception of the good life" (p. 239).

Libertarians reject the liberal commitment to welfare rights in health care on the ground that, in a pluralistic and multicultural society, there can be no overlapping consensus on a substantive notion of equality or fairness. Liberal communitarians also believe that we cannot justify a criterion that specifies basic medical services that society should guarantee as a matter of justice, but rather than opt for a minimalist political conception they argue for a richer political conception that incorporates certain substantive ideals of the person and of democratic deliberation. Libertarians believe the liberal account goes too far; liberal communitarians believe that, in some respects, it does not go far enough. What might a liberal political conception look like and can it be the object of an overlapping consensus in a pluralistic, multicultural society?

PLURALISM AND RAWLSIAN POLITICAL LIBERALISM

Perhaps the most well-known and sophisticated liberal theory of just health-care is the one by Norman Daniels that builds on the early work of John Rawls. Though Rawls offers no theory of just health-care himself, Daniels believes that Rawls's principle of equal opportunity can be extended to provide a moral foundation for a right to health care. This might at first seem problematic, for as it is usually understood, Rawls' principle has to do with the impact of *social* structures, whether just or unjust, on opportunity, and much disease is the result of a natural lottery rather than social structure.[13] But diseases, no less than social structures, can preclude an individual from being able to compete with others for desirable social positions under conditions of fairness, Daniels argues, so we should think of equal opportunity as being concerned to counteract the opportunity-limiting effects of both sorts of impediments.

In the original formulation of his theory, Daniels pays little attention to the great diversity in beliefs about philosophical, religious, and moral matters characterizing democratic societies and to the implications of such diversity for a theory of just health care. Rawls himself recognizes the failure to take pluralism seriously as a shortcoming of his book *A Theory of Justice*: "Justice as fairness is presented there as a comprehensive liberal doctrine . . . in which all the members of its well-ordered society affirm that same doctrine. This kind of well-ordered society contradicts the fact of reasonable pluralism" (Rawls, 1999, p. 614). Rawls rectifies this shortcoming in his later work where he considers the justification of a conception of justice as a political enterprise whose aim is to show that it can be freely endorsed by citizens with different reasonable conceptions of the good from their particular perspectives.

According to Rawls, a liberal political conception of justice is characterized by three main features: (*1*) It consists of principles for evaluating the basic structure of social institutions; (*2*) the reasoning about matters of justice that it licenses does not rely on, but is independent of, comprehensive moral or religious views; and (*3*) it can be constructed out of certain key ideas that are already accepted by most people who share a democratic culture, such as the idea that society is a fair system of cooperation and that the terms of cooperation must be ones that free and equal persons can accept.[14] Justice as fairness—according to which the basic structure of society must maximize the long-term expectations of the least advantaged members of society, given background institutions that guarantee equal basic liberties and fair equality of opportunity—expresses and elaborates these key democratic ideas. In Rawls's view, this is a political conception of justice that can be justified to reasonable individuals with different systems of moral and other beliefs. But justice as fairness, Rawls now emphasizes, is not the only admissible liberal political conception:

The content of public reason is given by a family of political conceptions of justice, and not by a single one. There are many liberalisms and related views, and therefore many forms of public reason specified by a family of reasonable political conceptions. Of these, justice as fairness, whatever its merits, is but one. (Rawls, 1999, p. 581)

The principles of every liberal political conception must specify and give priority to certain basic rights, liberties, and opportunities, and must assure "to all citizens adequate all-purpose means to make effective use of their liberties and opportunities" (1996, p. 6). But justice as fairness is only one way of understanding these requirements. Other reasonable liberal political conceptions include "Habermas's discourse

conception of legitimacy . . . as well as Catholic views of the common good and solidarity when they are expressed in terms of political values" (Rawls, 1999, pp. 582–83).

An important question for Daniels' view, if he accepts the recasting of the problem of just health care in the terms of Rawls's later work, is whether there are reasonable political conceptions that are significantly different from justice as fairness with respect to the principle of fair equality of opportunity. Justice as fairness may have, as Rawls claims in *Political Liberalism*, a special place among the family of reasonable political conceptions in that it is the *most* reasonable political conception that can be developed from certain key ideas implicit in the public culture of a democratic society. But Rawls acknowledges that it is not the only reasonable political conception that meets this condition and that justice as fairness, with its principle of fair equality of opportunity, expresses only a particular, "egalitarian form" or variant of political liberalism (Rawls, 1996, p. 6).

If we take this to suggest that there are reasonable liberal conceptions that do not contain the principle of fair equality of opportunity or do not give it the same weight that it has in justice as fairness, then it cannot be claimed that reasonable people (in Rawls's sense) will necessarily converge on a Daniels-type theory of just health care. In fact, reasonable people might converge on some other theory that contains a different conception of equal opportunity than the one Rawls advances in *Theory of Justice*, so that Daniels's equal opportunity account is only one of a number of competing accounts, each of which can lay claim to being a liberal theory of just health care. The question then arises whether there is a liberal argument for a right to health care that does not rely on the principle of fair equality of opportunity and that reasonable people cannot reasonably reject. Putting the question another way, are there any elements of liberal political conceptions *gen-*

erally upon which we can draw to ground such a right? A possible alternative to Daniels' approach is to argue for such a right from the general requirement that a liberal political conception of justice include measures to ensure for all citizens "adequate all-purpose means to make effective use" of their freedoms. On this view, health is conceived as a material precondition of the effective use of a wide range of freedoms, and health *care* is a right because it maintains or restores health, or where this is not possible, helps to ameliorate the effects of disease. It might also be argued that this generic liberal argument for a right to health care better accommodates the fact of reasonable pluralism than does Daniels's fair equality of opportunity argument.

Whatever the merits of this proposal might be, Daniels remains committed to his equal opportunity account, even though, like Rawls, he now takes the fact of pluralism more seriously than he did in the early formulation of his theory in *Just Health Care* (1985). The fair equality of opportunity view, earlier argued for on philosophical grounds, is now defended as the appropriate political conception for a democratic society characterized by a diversity of religious, philosophical, and moral doctrines.

This task is undertaken in chapter 4 of *From Chance to Choice: Genetics and Justice*, written by Daniels, Allen Buchanan, Dan Brock, and Daniel Wikler (2000; see also Daniels, 1990). Though a right to health care can be defended in various ways, it is the impact of disease and impairment on equal opportunity that for them has the greatest appeal as the foundation of such a right. But the authors also acknowledge that in a pluralistic society there may be various conceptions of equal opportunity, some more expansive than fair equality of opportunity. Two views of this sort are discussed at some length: In one, the target of egalitarian concerns is *welfare*, in the other, "positive freedom or *capability* of people to do or be what they choose" (Daniels, 1990, p. 273). The prob-

lem with these more demanding views, they claim, is that they derive from comprehensive moral or philosophical doctrines that not all reasonable people can accept.

A less demanding principle than fair equality of opportunity is the nondiscrimination view, which requires only the elimination of legal and informal barriers to access to desirable social positions. However, this weaker principle, they argue, does not adequately express a feature of the conception of equal opportunity that has considerable appeal in our public culture, namely, that competition for jobs or offices should not be unfairly distorted by one's initial social starting place, by one's family of origin, one's social class, and so forth. Working with this set of conceptions of equal opportunity, Daniels and colleagues attempt to show that there can be an overlapping consensus among reasonable people on a political conception of just health care that bases a right to health care on the principle of fair equality of opportunity, interpreted in terms of a notion of normal species functioning.[15] Proponents of the more expansive conceptions of equal opportunity can *at least* accept this, and proponents of the weaker conception can be shown to be unreasonable in so restricting the scope of the demands of equal opportunity.

Of course, an overlapping consensus on a political conception of just health care, or justice more generally, might not include everyone in the society, but universal inclusion is not a requirement of the Rawlsian project and it does not necessarily count against it or against a political theory of just health care defended along these lines, that some members of society are left out. For example, individuals who have immigrated to liberal democratic societies from authoritarian or tribal societies might not accept key elements of a public, democratic culture, at least for a time. (Arguably, this is true of certain cultural groups in which women are socialized to be self-effacing and unconditionally obedient to their husbands or other male relatives.) They may retain conceptions of justice and equality that are the product of their native cultures, conceptions rooted in particular moral, religious, and philosophical belief systems. To the extent that they do not accept certain fundamental intuitive ideas present in the democratic political culture, they will have no reason to support a political conception of justice constructed out of these ideas. Or rather, they will have no reason of the *right type*, for it may be in their self-interest to comply with the norms of the democratic society if the state uses its coercive power to enforce obedience.

To the question, Why should we comply with democratic principles when our own conceptions of justice and equality do not recognize their validity? all that can be said is, this is how we do things here, and as long as you live here, you have to play by the rules. One would like to be able to show such individuals that they have reasons of a different sort for compliance, that it is not just because the superior power of the state leaves them no choice, but in Rawls's account this is not possible until they have assimilated fundamental normative ideas of the political culture.

Let us then confine the discussion to a pluralistic society of a certain sort, a society in which convergence on a liberal political conception of justice for the right reasons is possible among different cultural groups and adherents of different comprehensive doctrines. And let us suppose further that there will be a consensus in this society that health care is a requirement of justice because it is necessary to ensure fair equality of opportunity. It is still possible, indeed likely, that people's diverse cultural backgrounds and particular normative commitments will lead them to disagree about which scheme of medical and health services promotes fair equality of opportunity. Though Emanuel presents this as a serious problem for the liberal account,[16] it is not clear why a proponent of the fair equality of opportunity view cannot accept disagreement on this level, indeed why he cannot welcome this sort of disagreement, as long as it is constrained by basic agreement

on the principle itself.[17] It need be no embarrassment to the liberal account that, given a reasonable pluralism, there will be a number of *sufficiently just* schemes of medical and health services, each of which can plausibly be regarded as living up to the principle of fair equality of opportunity. Different just health and medical schemes might assess differently the impact of particular medical services and technologies on the range of opportunities we enjoy. They might also assign different relative weights to categories of care: mental versus physical, preventive versus acute, and acute versus long-term care.

Of course, this does not show that Daniels' view is correct or that the reasoning by which he defends it, in both his early and more recent work, is sound. Engelhardt, for example, believes that in a pluralistic society there can only be consensus on a process of peaceable negotiation for resolving disputes, not on a substantive criterion. The point is a more modest one, namely the liberal account can allow a range of views about the importance of different medical and health services, and hence about what justice specifically requires in the realm of health care. The range is narrower than on some other accounts—for example, Engelhardt's and Emanuel's—but some measure of local variation can be accommodated.[18]

CONCLUSION

My main intention in canvassing the libertarian, liberal communitarian, and liberal responses to the fact of pluralism, and multiculturalism as an aspect of pluralism, has not been to advocate for one of them in particular. Too many important issues have been left unsettled to reach a conclusion about which is the better theory. Rather, I hope to have indicated the main issues that must be addressed by a theory of just health care for a pluralistic, multicultural society. I have assumed throughout that a theory of just health care must meet certain requirements, that the goal is not to provide the most philosophically compelling account of justice, but rather a conception of justice that reasonable people with diverse moral, philosophical, and religious belief systems can freely endorse despite their disagreements about other matters. In this sense, a theory of just health care that takes pluralism seriously must be political.

If we understand the task of constructing a political theory of justice the way John Rawls does, then an objection to Engelhardt might be that the fundamental intuitive ideas embedded in the public, democratic culture furnish us with sufficient materials for working up a more robust theory of just health care than the procedural one that Engelhardt defends. But we might not understand the task this way, and even if we do, these ideas may be too thin to support anything more than a libertarian solution. These are complex issues that I have not tried to resolve. Emanuel believes that, because of pluralism, any principle for determining what society should guarantee to citizens as a matter of justice, even if generally agreed upon, will be so abstract as to be of little practical use. The questions that pluralism and, secondarily, multiculturalism pose for a theory of just health care might therefore be formulated in the following ways: (1) What political conception (or conceptions) of just health care can secure the uncoerced allegiance of reasonable people—people who are committed to their own conceptions of the good but who recognize that they live in a pluralistic society and are concerned to live with one another on fair terms? And (2) Will this conception include a substantive and practically useful principle of health care entitlement?

Acknowledgment

I want to thank Arthur Kuflik for spending many hours with me discussing the issues in this chapter and for helping me clarify and organize my thoughts on different approaches to a theory of justice for health care.

NOTES

1. The notion of respect for cultural diversity is continuous with a familiar feature of liberal political thought, namely religious toleration.

2. See Ronald Bayer's helpful discussion of multiculturalism in "AIDS Prevention and Cultural Sensitivity: Are They Compatible?" *American Journal of Public Health* 84, no. 6, June 1994: 895–98.

3. This point is made by Amy Gutmann, "The Challenge of Multiculturalism in Political Ethics." *Philosophy and Public Affairs* 22, no. 3, summer 1993: 171–206.

4. Here I follow Joseph Chan, "Legitimacy, Unanimity, and Perfectionism." *Philosophy and Public Affairs* 29, no. 1, winter 2000: 3–42.

5. Rawls (1996) introduces the idea of an overlapping consensus on pp. 38–40 of *Political Liberalism.*

6. *Reasonable pluralism* is to be distinguished from *pluralism as such* and refers only to a pluralism of reasonable conceptions. Rawls discusses the latter notion in *Political Liberalism,* pp. 58–66.

7. The distinction between a substantive *principle* that determines an overarching set of medical services and substantive *ideals* incorporated into the political conception is discussed more fully in the section titled "a Liberal Communitarian Response to Pluralism."

8. What would Engelhardt say to a person who would rather force his views on others and who answers his critics this way: "To be sure, I cannot rationally convince you that I am right, but then you can't rationally convince me that you are right either"? The notion of rational justification that Engelhardt employs here seems to be something like rational *proof*, and it is questionable whether this is an appropriate way to understand how rational justification works in ethics.

9. The literature is vast. See, for example, Malcolm MacLachlan, *Culture and Health Care* (New York: John Wiley, 1997).

10. Whether diseases are social constructions determined by our positive or negative evaluations or whether they have some more "objective" basis is a long-standing controversy in the philosophy of medicine. For two opposing views, see Christopher Boorse, "On the Distinction between Disease and Illness," *Philosophy and Public Affairs* 5, no. 1, 1975: 49–68, and Peter Sedgwick, "Illness-Mental & Otherwise," *Hastings Center Studies,* 1, no. 3, 1973.

11. The discussion in this paragraph closely follows Harry Brighouse, "Neutrality, Publicity,

and State Funding of the Arts." *Philosophy and Public Affairs* 24, no. 1, winter 1995: 35–63. I should note that I merely mention these as grounds of the appeal and do not take a position on the merits of the argument for neutrality.

12. Emanuel (1991) distinguishes among four conceptions of the good, each of which endorses a different scheme of health-care services. The *physical* conception justifies giving priority to the use of aggressive life-saving treatments for all patients; the *relational* conception favors an age-based scheme in which elderly patients receive palliative rather than life-saving care; the *autonomous* conception supports a system that focuses on providing medical care that has a reasonable prospect of enabling patients to live independent lives; and the *utilitarian* conception endorses the use of cost-effectiveness as the criterion for determining which services to provide and to whom (Emanuel, 1991, *The Ends of Human Life*, pp. 126–144).

13. Both the incidence and the distribution of disease are heavily influenced by socioeconomic factors that shape a person's relative social advantage. Recently, a number of bioethicists have called for greater attention to the social determinants of health, which, research has shown, do more to explain health differences between advantaged and disadvantaged members of society than do disparities in access to medical care. See, for example, James Hurowitz, "Toward a Social Policy for Health," *New England Journal of Medicine* 329, no. 2, July 8, 1993: 130–33.

14. See Rawls, (1999), "The Idea of Public Reason Revisited."

15. The normal species functioning interpretation of the principle of fair equality of opportunity is presented in chapter 4 of Daniels et al., *From Chance to Choice*, as well as in Daniels' (1981), "Health-Care Needs and Distributive Justice," and Daniels (1985) *Just Health Care.*

16. See chapter 4 of Emanuel (1991), *The Ends of Human Life.*

17. Here is where democratic political processes play an important role. Democratic deliberation is arguably the most appropriate way for citizens collectively to reach agreement on the specific requirements of the principle. Amy Gutmann and Dennis Thompson, in *Democracy and Disagreement* (1996), put democratic deliberation at the center of their attempt to solve the problem of reasonable pluralism.

18. See Daniels (1992), in which he offers this reply to Emanuel in his review of Emanuel's *The Ends of Human Life.*

REFERENCES

Bayer, R. (1994). AIDS prevention and cultural sensitivity: Are they compatible? *American Journal of Public Health* 84 (6), 895–98.

Boorse, C. (1975). On the distinction between disease and illness. *Philosophy and Public Affairs* 5 (1), 49–68.

Brighouse, H. (1995). Neutrality, publicity, and state funding of the arts. *Philosophy and Public Affairs* 24 (1), 35–63.

Chan, J. (2000). Legitimacy, unanimity, and perfectionism. *Philosophy and Public Affairs* 29 (1), 3–42.

Daniels, N. (1981). Health-care needs and distributive justice. *Philosophy and Public Affairs* 10 (2), 146–79.

Daniels, N. (1985). *Just Health Care.* Cambridge: Cambridge University Press.

Daniels, N. (1990). Equality of what: Welfare, resources, or capabilities? *Philosophy and Phenomenological Research* 50 (Suppl), 273–96.

Daniels, N. (1992). Review of *The Ends of Human Life. Hastings Center Report* 22 (6), 41–42.

Daniels, N. (1996). Reflective equilibrium and justice as political. In Daniels, *Justice and Justification.* Cambridge: Cambridge University Press, pp. 144–75.

Daniels, N. (2000). With Allen Buchanan, Dan W. Brock, and Daniel Wikler. *From Chance to Choice: Genetics and Justice* Cambridge: Cambridge University Press.

Emanuel, E. (1991). *The Ends of Human Life: Medical Ethics in a Liberal Polity.* Cambridge, MA: Harvard University Press.

Engelhardt, Jr., H.T. (1974). Disease of masturbation: Values and the concept of disease. *Bulletin of the History of Medicine* 48 (2), 234–48.

Engelhardt, Jr., H.T. (1991). *Bioethics and Secular Humanism: The Search for a Common Morality.* London: SCM Press.

Engelhardt, Jr., H.T. (1999) Freedom and moral diversity: the moral failures of health care in the welfare state. In J. Arras and B. Steinbock (eds.), *Ethical Issues in Modern Medicine*, 5th ed. Mountain View, CA: Mayfield, pp. 642–51. Reprinted from (1997). *Social Philosophy and Policy* 14 (2), 180–96.

Gutmann, A. (1993). The challenge of multiculturalism in political ethics. *Philosophy and Public Affairs* 22 (3), 171–206.

Gutmann, A. and Thompson, D. (1996). *Democracy and Disagreement.* Cambridge, MA: Harvard University Press.

Hurowitz, J. (1993). Toward a social policy for

health. *New England Journal of Medicine* 329 (2), 130–33.

MacLachlan, M. (1997). *Culture and Health Care*. New York: John Wiley.

Rawls, J. (1971). *A Theory of Justice*. Cambridge, MA: Harvard University Press.

Rawls, J. (1996). *Political Liberalism*. New York: Columbia University Press.

Rawls, J. (1999). The idea of public reason revisited. In *John Rawls: Collected Papers*. Cambridge, MA: Harvard University Press, pp. 573–615.

Sedgwick, P. (1973). "Illness-Mental and Otherwise," *Hastings Center Studies* 3 (1), 19–40.

Taylor, C. (1993). *The Politics of Recognition*. In A Gutmann (ed.), *Multiculturalism and the Politics of Recognition*. Princeton, NJ: Princeton University Press.

4

Utilitarian Approaches to Justice in Health Care

Matti Häyry

Utilitarianism, as an ethical tradition, insists first, "that action is best which procures the greatest happiness for the greatest numbers" (Hutcheson, 1725) and, second, that "justice is a principle which proposes to itself the production of the greatest sum of pleasure or happiness" (Godwin, 1793). When these principles are applied to the problems of justice in health care, the self-evident norm seems to be that all traditional and common-sense accounts of equity, fairness, and deserts should be overridden by straightforward calculations of utility, or the net good produced by medical decisions and public policies.

My purpose in this chapter, however, is to show that there is more than meets the eye in utilitarian responses to health care provision. Although the idea of adding and subtracting utilities and disutilities has been popular in health administration, this is by no means all there is to "procuring the greatest happiness for the greatest numbers."

ALL APPROACHES ARE UTILITARIAN, AREN'T THEY?

In one sense, all approaches to justice in health-care provision are utilitarian. The primary problem is that resources are limited, and that all possible life-saving and health-enhancing treatments cannot be extended to everyone. Because difficult choices between individuals and groups must be made, no one can, knowingly and seriously, propose policies that would be inefficient, that is, which would simply throw away scarce resources to no one's benefit.

Even those who prefer individual liberty to the well-being of the population as a whole (Nozick, 1974) are likely to oppose public-health policies that are not aimed effectively at the general good. Although these "libertarians" can question attempts to redistribute welfare by state coercion in the first place, they do not presumably want to see their tax dollars wasted if they are collected anyway and if the alternative is to do some good with them.

There is also another sense in which many current approaches to justice in health care are utilitarian. One of the basic tenets of utilitarianism is that individuals should be treated impartially when laws and public policies are framed. Those making decisions that can have an impact on the lives of others should not favor their relatives or friends, or deny people's access to health care on account of their skin color, gender, or ethnic origin. This idea, which was strongly advocated by the utilitarians of the eighteenth and nineteenth centuries (Bentham, 1789; Godwin, 1793; Mill, 1861), is now widely shared regardless of political or ideological persuasions.

THEN WHAT IS WRONG WITH UTILITARIANISM?

Many ethicists believe, however, that utilitarian approaches to health care can be unjust, or otherwise immoral. Justice, some of them argue, demands that individuals get what is their due, or what they can reasonably expect. Others contend that justice as efficiency and impartiality is not enough—that, for instance, caring for the vulnerable is more important than being effective or fair. Utilitarianism, these theorists contend, is a cold, calculating doctrine that ignores special relationships between people and neglects the needs of those who are worst-off (Rawls, 1972; B. Williams, 1973; MacIntyre, 1981; Maclean, 1993).

The question is, how can this be true if utilitarians have always endeavored to promote the greatest happiness of humankind?

The simplest answer can be found in the definitions utilitarians have given to the concept of "happiness." The early champions of the theory defined happiness as pleasure (Bentham, 1789; Godwin, 1793; Mill, 1861; Sidgwick, 1874), thereby alienating all the good Christians who believed that hedonism is an invitation to indecency and sin rather than a respectable theory of value. Twentieth-century utilitarians did

not help much by equaling happiness with contentment, enjoyment, the fulfillment of desires, or the satisfaction of preferences (Smart, 1961; Brandt, 1979; Hare, 1981). Demands to aggregate these experiences and states seem to miss all the higher aspects of human perfection and human flourishing.

Concrete and measurable units of value are, however, indispensable in theories designed to be as "scientific" as possible. The satisfaction of preferences resulting from a course of action can, at least in principle, be studied empirically, and then compared with the preference satisfaction resulting from other courses of action, so as to reach the right decision.

Incidentally, the exact calculation of the net good in each situation is not a necessary element of all utilitarian approaches to justice in health care. But the point here is that many people have believed that it is, and they have founded their critical remarks on this belief. Besides, the idea of counting utilities provides a bridge to the quantification of the quality of human life, which many theorists see as the paragon of utilitarianism in health-care provision. An examination of the best-known quality-of-life indicator, the *quality adjusted life year*, or QALY, can be used to identify the strengths and weaknesses of this notion.

QALYs—A UTILITARIAN APPROACH TO JUSTICE IN HEALTH CARE?

The motivation for the development of quality-of-life measures in health economics has been—and is—that survival rates and other medical indicators draw an inadequate picture of the effects of medical interventions (Edgar, 1998). After an operation, one patient can live an active life, and another patient can be permanently confined to bed. Similarly, some treatments can ensure that the patient experiences no pain or distress afterwards, others can have agonizing side effects. The QALY method was designed in the 1970s to account for the intuition that individuals typically prefer ability to disability and contentment to distress and pain.

The QALY unit stands for one life year in good health without disability or distress. If a patient is expected to live five years after an operation enjoying this level of health, the value of the treatment is five QALYs. But if the treatment, although resulting in five years of survival, leaves the patient disabled or distressed, then its value is diminished. The ratio of the reduction can be counted by using a matrix devised by the inventors of the method, who interviewed physicians, health administrators, and patients to arrive at their figures (Rosser and Kind, 1978; Kind et al., 1982). For instance, the ratio for a state where an individual is unable to work and suffers from severe distress is, according to their calculations, 0.700, which means that five years in this condition produces only 3.5 QALYs, as opposed to the 5 QALYs of the five good years. (For a clear and concise exposition and assessment of the QALY method, see Edgar, 1998.)

The QALY model could, in principle, be employed to compare the benefits individual patients can expect from different treatments. It is possible that one alternative would produce five years of good health and another six years of inferior health, in which case the QALY value of the shorter life after the treatment would be greater than that of the longer life. But this result is not very interesting, because it is based, at best, on the typical responses people have toward different levels of disability and distress. The individual patients can simply be asked whether they would rather have five good years or six bad years, and whatever their decision, it cannot be overruled by an appeal to other people's attitudes.

The situation can, however, be different at the societal level. If the task of public-health authorities is to maximize the health of the population, then the QALY method can arguably be employed to allocate scarce medical resources to treatments and policies that are the most effective in terms of the quantity and quality of continued human life.

One of the creators of the model, Alan Williams, argued that this is exactly what should be done. Williams suggested (1985) that the cost-effectiveness of various treatments can and should be assessed by calculating the cost per QALY incurred by them. He examined three different treatments for kidney failure and estimated that, whereas hemodialysis in hospital and at home cost, on the average, £14,000 and £11,000 per QALY produced, kidney transplantation is the most cost-effective treatment at only £3,000 per QALY. One reading of this result is that health authorities, faced with the choice between a group of patients who can benefit from kidney transplantation and a group who cannot, ought to prefer the former, because more QALYs will be produced by allocating scarce resources to their treatment.

A large-scale attempt to allocate health resources along the lines sketched by Williams was made in Oregon, where a statewide rationing plan was drafted in the late 1980s (Daniels, 1991; Dougherty, 1991; Hadorn, 1991; Stason, 1991).

A CLASSICAL UTILITARIAN DEFENSE OF THE QALY MODEL

The QALY model can be defended both on contractarian (Menzel, 1990) and on utilitarian grounds. Williams (1988), taking the latter route, has argued that the strength of the approach lies in its impartiality, or egalitarianism. It does not judge people on their worth, deserts, social status, age, gender, or other factors that are irrelevant in provision of a just health-care system. It calculates the cost-effectiveness of treatments, and indicates the areas in which the health of the population can best be enhanced by the available resources.

It is not, by the way, necessary to confine the application of the QALY model to medical measures alone. If more QALYs can be more economically produced by improvements in sanitation, or by investments in education, or by paying attention to environmental issues, then this ought to be done. Exotic life-saving treatments are not the only way to add to the length and happiness of human lives.

All this is perfectly in line with the ideas of the classical utilitarians. Anti-favoritism was a paramount feature in the thinking of William Godwin (1793), who scandalized his contemporaries with an example involving a known benefactor and a family member. The benefactor's house is on fire, and a bystander can save either the master of the house or the master's valet, who, however, happens to be the bystander's own father. Godwin argued that, because more good to humankind can be accomplished by saving the benefactor, justice requires that he should be saved instead of the valet. There is no magic, he retorted to his critics, in the pronoun "my" that could overturn the demands of "impartial truth" and "pure, unadulterated justice."

In all fairness to Godwin, it must be noted that his own ultimate position was anarchistic—he believed that people can best get along with each other without state coercion or intervention. The idea of public health authorities making decisions on behalf of other citizens would probably have been alien to his way of thinking.

Jeremy Bentham (1789), in turn, contended that all legislation and public policies ought to be aimed at the greatest happiness of the greatest numbers. He also argued that "happiness" should be defined as pleasure and lack of pain, and that only quantitative factors should be taken into account when alternative courses of action are assessed. In Bentham's hedonistic calculus, pleasures and pains are compared by their intensity, duration, certainty or uncertainty, and propinquity or remoteness, and actions by the fecundity and purity of the experiences they produce, and by the number of individuals who experience them. By the "fecundity" of a pleasure or a pain, Bentham meant the "chance it has of being followed by sensations of the same kind," and by "purity" the chance it has of not

being followed by experiences of the opposite kind.

Because the QALY model is designed to measure the quantity and quality of people's lives with or without medical interventions, it can be seen as a refined version of Bentham's calculus in the context of health care. And if resources are scarce, the classical utilitarian duty seems to be to allocate them where they can be expected to produce the greatest amount of QALYs.

A THEOLOGICAL UTILITARIAN CRITIQUE OF THE QALY MODEL

The QALY model has, however, been criticized on grounds that can, despite their initial appearance, be construed as utilitarian. The first argument against the QALY method is that it ignores the value of life, or the value of saving lives as such. An expensive treatment can save a patient, whose life quality will afterwards be very poor. If the resources needed for this operation are allocated to other purposes, they can enhance the life quality of thousands of others, thereby making it more QALY-effective to let the patient with the expensive needs die. But this, it can be argued, is immoral and unjust, because saving lives is surely more important than improving life quality.

One utilitarian response to this is that life is valuable only as a means to good experiences, and that survival without proper life quality is not in itself a goal worth pursuing (Crisp, 1989). But more interestingly, the policy of saving lives whatever their quality can also be given a utilitarian justification.

George Berkeley, better known in the history of philosophy for his immaterialism, sketched (1712) a view that can be called "theological utilitarianism" (Albee, 1902; M. Häyry and H. Häyry, 1994), and other British moralists of the eighteenth and nineteenth centuries (Gay, 1731; Brown, 1751; Tucker, 1768–77; Paley, 1785; Stephen, 1873) developed the doctrine further (Albee, 1902; Häyry, 1994).

The gist of this theory is that we can tell, by observing the human nature and the nature of the world, that God is a utilitarian who wants all His creatures to be as happy as possible. Human beings, in their turn, have an obligation to act in accordance with God's wishes, that is, to aim at the greatest happiness of the greatest numbers.

There are, in principle, two ways in which people can accomplish this. The first is to calculate in each situation which course of action would maximally promote the human good. But this, as the theological utilitarians unanimously pointed out, is a problematic approach. Both our knowledge and our understanding are limited, which means that we can never foresee accurately all the consequences of our actions. And even if we could foresee them, their assessment would be too time-consuming to serve any practical purposes. Besides, a morality based on probabilities assessed by fallible individuals is clearly inferior to a morality based on certainty.

This is why the theological utilitarians preferred another way of obeying God, which is to observe the rules and commandments God has given to humankind through revelation and tradition. Among these is the prohibition of killing, which can also be interpreted as an imperative to saves lives whenever possible.

In the discussion concerning QALYs and their applicability to resource allocation, the theological utilitarian line of argument is relevant in two respects. First, it shows that the strict duty to prefer survival to life quality, usually known as the *sanctity-of-life doctrine* and associated with "deontological" and "teleological" types of thinking (Kuhse, 1987), can also be given a utilitarian reading. The question is not whether you are a utilitarian or not, but, rather, whether you believe that a divine being has laid down principles that rule out the application of the QALY method in the allocation of health-care resources.

Second, however, theological utilitarians also raised another important issue, namely our limited capacity to assess the consequences of our actions. This critique goes straight into the heart of the QALY model, and also undermines all other attempts to calculate the value of lives in terms of their duration and their objective or subjective goodness. Health authorities do not know for certain what the consequences of their decisions are, and they know even less about the way other people experience these consequences. I will return to these questions toward the end of this chapter, but let me first recount a more contemporary utilitarian argument against the use of QALYs as a measure of justice in health-care provision.

A LIBERAL UTILITARIAN CRITIQUE OF THE QALY MODEL

John Harris, who has no faith in the sanctity-of-life doctrine (1980, 1985), has argued that the QALY method is unjust on at least two accounts. The first is that its application is inevitably discriminatory, especially when it comes to comparing old people to the young. On the average, the remaining life span of neonates is longer than that of old-age pensioners. Therefore, regardless of the quality of life enjoyed by the individuals involved, neonates should be preferred to the elderly in a standard QALY approach, and more resources ought to be allocated to their care—which can be seen as "ageist."

It has been suggested (Edgar, 1998) that this implication can be avoided by giving more weight to the remaining life years of the elderly. Although this is a feasible solution, it gives rise to new questions. If the model is supposed to be impartial, what justifies the extra weight given to some groups of people and not to others? If survival in good health should be maximized, then why prefer alternatives that contradict this goal?

Harris's second argument is based on the intuition, or insight, that, from an individual's perspective, a life is a life whatever its length or character. There is no reason why I should prefer a better life for someone else to a poorer life for myself. If I desire to live, then it is this desire that gives my life its worth. The other person's situation is, of course, similar. But as there is no reliable way to compare the strength of our respective desires to live, no authoritative choices can be made between us by comparing the values of our remaining lives.

At first glance, Harris's argument seems to be directed against utilitarianism in its entirety. If impartiality is paramount, as Harris himself seems to concede in the case of ageism, then what magic is there in the pronoun "I" that could overturn the demands of "impartial truth" and "pure, unadulterated justice" (Godwin, 1793)?

UTILITARIANISM VERSUS EGOISM

One answer to this question can be found in the work of Henry Sidgwick (1874), who summarized the utilitarian case against other moral doctrines in a way that also exposed the limitations of the view itself. His starting point was that ethical theories should conform to certain basic intuitions, namely those of justice, prudence, and the universality of goodness. Justice requires that "whatever action any of us judges to be right for himself, he implicitly judges to be right for all similar persons in similar circumstances." Prudence dictates that "one ought to have impartial concern for all parts of one's conscious life." And the universality of goodness means that "the good of any one individual is of no more importance from the point of view of the universe than the good of any other."

According to Sidgwick, utilitarianism, which states that we should always aim at promoting the general good, is a sound moral theory because it can accommodate all these basic intuitions. But the problem is that a rival doctrine, namely *rational egoism*, can also accomplish this, given that the universality of good is not interpreted too strictly. Egoists can universalize their views by admitting that, whereas it is their own duty to maximize their own happiness, others, too, are entitled or obliged to maximize their own good. Egoists can be

prudential and value all parts of their lives equally. And they can argue that, whereas from the point of view of the universe their good is no more important than the good of others, from their own point of view their happiness outweighs the happiness of others.

This line of argument would fully justify Harris's position in the QALY debate. Health authorities would be free to hold that for them the maximization of QALYs among the population is paramount, and I could counter this by noting that for me it is not. The only minor difficulty is that Harris would in this case be an egoist, which would make his criticism of the QALY model nonutilitarian.

UNCERTAIN QUALITIES, FIRM NUMBERS

Another response to Godwin's question regarding impartiality and justice is to say that it would be all right to apply the QALY model to resource allocation, if we could be certain that QALYs measure what is important in our lives. But they do not, because the figures arrived at by the inventors of the method are arbitrary, and because this arbitrariness cannot be properly rectified by any methods currently known to social science or psychological research.

This response is more in line with the basic utilitarian credos. It does not deny the status of the greatest happiness of the greatest numbers as the ultimate aim of health policies. Instead, it reintroduces to the discussion the epistemic concerns first raised by the theological utilitarians, and also emphasized by the proponents of "rule utilitarianism" in the twentieth century (Harrod, 1936; Ewing, 1953; Toulmin, 1953; Nowell-Smith, 1954; Stout, 1954; Brandt, 1959; Harsanyi, 1982). And, even more importantly in our present context, the response seems to be compatible with other views presented by Harris—especially with the startling solution he has proposed to the allocation of scarce resources in organ transplantation.

In his famous essay "The Survival Lottery," Harris (1975) argues that a reasonable way to attain organs for transplantation would be to arrange a nationwide "lottery" where suitable donors are selected. Every time two or more people would die unless a new organ can be found for them, a computer identifies an individual whose tissue type is compatible with theirs. This individual is then called up and killed in order to save the lives of those in need of the organs.

The difference between this model and the application of the QALY method seems to be, in Harris's view, that while measurements concerning the quality of life are open to dispute, the simple computation of lives is not. I can argue that my remaining life is as valuable as the life of anyone else, and I can use this argument to reject proposals to prioritize treatments on the basis of QALY assessments. But because two lives are twice as valuable as one, I cannot resort to this argument in the organ transplantation case. Numbers count—that is, the maximum number of lives should be saved by good health policies.

MURDERING TO SAVE LIVES?

The lottery model presented by Harris has been criticized (Maclean, 1993) on the grounds that killing innocent persons equals murdering them, and murder is never morally acceptable. Although this is perfectly true, the question, from the utilitarian viewpoint, is how to define "murder" in a way that includes the killing of suitable organ donors but excludes other decisions that lead to the death of innocent persons, yet are generally accepted. Harris defends the lottery by noting that if the authorities refuse to take the life of the donor, they decide, in effect, to take the lives of those who need the organs. This defense is, of course, based on the assumption that acts and omissions are morally equivalent if their consequences are relevantly similar. But this assumption is widely shared among contemporary utilitarians (Glover, 1977; Singer, 1979; Harris, 1980).

We need not, however, take the word of the utilitarians for it, or rely on the moral symmetry of acts and omissions. Health authorities are often expected to act in ways that are aimed at saving the lives of the many at the expense of the lives of a few. Vaccination programs, which are designed to improve the survival rates of the population as a whole, are usually accepted, although they are known to be fatal to a fraction of the population. An example of this is the smallpox vaccination conducted by the health authorities of the City of New York in 1947. The safety of a city of 8 million was secured, but the human costs were 45 known cases of postvaccinial encephalitis—inflammation of the brain—with four deaths (Last, 1987). The health authorities actively did something that resulted in the loss of four lives. Does this make them killers? Does it make them murderers? If not, what is wrong with Harris's transplantation lottery?

Some ethicists have contended that acceptable and unacceptable cases of allocating the loss of lives can be distinguished by devices like the "doctrine of the double effect" (Callahan, 1970; Foot, 1978)—but this solution remains contested (H. Häyry and M. Häyry, 1989). Others have argued that ethical dilemmas in health-care provision should be solved by considering what is rational (Harris, 1975, 1998), or reasonable (Rhodes, 1998, 1999), or emotionally acceptable (Warnock, 1985; Maclean, 1993). All these proposals can, however, be questioned if their purpose is to guide the decisions of autocratic health authorities (Häyry, 1999, 2001a, 2001b; Takala and Häyry, 2000).

TAKING UNCERTAINTY SERIOUSLY

Regardless of the definition of "murder" in the context of medicine and health care, however, the "utilitarianism of lives" advocated by Harris can be challenged on broadly the same grounds he himself employs to reject the QALY model. If the value of my life is, to me, incommensurable, then why should I be committed to the idea that any two lives should be preferred to mine? Although these lives, too, may have incommensurable value to other people, no moral arithmetic can compel me to regard them as more important. Harris himself argues that a life is a life, whatever its quality seen from the outside. Following the same logic, incommensurable value is incommensurable value, no matter how many times it is multiplied.

Furthermore, it can also be argued (Gillon, 1985; M. Häyry and H. Häyry, 1990) that the saving of lives should not always be preferred to the improvement of life quality. If an entire nation's quality-of-life budget could be spent on the prolongation of one person's life by one day, it would not seem rational, or reasonable, or emotionally acceptable, to hold onto the utilitarianism of lives.

This does not, however, necessarily mean that the greatest happiness of the greatest numbers should be abandoned as the ultimate goal of health policies. It only means that the uncertainty of our judgments concerning the good of others, and the conflicts that occur between the interests of individuals and groups, ought to be taken seriously into account.

Justice in health-care provision has to do with the allocation of scarce resources between individuals and groups whose basic needs and interests are occasionally opposed to each other. These needs and interests are personal, and they vary from one individual to the other, which is why sound health policies cannot be based on the views of experts who believe they know what the population craves. A more sensitive method for identifying people's actual needs and interests is necessary. In addition, conflicts between people's needs and interests are possible, and justice—in the utilitarian sense at least—requires that these should be solved without producing or allowing unnecessary suffering.

JUSTICE AND AUTONOMY

Many attempts besides the QALY model have been made to define "scientifically"

what individuals want, or what makes their lives good (Häyry, 1991). But all these attempts beg the same question. How can we define objectively something that is, essentially, also subjective?

One route open to utilitarian and nonutilitarian ethicists alike is to ask the individuals themselves what they want. By giving full weight to the wishes of actual and potential patients, public-health authorities act justly—both in that the individuals' right to self-determination is respected, and in that resources are not wasted in medical interventions that are, from their own viewpoint, futile.

The utilitarian justification for this policy can be found in the work of John Stuart Mill (1859). He argued that if people's liberty—that is, their right to make choices regarding their own thoughts, actions, and lives—is protected, they will become more effective and more creative than they would otherwise have been. This, according to Mill, will in the end promote the greatest happiness of humankind, and legitimate the evil consequences of the bad choices people inevitably sometimes make.

In health-care provision, this means, for instance, that if individuals genuinely wish to die rather than protract their lives, which they see as miserable, they should be allowed to die—and perhaps physicians or other suitable health professionals ought to help them to die quickly and painlessly, if that is what they want. In social policy more generally, the respect for individual liberty should imply that mature adults who are adequately informed should be allowed to use whatever drugs they choose. Paternalistic policies that permit the use of tea, coffee, alcohol, and tobacco, but prohibit the use of marijuana, cocaine, and heroin, cannot be easily defended within the Millian, "liberal utilitarian," framework.

It must be added, however, that the concepts of "liberty" and "autonomy" have been given many readings in the contemporary discussion. In the context of genetic knowledge, at least, it has been argued both that autonomy entails a duty to know about one's hereditary ailments (Rhodes, 1998), and that it grants us the right to remain in ignorance (Takala, 1999; Takala and Häyry, 2000).

JUSTICE AND DEMOCRACY

Respect for autonomy does not, however, in its utilitarian form, offer solutions to situations where the needs and interests of individuals are in conflict. If two groups of people compete for the same medical resources, be they lifesaving, health-promoting, or quality-of-life-improving, appeals to their self-determined wishes do not necessarily help the public authorities in their task to allocate the resources justly, or fairly.

One possibility in these situations is to rely on democratic decision making. The utilitarian justification for this can be derived from the writings of John Stuart Mill (1861, 1863), who partly founded his views on the empiricist psychology advocated by his father, James Mill (1829). The crux of the justification is that people who are governed by despotic leaders, however benevolent these may be, become incapable of formulating their own views on public matters and have to settle for the passive pleasures of submission and obedience, instead of pursuing the "higher" and active pleasures of participation in the public life. The inability to formulate and to express original views is detrimental to the general good, because it is highly doubtful that despots could always arrive at the best solutions by themselves. And even if they could manage this, they would doom their subjects to passivity, which does not contribute to their highest attainable happiness.

The implication here is that it is not for the inventors of the QALY model, or their critics, to judge whose lives should be saved, whose health promoted, or whose quality of life improved, if everyone cannot be benefited equally. Decisions regarding allocation ought to be made by all the people whose lives are, or can be, influenced

by them. From the utilitarian point of view, there are two reasons for this. The first is that when everyone participates in the formulation of the policies, it is more probable that the chosen policy is the right one in view of the general good. This is based on James Mill's idea that the truth forces itself to the center of our attention, if it has been properly expressed, either mentally or in social discourse. The second reason is that if people participate in the formulation of health policies, their lives become better even if their every medical need cannot always be met. John Stuart Mill believed that this improvement is due to the activity of participation itself. Another plausible interpretation is that individuals can accept more readily the consequences of even bad political decisions if they have been given the opportunity to take part in making them (Häyry and Takala, 1998).

UTILITARIANS AND UTILITARIANS

Utilitarianism in health-care provision has usually been linked with the idea of calculating the benefits and costs of alternative policies in terms of survival, health, life quality, and financial resources. This is a perfectly sound view, and supporters of this type of utilitarianism include some of the champions of the QALY model, most notably Alan Williams, and the proponents of the lifesaving policy advocated by John Harris. They believe that, first, it is the main task of the public-health authorities to promote the greatest medical good of the population, and, second, that the medical good of the population can be defined in a way that makes this goal attainable by relatively simple maximizing policies.

Depending on the definition of the good to be achieved, these "dogmatic utilitarians" can believe that it is the duty of the authorities to maximize QALYs (A. Williams, 1988), or to keep alive as many people as possible, if this is what they wish. There are, of course, numerous other alternatives to choose from, and each definition supports a different utilitarian view regarding the obligations of politicians and health-care providers. But justice, according to all these theories, prevails when health policies are guided by such norms.

As I have shown in the above, however, utilitarian approaches to justice in health care are not confined to views like this. A long tradition, which started with the theological utilitarians, accepts the goal, the greatest happiness of the greatest numbers, but questions our ability to define once and for all what human happiness consists of. "Skeptical utilitarians" can believe that the good to be aimed at should be defined democratically, or in a manner that allows each citizen to participate in the discussion concerning values and their priorities in the society in which they live.

This approach has some "communitarian" innuendoes. It recognizes the fact that the views individuals hold are, to a large extent, determined by the views held in their societies and communities more generally. This is why solutions accepted in one society are not necessarily acceptable in others. But the difference between skeptical utilitarians and genuine communitarians is that the former still believe in the maximization of happiness as an ideal that can, in theory at least, justify radical reforms, whereas the latter see the traditions of communities as the conservative cornerstones of justice and morality (MacIntyre, 1981).

UTILITARIANS AND NONUTILITARIANS

Those who oppose all utilitarian approaches to justice in health care can argue, and rightly I believe, that even the skeptics must, in the end, condone solutions that are not necessarily acceptable to rational and reasonable individuals who value sufficiently their own existence and ideals. Theoretically, if not in practice, the following type of situation has to be faced (McCloskey, 1963; B. Williams, 1973; Primorac, 1978; Ten, 1987; Häyry, 1992, 1994). Democratic processes that truly reflect the autonomous choices of individuals, and that promote the greatest happiness of the greatest numbers defined by those choices, can command me to sacrifice my life, or the lives of people I care for or am responsible for, in order to save the lives of other people whom I know nothing about. In cases like this, all utilitarians must believe that it is my duty to submit to the general good, and prefer the general good to my own good, and to the good of my family, friends, and dependents.

As far as I know, other ethical theories fare no better in these situations—they cannot provide universally acceptable solutions to them either. But perhaps that is the point. Perhaps justice in health care, and in other areas of life, implies the admission that not all problems have unequivocal solutions. I do not know whether this view makes me an ultraskeptical utilitarian, or a nonutilitarian who still thinks that the greatest happiness of the greatest numbers would be nice. But I do believe that the difference between these two positions is, in practice, well-nigh imperceptible. The champions of both views can approve the attempts of health economists to develop new and improved quality-of-life measures that take people's differences and conflicting viewpoints better into account. And they can both criticize such attempts, if they are poorly grounded or yield intuitively unacceptable norms.

In the name of my own intellectual integrity, I must confess that I cannot be a genuine utilitarian. But in the name of the greatest happiness of the greatest numbers, which I believe to be a laudable ideal, I think I will continue to defend the skeptical utilitarian approach to justice in health care.

REFERENCES

Albee, E. (1902). *A History of English Utilitarianism*, New York: Macmillan.
Bentham, J. (1789). *An Introduction to the Principles of Morals and Legislation.* Edited by J. H. Burns and H.L.A. Hart and re-

printed with a new introduction. London and New York: Methuen, 1982.

Berkeley, G. (1712). *Passive Obedience*. Reprinted in A. C. Frasier (ed.), *The Works of George Berkeley*, 2nd ed., Vol. 3, Oxford: Oxford University Press, 1912.

Brandt, R. B. (1959). *Ethical Theory: The Problems of Normative and Critical Ethics*. Englewood Cliffs, NJ: Prentice-Hall.

Brandt, R. B. (1979). *A Theory of the Good and the Right*. Oxford: Clarendon Press.

Brown, J. (1751). *Essays on the Characteristics*. London.

Callahan, D. (1970). *Abortion: Law, Choice and Morality*. London: Macmillan.

Crisp, R. (1989). Deciding who will die: QALYs and political theory. *Politics* 9, 31–35.

Daniels, N. (1991). Is the Oregon rationing plan fair? *JAMA* 265, 2232–35.

Dougherty, C. J. (1991). Setting health care priorities: Oregon's next steps. *Hastings Center Report* 21(3), 1–10.

Edgar, A. (1998). Quality of life indicators. In R. Chadwick (ed.), *Encyclopedia of Applied Ethics*, Vol. 3. San Diego: Academic Press, pp. 759–76.

Ewing, A. C. (1953). Suppose everybody acted like me. *Philosophy* 28, 16–29.

Foot, P. (1978). *Virtues and Vices and Other Essays in Moral Philosophy*. Berkeley and Los Angeles: University of California Press.

Gay, J. (1731). Preliminary dissertation concerning the fundamental principle of virtue or morality. In W. King, *Essay on the Origin of Evil*. Partly reprinted in D. D. Raphael (ed.), *British Moralists 1650–1800: Vol. I. Hobbes–Gay*. Indianapolis, IN, and Cambridge: Hackett Publishing, 1991.

Gillon, R. (1985). Justice and allocation of medical resources. *British Medical Journal* 291, 266–68.

Glover, J. (1977). *Causing Death and Saving Lives*. Harmodsworth, UK: Penguin Books.

Godwin, W. (1793). *Enquiry Concerning Political Justice and Its Influence on Modern Morals and Happiness*. Edited by I. Kramnick. Harmondsworth, UK: Penguin Books, 1985.

Hadorn, D. C. (1991). The Oregon priority-setting exercise: Quality of life and public policy. *Hastings Center Report* 21(3), 11–16.

Hare, R. M. (1981). *Moral Thinking: Its Levels, Method and Point*. Oxford: Clarendon Press.

Harris, J. (1975). The survival lottery. *Philosophy* 50, 81–87.

Harris, J. (1980). *Violence and Responsibility*. London: Routledge & Kegan Paul.

Harris, J. (1985). *The Value of Life*. London: Routledge & Kegan Paul.

Harris, J. (1998). *Clones, Genes, and Immortality*. Oxford and New York: Oxford University Press.

Harrod, R. F. (1936). Utilitarianism revised. *Mind* 45, 137–56.

Harsanyi, J. C. (1982). Some epistemological advantages of a rule-utilitarian position in ethics. *Midwest Studies in Philosophy* 7, 389–402.

Häyry, H. and Häyry, M. (1989). Utilitarianism, human rights, and the redistribution of health through preventive medical measures. *Journal of Applied Philosophy* 6, 43–51.

Häyry, M. (1991). Measuring the quality of life: Why, how and what? *Theoretical Medicine* 12, 97–116.

Häyry, M. (1992). A defence of the utilitarian theory of punishment. In W. Cragg (ed.), *Retributivism and Its Critics. Archiv für Rechts- und Sozialphilosophie*, Beiheft 47, Stuttgart: Franz Steiner Verlag, pp. 129–147.

Häyry, M. (1994). *Liberal Utilitarianism and Applied Ethics*. London and New York: Routledge.

Häyry, M. (1999). What the fox would have said, had he been a hedgehog: On the methodology and normative approach of John Harris's Wonderwoman and Superman. In V. Launis, J. Pietarinen and J. Räikkä (eds)., *Genes and Morality: New Essays*. Amsterdam and Atlanta: Rodopi, pp. 11–19.

Häyry, M. (2001a). Abortion, disability, assent and consent. *Cambridge Quarterly of Healthcare Ethics* 10, 79–87.

Häyry, M. (2001b). But what if we *feel* that cloning is wrong? *Cambridge Quarterly of Healthcare Ethics*, 10, 205–08.

Häyry, M. and Häyry, H. (1990). Health care as a right, fairness and medical resources. *Bioethics* 4, 1–21.

Häyry, M. and Häyry, H. (1994). Obedience to rules and Berkeley's theological utilitarianism. *Utilitas* 6, 233–42.

Häyry, M. and Takala, T. (1998). Genetic engineering and the risk of harm. *Medicine, Health Care and Philosophy* 1, 61–64.

Hutcheson, F. (1725). *An Inquiry into the Original of Our Ideas of Beauty and Virtue, Treatise II*. Partly reprinted in D. D. Raphael (ed.), *British Moralists 1650–1800: Vol. I. Hobbes–Gay*. Indianapolis, IN, and Cambridge: Hackett Publishing, 1991.

Kind, P., Rosser R. M., and Williams, A. (1982). Valuation of quality of life: Some psychometric evidence. In M. W. Jones-Lee (ed.), *The Value of Life and Safety*, Amsterdam: Elsevier/North Holland, pp. 159–70.

Kuhse, H. (1987). *The Sanctity-of-Life Doctrine*

in Medicine: A Critique. Oxford: Oxford University Press.

Last, J. M. (1987). *Public Health and Human Ecology*. Ottawa: Appleton & Lange.

McCloskey, H. J. (1963). A note on utilitarian punishment. *Mind* 72, 599.

MacIntyre, A. (1981). *After Virtue: A Study in Moral Theory*, 2nd ed. London: Duckworth.

Maclean, A. (1993). *The Elimination of Morality*. London and New York: Routledge.

Menzel, P. (1990). *Strong Medicine: The Ethical Rationing of Health Care*. New York: Oxford University Press.

Mill, J. (1829). *Analysis of the Phenomena of the Human Mind*. London.

Mill, J. S. (1859). *On Liberty*. Reprinted in R. Wollheim (ed.), *Three Essays*. Oxford and New York: Oxford University Press, 1975.

Mill, J. S. (1861). *Utilitarianism*. Edited by G. Sher and reprinted with an introduction. Indianapolis, IN, and Cambridge: Hackett Publishing, 1979.

Mill, J. S. (1863). *Considerations on Representative Government*, 3rd ed. London: Longman, Green, Longman, Roberts & Green, 1865.

Nowell-Smith, P. (1954). *Ethics*. Harmondsworth, UK: Pelican Books.

Nozick, R. (1974). *Anarchy, State, and Utopia*. Oxford and New York: Basil Blackwell.

Paley, W. (1785). *Principles of Moral and Political Philosophy*. Partly reprinted in D. D. Raphael (ed.), *British Moralists 1650–1800: Vol. II. Hume–Bentham*. Indianapolis, IN, and Cambridge: Hackett Publishing, 1991.

Primorac, I. (1978). Utilitarianism and the self-sacrifice of the innocent. *Analysis* 38, 194–99.

Rawls, J. (1972). *A Theory of Justice*. Oxford: Oxford University Press.

Rhodes, R. (1998). Genetic links, family ties and social bonds: Rights and responsibilities in the face of genetic knowledge. *Journal of Medicine and Philosophy* 23, 10–30.

Rhodes, R. (1999). Abortion and assent. *Cambridge Quarterly of Healthcare Ethics* 8, 416–27.

Rosser, R. M. and Kind, P. (1978). A scale of valuation of states of illness. Is there a social consensus? *International Journal of Epidemiology* 7, 347–88.

Sidgwick, H. (1874). *The Methods of Ethics*, 7th ed. London: Macmillan, 1907.

Singer, P. (1979). *Practical Ethics*. Cambridge: Cambridge University Press.

Smart, J.J.C. (1961). *An Outline of a System of Utilitarian Ethics*. Reprinted in J.J.C. Smart and B. Williams (eds.), *Utilitarianism: For and Against*. Cambridge: Cambridge University Press, 1973.

Stason, W. B. (1991). Oregon's bold medical initiative. *JAMA* 265, 2237–38.

Stephen, J. F. (1873). *Liberty, Equality, Fraternity*, 2nd ed., 1874. Edited by R. J. White. Cambridge: Cambridge University Press, 1967.

Stout, A. K. (1954). Suppose everybody did the same. *Australasian Journal of Philosophy* 32, 1–29.

Takala, T. (1999). The right to genetic ignorance confirmed. *Bioethics* 13, 288–93.

Takala, T. and Häyry, M. (2000). Genetic ignorance, moral obligations and social duties. *Journal of Medicine and Philosophy* 25, 107–13.

Ten, C. L. (1987). *Crime, Guilt, and Punishment*. Oxford: Clarendon Press.

Toulmin, S. (1953). *The Place of Reason in Ethics*. New York: Cambridge University Press.

Tucker, A. (1768–77). *The Light of Nature Pursued*. Edited by H. P. St John Milmay. London, 1805.

Warnock, M. (1985). *A Question of Life: The Warnock Report of Human Fertilisation and Embryology*. Oxford and New York: Basil Blackwell.

Williams, A. (1985). Economics of coronary bypass grafting. *British Medical Journal* 291, 326–29.

Williams, A. (1988). Ethics and efficiency in the provision of health care. In J. M. Bell and S. Mendus (eds.), *Philosophy and Medical Welfare*, Cambridge: Cambridge University Press, pp. 111–26.

Williams, B. (1973). A critique of utilitarianism. In J.J.C. Smart and B. Williams (eds.), *Utilitarianism: For and Against*. Cambridge: Cambridge University Press.

5

Aggregation and the Moral Relevance of Context in Health-Care Decision Making

David Wasserman

Much of the philosophical literature on "tragic choices"—choices about whom to save with limited resources—presents the dilemma of an individual agent, deciding which victims to rescue when there is not enough time, medicine, or gasoline to rescue all. The agent is a helicopter pilot or emergency room physician; the victims are all strangers, but identifiable ones—the agent can observe their fear and peril even if he does not know their names. In contrast, much of the economic and policy literature on tragic choices concerns decisions made by governments or institutions, at a greater temporal distance, about people who can be identified only by the fates they will suffer—decisions about how much to invest in highway safety, cancer research, or rescue helicopters. In this chapter, I will consider the question of whether these are fundamentally different kinds of choices that ought to be governed by different decision rules or distributional principles.

I will focus on the allocation of scarce health-care resources, where the differences between the two kinds of choices described above are generally thought to support different decision rules. Thus, of the institutes included in the National Institute of Health (NIH), fewer than half are devoted to diseases that would generally be regarded as life-threatening. No one seriously suggests that those institutes receive the entire NIH budget until the life-threatening diseases they study are eradicated. At the same time, most people would regard it as acceptable, if not mandatory, for a doctor in a short-staffed emergency room (ER) to treat a small number of people who would otherwise die rather than a larger number of people who would otherwise lose an arm or suffer other nonlethal harms.[1] In allocating health-care resources, it clearly seems more acceptable to trade off death against lesser harms when the decision concerns harms that will be incurred in the future by individuals who are not currently identifiable than when it concerns harms that will be incurred in the present and close at hand by identifiable individuals.

Yet the decisions made in those two contexts, and the responsibility of the decision makers for their consequences, are quite similar. In both contexts, some individuals will suffer harm because they have been denied the resources to prevent it. Regardless of whether the harm is imminent or remote, its victims identified or unidentified, it comes to its victims in the same way, from a disease that the decision maker could have treated or developed the means to treat. And though it is not certain that some people will lose their arms or lives unless the research makes a treatment available, it is also not certain that some people will lose their arms or lives unless they receive an available treatment—spontaneous recovery is possible in either setting. The moral difference, if any, between the two contexts must lie elsewhere.

In this chapter I examine a variety of explanations for the differing acceptability of aggregation in these two contexts. By "aggregation" I mean the interpersonal cumulation (strictly additive or not) of harms and benefits of varying magnitude to resolve conflicts over scarce resources. As such, aggregation is an essential feature of consequentialism, but some forms of aggregation are accepted in some contexts by most non-consequentialists.

Explaining the varying acceptability of aggregating harms in the two contexts is complicated by the multiplicity of differences between them:[2]: between treatment decisions made by physicians or other health-care providers about identified individuals with imminent medical needs, and funding decisions made by legislators or health-care bureaucrats that will affect currently unidentified individuals whose medical needs have not yet arisen. At least three different factors are contrasted: the imminence of the harm, the social role or institutional status of the decision makers, and the identifiability of the claimants.

These different factors overlap, but only partially. Decision makers tend to discount future medical needs, but they also tend to favor currently identifiable people over currently unidentifiable ones, regardless of whether their needs are imminent. The distinction between future and present seems to lose some of its moral significance when it is divorced from certainty about outcome (which is admittedly hard to do): Our willingness to discount future harms may reflect a resilient optimism as much as a preference for the present. And although it is easier to identify people who are now afflicted than people who will be, we can often, and increasingly, identify individuals now who will have medical needs in the future. In the case of late-onset genetic diseases, for example, those who are certain or likely to have the disease will be identifiable long before they need medical attention (whether their "conditions" arise now or later depends on whether we regard their conditions as having a latent phase). In practice, identifiability and agent-type are associated, because institutions typically decide on long-term projects and policies with unknown effects on specific people. But individuals can make decisions under similar uncertainty, and institutional decisions sometimes involve identifiable victims and beneficiaries.

It is not clear what role these different factors play in the perceived acceptability of different distributional rules, and what moral significance, if any, they have. Philosophers who have defended the moral relevance of context have not been clear about whether context is defined by the imminence of harm, the identifiability of the victims, the social role of the rescuer, or some combination of factors. I will attempt to tease apart these factors in reviewing several proposed justifications and question whether any of the factors can bear the moral weight assigned to them.

SHOULD CONTEXT MATTER?

To some commentators, it has seemed obvious that these factors can only explain, not justify, the use of different distributional rules. The two kinds of choices are essentially the same, differing only in the clarity with which they reveal the tragic necessity of letting some people die or suffer in order to rescue others. Guido Calabresi and Philip Bobbitt distinguished first-order determinations, about "how much [of a good] will be produced, within the limits set by natural scarcity," and second-order determinations, about "how shall get what is made" (p. 19). Although they appeared to have a different subject matter, first-order determinations were really just like second-order determinations operating "at a higher level of generality" (1978, p. 134):

For example, imagine two people, one in need of tragic good A and the other in need of tragic good B. If the production of A for the first person necessarily means that no B can be produced, then a decision to concentrate societal resources on A operates as a second-order allocation between the one in need of A and the one in need of B. (Calabresi and Bobbitt, 1978, p. 221)

Calabresi and Bobbitt believed that it was easy to overlook this obvious truth, however:

And yet a first-order determination does not really seem to us to be merely a broader second-order decision. A decision as to how many iron lungs will be built is simply not perceived as the same kind of decision as one which determines who will actually be granted the use of such a machine. (1978, p. 135)

Several philosophers have argued, however, that these two kinds of decisions *should not* be perceived as being the same because they are different in morally relevant respects. Although both involve trade-offs among the interests of different people, there are moral reasons for making the trade-offs differently in different contexts. Moreover, those reasons are not the consequentialist ones that Calebresi and Bobbitt would readily acknowledge, which rest on no moral principle other than the maximization of good consequences or the minimization of bad ones.[3]

Frances Kamm maintains that, whereas it is objectionable to save any number of arms rather than one life when "choosing whom to aid 'here and now,'" it is acceptable to trade lives for arms "in making such macro decisions as whether to invest in research to cure a disease that will kill a few people or in research to cure a disease that will kill no one but will wither an arm in many" (Kamm, 1998a, p. 942). The "principle of public investment" for research funding "should not govern how we distribute in an emergency room, for example, if one hundred people come in with arms falling off at the same time as one comes in with a fatal condition" (Kamm, 1998b, p. 973).

What kinds of justification could a nonconsequentialist offer for the relevance of context to the distribution of scarce medical resources? Kamm may well be correct as a descriptive matter that in allocating funds to "an institution like an emergency room," public policy recognizes that a morality with strong constraints on aggregation holds sway "in some areas of life, however small" (Kamm, 1998b, p. 973).[4] The question, however, is why public policy *should* recognize such "deontic preserves." Without some argument for the moral relevance of context, the designation of such preserves seems ad hoc or conventional, an expression of ambivalence or sentimentality rather than moral principle.

A context-sensitive morality, as I will call it, must not only explain, but justify, the greater acceptability of aggregation in decisions that will affect currently unidentifiable individuals at some future time. Many deontologists acknowledge that it is easier to treat people as mere objects or means when they are anonymous and remote in space and time. But the fact that it is easier to aggregate in those contexts hardly makes it more acceptable to do so. In explaining differing constraints on aggregation, the question a context-sensitive morality must answer is why a rule that is unacceptable in choosing among identified individuals, or present harms, should be acceptable in choosing among unidentified individuals or future harms.

That is a distinct question from the one raised by choices *across* contexts, between harms that differ in immediacy or victims who differ in identifiability. Several philosophers (e.g., Fried, 1970) have commented on the apparent preference for imminent needs and identifiable individuals reflected in such choices (e.g., in the decision to save a trapped coal miner with funds that could prevent many later mining disasters). A context-sensitive morality, however, must explain why different rules apply in choosing between harms that are *equally* imminent and victims who are *equally* identifiable. A complete explanation is unlikely to be supplied by an account of the preference for imminent harms or identifiable victims. If, for example, decision makers simply gave more weight to harms that were imminent or victims who were identifiable (or discounted harms or victims who were not), it would still be necessary to explain why our balancing of the competing interests came out differently when *all of them* had that extra weight, as opposed to when *none of them* had.

In this regard, it is instructive to consider Kamm's suggestion that it may be acceptable to save one life now rather than many lives in the future because of our "special horror" at letting someone die when we have the means to save him:

[W]e seek to avoid having to stand by doing nothing *at a time when we have resources that could be used*. If we aid now, we will not have resources in the future. In the future, it will not be true that we stand by not helping *when we have the resources* with which to help. (Kamm, 1993, 141–142)

Kamm may be correct that there is a special horror in standing by when we have the resources to help. But this would not explain (nor is it offered to explain) our greater willingness to trade lives against lesser interests in the future than in the present. It is still necessary to explain why the special horror of letting one person lose his life prevails over the special horror of letting many people lose an arm here and now, whereas the mere horror of letting one person lose his life does not prevail over the mere horror of letting many people lose an arm there and then.[5]

What are the prospects for developing a context-sensitive morality along the lines I have suggested? I will look at three explanations for the varying acceptability of aggregation, which emphasize different factors among those usually conjoined in the here-and-now and there-and-then. The first stresses the imminence of harm or need; the second, social or professional role; the third, uncertainty about identity. I will not choose among these competing explanations, in part because they have not been articulated fully enough to permit an informed choice. I will, however, attempt to develop the explanation based on identifiability, because it strikes me as the most promising, and the one that most closely accords with the intuitions supporting a context-sensitive morality. But in the end, I find even that explanation inadequate.[6]

THE IMMINENCE OF HARM

Kamm's explanation for our refusal to count arms against lives in the here-and-now emphasizes the imminence of the victim's harm. Kamm suggests that agents have duties toward people who "confront" them with their imminent needs that they lack toward people who do not confront them this way (Kamm, 1998b, p. 973). These duties may preclude them from engaging in certain kinds of trade-offs, in particular, from aggregating lesser harms against death. Even the relatively limited contact between the rescuer and prospective victims on the high seas or in an emergency room creates a duty to rescue each victim; one's limited resources create a conflict among those duties that cannot be resolved by maximizing the number of weighted duties that will be fulfilled, or by minimizing the number of weighted violations. The agent deciding what resources to produce is not, as a general matter, encumbered by such duties, so she can trade off lives for arms or focus on diseases that affect the most productive members of society. The agent has no duty to stock up for the kind of encounters that constrain the trade-offs she can make:

> Suppose I have a car and a seriously ill person asks me to take him to the hospital: I have a duty to do this. But I do not have a duty to buy a car so that when I face a seriously ill person, I can take him to the hospital. (Possibly, I might even refrain from buying a car just so that I will not be put in the position of having to take people to the hospital when they confront me.) (Kamm 1998b, p. 973)

Kamm offers this example to illustrate that "we may have a duty to behave in a certain way if we have a resource, but not necessarily to see to it that we have that resource" (1998b, p. 973). It is doubtful, however, that those who reject Kamm's claim of context-sensitivity would deny this, or more broadly, that they would embrace the absurd proposition that we have a (present) duty at t1 to satisfy the condition of any conditional (future) duty at t2. (Surely there are duty-triggering conditions at t2 that we have a duty *not* to bring about at t1; e.g., a duty to aid a friend if he is badly hurt.) They may, however, accept the more plausible proposition that Kamm earlier ascribes to them: "that we have a duty at t1 (when doing research and development) to make it possible for us to fulfill the duties we will have at t2 (in the emergency room)" (Kamm, 1998b, p. 973). There are many duties we can anticipate having at t2—to feed, clothe, and shelter our children, for example—that do not appear to be conditional on our having the resources to satisfy them, or (if "ought" implies "can") that impose a duty at t1 to ensure that we have those resources. What opponents of Kamm's context-sensitivity would deny is that such "anticipatory duties," as I shall call them, are governed by different rules in the event of conflict than are duties to aid here-and-now.

Kamm's example is simply not relevant to this issue, because its point is to deny that she has *any* anticipatory duties toward the strangers at her doorstep. Her example addresses the concern that morality demands too much, by suggesting that while we acquire a duty to aid needy individuals when they confront us, we do not have to anticipate their arrival. It also suggests that there is an element of fortuity in the moral obligations we incur. But it cannot do the work Kamm requires of it, as it does nothing to explain why the duties we undeniably *do* have in some circumstances, to some individuals, to anticipate their future needs should have different constraints on trade-offs than the duties we have toward individuals who confront us with their imminent needs.

If we consider individuals toward whom the agent does have an anticipatory duty, it is by no means clear that the imminence of their needs plays the constraining role Kamm ascribes to it. Thus, imagine that 21 small children live with a caretaker in his isolated cabin. All but one of the children will lose their legs during the coming winter if the caretaker does not produce a certain drug he does not have; but that one child, whom the caretaker can identify, will lose his life if he does not produce a different drug. Alas, both drugs are made from the same plant, and the caretaker has only enough to produce one medication or the other (there is, of course, no time to get more from outside). It seems clear that if the agent should favor life over limbs in the emergency room, he should favor life over limbs in these circumstances. And yet this would involve a duty to produce or procure resources at t1, not merely to use the resources that he has at t2.

This example suggests that the same distributional rules apply regardless of the imminence of the competing needs when the agent has a prior duty of care to each of the needy individuals.[7] Is there some other aspect of the here-and-now that mandates stronger constraints on aggregation? The cabin case introduces into macro, or production, decisions two factors more often associated with micro, or distribution, decisions: The agent has a special relationship with each of the claimants, and each is identifiable at the time the decision is made. Can either factor account for the restrictions on aggregation typically found in micro contexts?

SPECIAL RELATIONSHIPS AND PROFESSIONAL ROLES

An account based on special relationships would regard the morally relevant difference between the here-and-now and the then-and-there not as the decision maker's knowledge of the victims in the former setting, but as her constraining duties toward them. Thus, Brock observes that while those making decisions at macro-levels

are typically government legislators, health officials, or health plan administrators, prioritizing different patients for needed treatment is typically done by physicians. A common objection to "bedside rationing" done by physicians is that physician's commitments are and should be to the individual patients whom they are treating, and not to broader social goals. (Brock, 2000, pp. 14–15)

Without some non-consequentualist justifications of why different constraints are attached to different social roles, however, this explanation merely provides a descriptive account of the operation of those roles. Why should physicians have duties toward their patients that preclude them from making certain trade-offs when their interests conflict? Why should public officials be permitted or even required to make those trade-offs? Not only are a physician's patients strangers in many morally relevant respects, but it is not clear why we should recognize the social role of the physician in the first place—we might have morally impoverished lives without friends, but it is by no means clear that our lives would be morally impoverished if our medical needs were met by health-care bureaucrats instead of physicians.[8]

Moreover, constraints on aggregation appear to vary less with the social or professional role of the decision maker than with the identifiability of the affected individuals. Consider the allocation of funding by a government agency with a general duty to support health-promoting research but no special relationship with, or duty toward, individuals facing particular health threats. Assume that the agency can support only one of two research programs: Program *A* has a very good chance of finding a cure within 10 years for a lung disease that would otherwise kill 50 people; Program *B* has a very good chance of finding a cure within 10 years for a circulatory disease that would otherwise cause 1,000 people to lose a leg. Assume (however improbable this may be) that all the 1,050 people who will be affected by this decision are asymptomatic but identifiable through medical testing. The 50 individuals virtually certain to lose their lives would have as much reason to feel abandoned by the selection of a research program for a limb disease as a person left to die in the emergency room. It would attenuate the sense of abandonment if the research program had only a slight chance of success, but no more so than it would if there were only a slight chance of saving the patient in the emergency room. (In both cases, there might also be some chance of survival from spontaneous recovery or the independent discovery of a cure.) The fact that the victims are abandoned by government researchers rather than private physicians does little or nothing to blunt their complaint. Identifiability thus appears to impose the same constraints on production as on distribution regardless of whether the agent has any special relationship with the claimants.

Further, when the claimants are *not* identifiable at the time the production decision must be made, there appear to be looser constraints on aggregation even when the decision maker is a physician who has, or is likely to have, a professional relationship with many or all of them. Thus, an emergency room physician not only has a duty to treat the patients who appear on her doorstep, but also a duty to make sure she has the resources necessary to treat those likely to appear at her doorstep. Her duty to make resources available for some of the patients she expects may conflict with her duty to make resources available for others—if, say, she does not have enough funds or time to obtain medicines for the full array of conditions she expects to see on her shift. Arguably, the physician may use her limited funds to order medication that would save many limbs rather than medication that would save one life, while she must allocate fungible resources like her own time to save a few lives rather than many arms once the ambulances arrive. Counting arms against lives in procurement decisions seems permissible regardless of whether the physician has, or is likely to have, a professional relationship with the as-yet unidentified claimants. It would seem no less permissible to count arms against lives in a one-physician town, where (almost) anyone coming into the emergency room on that shift was likely to be the physician's patient.

The explanation in terms of the agent's role-morality might be recast to emphasize the role of institutional decision makers, rather than of physicians and other professionals. Instead of asking why the latter are exempt from the demands of consequentialism—a question that treats consequentialism as the moral default—this account would begin by asking why institutional agents are subject to those demands; why they are permitted or required to trade off the interests of unidentifiable individuals in ways that would be unacceptable for a conscientious physician choosing among identifiable individuals. Such an account would not treat the emergency room as a special domain protected from the reigning consequentialism, but as a setting where the duties to individuals governing most of our moral lives were not preempted or overridden by the imperatives of institutional decision making. But even if such an account could be developed—and it would clearly take a lot of work—an explanation based on the role-morality of institutional agents would not conform to our victim-centered intuitions.

IDENTIFIABILITY AND THE COMPLAINT ACCOUNT

Intuitively, then, identifiability appears to be the most important factor in distinguishing contexts. But identifiability comes in different forms: The victims of a life-or limb-threatening disorder may be identifiable to different people, to varying degrees, with varying effort. For the remainder of this chapter I will treat an individual as identifiable with respect to a given harm if anyone—the individual, the decision maker, or a third party—could, with reasonable effort, determine that he would suffer that harm before an irrevocable allocation decision must be made. I use the phrase "reasonable effort" to bracket the issue of how much effort is necessary. Surely we would not treat prospective victims as identifiable in a morally relevant sense if their identification would be so costly that it would dramatically reduce their odds of survival.

It is, of course, one thing to claim that identifiability plays a significant role in our intuitions about trade-offs, quite another to justify that role. One way of accounting for the moral significance of *un*identifiability would be in terms of the defense it offered to a complaint about the decision to favor arms over life. On this account, it would be presumptively correct to accord priority to a life over any number of arms; it would be reasonable for an individual to reject a principle that let him die in order to save 20 arms. This account is similar to what Scanlon, following Parfit, calls the "complaint model": "a person's complaint against a principle must have to do with its effects on him or her, and someone can reasonably reject a principle if there is some alternative to which no other person has a complaint as strong" (Scanlon, 1998, p. 229). The individual who stands to lose his life as the result of a micro-decision allocating scarce resources to limb saving can complain about the lethal effect on him of that decision; no one who stood to lose his or her limb as a result of the alternative decision to allocate scarce resources to life saving would have as strong a complaint.[9]

The question for this account is why an individual who stands to lose his life as a result of a macro-decision, made in unavoidable ignorance of who would die, would not have a complaint as well. After all, the decision makers knew that if they made a macro allocation to fund research on the limb-threatening disease, someone would lose his life who would have lived if they had instead funded research on the life-threatening disease. Cannot the person who ends up losing his life invoke the effects of that decision on him, and claim that no one would have had as strong a complaint if the decision makers had instead favored life over arms? The answer given by this account is that if the individual who loses his life would have endorsed the decision favoring arms over life and has no reason now, after his identity is known, to regard that endorsement as unreasonable in light of the information available at the time the decision had to be made, he lacks any basis for complaining about that decision. (He may have some basis for complaint if he is far more "death-averse" than most people, but I will set aside this complication.).

The "complaint account" begins with the simplifying assumptions that no one has any way of knowing who will be afflicted by either disease, so that everyone can be regarded as at risk of one or both of the diseases—a small risk of a life-threatening disease and a much larger risk of a limb-threatening disease (whether the risk is actual or merely "epistemic" does not matter), and that everyone has the same risk-preferences, so that the decision to fund research for the latter could be justified in terms of what Charles Fried (1970, pp. 177–82) has called the individual "risk-budget." Although the assumption of uniform risk preferences is unrealistic, it is rea-sonable to assume that there is some trade-off between risk to life and risk to limb that virtually everyone would be willing to make. Only a person obsessed with death to the exclusion of all lesser harms would reject any increase in the risk of death for some much greater reduction in the risk of arm loss.[10] If an individual now facing death has no reason to reproach himself for his own moderate risk-preferences, a person now facing death as the result of a collective decision to budget risks the same way has no reason to reproach the decision makers (unless he has some reason to think that collective decision makers should be more averse to lethal risks than the individuals facing them).

This account treats the counterfactual endorsement of the person disadvantaged by a social decision as having normative significance. In this respect, it resembles a hypothetical argument seeking to justify a proposed scheme of social cooperation in terms of the consent that the affected individuals *would have* given. But the appeal to counterfactual endorsement in the complaint account is quite different, because it is offered to justify a decision that has actually been made, and made irrevocably. The individual facing death as the result of a micro-allocation to limb-saving research is not being asked to endorse, on the basis of his hypothetical consent, a present decision that would disadvantage him. He is in a very different posture than Dworkin's poker player, asked to relinquish a good hand in unanticipated circumstances, on the basis of a rule that he would have, but had not in fact, agreed to (Dworkin, 1974, p. 18). The individual with the life-threatening disease has been dealt a bad hand in clearly anticipated circumstances, and he cannot relinquish it—it is impossible to deal again. Indeed, if there *were* a present choice to be made—if the limb-saving medication could still be converted into the life-saving medication (a variation I discuss below)—he would not have to endorse an adverse decision: His society would then face a micro-allocation between identifiable victims, in which his life would, per Kamm, prevail over any number of limbs; the fact that he would have chosen a macro-allocation favoring limbs over life would *not* preclude him from demanding that the society now favor life over limbs. But as things stand, there is no possibility for conversion—the decision favoring limbs over life was irrevocably made at a time when he could not be identified as a victim. The only question is whether he now has grounds to complain about that decision; the complaint accounts holds that he does not.

This non-consequentialist account of identifiability suggests that decision makers are only permitted to trade off life for arms because no one can complain, and that they should take reasonable steps to deny themselves that permission by giving individuals the information they need to reject the trade-off. This might seem to offer an insufficiently robust justification for choosing limbs over life in macro-allocations. The complaint account might also seem too weak in treating that choice as permissive rather than required. It is not clear that the decision makers are compelled to make that choice by the strength of the complaints they would face if they made the opposite choice. Had they chosen life over arms instead, those who subsequently lost their limbs would not appear to have a complaint. They would not, per Kamm, have had a complaint in a micro-setting, where it was, or could be, known that *their* arms would be sacrificed to save the life of an identifiable person, so it is difficult to see how they would have a complaint in a macro setting, where they could not have known that it was their arms that would be lost.[11]

The defender of a complaint account of identifiability might respond that the justification for choosing limbs over life in macro-settings *should* be no more robust than their account makes it out to be—that choice *is* merely permissible, not mandatory. She might insist that the choice of limbs over life is just one acceptable option

in the face of ignorance about identity. Such ignorance is a regrettable fact about social decision making; it does not enjoy the privileged status of the stipulated ignorance in the original position. It is not needed to prevent bias or partiality. An identified individual who demands life-saving treatment for himself rather than limb-saving treatment for a large number of other identified or identifiable people is hardly engaged in special pleading, for which ignorance would be a desirable prophylactic. He is not at all like an individual so inured to privilege he cannot recognize the unfairness of the social arrangements responsible for his advantage. His demand is endorsed by the rest of us, who are not afflicted with either the life-or limb-threatening injury.

Still, the complaint account relies on a peculiar kind of ignorance to defend the macro-allocation. From the decision maker's point of view, if not the victims', things did not turn our any differently than expected—it was virtually certain that someone would die, and the person who in fact died was as likely a victim as anyone else. For this reason, the decision to favor arms over life cannot be treated like a justified mistake—the best choice in light of the available information, but not in light of complete information—because it is not a mistake at all. The incidence of life- and limb-threatening disease is just as expected, and the death of this individual, or of any individual in the society, was a foreseeable outcome.

The peculiarity of the kind of ignorance involved, and the uncertain moral status of that ignorance, are suggested by a hypothetical in which it is becomes possible to defer the choice between life- and limb-saving treatments to a point at which the victims are identifiable. Suppose an emergency room (ER) expects an average of 50 patients a day with a limb-threatening injury and only one with a life-threatening injury. Suppose also the medicine for the latter injury costs 50 times as much as the medicine for the former, and that the ER, which must purchase its medicine every morning, has funds for one or the other but not both. With its limited funds, it obtains the medication for the limb-threatening injury rather than the life-threatening one. This might seem like a reasonable decision if the injuries were truly adventitious, so that there was no way of knowing at the beginning of the day who was going to need either kind of medicine.

But what if a process is developed to convert the limb-saving medicine into the life-saving medicine in a few minutes? If one patient with the life-threatening injury arrived at the ER at the same time as 50 patients with the limb-threatening injury, it would be too late to convert. If, however, the technicians were dispatched to get the victims and phoned in to the ER when they were a few minutes away, there would be time. Should the ER physician begin the conversion process if she knows, or could learn, the identity of all 51 patients?

The problem is not one of line-drawing, of deciding when identification becomes clear or detailed enough, or whether there is enough time for the conversion. It is that the information the ER receives from the field is not the sort that would normally require it to alter its preparations. The proportion of people with the two injuries is exactly what the ER estimated, and there are no details about the individual victims that would arguably support a change in priority (e.g., that those with the limb-threatening injury had maliciously inflicted the life-threatening injury). For this reason, it might seem perverse to require the ER to make a frenzied last-minute conversion. But it might also seem perverse to require the ER to maintain its initial purchasing policy if it was very likely that most of those with life-threatening injuries would be identified in time to convert the medication. Why not simply anticipate their likely identification by purchasing the life-saving medication in the first place? And yet at the time the purchase is made, the injured are still not identifiable, and the en-

tire at-risk population might well prefer that the ER purchase the limb-saving medication. I do not believe there is an obvious solution to the ER's dilemma; it merely highlights the uncertain moral significance of identifiability.

The Limits of the Complaint Account

A broader concern is that the complaint account of identifiability lacks generality; it does not apply in many settings where it would seem appropriate to favor limbs over life. Thus, for example, it might be acceptable for the government to fund research on a rare limb-threatening disease rather than a still rarer life-threatening disease, where no one in the population was known to be at disproportionately greater risk of either, even if the risk of the limb-threatening disease was so low that most people would rather incur that risk than the still-lower risk of the life-threatening disease. If those who end up with the fatal disease would have agreed to fund research on the limb-threatening disease, it would not have been on prudential grounds; if they are now precluded from complaining, it is not because they would have endorsed that decision *ex ante* on the basis of their risk-budgets.

Moreover, the choice of limbs over life would appear to be no less acceptable if it were possible to identify all and only the limb victims in advance, even though that would block the application of the complaint account. Consider a case in which those who face limb loss are known at the time the decision must be made, but the smaller, nonoverlapping group who face death is not. If it is acceptable to chose limbs over life when the identities of the limb-victims are unknown, it might seem at least as acceptable to choose limbs over life when the veil is partially lifted so that their identity, but not that of the life-victims, is known. But once the limb-victims are known, everyone else will lack a self-interested reason to chose limbs over life; they will have nothing to gain, and much to lose, from that choice. Thus, the decision makers could not presume the universal acceptability of the limb-saving policy at the time it was chosen. If that choice is justified, it can only be because the complaint the limb-losers would have about the choice of life over limb would be greater than the complaint everyone else would have about the choice of limb over life. But that leaves the question of how the strength of the competing complaints is assessed.

Finally, it often seems acceptable for the government to choose limbs over lives when neither group of victims is identifiable when the choice must be made, but it is known that nonoverlapping groups of people are at *risk* for the two diseases. Many people, much of the time, know enough about the risks they face to know that they sometimes differ substantially from the population averages. Nevertheless, uncertainty appears to loosen the constraints on aggregation even when some individuals are (known to be) at greater risk than others. Thus, even if it was known that people on the East Coast were at comparatively greater risk of a limb-threatening disease than people on the West Coast of a life-threatening disease, it would still appear acceptable for the federal government to devote a significant share of its budget (the same share as it would in the absence of such demographic knowledge?) to research the limb-threatening disease—as long as the (known) risk of death to individual West Coasters was, however disproportionate, still small in absolute terms, and as long as disparities in risk were not correlated with suspect classifications: race, ethnicity, gender. It seems, for reasons still obscure, more appropriate to aggregate the risks of greater and lesser harms than the actual harms. An explanation in terms of the distinction between aggregating risks and aggregating harms would have to treat certainty as categorically different from, or discontinuous with, mere risks, a view that seems at odds with a probabilistic understanding of risk. That view may be defensible, but it has yet to be defended by the proponents of context-sensitivity.

NOTES

1. Similarly, in determining the NIH budget, it would be considered appropriate to take account of such indirect consequences of disease as lost productivity. In contrast, it would be considered highly inappropriate for the emergency room physician to consider the impact on productivity of her treatment decisions. The appropriateness of taking into account such indirect effects thus appears to vary with context (Brock, 2000); this difference might well have the same explanation as the difference in aggregating harms of varying magnitude. But as I can find no plausible explanation for the latter, I will not explore this possibility further.

2. Discussion of these explanations is also complicated by the variety of terms used to make much the same vague distinction between contexts: distribution versus production; second-order versus first-order determinations; micro- versus macro-decisions; decisions about the here-and-now and the there-and-then. Calebresi and Bobbitt (1978) use the first two pairs of terms interchangeably; Kamm (1993, 1998a, 1998b) and Brock (1998, 2000), the latter two. I will use all four pairs of terms interchangeably, except where one pair is specifically called for.

Nord (1999, p. 7) offers a tripartite distinction, between the budget level, at which treatment and prevention capacity are decided; the admissions level, at which it is decided who will be admitted to a service "given the capacity to treat that has been decided for that service;" and the bedside or clinical level, at which it is decided "how to treat those individuals who are admitted." Decisions on the budget level are generally made by legislators or bureaucrats about individuals unknown to the decision makers; admissions and bedside decisions are generally made by health professionals who have at least some knowledge of and personal contact with the affected individuals—much more at the bedside level (Nord, 1999, p. 138).

3. For example, it is argued that institutions do a better job than do individuals at certain kinds of aggregation, or that having individuals aggregate in those ways would have other undesirable effects, such as undermining trust. These arguments are countered by equally consequentialist ones—for example, that individual agents must make finely grained judgments of marginal utility in order for policies to work (Goodin, 1990; Ubel, 2000).

4. Specifically, Kamm claims that the morality that holds sway in the emergency room and other micro settings is Sobjectivity 3, which, to oversimplify, permits the aggregation of lives, and of "relevant" lesser interests like arms, in choices among equal numbers of lives. Macro settings are governed by Sobjectivity 4, which, to oversimplify, permits lives to be outweighed by a sufficiently large number of "relevant" lesser interests. Kamm's other Sobjectivities (1, 2, and 5) involve various combinations of objective and subjective elements, but Kamm does not believe that they are adopted by common-sense morality in resolving conflicts about the allocation of scarce resources. As Kamm states: "I believe that the combination of Sobjectivities 3 and 4 represent common-sense morality's solution to the distribution of a resource that is not divisible between groups needing it when the probability of success in helping each group is equal" (1998a, p. 942).

5. Perhaps Kamm might contend that the horror in standing by was "special" only when it was death that we could prevent, not some lesser harm, and only when we could still avoid that harm. That horror would not be evoked by the loss of limb, and it would not operate as a thumb on the scales when we were choosing between the future loss of life and limb, because at that future time we would lack the resources to aid. But this would offer more of a psychological than a moral explanation: Kamm might experience greater horror at letting a child die whom she still had the means to save (but only by letting 20 other children lose an arm) than at letting a child die whom she no longer had the means to save (because she had chosen to save the arms of 20 other children), but it is not clear why that greater horror would give her any moral reason to decide differently, *if* the decision to aid the 20 children would have been the right one. Why shouldn't she regard that horror as a distorting influence, against which she should bind herself in advance?

Moreover, the explanation would lack sufficient generality. The special horror of standing by and letting someone die cannot explain the constraint on choosing between two imminently imperiled lives on the basis of their value to others—regardless of which life we chose, we would feel the same horror at standing by while the other was lost. Nor could it explain why the constraints on aggregation vary in choosing between arms and fingers, as well as lives and arms. If there were no special horror in standing by and letting someone lose his arm when we have the resources to prevent it, there would be no more reason to chose an arm over 20 fingers here and now than there and then.

6. Another explanation might begin with the one form of aggregation that seems appropriate in almost all contexts: counting lives (at least lives directly saved) against lives, or more generally, interests of equal magnitude against each other (when the threats to those interests are equally imminent). Although it may be objectionable to count the certain loss of arms against the certain loss of life in the emergency room, it is not only appropriate, but mandatory, to count lives against lives, and to choose the greater number in that setting. Kamm (1993, 1998a, 1998b) and Scanlon (1998) have argued that we are required to do so not to produce the best outcome but to act fairly. To fail to alter the decision rule when a standoff among equal interests is broken by an additional interest of sufficient magnitude on one side—a life, or arguably an arm—is to slight the latter interest and treat its bearer unfairly. If this fairness justification for choosing the greater number were tenable, an argument could perhaps be made that it could be extended to the aggregation of lesser interests against greater in macro- but not micro-contexts. But I do not believe the fairness justification is tenable, and I do not see how, even if it were, it could be selectively extended to the aggregation of lesser interests in macro contexts.

7. Indeed, it would be peculiar if imminence played a significant role for Kamm in establishing the rule for distributing health resources, for she elsewhere assigns "urgency"—how soon an individual will suffer adverse consequences if he does not receive a health resource—a relatively minor role in the distribution of scarce health resources (Kamm, 1993, pp. 268–69).

8. It is unlikely that any attempt to treat physicians as "special-purpose friends" would be more successful than Charles Fried's widely criticized attempt (1977) to treat attorneys that way.

9. Scanlon (1998, pp. 240–41) believes that the complaint model could be stretched to give each of the individuals with a significant lesser interest a grievance, but he does not suggest how this could be done.

10. This account also makes two other assumptions: First, the individual now facing the lethal harm was not involved in the actual decision to incur that risk (although the decision accorded with his risk-budget); second, he has no procedural grievance about not having been involved. The first assumption is needed because the acceptability of a decision to favor arms over life in macro settings cannot rest on each individual's actual agreement to it; the second assumption is needed because an objection to that decision cannot rest on a procedural flaw that could have been avoided and would, by stipulation, have had no effect on the allocation actually made.

11. It might be argued that a macro-allocation favoring life over arms is objectionable because the decision makers in a democratic society are obliged in such settings to defer to the risk-preferences of (a majority of) its members. But in that case, a complaint could be made by any member of that society ex ante, alleging a violation of democracy, not an error in distributive priorities. The only complaint the victims of the limb disorder would have special standing to make would be the oblique one that they had been harmed by a decision unfair to the population as a whole. More important, this account would have to explain why a society should not defer to the risk-preferences of a majority of its members *after* the veil is lifted—why should a single identified person facing death be able to veto the majority-favored allocation of resources to limb-saving? The recourse to democratic decision making merely seems to defer or displace the question of why identifiability is morally relevant.

REFERENCES

Brock, D. (1998). Aggregating costs and benefits. *Philosophy and Phenomenological Research* 58, 963–68.

Brock, D. (2000). *Separate Spheres and Indirect Benefits*. Draft prepared for World Health Organization meeting on Fairness and Goodness, Trivandrum, India, March 12–15, 2000.

Calabresi, C. and Bobbitt, P. (1978). *Tragic Choices*. New York: Norton.

Dworkin, R. (1974). The original position. In N. Daniels (ed.), *Reading Rawls: Critical Studies of Rawls' Theory of Justice*. New York: Basic Books, pp. 1–53.

Fried, C. (1970). *An Anatomy of Values*. Cambridge, MA: Harvard University Press.

Fried, C. (1977). *Right and Wrong*. Cambridge, MA: Harvard University Press.

Goodin, R. (1990). Government house utilitarianism. In L. Allison (ed.), *The Utilitarian Response: The Contemporary Viability of Utilitarian Political Philosophy*. London: Sage.

Kamm, F. (1993). *Morality, Mortality. Vol. I: Death and Whom to Save From It*. New York: Oxford University Press.

Kamm, F. (1998a). Precis of *Morality, Mortality. Vol. I: Death and Whom to Save From It. Philosophy and Phenomenological Research* 58, 939–45.

Kamm., F. (1998b). Replies. *Philosophy and Phenomenological Research* 58, 969–75.

Nord, E. (1999). *Cost-Value Analysis in Health Care*. New York: Cambridge University Press.

Rawls, J. (1971). *A Theory of Justice*. Cambridge, MA: Harvard University Press.

Scanlon, T. (1998). *What We Owe to Each Other*. Cambridge, MA: Harvard University Press.

Ubel, P. (2000) *Pricing Life: Why It's Time For Health-Care Rationing*. Cambridge, MA: MIT Press.

6

Why There Is No Right to Health Care

Bernard H. Baumrin

The rhetoric of rights dominates discourse about the distribution of health care. Interested parties invoke the right to health care as justification for insisting on expanded access, enriched benefits, and limitless entitlements to special services. Such expansionist attitudes go back at least to the proclamation of the World Health Organization's Preamble to its Constitution on July 22, 1946, where it declared:

Health is a state of complete physical, mental and social well-being and not merely the absence of disease or infirmity.

The enjoyment of the highest attainable standard of health is one of the fundamental rights of every human being without distinction of race, political belief, economic or social condition.

Moreover, as recently as 1997 the Council of Europe declared in its Preamble to its Convention for Protection of Human Rights and Dignity of the Human Being with Regard to the Application of Biology and Biomedicine:

Resolving to take such measures as are necessary to safeguard human dignity and the fundamental rights and freedoms of the individual with regard to the application of biology and medicine.

Such claims to the existence of preexisting fundamental and human rights to health care and health benefits have fed the fire of asserting unqualified entitlements to the concern and care of others. Ordinary people, and medical-care professionals, are called upon to satisfy these claims and feel justifiably uneasy about their failure to pitch in adequately to alleviate the suffering of those in need of various forms of health care—medications, rehabilitative services, long-term care for the disabled, nutritional supplements, prosthetics, and so on. If there were a fundamental right to health care such unease would be fully justified.

In this chapter I take up the claim that there is such a fundamental right to limitless health care and try to show that it has no theoretical legs and is merely an incoherent rhetorical flourish, which, when fully examined, is unsupported and unsupportable, and should be replaced with appeals to a very circumscribed set of quite limited statutory entitlements. Further, arguments for new statutory entitlements should be understood as competing with other claims (e.g., for education, housing, welfare, water, electricity) for the just distribution of limited public resources on discretionary expenditures.

RIGHTS AND CANS

Claims about morality are either true or not true. That is not a controversial claim, but that some are actually true is controversial. One such claim is "ought implies can"—a justly famous dictum of Immanuel Kant's. Every proper instance seems also true.

To have an obligation to do x means that I must be able to do x.
If I'm not able to do something I can't have an obligation to do it.
One cannot have an obligation to do the impossible.

There is something about the logic of *ought* and *obligation* that requires it to be linked to the modality of possibility. There is another interesting, though less talked about, feature of this logic, namely "that no one *ought* to do what has to/must be." That is, if something will occur, will be, no matter what, then an agent related to this inexorable future event/occurrence cannot properly be said to be obliged to do something that will bring the event about, for whether one does or doesn't do it the event will occur without the agent's intervention. "Ought," we all know, only applies when the doing or not doing will make a difference.

So, if I *ought* to do something x, then it must follow (1) that I *can* do it (or at least I can *try* to do it) and that my success or failure could make a difference. (2) If I could not make a difference then I am under no obligation to try to do it.

My second point about the language of ethics is about the term "right" in the sense of having a right. Rights are created either (1) naturally (as the right to life) or (2) contractually by voluntary undertakings (as the right to repayment) or (3) legislatively (as in the right to bear arms or engage in the free exercise of religion or speech). Where there are no contracts or no legislation pertaining to some matter, there are no rights, except natural rights, if there are any, which are always with us.[1]

A second linguistic feature of talk about rights holds that there is a relation, a sort of complementarity or reciprocity, between rights and obligations, such that if someone has a right to repayment then someone else has a duty to repay. For every such right there is a reciprocal duty or duties, so that it has often been said "no duties, no rights." This has become known as the *correlativity thesis*. Whether this thesis holds in every case will not concern us for the moment. One can easily see that for either natural or legislative rights, the correlative duties fall very broadly, whereas for contractual rights the duties adhere very narrowly. If Jones owes me 10 ducats, then Smith has no duty to pay those ducats to me, whereas if Jones has a duty not to kill me, then Smith probably has the same duty, and if general legislation gives me a right to park in Bradmoor Road then everyone has a duty not to prevent me from doing so.

Of course, when one has a duty, one has an obligation, and hence one ought (either to pay, or refrain from killing, or from interfering with, etc.), and that connects up with our first point. Clearly, it is pretty easy not to kill someone (one just *can not* do it) or refrain from stopping me from parking on Bradmoor (e.g., by not being on Bradmoor, or walking on by). These negative duties are easy to fulfill; one simply *can* do them, can fulfill them, and so we can readily see that *duties* easily connect to *oughts* through *cans*.

So when we say that "ought implies can" we are in effect saying that the right that establishes the ought is contingent on some agent's ability (in general) to accomplish the task. There are, however, two complications worth attending to. (*1*) whereas all negative duties can be fulfilled by abstention, positive duties may run afoul of the facts, and (*2*) in the case of contractual duties, impossibility may frustrate the actual fulfillment of the duty (Jones has lost all his ducats, and the ability to get any more). We need to deal with these two kinds of case. In the later we would not want to say that because Jones is broke he does not still have the duty to repay, so his not being able does not erase the duty; it just puts it on hold; even if it is never fulfilled, the duty remains (an albatross about Jones's neck). Many of our duties are like this—waiting, as it were, patiently for the situation to be right, to repay, to make amends, to make happy, and so forth.

The unfulfilled duties circle like a little airy crown around each head waiting for the propitious moment to be plucked into fulfillment. If the will is there, only the local facts prevent immediate satisfaction. There is nothing in the nature of things that prevents their satisfaction. My own crown of unfulfilled duties is already vast, and with each passing day it grows ever larger no matter how much I try to trim it down.

But also when I said above that positive duties may run afoul of the facts, I was talking not about contractual duties only, but of duties of a more general nature. Some of these are opportunistic duties like the positive duty to give aid, which generally only occurs when one is situationally in a position to do so (e.g., to save someone apparently drowning, to help a less able person cross the street). Naturally, there may be no positive duty to give aid; there may only be the *belief* that such a positive duty exists. These duties are really unlike contractual duties. They are more seriously voluntary and may always be above the demands of duty proper. They may be nice things to do, but there is no duty to do them. We will return to this point shortly.

CANS AND THE RIGHT TO HEALTH CARE

I hope by now to have warmed you to my subject on the right to health care. First, we need to determine which kind of right this candidate right is. Is it natural (like the right to life) and merely requires that persons abstain from injuring another? It seems clearly *not* this, for the duty to provide health care is a positive duty and falls on very few, and natural rights (and their appended duties) fall on everyone.

Is the right to health care contractual? There is a line in the Hippocratic Oath to the effect that "whatever houses" the physician may visit he "will come for the benefit of the sick" and another to use his art "for the benefit of the sick . . . [and to] keep them from harm and injustice." On a very broad reading, these parts of the Oath might be used to subscribe to the view that each physician has a duty to the whole of humankind to heal. But at most, this could only support the view that Hippocratic Oath takers (and others who have subscribed to similar undertakings voluntarily) collectively have a duty to the whole of humankind, and clearly those few could not provide sufficiently. Moreover, here the right to health care would be as amorphous a halo of expectations as is my crown of unfulfilled duties. For just as I cannot do all I should, here all that should be done by physicians to heal cannot be done. After all, illness is boundless. Is this all that is potentially meant by a right to health care—that there are well-founded expectations that Hippocratic physicians have voluntarily sworn to heal the sick? We will return to this.

Finally, is the right to health care merely a legislative creation? Two initial difficulties exist: First, legislation is notoriously national. A legislated right to health care in Switzerland does not create a right to health care on anyone in France or Italy. So for there to be a general right to health care (a right that everyone can claim to have), it must be legislated generally (e.g., by the United Nations and therewith apply to all member states). The first difficulty remains, as not all states are member states, and so it is still a limited right. Even if they were all member states, the United Nations itself does not provide the means; it only creates the "right," and without the means the duty is empty. Even if it were supposed that the United Nations created the universal right to health care (however defined) it would at most create the duty of the member states to provide health care for all, but no state believes itself so obliged, nor is it able, to provide health care for everyone (i.e., of every nation), so that "right" is not attended with fulfillable duties, and without fulfillability (invoking now "ought implies can") there is no genuine duty, and if no genuine duty no genuine right. Mere talk of rights does not create real duties—it takes more.

If, as seems likely, no one would claim there is a natural right to health care (and the appended duty that there be physicians from the beginning of human time) that leaves us the two viable candidates—the voluntary duty physicians create by oath or other undertaking and which at most they can only try to fulfill, or the legislatively created right (either by individual states for their own nationals or by the United Nations for everyone). Assuming, for argument's sake, either construction: Are the rights created by legislation real if they cannot be fulfilled (i.e., such rights, being positive, require the wherewithal for their fulfillment if the obligations created are to count)? If they cannot be fulfilled, then there is no obligation, no ought, and if no obligation then no right.

In order actually to answer this question, to give more than a pro forma philosophic gloss, we need to specify what counts as health care. It is not enough to have some airy notion of what physicians or nations are obliged to do. The former may think the obligation is fulfilled by merely keeping office or clinic hours open to all comers,

and the later may think its duty fulfilled by creating a national health service that provides minimal emergency care, or a little less or a little more than that.

Specifying the meaning of health care in this context is made more difficult by the realization that each inclusion of a form of care raises the cost (in human energy and material) very significantly, so significantly that single entries may make fulfillment impossible—for example, depth psychology therapy (if everyone had such care, a very significant part of the population would be psychiatrists). Suppose we create a small but seemingly satisfactory service list:

List 1
Emergency trauma care
Epidemic disease treatment and prevention services
Acute illness treatment and recuperative facilities
Obstetrics

I have left off list 1:

List 2
All chronic care
Psychological services
Rehabilitative care
Cosmetic surgery and care
Reconstructive care (including transplants)

I have left off lists 1 and 2:

List 3
well care
dental care
nutrition

There are, of course, many more items omitted from these lists. Suffice it to say that any item from list 2 above would outstrip the resources of the best-intentioned, best-endowed nation (and even if one could accommodate one item on list 2 for the general population, surely that would do it). Not only is illness boundless but the desire for care is boundless as well. We not only have infection, disease, trauma, malnutrition, but also corns, rashes, sniffles, boils, depression, insomnia, baldness, infertility, impotency, flutters, chills, sweats, spasms, and the endless desire to be better, or normal, or just different. Every departure from the desired, we have learned, can be medicalized even if it shouldn't be.

Suppose, then, we limit the meaning of health care in the phrase "the right to health care" to list 1 (suitably amended to cover any obvious omissions). Is that what the right to health care is intended to mean, or have we thus perverted it significantly? Surely if the Hippocratic physician were to define what he thought he had taken an oath to provide it would be to something like list 1, minus the personal provision of recuperative facilities and would think of himself as misunderstood if it were demanded that he provide, as obligatory, the items on list 2. Nations, conversely, might very well be expected to provide most, perhaps all, the items on list 2. So it really turns out that we are talking about at least two different rights, and if we do not specify the origin (the basis) of the right to health care, we introduce a fatal confusion into the discussion. If health care is restricted to list 1, then it could very well be an obligation physicians have undertaken and/or nations have undertaken, at least for their own citizens. Then we need only look to the resources, actual or obtainable, to see whether there is a genuine right (because there is a fulfillable duty) of either of these narrower sorts.

With respect to an oath-created right, the collective responsibility (of all oath takers) would need to be recognized by those who thus have created the obligation. It would clearly not be enough for the right to be assumed by those who claim it and the obligation to be merely imputed. So it still remains to be seen whether the oath takers believe that they are creating a right to health care in the general population or merely going through some ritualized behavior. My own limited experience indicates that the majority of oath takers believe they are performing a near meaningless ritual, and even more physicians (and other health-care providers do

not even do that). So if there is a general obligation to provide the care on list 1, it falls on such a small number of providers that it cannot be said on that ground to create an effective right in the general population for health care even if restricted only to items on list 1.

We should now look to state-created rights to health care through legislation as it applies just to list 1. Pretty clearly, most states (nations) do not provide the resources even if they provide the legislation. So in those states there is no effective obligation, hence no real right. In some nations (e.g., the United States) there is no general legislation, hence no right of this sort, though there is a general expectation, multibased, that local governments will secure the health care on list 1, somehow, and that the federal government will assure that it is available to those unable to arrange for their own care under targeted legislation like Medicare and Medicaid. Thus, though there is no real right, there is an ill-founded obligation resting in the breach that serves the social purpose of a real right. So widespread is the general expectation that the government, national or local, or hospitals, or doctors, already have some unspecified obligation to provide various forms of medical care that the invocation of a right to health care falls on ready ears. However, in the absence of the foundations discussed above, the invocation is merely rhetorical. Philosophers and bioethicists who enter into this game of supposing that "what ought to be is," do no service to the larger community.

In those nations (e.g., the United Kingdom) where there is both legislation and resource distribution to secure the mandate of that legislation, there is a real right to health care established by the mandate of the legislature despite the inadequate resources devoted to its satisfaction. The population is entitled to the care on list 1 (suitably modified to include what I have inadvertently omitted), but that right does not extend to items like those on list 2. For the right to extend beyond list 1, adequate resources must be made available (presumably after the resources to satisfy list 1 actually have been provided). In fact, the struggle for the expansion of health-care services in such nations is the jockeying among patients and providers to move items from list 2 (or even from list 3) onto List 1 and, thereby, effectively obliging the government to supply the resources as part of the national mandate.

In this brief chapter I have said nothing nice about anyone. And in this conclusion I will not be saying anything nice either. Philosophers have acted no better than populist lobbyists in elevating the notion of a right to health care to the status of objective fact. There is no such right in general and, in particular, it is to be found only within the confines of a few medically enlightened nations. Even here it is a niggardly thing, graced with fine words but in practice an impoverished provision. I believe that the competition to expand health-care services to meet health-care expectations will be the main social battlefield of the 21st century. As life's horizon extends for some, all others will feel cheated for being left behind, and left behind by their own national guardians.

NOTE

1. There are quasi-rights, relationships that look like rights, that are not parasitic on these three—like debts of gratitude; social expectations not actually legislated; and similar sorts of claims that people have on one another. Most are more matters of etiquette, and some depend largely on implied contracts, both linguistically and nonlinguistically based.

7

Specifying the Content of the Human Right to Health Care

Kristen Hessler and Allen Buchanan

Recent writing on the human right to health care is characterized by two trends. First, human rights scholars and health professionals emphasize that health is a complex good, promoted and protected by much more than services provided by medical professionals.[1] This has prompted recognition that the human right to health care is not confined to entitlements to medical care alone. Second, and relatedly, some writers have attempted to delineate a universal, determinate standard defining the precise scope and content of the human right to health care (Toebes, 1999). We argue in this chapter that, whereas the first trend is an important step forward, the second is misguided.

We proceed by first exploring the meaning of a human right to health care, considered in the context of the importance of health as a component of general well-being. We then consider some arguments against the claim that health care is a human right, and we show that those arguments fail. We then briefly survey three dif-

ferent accounts of health care as a human right. On the basis of those accounts, we demonstrate that a human right to health care is necessarily vague, and that the appropriate forum for specifying its content is through appropriate democratic political procedures, and not by moral or political theory alone.

HUMAN RIGHTS

"Human rights" are those moral rights that all people possess. International human rights documents, like the Universal Declaration of Human Rights, reflect the efforts of the international community to make the protection of these rights binding under international law. As the rights of all persons as such, human rights are importantly egalitarian. Hence, the first article of the Universal Declaration of Human Rights proclaims, "All human beings are born free and equal in dignity and rights," and the preamble of each document comprising the International Bill of Rights states that "recognition of the inherent dignity and of the equal and inalienable rights of all members of the human family is the foundation of freedom, justice and peace in the world." More substantially, international human rights documents enumerate specific rights that all persons have, including rights to life, rights to be free from torture or arbitrary arrest, to marry and to start a family.

Two features may be taken as essential to all human rights claims. First, the claim that health care is a human right is much stronger than the claim that health care is a good thing, or that it is desirable that all people have health care. One does not have a right to all those things that might increase one's well-being; for instance, one does not have a human right to possess a sense of humor. Rather, human rights are moral entitlements: "*A* has a right to *X*" means "*A* is morally entitled to *X*." As such, *A*'s possessing human rights entails that some other agent, or group of agents, has obligations to *X*. These obligations may include providing *A* with *X*, or, more minimally, refraining from depriving *A* of *X*. Second, human rights are universal rights, in the sense that they "are held by people simply as people" (Nickel, 1987, p. 3). Thus, at a sufficiently abstract level of description at least, the human rights attributable to any one person will be attributable to all people.

RIGHT TO HEALTH CARE, RIGHT TO HEALTH

In the United States, discussions about a right to health care often are focused explicitly on rights to medical care—that is, services provided by medical professionals to individuals (Toebes, 1999, p. 246). However, in a global context, it is clear that such services are only a small component of the health-related services that make a difference to people's health. Public-health services are at least as important as medical services, and in many places much more important, to improving the health of large numbers of people.[2] Even more general fac-

tors like poverty and fertility rates affect the health of entire populations.[3]

Unsurprisingly, poorer countries fare worse on all sorts of health measures than do richer ones. One obvious reason for this is that richer countries have more money to spend on medical care, but no less important is the fact that citizens of richer countries have better access to healthy environments and adequate nutrition. The broad range of factors that influence the health of individuals and entire populations indicates that health is a complex good.

This raises a thorny terminological issue in human rights literature. Given the complexity of health, many have thought that the right to health care is too narrow and have favored using the term "right to health" instead. Support for this usage comes from the major human rights documents, which more often assert a "right to health" than a "right to health care." For example, the International Covenant on Economic, Social and Cultural Rights includes the "right of everyone to the enjoyment of the highest attainable standard of physical and mental health,"[4] whereas the Universal Declaration of Human Rights embeds a right specifically to medical care within a broader right to health and well-being.[5] However, the problem with asserting a right to health, as opposed to asserting a right to health care, is that it seems too demanding. A *right to health care* implies, on its face, a right to certain services; by contrast, a *right to health* seems to imply a right to be healthy, which is an impossible standard. Some severely ill or impaired individuals will never be healthy, no matter how many resources are expended on them. Moreover, seriously pursuing health for everyone would be so draining on social resources as to leave little, if any, room for the pursuit of other social goals.

However, despite this objection, there are two reasons to search for an acceptable interpretation of the "right to health" rather than to reject the term entirely. One is that, as we mentioned, major human rights treaties assert a right to health. It would be a serious cost to reject all articles in human rights treaties that assert a right to health, especially if an acceptable understanding of that locution were available. Second, given that it is undeniable that factors other than access to medical care have a significant impact on health, the notion of a right to health is valuable. A right to health *care* seems too narrow to cover factors like healthy environmental conditions or good sanitation facilities. This suggests that the "right to health" may be a useful label for a wider category than that of rights to medical care. Such an understanding is consistent with current usage of these terms, as many human rights treaties assert specific rights to certain kinds of medical care or public health services as a part of the general right to health.

There are two ways to understand a right to health as including the right to health care. One is to see the right to health as shorthand for a longer list of specific entitlements, including the subset of entitlements that comprise the right to health care. To a certain extent, we accept this description. We use the term "right to health care" in this chapter to refer to rights to services rendered by health-care professionals to individuals or to populations. Thus, the right to health care includes curative and preventive services provided to individuals—such as therapy for illness, health screenings, and prenatal care—as well as population-based services like immunizations. The right to health care, on our understanding, does not include rights to clean water, adequate sanitation, or the careful placement of toxic waste. In this sense, the right to health care picks out a subset of the entitlements that comprise the broader right to health.

However, this should not blind us to the other, more foundational, way of understanding the right to health as including the right to health care. The right to health asserts that the basic human interest in health is so important as to justify asserting a so-cial obligation to satisfy that interest. It is because health is so important to human beings that rights to health care are so important. However, it is also with an eye on the importance of the basic human interest in health that we see that, in some circumstances, health care is less important than other contributors to health, like sanitation or clean water. In this way, rights to health care and rights to healthy environments are best seen as parts of the right to health, in the sense that they are different kinds of claims that are both justified by reference to the basic human interest in health.

ARGUMENTS AGAINST A HUMAN RIGHT TO HEALTH CARE

Typically, arguments against a right to health care are only one application of more general arguments against the whole category of social and economic rights. Maurice Cranston argues, for example, that civil and political rights are universal human rights, but that social and economic rights are not. The major difference, in his view, is that civil and political rights can be implemented very easily, via simple legislation; but social and economic rights cannot. "The traditional 'political and civil rights' can . . . be readily secured by legislation; and generally they can be secured by fairly simple legislation. Since those rights are for the most part rights against government interference with a man's activities, a large part of the legislation needed has to do no more than restrain the government's own executive arm" (Cranston, 1973, p. 66). Because social and economic rights require expenditures that many poor nations cannot afford, Cranston believes they are not universal human rights at all.

However, Cranston is mistaken in his characterization of civil and political rights. The issue of limited public resources arises for civil and political rights as well as for social and economic rights.[6] The implementation and enforcement of civil and political rights cost money. As one observer noted: "The need for expenditure is clearly evident in rights such as that to a fair hearing before an independent and impartial court; funds will be required not only for the buildings and personnel which constitute a court system but also for the provision of legal aid and interpreters where these are required" (McBride, 1997, p. 128). Further, it would be difficult to disagree with the Human Rights Committee's assertions that the prohibition of torture entails positive obligations to supervise the treatment of prisoners and to establish complaint procedures, and that upholding the right to free assembly requires states to ensure that demonstrations are not suppressed (McBride, 1997, p. 128–29).[7] This shows that expenditures of money must be made in implementing civil and political rights, as in implementing social and economic rights. If one is willing to recognize civil and political human rights as human rights, then the fact that social and economic rights require state expenditures does not imply that they are not human rights.

Cranston has another objection to social and economic rights. This is that such rights are not of "paramount importance," or morally urgent. According to Cranston, "A human right is something of which no one may be deprived without a grave affront to justice" (Cranston, 1973, p. 68). In Cranston's view, civil and political rights, like the right against torture, pass the test of paramount importance: "[T]he use of torture at the pleasure of a despot is precisely the kind of thing which declarations of the Rights of Man are meant to outlaw, and which the United Nations at its inception was expected to banish from the earth. This is a matter of moral urgency, which is far removed from questions of holidays with pay" (Cranston, 1973, p. 71). Holidays with pay, and other social and economic rights like rights to health care, are in Cranston's view merely goals, and not matters of moral urgency. Thus, in his view, they are by definition not universal human rights.

Cranston spells out this objection in two

different ways. First, he argues that the difference between civil and political human rights on the one hand, and economic and social rights on the other, is analogous to the distinction between duty and charity. In his view, no one can be morally obligated to provide *charity* for another (indeed, this is what makes it charity); but because economic and social rights are really just charity for the worst-off, no one can be obligated to uphold them, and therefore they are not really rights at all. The problem with this formulation of Cranston's objection is that he does not *argue* for his characterization of social and economic rights as charity. Cranston cannot simply label them charity, for that would be begging the question (Buchanan, 1987). As we have seen, government expenditure is as necessary for civil and political rights as for social and economic rights, so the fact that government expenditure is required to achieve social and economic rights cannot hold up as a justification for labeling them charitable goals as opposed to human rights.

The second and related development of Cranston's second objection is that there is no readily identifiable duty-holder who is responsible for upholding social and economic rights, and therefore that these are not really rights at all.

They [economic and social rights] are rights to be given things, things such as a decent income, schools, and social services. But who is called upon to do the giving? Whose duty is it? When the authors of the United Nations Covenant on Economic and Social Rights assert that "everyone has the right to social security," are they saying that everyone ought to subscribe to some form of world-wide social security system from which each in turn may benefit in case of need? If something of this kind is meant, why do the United Nations Covenants make no provision for instituting such a system? And if no such system exists, where is the obligation, and where the right? (Cranston, 1973, p. 69)

The problem with this argument is that Cranston seems to assume that there can be no rights to anything that cannot readily be provided by identifiable parties. But surely this does not distinguish neatly between civil and political rights and social and economic rights. To ensure the enjoyment of civil and political rights, stable, rights-respecting institutions must be developed and staffed by individuals trained to uphold them and to hear grievances. In many places, such institutions do not currently exist and cannot be established overnight (or via "simple legislation") (McBride, 1997, pp. 129–34). But more importantly, it is simply false that no rights exist to goods that cannot be immediately provided. There is no incoherence in understanding human rights as entitlements to be progressively achieved. This concession does not give up on the project of human rights; it merely implies that enjoyment of human rights will not be achieved quickly.

JUSTIFYING A HUMAN RIGHT TO HEALTH CARE

As we have seen, Cranston failed to establish that human rights must consist of only civil and political rights. Civil and political rights are neither costless nor obviously more "morally urgent" than other human rights. However, though Cranston has not given us good reason to deny the existence of a human right to health care, we have yet to see a positive argument that health care is a human right.

To assert the existence of a human right to health care is to make a very strong moral claim: that everyone in the world, regardless of nationality, culture, country of citizenship, or any other distinguishing feature, can claim a moral entitlement to certain medical services and public-health measures. In the sections that follow we discuss several ways of justifying this claim, paying particular attention to how each account specifies the scope and content of the human right to health care. In evaluating these accounts, we focus on two main questions. First: Does the account securely justify the existence of a human right to

health care? Second: Does the account provide us with the theoretical resources to determine in practice what kinds of health care must be provided to secure enjoyment of the human right to health care?[8]

Health Care as a Basic Need

One account of human rights is that they are generated by a set of basic needs shared by all people. The universality of human rights on this view derives from the universality of human needs. The main difficulty with this approach is that "basic needs" are difficult to define. The most basic human needs are those things essential to survival. However, if we take this to imply that the human rights to health care is an entitlement to all and only that health care necessary for survival, we will find that this account is both too narrow and too broad. It is too narrow because health care is important not just for saving or extending lives in dire situations, but also for making people healthier, or more comfortable, or for removing barriers to important opportunities. It is too broad because it is literally impossible to provide all people with all health care they need to survive. Given the great cost of some medical care, especially very advanced technology like kidney dialysis machines or organ transplants, and even the expense of public health, limitations on resources will severely constrain the fulfillment of a right to health care, if that right is understood as the right to all care needed to survive.

To be plausible, then, a basic needs justification of human rights requires qualification. David Ozar's account of "basic needs" identifies such needs as those necessary for minimal security. His definition of "minimal security" is "the condition of a person who has sufficient resources to assure survival not only in the present moment and for one additional moment into the future, but for several more moments into the future as well, so that it is reasonable and possible for the person to devote some part of his or her energy and attention to ends other than survival" (Ozar,

1983, p. 302). This is a morally significant threshold, in Ozar's view, because without the freedom to attend to ends other than survival, a person cannot live a life that fulfils distinctively human capacities. Basic needs are those which, when satisfied, would place one at or above the level of minimal security. Basic health care, then, is "such health care as will place a person at the level of minimal security with regard to health care" (Ozar, 1983, p. 307).

Exactly what sorts of health care count as basic, on this account? Ozar indicates that this category includes such things as emergency medical care, treatment to prevent illnesses from becoming life-threatening, and some care for conditions that are not life-threatening, like physical therapy or the relief of pain.[9] Notice that these descriptions are vague and suggestive. This is true for at least three reasons. First, as Ozar notes, the development of medical technology continues to result in new treatments becoming available. This has the result that any specific list of basic health-care services must be dated (Ozar, 1983, p. 304). Second, the threats to people's health vary from place to place: Malaria is a serious health problem in many places, but not in Tucson, Arizona. So both malaria treatment and prevention are basic health needs in some areas but not others.

These first two sources of indeterminacy about the content of the human right to health care are in principle resolvable. However, the category of basic health care is still fuzzy, even given Ozar's analysis. As he points out, his analysis does not tell us whether American citizens have a right to what he calls "life-maintaining care"— which maintains "the lives of persons who, according to our best judgments about their conditions, have lost the capacity to ever maintain their lives without assistance" (Ozar, 1983, p. 308). We could add that Ozar's analysis does not tell us whether those who suffer from kidney disease have rights to publicly funded dialysis, or whether all children have a right to some set of immunizations. This third source of

indeterminacy about the content of the right to health care indicates that the concept of basic health care is not well-defined enough to specify the content of the human right to health care.

A more basic question is whether Ozar's account securely justifies the existence of a human right to health care in the first place. According to his account, people have human rights to those things necessary for minimal security—that is, to those things necessary to assure survival for several "moments" into the future. It does seem plausible that guaranteed access to some health care is necessary to assure my survival in the event that I am the victim of some fairly common mishap: an accident, for example, or a bout of malaria. However, to assure my survival for some significant time, very much health care might be required; for example, I might need a heart transplant. But surely the right to health care does not require everyone to receive heart transplants as needed. Because donor hearts are scarce, and because a social guarantee of a heart transplant for everyone as needed would be prohibitively expensive, it would be impossible to guarantee heart transplants to all who need them to survive for a significant time. From this we can conclude that the right to health care is not really the right to anything necessary to ensure anyone's survival for a significant time.[10] If that is so, then we have good reason to reject Ozar's account as too broad.[11]

Health Care and Human Dignity

The view that human rights are those moral entitlements that respect human dignity is implied by the language in some prominent human rights documents. The International Covenant on Civil and Political Rights, for example, asserts that "[human] rights derive from the inherent dignity of the human person." Similarly, the United Nations' Charter asserts that one of the UN's missions is "to reaffirm faith in fundamental human rights, in the dignity and worth of the human person, in the equal rights of men and women and nations large and small." Jack Donnelly endorses this view: "Human rights are 'needed' for human dignity, rather than health, and violations of human rights are denials of one's humanity rather than deprivations of needs. We have human rights not to the requisites for health, but to those things 'needed' for a truly human life" (Donnelly, 1985, p. 31; Donnelly, 1989, p. 17).

This view avoids the problem of having to come up with a plausible list of basic human needs. However, the real work of this approach is to generate a compelling characterization of human dignity, and its material conditions, in order to get a sense of the scope of human rights. Thus, we might understand "human dignity" as "conditions fitting or suitable for human beings." Unfortunately, this understanding is so close to the meaning of human rights—"the moral entitlements of all human beings as such"—that it sheds little or no light on the concept of a human right. It is probably as a consequence of this fact that Donnelly is led to assert that "human rights doctrines rest on something very much like an equation of having human rights and being human" (Donnelly, 1985, p. 33). The defects of this kind of analysis for our purposes are obvious; starting with the concept of human dignity does not set us very far along the road toward justifying the claim that health care is a human right, not to mention toward ascertaining what kinds of health care are necessary for fulfilling that right. The appeal to human dignity has a broad resonance, but this is purchased by its vagueness.

Health Care as a Basic Right

Henry Shue has argued that certain human rights are basic, in the sense that their enjoyment is necessary for the enjoyment of any other right (Shue, 1996, p. 19). For example, if one does not enjoy the right to physical security (in Shue's phraseology: the right "not to be subjected to murder, torture, mayhem, rape or assault") (Shue, 1996, p. 23), then it is impossible for one

to enjoy other, nonbasic rights like the right freely to assemble. Shue writes (1996): "[T]he substance of a basic right can have its status only because, and so only if, its enjoyment is a constituent part of the enjoyment of every other right, as . . . enjoying not being assaulted is a component part of the enjoyment of anything else, such as assembling for a meeting" (p. 67). Shue argues for three main categories of basic rights: rights to security; rights to subsistence; and certain liberty rights, including rights to political participation. He includes health care and public health as components of the basic right to subsistence. Thus, Shue places health care and public-health measures in a privileged class of human rights—basic rights—which in his view deserve first attention. If Shue's arguments are good ones, then anyone who accepts human rights at all should accept that health care, including public-health measures, is a human right of particular importance.

However, Shue's arguments support a much wider class of basic rights than he realizes. Basic rights are those whose enjoyment is necessary to the enjoyment of any other rights. According to this account, health care is a basic right because it, like freedom from assault, is necessary for the enjoyment of any other right. In the argument quoted above, Shue states that basic rights are *constituent parts* of nonbasic rights: One does not enjoy the right to assemble, for example, if one does not enjoy the right not to be beaten for joining certain assemblies. But consider his argument that political participation is a basic right. In his view, the content of the basic right to political participation includes "genuine influence upon the fundamental choices among the social institutions and the social policies that control security and subsistence and, where the person is directly affected, genuine influence upon the operation of institutions and the implementation of policy" (Shue, 1996, p. 71). In support of his claim that participation is a basic right, Shue (1996) argues:

It is not possible to enjoy full rights to security or to subsistence without also having rights to participate effectively in the control of security and subsistence. A right is the basis for a certain kind of demand: a demand the fulfillment of which ought to be socially guaranteed. Without channels through which the demand can be made known to those who ought to be guaranteeing its fulfillment, when it is in fact being ignored, one cannot exercise this right. (p. 75)

In this argument we see that the sense in which a basic right must be necessary to the enjoyment of all other rights is not as narrow as it might have appeared at first. For enjoying a right to effective political participation is not *logically* a constituent of enjoying rights to security and subsistence; if participation is required for the enjoyment of all other human rights it is because of empirical facts about the tendencies of nonparticipatory governments to ignore the interests of their citizens.

Moreover, we can show in a different way that, on Shue's view, the scope of basic rights must be vast indeed. Shue (1996) argues that the right to participation is no mere formal requirement; rather, "for a right to the liberty of participation to be of any consequence, the participation must be effective and exert some influence upon outcomes" (p. 71). However, the conditions for effective political participation are themselves extensive. For example, surely some kind of education is necessary to render people's participation effective, as are free deliberation among citizens, which requires a free press and rights to free speech and free association. Indeed, the class of basic rights threatens, on this kind of expansion, to include nearly all human rights.

In this way, basic rights are much more extensive, by his own argument, than Shue realizes. The more extensive the class of basic rights becomes, the less that class can accurately be described as a set of core rights deserving first priority among all human rights. Instead, we begin to see a complex interdependency among the entire corpus of rights, with no clear priority

attached to one small subclass of rights. While this view of human rights might support the claim that health care is a human right because it is a basic right, we would need arguments different from Shue's to bear out that claim.

Finally, if we could show that some health care is necessary for the enjoyment of other rights, we would still be left with problems determining the content of the human right to health care. It is a reasonable assumption that healthy people have an advantage when it comes to enjoying their human rights; but this does not tell us how to decide which health-care services to provide when we face a limited budget, nor how to balance health against other necessary conditions for enjoying other human rights, nor even which aspects of health are most important to enjoying other human rights. So the thesis that health care is necessary to securing people's abilities to enjoy other human rights does not eliminate the need to specify further the content of the human right to health care.

JUSTIFYING THE HUMAN RIGHT TO HEALTH CARE

As we have seen, neither the basic needs approach, nor Shue's basic rights approach, nor the human dignity approach to human rights provides a clear account of a human right to health care that offers some guidance for understanding its content. We suggest instead that human rights should be understood as moral claims grounded in *basic human interests*. These are interests that are universally shared by all (or nearly all) human beings, and they are the kinds of interests that justify assigning obligations to others, or to society generally, to secure or protect those interests. The interest in developing a sense of humor, though it may be important to human well-being for some individuals, and may at least be beneficial for most, is not as important for well-being as adequate food, shelter, or access to immunizations. Because some interests are so important for virtually all human beings, they ground obligations on others to help see that they are satisfied. Ultimately, what grounds human rights, including the corresponding obligations, is something fundamental to morality: equal consideration for all persons.

We can say, on this account, that health care is a human right because being healthy is a universal interest, common to all people, that grounds duties in others. The basic human interest in health grounds negative duties—duties not to make anyone sick—and, especially for governments, positive duties—duties to protect and/or to promote the health of others.

One advantage of this account is that it places all human rights on the same footing. People have a human right to health care because they have a basic interest in health, which justifies assigning responsibilities to society to ensure that this interest is met. Similarly, people have a basic interest in security, and in being able to express freely their deeply held views. Both interests are components of overall well-being. Thus, when different human rights conflict, this view refers us back to consider how the interests that ground the conflicting rights contribute to human well-being. This provides at least the possibility of a principled method for resolving such conflicts.

However, the specification problem still looms. The fact that the human right to health care is grounded in the basic human interest in health does not imply anything about the specific content of the right to health care. For example, it does not specify whether that right includes a right to access to abortions, or how to decide which health services to provide when resources are limited. We address this question in the next section.

THE CONTENT OF THE RIGHT TO HEALTH CARE IN INTERNATIONAL LAW

The vagueness of the right to health care creates some difficulty for implementing the right to health care—that is, for ensuring that people enjoy this right. If it is not clear what the content of a human right is, implementing that right through international human rights law, and monitoring nations' compliance, will be correspondingly difficult. In response to this problem, some observers have attempted to specify the scope and content of the right to health care for legal purposes. Brigit Toebes, for example, concludes her extensive study on the human right to health in international law with an account of its core content:

Irrespective of their available resources, States have to provide access to maternal and child health care, including family planning; immunisation against the major infectious diseases; appropriate treatment of common diseases and injuries; essential drugs; and adequate supply of safe water and basic sanitation. In addition, they are to assure freedom from serious environmental health threats. (Toebes, 1999)

Toebes's aim is to give an account of the content of the human right to health care that is universally applicable to all nations. However, in pursuing this goal, she ignores several important parameters of difference among nations. First, Toebes ignores the particular circumstances of individual states in her prescription for which health-related services they should provide. Her qualifier—that states (nations) are obligated to provide health care as she defines it, "[i]rrespective of their available resources"—is much too strong. On her view, states would be considered in violation of human rights legal standards if they could not afford to provide all the services that she includes in the right to health care. But surely there is something perverse about a system that would criminalize states essentially for their poverty. If all states had something like a fair share of the world's resources, then requiring them to spend some fixed sum (at least) on health-care provision might be justifiable. But without such attention to global distributive justice, disregarding a nation's available resources is inexcusable.

Second, Toebes's specification of the content of the human right to health care ignores the fact that different health-related problems in different countries may well require different health services. Any attempt to specify a single, universal standard for the human right to health care must depend on the premise that all health problems in all countries can be equally well addressed by the universal package of health services. But a very limited set of services is all that most nations can ensure, and no very limited set of services can adequately address the diverse health needs of different nations.

Third, Toebes also ignores cultural differences that might be relevant to the implementation of a right to health care. For example, the International Conference on Population and Development was boycotted by several Moslem nations because the draft statement issued by the UN in preparation for the conference included access to family planning as a strategy for population control. In reporting on this boycott, David Thomasma notes that at its root is a fundamental objection to the preparatory statement, namely that "the very idea of intervening in reproduction to control population growth is seen as Western-influenced scientific bigotry—blasphemy even—that denies the power of God. This is a fundamental objection to scientific advancement and to the objectification of human processes for manipulation and control" (Thomasma, 1997, p. 297). If Thomasma's analysis of the boycott is correct, this is an example of the cultural differences among nations that affect how human rights should be implemented within nations.

These differences among states—differences in resource levels, health-related problems, and culture—combine to recommend *against* the project of incorporating into international human rights law a universal, determinate specification of the content of the human right to health care. However, to implement and enforce the human right to health care in international law, we need some account of how it should be specified. Without such an account, we are threatened by two undesirable consequences: Either states will be free to claim almost any arrangement as a fulfillment of the human right to health care, or the international monitoring bodies will be tempted to enforce one single standard on all states, regardless of their differences.

Currently, the content of human rights in international law is specified mainly through the operation of international institutions, with some contribution from national governments. For example, one international institution that contributes to this process is the Human Rights Committee, a UN organization that monitors the reports of state representatives and nongovernmental organizations (like Amnesty International) on human rights enjoyment within those countries that have ratified the International Covenant on Civil and Political Rights (ICCPR). As a part of this process, countries are permitted to present their understandings of the content of human rights, and the UN committee issues judgments on how well particular nations have implemented human rights. This process contributes to the specification of human rights law, for in making its judgments the committee must clarify its understanding of the provisions of the ICCPR.

Whereas specifying human rights is an essential process in human rights implementation, we should ask whether the authority for specifying such rights properly lies with international institutions, or whether it should lie elsewhere, or whether there should be a division of labor regarding the tasks of specification. The most obvious justification for granting this authority to international institutions is that large segments of human rights are best viewed as rights against the state. Rights against torture and arbitrary imprisonment, as well as rights to health care, impose obligations on the state. Accordingly, states should not be allowed to specify the content of human rights for themselves, for this would allow them to judge the extent of their own obligations. On this view, the best human rights protection must come from supra-national institutions.

However, if all human rights are specified through international institutions, it is unlikely that the local differences that we mentioned earlier—which include differences in levels of resources, existing health problems, and culture—will be taken adequately into account. Our discussion of the vagueness of the human right to health care has thus led us to an institutional question relating to all human rights: What institutions can specify the content of human rights in such a way that differences among states are taken adequately into account?

We propose that the virtues of democratic governments suggest that they are better suited than international institutions in protecting the human rights of their own citizens than are international institutions, and also that they might be able to do so in a way that adequately accommodates local differences. Briefly, those virtues are as follows: First, through contested elections, democratic procedures allow people to assert their interests in the political arena. Moreover, through majoritarian decision procedures, democratic government embodies equal consideration for the interests of all citizens (Christiano, 1994). Therefore, insofar as human rights are grounded in basic human interests, there is an important connection between democratic politics and human rights.

Second, democracy is (at least in theory) the system of government that is most closely allied with the interests of the governed; to the extent that this ideal is realized in practice, democratic governments have little impetus to violate the human rights of their citizens. Third, participatory political procedures are most likely to bring out the knowledge that citizens have of their particular human rights problems, and of solutions that would make the most sense for those problems. These virtues provide grounds for exempting democratic governments from the general authority of international institutions to interpret human rights law. On our view, then, states that function democratically should have

some authority to interpret human rights law for implementation within their borders.

Democratic states should not have absolute interpretive authority, however, even regarding the human rights of their own citizens. One reason is that human rights, while vague, are not meaningless. The human right to health care asserts that all people have the right to health care sufficient for their health and well-being. While this broad statement leaves many particular questions unanswered, it is determinate enough to provide the grounds for criticizing a system in which only members of a certain class, or race, have access to any health-related services. Some situations clearly violate human rights, even in their vague form. For that reason, international human rights bodies should have a role to play in supervising the implementation of human rights in both democratic and non-democratic states.

At this point, one might raise the objection that this account seems circular. The appearance of circularity is suggested by the fact that we have argued that human rights require interpretation in order to be implemented and enforced, but also that the international community should supervise the implementation of human rights even within democratic countries. To do this, it would seem that international institutions would have to solve the specification problem. However, if they could do so, then there would be no need for specifying human rights at the national level through democratic institutions.

Our reply to this objection is to note the restricted way in which international institutions should supervise the implementation of human rights within democratic countries. We suggest that the role of international institutions should be limited to two functions. First, they should specify *minimal* conditions for effective democratic procedures within states. These conditions must be designed to ensure that democratic procedures work as they should, so they will include a well-functioning electoral system, wide freedom of speech and association, and the like. Second, international institutions should review national health-care situations and point out any obviously inadequate policies. For neither of these tasks must the specification problem be solved; therefore, objection that our account is circular is unfounded.

CONCLUSION

We conclude by acknowledging two limitations of our argument in this chapter. First, a thorough treatment of the human right to health care must acknowledge problems of international distributive justice. In our presentation here, we have worked within the assumption that nations have widely diverse levels of resources, such that some nations do not have enough resources to spend on their legitimate needs. We have relied on this assumption for the limited purpose of pointing out the fruitlessness of holding poor nations responsible for providing the same protections for all human rights that richer nations are capable of providing.

However, two reasons exist to go beyond this assumption in the search for a complete theory of human rights and their correlative obligations. First, on many plausible theories of distributive justice, the radical inequality of the international distribution of resources is seriously unjust. Second, to the extent that the human right to health care has determinate content, it justifies holding the international community responsible for providing health care adequate for the health and well-being of populations whose governments are too poor to do so. Both of these premises would lead to an examination of *international* duties for human rights protection.

Moreover, the human right to health care exists within a framework of human rights more generally. Accordingly, research on the human right to health care should shed light on how to make sense of the human right to health care within that framework. The most illuminating research is likely to involve sustained attention to the basic human interest in health. Important questions

in this area include how that interest can be satisfied in different circumstances, and how that interest is related to other basic human interests that ground other human rights. Understanding human rights as grounded in basic human interests provides a framework for understanding the interdependence among health care and other human rights, and for beginning to provide an account of how to make implementation decisions about these rights, even when they conflict.

NOTES

1. See, for example, Audrey Chapman's "Introduction" in Chapman, 1994, p. 9: "Clearly there are areas of the world in which the most valuable steps toward improvement of health care are not medical services but public health protection. Poor countries with limited resources would better improve health standards by investing scarce resources in clean water and environmental clean-up rather than by offering curative health care to a small fraction of the population. Moreover, even within an advanced industrialized country, health status will continue to deteriorate and health care costs will continue to escalate unless there is greater attention to promoting more favorable health conditions."

2. The World Bank divides public health into three categories: population-based services, like immunizations; efforts to promote healthy behaviors, like antismoking campaigns; and efforts to provide healthy environments, including adequate public sanitation and clean water supplies. (See World Bank, 1993, p. 72, and more generally chap. 4, "Public Health.")

3. For example, see the World Bank's correlation between fertility rates and life expectancy in sub-Saharan Africa and Latin America and the Caribbean (World Bank, 1993, p. 30); and charts relating national income with fertility, infant mortality, and life expectancy (p. 236).

4. International Covenant on Economic, Social and Cultural Rights, G.A. res. 2200A (XXI), 21 U.N. GAOR Supp. (No. 16) at 49, U.N. Doc. A/6316 (1966), 993 U.N.T.S. 3, entered into force January 3, 1976. Article 12.

5. Universal Declaration of Human Rights, Article 25.

6. For extended treatment of this point, see Holmes and Sunstein, 1999.

7. The Human Rights Committee is responsible for monitoring the implementation of civil and political rights within nations.

8. We do not discuss Norman Daniel's ac-

count of the importance of health care for preserving equality of opportunity. Although this important account may be suitable for grounding a human right to health care, the account was not explicitly developed in these terms. Because it would take a lengthy analysis to ascertain the implications of Daniels's account for the human right to health care, and then to assess its adequacy in that regard, we leave this analysis for another day. (See Daniels, 1985.)

9. Ozar is guilty in this particular study of narrowly focusing on medical care and avoiding the issue of public-health needs.

10. We assume here that we cannot have rights to things that are impossible to guarantee. (In contrast, there is no problem asserting rights that, for contingent reasons, cannot currently be honored but that could plausibly be honored in the future. Such rights are ones to be progressively realized.) Probably the best that can be guaranteed is an equal or fair chance at receiving a heart transplant.

11. Ozar's account is probably also too narrow. We might believe it is possible that a right to health care includes the right to a cure for painful conditions that limit the extent to which sufferers can take advantage of important opportunities (along the lines of Norman Daniels's account of the importance of health care. See Daniels, 1985). Ozar's account seems to rule out this possibility on principle, because curing such conditions is not necessary for continued survival.

REFERENCES

Buchanan, A. (1987). Justice and charity. *Ethics* 97, 558–75.

Chapman, A. (1994). *Health Care Reform: A Human Rights Approach*. Washington, DC: Georgetown University Press.

Christiano, T. (1994). *Rule of the Many*. Boulder, CO: Westview Press.

Cranston, M. (1973). *What Are Human Rights?* New York: Taplinger Publishing.

Daniels, N. (1985). *Just Health Care*. New York: Cambridge University Press.

Donnelly, J. (1985). *The Concept of Human Rights*. London: Croom Helm.

Donnelly, J. (1989). *Universal Human Rights in Theory and Practice*. Ithaca, NY: Cornell University Press.

Holmes, S. and Sunstein, C. (1999). *The Cost of Rights: Why Liberty Depends on Taxes*. New York: Norton.

McBride, J. (1997). Reservations and the capacity to implement human rights treaties. In J.P. Gardner (ed.), *Human Rights as General Norms and a State's Right to Opt Out: Reservations and Objections to Human Rights Conventions*. London: The British Institute of International and Comparative Law.

Nickel, J. (1987). *Making Sense of Human Rights*. Berkeley: University of California Press.

Ozar, D. (1983). What should count as basic health care? *Theoretical Medicine* 4, 129–41. Reprinted in P. Werhane, A.R. Gini, and D.T. Ozar (eds.), *Philosophical Issues in Human Rights*. New York: Random House, 1986.

Shue, H. (1996). *Basic Rights*, 2nd ed. Princeton, NJ: Princeton University Press.

Thomasma, D. (1997). Bioethics and international human rights. *Journal of Law, Medicine and Ethics* 25, 295–306.

Toebes, B. (1999). *The Right to Health as a Human Right in International Law*. Amsterdam: Hart/Intersentia.

World Bank (1993). *World Development Report 1993: Investing in Health*. New York: Oxford University Press.

II

RATIONING AND ACCESS
IN TODAY'S WORLD

The chapters in this section examine issues of justice in today's world. Today's world—the real, actual world—often seems unjust, a world in which some people are better off than others, some people are treated better than others, some entire countries fare better than others, while other people, both individually and as nations, have more health problems and poorer health status. Regional and national boundaries mark off different economic systems, forms of government, and political practices. These in turn shape different systems of health care, as well as different systems of education, law, and other institutions that also often seem unjust in their objectives and operations. In an ideal world, these institutions would be fair, never promoting the welfare of some persons at the expense of others nor privileging some individuals when others might be equal claimants for the allocation of a privilege or a good. But the fact remains that almost everywhere in the real world, some patients get better treatment than others, some hospitals and health-care institutions get more funding than others, and some often marginalized groups of people—the poor, the disabled, the elderly, children—get worse health care support than more powerful or influential groups. In short, the lofty ideals and ambitious conjectures of theoretical discussions of justice, like some of those espoused in the first section of this volume, do not square with the frayed and grimy realities of the actual world.

This lack of fit between theoretical and practical discussions of justice often invites claims that philosophical constructions are of no real value, or that head-in-the-clouds theorizing about matters like justice has no relevance to the real world. Such claims exhibit an extremely common failure in everyday reasoning about issues of justice: the failure to distinguish between what is known as ideal theory and what is called "partial-compliance theory." The former—ideal theory—provides an account of what justice might (and should) be were all the background institutions in the world it describes just. The latter—partial compliance theory—offers a second, less lofty but often more practical account of the real world. Ideal justice theory assumes that all citizens equally have enjoyed the same degree of justice (whatever the state has achieved), whereas partial compliance theory observes that, in most societies, the achievement of justice has been unsystematic and uneven and that some people have benefited more than others. Some people or groups may have been disadvantaged historically, over long periods of time; some current policies may operate inequitably, introducing new injustices. Departures from ideal justice may vary in degree: Some situations or systems may be slightly unjust, others grossly so. The central problem for partial compliance theory is what to do in an imperfect world: Not only may people disagree about what an ideal theory of justice would require, but attempts to achieve greater justice (however it is seen) may reinforce or exacerbate existing injustices. Consequently, partial compliance theory recommends certain policies and constraints that seem to be objectionable from the perspective of ideal justice theory.

In the real world, the degree of injustice in background institutions can vary from one locality or background situation to another. The justice of health-care systems is often described in terms of national systems: In this volume, for example, background situations relevant to the justness or unjustness of health care include those of the United States (a country without universal health insurance); the United Kingdom and Australia (countries with universal but two-tiered health care involving a public and a private sector); Scandinavia and Italy (countries with highly egalitarian, universal welfarist systems); and the developing world (in many instances, countries with seriously underfunded health care and gross inequities). The justness or unjustness of a situation in any country can be assessed in terms of many factors, including funding of hospitals and health-care institutions, insurance coverage of individuals, number and quality of procedures, health outcomes for individuals and groups, and much more. This section will focus on the situations—some described as just, others as unjust—in a variety of nations.

In the first selection in this section, Bruce Vladeck and Eliot Fishman, discussing the situation in the United States, argue that what appears to be an unjust distribution of health care is the price of the sort of constitutional and political system the United States has. America has not achieved a comprehensive, national health-care insurance or provider system. Is this a social cost of long-standing American political institutions, institutions that are hardly ever seriously questioned in American politics? Vladeck and Fishman offer an historical account to explain both what didn't happen in the U.S. (the establishment of universal insurance) and what did (Medicare, state-administered insurance, CHIP, Medicaid, and other programs) and they explain how the failure to achieve equitable access to health care in the United States is consistent with the retreat from active measures to promote distributive justice in many facets of American society.

Patricia Mann also explores the imperfect nature of the U.S. health-care system, particularly the gap between political ideals (which she believes America still has) and current political praxis. She sees the issues as a matter of "agency," the product of tension between ideals of distributive justice (fairness, equality) and the American perception of the individual as an autonomous economic and political agent. Each American could succeed, the myth goes, if he or she really tried; hence, support (read "handouts") for things like health care is unjustified. Those who are successful, this myth continues, should not be taxed to provide health care or other support for those who fail. Taking into consideration the views of Ronald Dworkin and Joyce Appleby, and the evident fact that some people have by nature more health problems than others, Mann challenges the misleading "macho autonomy binary" as-

sumption behind the dilemma and proposes a solution in her own "three-dimensional theory of agency."

Roger Crisp looks at the British National Health Service (NHS) and its apparent inability to treat all according to need. He asks in particular whether the NHS, in failing to treat all according to need, fails to satisfy its founding principle. Crisp's inquiry involves an exploration of what it is to "need" health care, and on what basis patients are or are not treated according to need. There is clear room for improvement in the NHS, he argues, if its underlying mandate is to be met.

Tony Hope, John Reynolds, and Siân Griffiths, also discussing the United Kingdom, explore practical real-world dilemmas as well, especially those about how to allocate health care when sufficient funds are not available. They describe a specific, concrete example, the Oxfordshire Priorities Forum, which has attempted to generate an ethical framework for making decisions about allocation on the basis of quality-of-life assessments, QALYs. Hope, Reynolds, and Griffiths examine the strengths and weaknesses of this approach, as evidence of the difficulty of making these triage decisions in real-world application of health-care allocation policy.

In his chapter on "Resources and Rights," Richard Tur also explores issues of justice in health-care resource allocation in the United Kingdom, where, as elsewhere, there are not enough resources in the form of life-saving procedures and drugs and other components of health care to go around. Tur focuses particularly on the processes of judicial review that are brought to bear on these situations. Courts of law decide what are sometimes heart-rending disputes over resources within a health care system like Britain's, disputes about cases which Tur vividly describes. Tur's interest lies in whether judicial review, by judges who are not elected, is the legitimate means for settling questions about the just allocation of health care in a democratic system.

The social realities of health in Australia are described by Mark Sheehan and Peter Sheehan, not just in individual terms, but as the outcome of complex social and individual factors. There are massive inequalities in health outcomes by income and social class, reflected, for example, in the astonishingly disparate life expectancies of indigenous and nonindigenous Australians. Sheehan and Sheehan appeal to Amartya Sen's "capabilities" analysis, as well as to other theoretical accounts, to scrutinize these disparities. The pattern of inequality in the social reality of health is hardly confined to Australia, they note, and they cite comparable figures for the United States and elsewhere that contribute to a disturbing picture of inequality.

In contrast, Tuija Takala argues that the Scandinavian health-care systems are fundamentally just. Their justness is a function of their strong commitment to solidarity, equity, and universality. Here Takala is appealing to an ideal theory of justice, but claiming that it can be reached and that such ideals can be actualized—or nearly fully actualized—in the real world. This does not mean that there are no tensions, and in a welfarist health-care system like the Scandinavian models Takala discusses, there are increasing tensions as a private health-care sector and individual choice are being introduced and as the system is pressed by growing demands on its resources.

In her report from Italy, Giovanna Ruberto also views her country's health-care system as essentially just. In using a structured network of regional agencies that are "completely patient-oriented," it provides the same comprehensive health care to poor and wealthy alike, without regard to income or tax contribution. She points out that in the World Health Organization's 2000 report on the health systems in 190 countries, Italy ranked second, surpassed only by France, and concludes that justice is compatible with excellent quality. However, Italy's system itself faces a number of

dilemmas as it confronts the limitations of its resources in light of rising costs, increasing demands, and bloated expectations. The problem is how to set goals and how to institute reforms with coherent direction and purpose. These problems, we might note, are faced by many other countries in the industrialized world.

Concluding this section, Baruch Brody explores further issues about rationing and access in today's world by examining clinical trials of new drugs—in this case, AIDS drugs—in developing countries. In many of these countries, background institutions and patterns of access to health care may be even more unjust than in the industrialized nations the previous chapters in this section have discussed. The specific issues that Brody addresses play out against developing-world backgrounds of extreme injustice: Can it be ethically acceptable to test AIDS drugs in populations when access to such drugs is beyond the financial reach of virtually all people affected, including virtually all of the subjects who have participated in the test? Although Brody's piece was written just before the pharmaceutical companies of the industrialized world lowered prices to African countries where rates of HIV infection are particularly high, the issues he explores remain urgent, and apply to many other drugs and technologies besides those for HIV/AIDS. Brody's question shows dilemmas of partial compliance at their most acute. How can a central component of health care—ethical testing of pharmaceuticals—be conducted where background conditions not only exhibit extreme scarcity but may also be grossly unjust? The rich can purchase drugs or travel to other countries while the poor have access to little or nothing at all in the way of adequate health care. Injustice is not found only in the poor nations; some rich nations exhibit patterns of injustice in health care as well, but the extreme scarcity that characterizes the developing nations' health systems may make these issues worse.

8

Unequal by Design: Health Care, Distributive Justice, and the American Political Process

Bruce C. Vladeck and Eliot Fishman

As recent events have so dramatically reminded us, American democracy takes place within a uniquely complex constitutional and legal framework. Every nation, of course, is different, but the United States may be more different than most in the way that a basic framework established more than two centuries ago has evolved, adapted, and been modified while maintaining certain remarkable continuities.

At the same time, the United States is the only modern industrial democracy without some form of universal health insurance. Indeed, in most of the United States, citizens have no right or legal guarantee of access to any medical care except evaluation and treatment by hospital emergency departments, if they can somehow contrive to find their way to one. We believe these two phenomena are causally related. That is our basic thesis: that inequities in health care in the United States arise from the fundamental constitutional and political structure of the American political system. That system does not make inequities inevitable, but it certainly makes ameliorating or eliminating them much more difficult than is the case in any other affluent society.

And this is an incredibly affluent society—perhaps more so than any other society in human history. Traditional economic appeals to scarcity as the root of inequities in American health care simply will not wash, given how much more this country already spends for health care than any other nation and how much living standards and wealth, at least for those in the upper half of the income distribution, have increased in the last decade.

To make our argument, we will consider the interrelationship among constitution, policy, and politics at three levels of the American system: in the failure to enact comprehensive national health insurance legislation; in the politics surrounding Medicare, the United States' single system of universal health insurance for part of the population; and in the operation of those health insurance programs for which responsibility is primarily devolved to the states, a long-standing and increasingly popular approach. We will not devote any of this chapter to describing or analyzing the extent of inequities in health care in the United States; there are abundant alternative sources for that information. (Commonwealth Fund, 1999; Kaiser Family Foundation, 2000; World Health Organization, 2000). But we will conclude with some observations on the implications of our analysis for competing strategies to redress those inequities.

NATIONAL HEALTH INSURANCE AND THE MADISONIAN DESIGN

In American politics, constitutional theory and constitutional interpretation are never just matters of objective analysis or dispassionate history. But a few aspects of the nation's basic governmental structure are largely indisputable. First, the Founding Fathers took the division of powers further than any other constitutional authors since, providing independent electoral bases for the national legislature and executive and lifetime tenure for federal judges within a structure that renders the three branches of government almost uniquely interdependent. Not only do Presidents and the Congress often have different political allegiances, but the House of Representatives and the Senate frequently march to different drummers, even when the same political party has a majority. The kind of unity of policy and politics possible in parliamentary governments in those instances in which one party has won a substantial majority, never mind the monolithic authority of majorities in the British system, can occur in the United States only when an electoral landslide is accompanied by chronological accidents in the terms of senators and Supreme Court justices, something so unlikely that it occurred for only four years, perhaps six, in the whole of the twentieth century.

In other words, a distinct bias toward inaction is built into the American political system. The Founding Fathers were apprehensive that a more plebiscitary type of democracy, at least as democracy was understood in the late eighteenth century, would unduly threaten the prerogatives of wealth and property ownership. They explicitly feared a "tyranny of the majority," and they explicitly advocated for a governmental structure that could take bold action only with great difficulty.[1]

Significant positive change in social policy has generally come more slowly—and much later—in the United States than in other democracies. And by most measures, the United States has been less willing to provide public support of social welfare measures than have other industrialized nations. Although among the most affluent, Americans are about the least heavily-taxed citizens of the First World; in direct correlation, they are also the least likely to benefit from public income support, family support, or health insurance programs. James Madison and his contemporaries got what they wanted.

Participants in the Constitutional Convention attended not solely as members of a sociocultural and political elite, but also as representatives of at least partially sovereign states. Much of the time and energy of the Convention was devoted to protection of the states' sovereignty and influence, and while the broad sweep of subsequent American history has been in the direction of nationalization of the economy, the culture, and political life, the governmental system is still profoundly shaped by these originating impulses.[2]

The significant and independent role of state governments in the formation and implementation of policy is the most obvious and important manifestation of the continuing role of subnational governments in the American political system. But there are other federal systems in the world, and in Canada and Germany, to name only the two most relevant examples, the subnational governments play a central role in the structure of national health insurance. What distinguishes the American political structure is the extent to which federal officials remain tied to subnational political forces and pressures.

Representation in the upper chamber of the American legislature (the Senate) is based on states, not on population, so that Wyoming's half-million residents elect as many senators as do California's 35 million. Thus, American public policy almost invariably tilts toward the interests of less-populated rural communities and the resource extraction industries on which many of them rely. Even in the House of Representatives, where seats are allocated to the states in proportion to population and where the Supreme Court has required relatively equal population distributions across districts, representatives are elected by local majorities in districts usually drawn by state legislatures under election laws and procedures administered by the states. Whenever policy issues counterpose the values of national uniformity with the ability to respond to the peculiarities of individual geographic communities, the local focus almost always wins out.

The United States is an especially large and heterogeneous country. Populations, cultures, and economic characteristics differ as widely as the nation's topography. So do health-care needs and the characteristics of health-care delivery systems. The interaction of so much diversity with a centrifugal political system further reinforces the difficulty of making dramatic, coherent, national policies. According to the famous and rarely disputed adage, in the United States all politics is local.

In other political systems, such centrifugal forces are counterbalanced by the role of political parties that in theory provide relatively coherent ideological positions with which voters can identify and around which elected representatives can organize. The Founding Fathers were largely opposed to the idea of creating stable, organized political parties (*Federalist Papers*, 1961). While most Americans have historically identified themselves as "Democrats" or "Republicans," American political parties have never displayed the unity or ideological discipline of their European counterparts. Because the United States has no nationally elected legislative officials, American legislators have always been mainly dependent on local majorities and ready to abandon their party leadership to respond to local imperatives.

But the distinctiveness of American political parties is ideological, not just structural. Indeed, one important school in the historical analysis of why America lacks comprehensive national health insurance pretty much starts and ends with the syllogism that: the United States is the only industrialized nation never to have had a major labor party; in the rest of the world national health insurance has been the product of labor party governments or the imminent threat of them; hence, there is no national health insurance in the United States. That syllogism, of course, begs the question of why there has never been a national labor party in this country.

The evolution of American political parties from early in the nineteenth century until very late in the twentieth century was dominated by sectional cleavages that cross-cut coherent ideological or class lines.[3] Prior to the Civil Rights Act of 1964 and the Voting Rights Act of 1965, the history of the Democratic Party was inseparable from the politics of the white supremacist South. Even when the Democrats attracted the allegiance of working people and progressive reformers, as they did briefly in the Wilson years and then more or less permanently since 1928, they were always constrained by the fact that a large portion of their national base was tied to the most conservative and localistic forces in American politics. Conversely, the dramatic realignment of Southern politics during the last four decades, combined with the evolution of campaign financing, may finally be leading American political parties to resemble the classic European model, reflected to a considerable extent in the 2000 elections.

Divided government, localism, weak national political parties—these are the structural elements of American government that have produced the most inequitable health-care system in the Western world. It could also be argued, rightly, that American political culture is itself substantially more conservative, more protective of the interests of private property, and more suspicious of governmental action and governmental intervention, than any other Western nation. Most important political phenomena—like American health policy—are overdetermined, in part because structure and culture interact and reinforce one another so strongly. But public opinion and even political culture are more malleable and more volatile than political structures, arguing for the greater importance of structural than cultural causes. And it is doubtful that a majority of Americans are ideologically opposed to more dramatic government action on health care. Although the extent of that support has waxed and waned in response to short-term forces, public opinion data in the United States for the last 50 years have usually shown widespread popular support for greater governmental intervention to reduce inequities in health care. Nevertheless, the conservatism of America's system appears to trump the flexibility of American public opinion on health-care issues.

Even a very cursory review of the history of national health insurance proposals in the United States bears out the effects of these forces. Notwithstanding the efforts of the American Labor League and some other early reformers, government intervention to assure access to health care for all Americans did not really arrive on the political agenda until 1935, when President Roosevelt's Advisory Committee on Social Security recommended that health insurance be a part of the basic package of protections extended to all Americans under a comprehensive national scheme of social insurance. Yet Roosevelt, who was perhaps the most extraordinarily pragmatic politician in the history of the American presidency, feared that opposition to health insurance from organized medicine would

jeopardize the entire package in the legislative process. At the time, Roosevelt was close to the peak of his extraordinary popularity, and his party commanded comfortable majorities in both houses of Congress. But that majority included a sizable fraction of Southerners, including a number of critical committee chairmen, whose willingness to support national pensions and cash assistance might be threatened if their local medical communities were mobilized in opposition. So health insurance was the only major recommendation of the Advisory Committee that was not included in the legislation proposed to, and ultimately enacted by, the Congress.

National health insurance thus became a major agenda in the unfinished business of the New Deal that the remaining New Dealers sought to advance after World War II ended. But by then they had lost their electoral majorities. Just as war-weariness and the yearning for a return to domestic agendas is often adduced as the explanation for the unanticipated success of the Labour Party in Britain's 1946 elections—which led immediately to the creation of the National Health Insurance—a similar desire for change in a more prosperous, less war-devastated nation ended the Democratic congressional majority in the United States in the same year and essentially doomed national health insurance in this country. President Truman's unsuccessful advocacy of the Murray-Wagner-Dingell health insurance proposal in 1948—the high-water mark of national health insurance efforts for the next generation—may have assisted in his unexpected reelection, but it did nothing to change a fundamentally unfavorable legislative balance of power.

Under another democratic system, of course, Truman's 1948 election would necessarily have altered the legislative balance of power. The Congress was controlled by a coalition of Republicans and conservative Southern Democrats from 1946 through 1964, and early in that period, after the defeat of Murray-Wagner-Dingell in 1948, the leading advocates of national health insurance both inside and outside the Executive branch concluded that movement toward greater equity in access to health care would have to come more incrementally, in the kind of smaller bites the Madisonian system seemed to make inevitable. After 1950, therefore, they decided to focus their efforts on a relatively modest proposal to provide hospital insurance for the elderly. The enactment of Medicare and Medicaid in 1965 is the signal exception to the general failure of the American political system to address widespread inequities in access to health care and will be discussed at greater length below.

Perhaps the only thing that surprises about the failure of the political system to enact major changes in the health-care system since 1965 is how close it came on two occasions. In 1972, a Nixon Administration that was preoccupied by reelection concerns and an ideologically fractionated Democratic Congress came remarkably close to actually enacting some form of national health insurance. In 1993, a newly elected Clinton Administration may have squandered its opportunity by moving too slowly, too obtusely, and with too little understanding of how to build a supportive coalition in the Congress. One of us was personally involved in the 1993–1994 Washington events, however, and believes the Clinton Administration never really came close to succeeding. In both 1972 and 1993–1994, there was widespread popular support for the national government doing *something* about reforming the health insurance system to improve access for all Americans, and a relatively popular President actively supported legislation to that effect. Still, the political system ultimately produced stalemate, just as it was designed to do.

THE POLITICAL ECONOMY OF MEDICARE

The politics of Medicare in America are the flip side of the politics of national health insurance. National health insurance always fails because our system disproportionately strengthens well-organized minorities and local interests, and because it has granted disproportionate power to a sizable ideological faction that opposes both redistribution and strong national government. These same structural forces have distorted Medicare politics and administration, and they threaten to destroy its basic social insurance structure.

Indeed, it is remarkable that Medicare got passed at all. That only happened because of the unique election landslide of 1964. Medicare was held up all through the 1950s and early 1960s by the effective veto power of senior Southern congressmen opposed to a big new federal program. However, thanks to the Goldwater nomination and the Kennedy assassination, the 89th Congress of 1965–1966 had an extremely large Democratic majority, by American standards, of 68 to 32 in the Senate and 295 to 140 in the House. The combined veto power of Republicans and Dixiecrats was temporarily suspended. But only partially—Wilbur Mills still chaired the Ways and Means Committee and he shaped the passage of both Medicare and Medicaid. Mills famously moved to include physician services in Medicare and to expand the Kerr-Mills program for the poor aged to welfare recipients of all ages in the Medicaid program. He intended these incremental expansions to forestall demands for national health insurance, a strategy that appears to have succeeded (Marmor, 2000, pp. 58–60).

Once Medicare was passed, the same old structural imperatives of American institutions took over. Medicare regularly draws the attention of the groups that are strongest in the Madisonian system: the wealthy, the geographically concentrated, and antigovernment legislators in the South and West entrenched in power by seniority and the safe seats of a regional ideology. This is so for three reasons. First, Medicare is the major source of income for multiple health and health-related industries, and the exclusive source of income for others, all of which are located in somebody's state or district (and most of whom are well-represented in the District of Columbia). Second, the more than $200 billion Medicare spends annually is a large pot of government expenditure to distribute among states and congressional districts. Third, Medicare is always vulnerable as a program that transfers money from younger to older and, to a lesser extent, from high income to low income Americans.

The growing interest in privatizing Medicare's benefits and administration do not derive from any demonstrable evidence that privatization would solve Medicare's problems. Furthermore, privatization is overwhelmingly unpopular with Medicare beneficiaries. But it draws strength from the ideological and structural forces arrayed against Medicare's redistributive character, and from distaste for the annual legislative fracas characteristic of special-interest and distributive politics. Medicare made it past America's political design in 1965 only because of an electoral/legislative anomaly. But America's political structure may, in the end, undo the work of that anomalous Congress.

Special-Interest Politics

The same basic elements of the Madisonian system—separation of powers, political localism, weak political parties—that combine to frustrate broad social reforms like national health insurance also work to produce a political system that revolves around the allocation and distribution of specific benefits to specific legislative districts, the enactment of generally inadequately enforced regulatory systems to respond to unavoidable public concerns, and deference to interests capable of making significant campaign contributions in a political system based on limited party loyalties and local television markets, in which candidates are eventually on their own. In the Madisonian game of factional conflict over government benefits—that is, special-interest politics—Medicare's annual $200

billion is a major prize or, more precisely, an enormous aggregation of small prizes. Medicare is the largest single source of income for the nation's hospitals, physicians, home-care agencies, clinical laboratories, durable medical equipment suppliers, and physical and occupational therapists, among others. Each of those groups works energetically to protect and advance its interests through the political process (Levitt et. al., 1998). The health-care industry is so big, however, and Medicare is so complicated, that it is necessary to understand some of the subtleties of the process in order to understand the political dynamics of Medicare and the ways in which those dynamics affect broader public policy concerns. A few examples help to illustrate that point.

Medicare accounts for as much as 40% of the income of the average U.S. hospital, but the hospital community is increasingly heterogeneous and internally fractious (Levitt et al., 1998). Medicare spends so much money on hospitals—more than half of its total outlays, if all hospital-delivered services are included—that at the highest levels of aggregation, hospital politics becomes indistinguishable from macrobudgetary politics, to the disadvantage of the hospital community. But most politics around Medicare occurs at levels far lower than that of the hospital community as a whole. The Balanced Budget Act of 1997, for example, contains no fewer than a half-dozen provisions increasing reimbursement for specific hospitals or, at most, for a mere handful; the Balanced Budget Refinement Act of 1999 contained a dozen more such provisions. A large part of the administrative resources of the Health Care Financing Administration (HCFA), which administers Medicare, are devoted to evaluating claims on behalf of particular hospitals, or small groups of hospitals, advanced by individual members of Congress. With every passing year, the prospective payment system (PPS), which Medicare employs to pay for acute inpatient hospitalizations, and which was touted by some of its initiators as a model of uniform, "scientific" national policy, looks less like a theoretical exercise in health economics and more like the loophole-infested Internal Revenue Code.

More broadly, PPS increasingly tilts toward particular classes of hospitals, especially teaching hospitals and those in rural communities. Teaching hospitals benefit from America's love of medical technology and the popular fascination with science, especially medical science. And while it is true that rural hospitals play an important role in their communities and are especially dependent on Medicare as a share of their total revenues, the basic Madisonian formula for representation in the U.S. Senate does them no harm, either.

Hospitals, doctors, HMOs, and Medicare contractors (that is, the insurance companies that provide Medicare with most of the administrative services necessary to operate its fee-for-service benefits) all have a major stake in Medicare policy and act as expected in the political system. Yet there are other service providers that essentially serve only Medicare customers. Literally thousands of home-health agencies, durable medical equipment suppliers, and firms that contract for therapy services, as the most notable examples, have been formed to do business with Medicare—a veritable Medicare–Industrial Complex. Individual entrepreneurs are the large majority of suppliers in most of these industries, although large, national publicly traded firms have become more important in the last two decades, as a buoyant stock market made equity capital easy to raise.

Nothing is more frustrating to Medicare administrators, nor more puzzling to outside observers, than the fact that the payment methods—and even levels of payment—are written into law, often at prices higher than a big buyer such as Medicare could obtain in the marketplace. Efforts to make Medicare a more "prudent purchaser" have been supported by administrations of both political parties for more than a decade. But Medicare suppliers occupy a political territory of classic dimensions in American political science: narrowly focused interest groups with an enormous specific stake in issues about which the rest of the body politic could not care less, seeking benefits of enormous importance to themselves that are almost invisible in the total aggregate of the federal budget. They thus have succeeded in resisting almost every effort to improve Medicare's purchasing by enlisting key members of Congress to defend their constituents from the depredations of the "big bad federal bureaucracy."

Medicare suppliers thus have built on the earlier successes of the more visible providers, such as hospitals and doctors, in turning the program from one that provides a legal entitlement to beneficiaries to one that provides a de facto political entitlement to providers. Part of that transformation dates to the attitudes of program administrators from the early days of Medicare when officials were concerned (astonishingly enough, in retrospect) that not enough providers would be willing to participate in the program; part of it stems from some truly misguided decisions by the federal judiciary over the years. Even though their only purpose is to sell services to a government program, and even though the government and its beneficiaries might be better off if there were fewer, larger, more efficient, and cheaper suppliers, these providers have acquired a kind of legitimacy in the political process that turns our conventional notions of the boundary between the public and private sectors upside down.

The analogy to defense contractors is not totally far-fetched. There are plenty of $400 toilet seats in the Medicare program. Medicare cannot deliver services to its beneficiaries without providers, and providers are major sources of employment, political activity, and campaign contributions in every congressional district in the nation. Although the average home-care agency is very much smaller than the average military base, efforts to close either one produce the same kinds of congressional responses.

Distributive Politics

Medicare spends money in just about every city and town in the United States. With the federal government reducing almost every other form of domestic spending, the geographic distribution of Medicare dollars has become a matter of increasing attention. The most dramatic recent example is the treatment of payment rates for capitated plans in the 1997 Balanced Budget Act. Congress sought to respond to the complaints of rural representatives that the adjusted average per capita cost (AAPCC) formula, based as it was on actual Medicare costs in specific counties, penalized lower cost (and therefore presumably more virtuous) rural counties as well as such low-cost metropolitan areas as the Twin Cities (Minneapolis–St. Paul) and Portland, Oregon. At the same time, however, Congress responded to the concerns of teaching hospitals by carving out costs associated with Medicare's teaching hospital payments from capitated rates; this was done so as to pay the money directly to the hospitals. Doing so by itself, however, would have produced significant rate reductions for HMOs in major urban communities on both coasts, so Congress also established a hold-harmless provision in which each county was guaranteed a rate increase of at least 2% per year. The result was, in essence, a series of simultaneous equations that could not be solved. The Balanced Budget Act of 1997 has produced the sought-after effect of substantial rate increases in rural counties, although it has not yet been accompanied by any increase in the availability of capitated plans in most of those communities. It has also produced modest rate increases in high-cost urban areas, but the Twin Cities and Portland have received almost no benefit.

There is no platonically ideal formula for allocating capitated payments across communities, especially since the dynamics of individual markets vary on a number of dimensions, only one of which is price. In fact, a strong case can be made against formula-driven administered prices as a fundamentally unsound way of setting capitated rates to begin with, a position that HCFA has long advanced in the face of considerable resistance from the HMO industry and Congress. But the health-policy debate increasingly consists of high-sounding arguments cloaking relatively narrow, traditional regional and local issues.

Redistributive Politics

The Madisonian system not only shapes Medicare's normal politics, but it also increasingly threatens Medicare's redistributive structure. Through an insurance mechanism, Medicare provides a set of service benefits to many people who otherwise would he unable to afford or obtain adequate access to health services. It has revolutionized access to health care for the elderly and the disabled and thus has contributed to the demonstrable improvements in health status and life expectancy of older Americans over the past 35 years. Medicare also has been an extremely powerful weapon for reducing poverty among the elderly and disabled.

Medicare does so at least in part by transferring income from workers to retired or disabled former workers. On average, each working-age person contributes something over $1,250 a year to provide about $5,000 in benefits to each Medicare beneficiary. (The astute observer may interject at this point that Medicare funds are not in fact actually transferred to Medicare beneficiaries but rather to providers that give them services—or as the more cynically astute observers might argue in the case of some managed care plans and some beneficiaries, providers that do not give them services. Certainly, unlike other Social Security programs, Medicare rarely puts cash into the hands of those who are described as its beneficiaries. But they benefit nonetheless.) Although hardly anyone will say it out loud, this transfer lies not far below the surface of many of the most bitter and contentious political fights about Medicare, especially in the past five years.

1965 Reconsidered

After roughly 30 years in which the miracle of 1965 managed to surmount it, the Madisonian political system is reasserting its discomfort with any governmental action that redistributes wealth from the better-off to the less well-off. In the last four years there have been efforts to transform the program from a defined benefit to a defined contribution (as proposed in the recent Breaux-Frist legislation and, before that, by Republicans and conservative Democrats on the Bipartisan Commission on the Future of Medicare); to encourage medical savings accounts (MSAs, popular with the House Republican leadership and resoundingly unpopular with Medicare beneficiaries); and to impose higher premiums on low-income and middle-income beneficiaries. Indeed, the insistence that Medicare and Social Security face a "crisis" because of aging baby boomers is rooted in visceral hostility to redistributive policy in all of its forms; the baby-boomer crisis disappears if the possibility of increased taxes on the more affluent is allowed into the discussion.

There is no question, from an economic point of view, that American society could afford to support Medicare indefinitely—indeed, to support a more generous Medicare program than the one we now have. The question is whether, politically, we want to do so. That question comes down to the extent of our willingness to require the better-off to subsidize the less well-off.

Nowhere is the redistributive dimension of Medicare politics more apparent than in the argument from urgency made by some proponents of radical change. They claim that it is imperative to do something soon, before a much larger share of the electorate is made up of Medicare beneficiaries or

people close to eligibility age, because at that point the politics of the issue presumably would change. In fact, the voting behavior of Medicare beneficiaries and their responses to public opinion polls do not differ substantially from those of 40- or 50-year-olds regarding Medicare policies. But the concerns of Medicare's critics in this regard mirror, almost precisely, the concerns expressed by Madison and his fellow Federalists when they were successfully campaigning for ratification of the Constitution they had drafted.

Arguments for privatization of Medicare do not rest on these exaggerated threats alone. They also draw extensively on the distaste of many policy analysts for the interest-group and distributive dimensions of Medicare's political economy described above. The tendency of politicians and the interests to which they respond to behave as politicians and interest groups generally do is advanced as a rationale for moving responsibility for Medicare's management out of the public sector altogether through some form of defined-contribution plan. Detractors argue that more rational or more effective administration of Medicare is virtually impossible unless it can be disentangled from the political process. This argument, of course, is most frequently made by those parties who, the rest of the time, are most busily engaged in interest-group and distributive polities. "Stop me before I sin again" might be the practical translation of this position.

STATE-ADMINISTERED HEALTH INSURANCE

Ever since the failure of the Clinton health reform effort in 1994, incremental, decentralized expansions of health coverage have dominated health-policy proposals for both Democrats and Republicans. The proposals have increasingly fallen into a specific pattern: benefits targeted at the poor or near-poor, administered by the states, and paid for by both state and the federal governments. And this is nothing new—with the obvious and important exception of Medicare (and with inroads into Medicare as well), a similar model has dominated public health insurance in the United States for 40 years.

This structure is a perennially effective legislative sell, but it also consistently falls short of its main legislative objectives. Enrollment, access to health care, or both are disappointing. (A few leading states that had often pioneered similar programs before participating in the federal equivalent are exceptions.) The states generally fail to enroll a substantial portion of the groups that are eligible under their own existing rules, and those rules themselves often exclude many who belong to the population ostensibly targeted by the authorizing federal legislation. These failures are most notable in the high proportion of the poor not eligible for or enrolled in Medicaid; the same pathology has also gotten a lot of recent attention in the Children's Health Insurance Program (CHIP) for the near-poor.

The early problems with CHIP should come as no surprise. Underenrollment, underfunding, and operational problems have plagued a series of state–federal health insurance programs beginning with the Kerr-Mills program for the elderly that preceded Medicare in the early 1960s, and continuing with (most notably) the original Medicaid program, the large Medicaid expansions of the late 1980s, the "Medicare Buy-in" (QMB/SLMB) program, CHIP, and in a variety of state-initiated health-insurance programs and "drug assistance" programs aimed at helping the elderly pay for prescription drugs.

The contrast with Medicare is striking. Medicare Part B (which covers physician expenses) was and is a voluntary program. Yet it enrolled 93% of the nation's senior citizens—17.7 million people—in its first year (Marmor, 2000, pp. 87–88). Both enrollment levels and access to health care have been an overwhelming success story in Medicare; they have been perennial problems in the state–federal programs.

Why the difference? Medicare differs from the Medicaid model in three relevant ways: It is administered by the federal government, its policies are part of national rather than state politics, and it covers all seniors rather than only the poor or near-poor. The problem with Medicaid and its policy cousins may arise from means-testing, from the lack of state administrative capacity, or from the lack of political incentives for states to advance these programs aggressively. The states may fall short because governors and state legislators find it politically unwise to spend taxpayer money on health insurance and especially health insurance for the poor, even when the federal government is picking up most of the tab. Or, it may be hard to enroll the working poor in a nonuniversal program, perhaps especially so for small state administrations.

State-Run and Means-Tested—A Brief History

The history of state-administered, means-tested health programs is a long saga of recurring troubles. It begins in 1960 when renewed political pressure for national health insurance for the elderly had been building for two years (Marmor, 2000, pp. 27–30). The Kerr-Mills bill of 1960 was a rearguard effort by conservative Democrats and Republicans to address that pressure without substantially increasing the scope of national government. It provided medical care to the indigent elderly using what is now Medicaid's structure: federal standards set a comprehensive package of benefits for the elderly poor (or those elderly whose medical expenses rendered them effectively poor), while the specific eligibility standards, coverage, and provider reimbursement levels were set by the states. States paid for the program with a federal match ranging from 50% to 80%, depending on state income levels. Kerr-Mills was widely regarded as a near-total disappointment. In its five years of existence (before it was replaced by Medicare), only five states established substantial programs, and they received almost 90% of the total funds. Eighteen states had no program in place at all.

In 1965, at the same time that Medicare largely supplanted the Kerr-Mills program for the elderly, Kerr-Mills was expanded into the Medicaid program both to continue to provide non-Medicare health benefits to the indigent elderly and to provide health-care coverage for two other poor populations—single-parent families and the disabled. These three populations were already eligible in principle for cash welfare payments, and Medicaid enrollment was largely a program for welfare beneficiaries until the late 1980s. The states had the option of making significant exceptions: States could enroll families poor enough for welfare but with two parents ("Ribicoff children") and individuals with incomes above Aid to Families With Dependent Children (AFDC) levels but with significant medical expenses that effectively brought them below the threshold ("medically needy").

Finally, a provision of the legislation required states to move toward comprehensive medical coverage of Medicaid enrollees. In short, the states were mandated to enroll their welfare population in Medicaid, although they had a substantial degree of latitude to set reimbursement rates and to expand eligibility beyond welfare. Medicaid was successful in important respects. Enrollment grew quickly, and there was immediate evidence that enrollees got more regular medical care (Davis and Schoen, 1978, pp. 62–67; Rowland et al., 1999). But Medicaid policy in the states very quickly became dominated by cost concerns. Most states stinted on reimbursement, and many did not take up the options to enroll "Ribicoff children" or the medically needy despite federal money to defray most of the expense. Many Medicaid recipients continued to rely on the same charity-care facilities that they had used before the program.

Medicaid's enactment coincided with a boom in enrollment in the older AFDC program, which in turn drove unanticipated increases in Medicaid enrollment.

Medicaid's rolls grew from 10 million people in 1967 to 24 million in 1976, paralleling similar growth in AFDC (Davis and Schoen, 1978, p. 56). Medicaid's expenses grew even faster, from $3.5 billion to $14 billion, as a result of the enrollment boom as well as rapid cost inflation in hospitals and nursing homes (Klarman, 1974; Davis and Schoen, 1978, pp. 56–62).

The states reacted to this growth by cutting back on coverage, reimbursement, and enrollment. In the early 1970s, states imposed a variety of limits on coverage for hospitalizations and physician office visits, and these limits were especially draconian in the South. Levels of Medicaid reimbursement for primary care were (and continue to be) held substantially lower than prevailing rates in most states: For example, in 1997 the average state paid 43% of the amount paid by private insurers for normal childbirth (Gruber et al., 1999). The result of limited reimbursement was limited access to mainstream providers, precisely the situation Medicaid was meant to resolve. Many Medicaid patients therefore continued to utilize traditional forms of charity care—clinics and/or safety net or public hospitals rather than private doctors' offices. And even though enrollment grew explosively, the states kept Medicaid as a program for welfare recipients only, despite the hopes of its sponsors in 1965. Medicaid did not enroll most poor children in most states, and the legislative requirement that states move toward comprehensive medical coverage for those who were enrolled was soon dropped (Davis, 1975, pp. 48–49). While Medicaid budgets grew dramatically in the late 1960s and early 1970s, this was in large part because of dramatic increases in AFDC enrollment, as the number of poor single-parent families exploded at the same time that AFDC enrollment rates went up from 60% to 90% among those who were eligible (Davis and Schoen, 1978, p. 59).

The dominance of cost concerns in the Medicaid program became glaring with the slow implementation of the Early and Periodic Screening, Diagnosis and Treatment program (EPSDT), passed by Congress in 1967. It provided Medicaid children coverage for well child visits and preventive care. Both the federal government, which failed to write regulations until 1971, and the states, which took years to implement the program, sought to avoid the relatively modest costs involved. A Democratic-majority Congress continued to push the program, but it took until 1976 for even a million children to get screening out of 12 million who were eligible (Davis and Schoen, 1978, p. 84). The only portion of Medicaid in which all states enthusiastically participated immediately after it was passed—Medicaid assumption of Medicare Part B premiums—was a net cost reduction for the states, saving the states the costs of providing care themselves for the indigent elderly (Davis, 1975, p. 41).

Just as Medicaid had boomed with AFDC enrollment in the late 1960s and early 1970s, it stagnated with the welfare rolls in the late 1970s and early 1980s, as states became increasingly stingy with both programs and as the federal government lowered eligibility requirements. Medicaid enrollment hit 22 million in 1975 and stayed at that level or below it for twelve years, until the federally mandated expansions of the late 1980s took effect, so that by 1987 only about 34% of the poor were covered by Medicaid (Morone, 1990). At the same time, Medicare's expenses and enrollment both continued to escalate rapidly.

The first substantial expansions to Medicaid eligibility began in the mid-1980s, mandating coverage of AFDC-eligible pregnant women and giving states a series of options to broaden eligibility to poor children, pregnant women, and seniors. As with optional eligibility expansions in the original 1965 legislation, most states were slow to take advantage. A series of Medicaid expansions between 1984 and 1990 followed a repeated pattern: Congress authorized a series of optional coverage expansions for poor and near-poor women and children; most states failed to take advantage of the options; Congress then made the coverage mandatory. Coverage of poor pregnant women and infants became mandatory in 1988, and mandatory Medicaid eligibility was expanded to a variety of poor or near-poor women, children, and seniors in 1989 and 1990. At this point most states did become more aggressive in their eligibility rules for pregnant women and infants, with many increasing eligibility beyond the federally mandated income maximum of 133% of poverty. And these expansions had a substantial impact: Enrollment grew from 23 million in 1988 to 36 million in 1996.

But the Medicaid expansions also introduced a massive new failure in the program. Millions of pregnant women and children were eligible for benefits but not enrolled. In 1996 only 58% of the uninsured children eligible for Medicaid under the expanded eligibility used it, whereas 77% of those children eligible for Medicaid under pre-expansion rules were enrolled—the latter figure is in line with other means-tested programs). This meant that *4.7 million children*, or 40% of all uninsured children, were eligible for free health coverage but were not taking advantage of it.

The problem of underenrollment spread to Medicaid's original welfare enrollment base with the abolition of the AFDC entitlement in 1997. With welfare reform causing millions of women to leave the welfare rolls that had previously provided an automatic link with Medicaid, many women lost Medicaid coverage for themselves and their children despite their continued theoretical entitlement. Welfare-related Medicaid enrollment in the 21 states with available data fell almost 40%, or 1.6 million, from June 1997 to December 1999 (Kaiser Commission, 2000). According to the Census Bureau, the number of children enrolled in Medicaid dropped about 400,000 between 1997 and 1998 (Alliance for Health Reform, 2000). A recent study concluded that a large majority of women and children who lose Medicaid coverage after leaving welfare remain uninsured; they do not obtain private health insurance (Garrett and Holahan, 2000).

Continuing the efforts to cover children that began in the mid-1980s, a bipartisan majority created the Children's Health Insurance Program (CHIP) in 1997, sending money to states to cover children from families with incomes up to 200% of poverty or higher. The program sought to provide more than $40 billion in federal matching funds over 10 years (Alliance for Health Reform, 2000). As of December 1998, some 40 states (including the District of Columbia) had begun enrolling children in CHIP programs. Medicaid and CHIP together should in principle cover up to two-thirds of the uninsured children in the United States (Kaiser Commission, 1999). But despite the CHIP legislation and earlier Medicaid expansions, 1998 Census Bureau data showed that the number of children lacking coverage grew substantially—from 9.8 million (13.8%) lacking coverage in 1995 to 11.1 million (15.4%) in 1998.

The CHIP program enjoyed a high profile when it was passed, but it soon became a high-profile problem. At least 2 million children are eligible but not enrolled in CHIP, in addition to the 4.7 million children who are eligible for Medicaid but not enrolled (Edmunds et al., 2000). Forty states did not draw down their full funding allotments for the first year of the program because of severe underenrollment problems, even though states were given three years to use each fiscal year's allocation to give them time to get programs up and running. The original legislation would have required those 40 states to forfeit their unspent funds to the 10 states that had spent their allotments, although recent legislation partially reduced that penalty.

By the beginning of 2001, all 50 states and the District of Columbia had begun enrolling children in CHIP programs. Medicaid and CHIP together should, in principle, cover up to three quarters of the uninsured children in the United States, and over 90% of the low-income uninsured.[4] But despite the CHIP legislation and earlier

earlier Medicaid expansions, restrained health cost inflation, and the best economic climate in a generation, 2000 Census Bureau data showed that the number of children lacking coverage has remained high. Child uninsurance initially grew substantially despite the new program—from 9.8 million (13.8%) lacking coverage in 1995 to 11.1 million (15.4%) in 1998. In 1999 child uninsurance fell almost back to its 1995 percentage, 13.9%, and in 2000 it fell further to 13%, lower than 1995 and somewhat higher than it was in 1992, seemingly a major accomplishment. But this was a result of increased employer-based coverage, as government health coverage remained at 17.9% of children, slightly lower than the percentage in 1997 before CHIP began and substantially lower than the pre-welfare reform 20.2% in 1995.[5] The 1999–2000 drop in child uninsurance is less than meets the eye: Whereas CHIP gains no more than replaced reductions in child Medicaid enrollment, the peak of the then-booming economy reversed some of the erosion in employer coverage that had declined throughout the early and mid-1990s—an achievement that is likely already a pleasant economic memory.

The QMB/SLMB, or "Medicare Buy-In" program seeks to reduce or eliminate out-of-pocket Medicare costs for the low-income elderly. As with the other Medicaid expansions of the mid-1980s, the program began as a voluntary state option, in which states could use their Medicaid program to pay Medicare cost-sharing fees for seniors whose incomes were low but above welfare eligibility levels (which for seniors means eligibility for the Supplementary Security Income program). And as with the other Medicaid expansions, voluntary state participation was minimal—only three states participated (Merrell et al., 1997). In 1988, the Medicare Buy-In program became mandatory in the ill-fated Medicare Catastrophic Coverage Act (MCCA). Although the new costs to states from the QMB program were supposed to be more than fully offset by savings from Medicare expansions, those savings did not materialize beyond the first year because most of MCCA was repealed in 1989 (Moon et al., 1998). Medicare Buy-In was then expanded again to give more limited financial benefits to higher-income beneficiaries with the Specified Low-Income Beneficiary (SLMB) program in 1990 and Qualified Individuals (QI) program in 1997, again with the costs shared between the states and the federal government.

These programs have been sharply limited by underenrollment problems. Nationally, approximately 85% of QMB and SLMB eligibles (3.3 million to 3.9 million people) were not receiving the Medicare Buy-In benefit in 1998 (Families USA, 1998; O'Brien and Rowland, 1999).[6] Many states do not make even minimal efforts to keep track of potential eligibles: Only 20 states bother to subscribe to data available monthly from the federal Health Care Financing Administration (HCFA), which identifies low-income individuals newly enrolled in Medicare, and among those states that receive the data, only 12 use it (Nemore, 1999). The minuscule enrollment for the modest benefits allocated to seniors in the 1997 QI program (reimbursing low-income seniors for the 1997 Balanced Budget Act's Medicare fee increases) is a particularly breathtaking example of the underenrollment problem: At the end of 1998, the first year of the QI program, only 1% of the money set aside for this program had been used, and only 3% of potential participants had been enrolled (Nemore, 1999).

As of 1998, some 18 states operated programs to cover some or all of prescription drug expenses for the poor elderly. (Six more states have authorized programs since.) These programs are not on the Medicaid model, because they are not federally mandated—they are in the pre-Medicaid model of voluntary state health-insurance initiatives, the kind that have been repeatedly folded into state–federal partnerships. Despite the fact that they are voluntary state initiatives, they also manifest both the underenrollment and the underfunding problems of other means-tested, state-run health coverage programs. These programs all have relatively generous income ceilings—between 150% and 250% of poverty—that would in principle incorporate a substantial minority of seniors (AARP Public Policy Institute, 1999). Yet only three of these plans have enrollment of more than 100,000, those of Pennsylvania, New Jersey, and New York. Most of the programs are tiny, whether because of state government disinterest, the stigma of means-tested benefits for moderate-income seniors, or a combination of both. Pennsylvania's program is the largest, with 236,000 beneficiaries in 1998. Yet this enrollment has been steadily dropping from its high of close to 500,000 in the late 1980s (Serafini, 2000). All of the state programs put together covered about 2% of Medicare beneficiaries in 2000.

Possible Causes

Two related problems emerge from this history of state-administered, means-tested health coverage: underfunding and underenrollment. Whereas the first is clearly an issue of conscious state stinginess, it is not clear that underenrollment results from state decisions as such, intentional or not. There are several plausible reasons that states do not enroll as many of the uninsured as they seemingly could. Nor is it clear that the federal government would be any more generous or effective in administering means-tested programs. Analysts have pointed to a variety of obstacles related to means-testing that link it to the underenrollment problem. One barrier to enrolling the working poor and near-poor is welfare stigma. Participants in the labor market and retirees are described as reluctant to participate in means-tested, "welfare" programs, and they are skeptical of the quality of care they will receive on "welfare insurance" (Rowland, 1999; Shaner, 1999; Alliance for Health Reform, 2000; O'Brien et al., 2000; Serafini, 2000).

Indeed, many working people may not even be aware that they or their children are eligible for public coverage: One study found that 6 out of 10 parents whose children qualify for CHIP or Medicaid do not believe the program applies to them, and that 82% of these parents said they would enroll their children if they knew they qualified (Holloway, 2000). The cumbersome enrollment process associated with income and asset verification may also limit enrollment: Lengthy asset tests, the necessity to provide citizenship and income verification, and the use of Medicaid applications in the CHIP and QMB programs may be keeping eligible individuals away from means-tested programs (Alliance for Health Reform, 2000).

In contrast, Medicare enrolled virtually its entire target population in its first year of operation. Analysts who blame the enrollment failures on the inherent administrative requirements and psychological barriers of means-testing can point to the advantages Medicare had on both counts: The Social Security system allowed almost automatic Medicare enrollment, with only a nominal step required for Part B participation. Medicare, moreover, is conceptualized as an earned social insurance benefit. Underenrollment has often been a problem for means-tested programs funded exclusively by the federal government, even programs with broad political support such as Head Start and the Women and Infant Children nutrition program (WIC). Means-tested programs must either enroll the (often isolated) nonworking poor, now increasingly cut off from cash welfare, or the skeptical working poor.

But if the difficulties of means-testing were overwhelming the good intentions of the states to enroll the eligible, operational differences between the states' programs would not make much of a difference. And there is striking evidence that states can do a much better job on enrollment. Vermont, a relatively poor state, has achieved near-universal coverage for children and 93.5% coverage for its whole population with means-tested public health insurance and effective marketing efforts. Notably, Vermont's governor is a physician who is ideologically strongly committed to universal health coverage. Enormous variations exist between states on both eligibility rules and outreach efforts. They seem to defy the traditional liberal concern about rural, conservative states, sometimes called the "Alabama problem." Two of the most successful CHIP programs have been in North Carolina and Alaska.

Means-testing may well make enrollment significantly harder than it is in a universal program like Medicare. But operational differences clearly do matter in making means-tested programs a success. The problem of eligible but not enrolled is therefore also an issue of either lack of policy innovation or lack of political will.

States are not doing as well as they might on enrollment, and they frequently focus predominantly on costs in their administration of means-tested health coverage. If governors and state legislators felt more was politically at stake, it is hard to believe they would not do better. But there is significant evidence that governors and legislators get little scrutiny in state elections for health-care policy in general, and even less for enrolling and covering low-income people. Although health care routinely appears in the top two or three issues in exit polling on national elections, it almost never does in state elections.[7] State elections are dominated by the issues of education, crime, and, importantly, taxes. The centrality of the tax issue helps to explain a striking disparity in national versus state elections in the country as a whole and particularly in states of the northeast. Republicans have achieved a thorough dominance of the nation's governorships in the last decade. Even New York, Massachusetts, Rhode Island, and Connecticut have Republican governors, although these states have become a virtual regional lock for Democrats in national elections. Republicans at the state level can run on tax cuts without raising the specter of cuts to middle-class entitlements. (Democrats have only recently rediscovered the middle-class issue of public education as a response to the dominance of taxes in state politics.) It is especially telling that the only health-care issue to get on the radar screen of elections in most states has been regulation of the HMOs that cover the insured middle class.

There is evidence that means-tested health coverage can be politically stronger at the national level than it has been in the states. The costs of Medicaid expansion and CHIP are considerably higher for the federal government than for the states, yet the legislation passed with substantial Republican support at the national level (and, in contrast, has fallen short on enrollment in a number of states with Democratic governors). It may be that virtually *any* health issue gets more traction on the national stage than on the state level.

The Political Allure of Devolution

Nevertheless, sending administrative power to the states is almost always appealing in American national health policy, and social policy generally. Whatever the merits of specific state-based programs, there is a more fundamental aspect of American political culture that drives the decentralizing tendency: the notion that state governments are closer to the people.

None of the usual American exceptionalism suspects—namely rugged individualism, the American aversion to politics and government in general, mistrust of the able-bodied poor—provides a clear explanation for why it is more attractive for state bureaucracies to run means-tested programs than for federal bureaucracies. Why should the American preference for health policies that are "mechanistic, self-enforcing, automatic solutions which might operate without further politics or even self-conscious deliberation at the political center" delegitimize national government and exempt state government? (Morone, 1990)

The connection between American resistance to political conflict and direct government action on the one hand and devolution to states on the other has to do with the way Americans and the American media think about state governments as opposed to the federal government. Small governing units seem clearly to be a legitimizer in and of themselves: The smaller the government, the less intimidating and foreign it seems as an institution. Indeed, debates over devolving social policy to the states, in their emphasis on the closeness of states to the people and the evils of Washington, seem to regard state government as not really government at all. This makes a certain amount of sense culturally. If most Americans were asked to name politicians or people in the government, how far down their list would they get before they got to their governor, never mind another state or local official? National government operates in the spotlight, the center of public life; state governments operate, largely ignored, at the periphery.

CONCLUSIONS

Despite the recent modest downtick in the number of uninsured Americans—in the context of an extraordinary period of economic growth and labor-market tightness— there is little reason to expect that the problems in equity of access to health care will subside any time soon. Certainly, neither of the major party candidates in the 2000 Presidential election proposed anything like measures that would be very much more than symbolic, and the closeness of the election outcomes dims even the chance of very modest, meliorative legislation, at least until 2005. Heightened partisan conflict can help crystallize substantive policy change when one party has a clear upper hand; but when popular support of the major parties is closely divided, the likelihood of substantive action falls dramatically.

The recent resurgence in the rate of growth in health-care costs also bodes badly. After several years in which states benefited from the windfall of reduced Medicaid enrollments due to welfare "reform," Medicaid costs have begun to increase sharply again, causing budget "crises" in Kansas, Ohio, and Texas, among other states. It seems certain that, as the economy slows and labor markets slacken, employers will be less and less willing to swallow increases in health insurance premium costs, causing some to withdraw from the market altogether while others seek to increase the share of the costs borne by employees. That developing increase in employee costs is a process that has significant equity effects, as lower-paid employees are much more hard-pressed to pay increased premiums than are their more affluent colleagues.

One predicts American political developments at one's peril, especially in the contemporary environment, which appears to be particularly volatile, unstable, and subject to unexpected turns of events. But while, as of this writing, the 2000 elections have barely ended, it may be possible to detect glimmers of trends that may, if they strengthen and continue, powerfully affect the future.

On the one hand, America's major political parties appear to be in the process of becoming more like classic political parties in the European sense. The partisan realignment of much of the South (and, though much less noticed and, because of the smaller populations, less significant, most of New England as well), the increased importance of corporate and individual "soft money," and the growing sophistication and success of the national party apparatuses in fund-raising and funds distribution, all tend to reinforce ideological homogeneity and party loyalty. Certainly, the two parties in Congress have rapidly become more ideologically unified, with both "Rockefeller Republicans" and "Blue Dog Democrats" becoming less and less numerous with every congressional election.

On the other hand, the heightened clarity of party conflict, to the extent it is apparent to the public at all, appears not yet to have increased public interest or participation in the electoral contest. Despite a very close contest and dramatically increased turnout by African-Americans, total voter turnout in the 2000 Presidential election appears to have been, at best, only marginally higher than the historically low level of 1996. Even though there may be more at stake, ideologically, in future elections it appears that fewer and fewer Americans will be bestirred to participate.

From the viewpoint of reducing inequities in access to health care, these trends could produce either very good or very bad news. An electoral sweep by a party (presumably the Democrats) committed to significant expansions in health insurance might produce a more dramatic and even more comprehensive set of measures than did the 1964 landslide. A similar sweep by a party holding opposing views would not only be a major setback to the cause of increased access to health insurance, but might propel major efforts to privatize and de-universalize Medicare, this nation's one semblance of comprehensive, universal insurance, which has produced a population group (Americans 65 and older) with fewer (though still significant) disparities in access to care than the rest of the population.

The structural obstacle course James Madison laid out for redistribution and majoritarian government remains intact. But his goal of limiting populist factionalism through America's sheer size and diversity seems increasingly overtaken by social and political change. In other words, for all the complexities and sophistication of Madison's design, elections still matter. In fact, they may matter more in the future than they have in the past. For those whose personal or professional agendas involve a significant commitment to the reduction in inequities in access to health care, the implications could not be more clear.

NOTES

1. The classic work on this subject is Robert Dahl, *A Preface to Democratic Theory* (Dahl, 1956).

2. See Federalist 10, 48, 49–51ff. (*Federalist Papers*, 1961). On the importance of state sovereignty to widely differing sides of the debate over the Constitutional Convention, compare Federalist Papers, Nos. 17 and 45 (*Federalist Papers*, 1961) and Banning, *The Sacred Fire of Liberty* (Banning, 1996) to Herbert Storing, ed., *The Anti-Federalist* (Storing, 1985).

3. Of the many analyses of the evolution of American political parties, this is the conclusion we find most accurate.

4. Peter Cunningham, "Targeting Communities with High Rates of Uninsured Children," *Health Affairs*, Web Exclusive, 2001, pp. w20–w29; Genevieve Kenney, Jennifer Haley, "Why Aren't More Uninsured Children Enrolled in Medicaid or SCHIP?" Urban Institute, 2001.

5. Robert Mills, "Health Insurance Coverage: 2000," Current Population Reports, Bureau of the Census, September 2001; 1988–1998 data available online from US Census Bureau, search under "Health Insurance Historical Table 3." As explained in the Mills report, the Census Bureau changed its questionnaire in 2000 to correct a flaw that was leading to an overestimate of the number of uninsured of about 8%. This new format has been employed only for 1999 and 2000 surveys, however, meaning that all pre-1999 years include this 8% over-estimate, while the last two years do not. To allow for comparisons between pre-1999 and post-1999 numbers, the Census provided uninsured estimates using the old methodology for 1999 and 2000 also, and I have used those here. Using the new methodology, the percent of children who are uninsured goes down to 12.6% in 1999 and 11.6% in 2000, and presumably would have been about 1%–1.5% lower for all the pre-1999 years as well. Note that the 17.9% figure for public coverage in 2000 would have been about 17.7% under the old methodology, and that the chart below on private and public coverage levels includes extrapolations of old methodology rates for 2000.

6. Because of the way HCFA and the states report QMB enrollment, statistics on QMB can lump together beneficiaries who are eligible for full Medicaid with those participating in the QMB program alone. Therefore, different modeling techniques produce varying statistics on enrollment. The General Accounting Office found only 2.4 million QMB-only enrollees in 1998, and a similar number in 1995 (GAO, 1999). But the Alliance for Health Reform estimated QMB enrollment at only 367,000 in 1995. (Alliance for Health Reform, 1997; O'Brien and Rowland, 1999). Families USA (1998) estimates QMB enrollment at 4.0–4.5 million, and Marilyn Moon et. al., (1998) find similar figures, pegging QMB enrollment at

78% of those eligible, but these authors explicitly include those enrolled in full Medicaid and the Supplementary Security Income program in their QMB count. SLMB enrollment is more consistently counted at about 200,000, or 14%–16% of eligibility.

7. Exit polls routinely ask voters to rank their "top issues" in deciding their vote. In national elections, either health care or Medicare ranked as one of the top three issue between 1992 and 1996 and a major issue in 1998: Health care was third in 1992 and 1994 and sixth in 1998, while Medicare ranked second in 1996. In 13 available exit polls in state elections from 1994 to 1998, health care was not listed by voters as an issue in 10 of them. It was fifth in California in 1994 and 1998 (with the latter score for a category called "Health care/ HMOs"), and was tied for sixth in Texas in 1994.

REFERENCES

AARP Public Policy Institute (1999). *State Pharmacy Assistance Programs*. New York.

Alliance for Health Reform, (1997). *Medicare and Medicaid Dual Eligibles*. New York.

Alliance for Health Reform (2000). *Health Coverage Update: Children's Health Insurance*. New York.

Banning, (1996). *The Sacred Fire of Liberty: James Madison and the Founding of the Federal Republic*. Ithaca, NY: Cornell University Press.

Commonwealth Fund (1999). *U.S. Minority Health*. New York.

Dahl, R. (1956). *A Preface to Democratic Theory*. Chicago: University of Chicago Press.

Davis, K. (1975). *National Health Insurance*. Washington D.C. New York: Brookings Institution.

Davis, K. and Schoen, C. (1978). *Health and the War on Poverty*. Washington, D.C. New York: Brookings Institution.

Edmunds, M., Teitelbaum, M. and Gleason, C. (2000). *All over the Map: A Progress Report on the State Children's Health Insurance Program*. Children's Defense Fund.

O'Brien E. and Rowland, D. (1999). *Medicare and Medicaid for the Elderly and Disabled Poor*. Kaiser Family Foundation.

EPIC Advisory Committee (1996). *EPIC Evaluation Report to the Governor and Legislature*, State of New York.

Families USA Foundation (1998). *Shortchanged: Billions Withheld From Medicare Beneficiaries*.

Federalist Papers (1961). New York: Mentor Books.

Garrett, B. and Holahan, J. (2000). Health insurance after welfare. *Health Affairs* 19 (1), 175–84.

General Accounting Office (1999). Low Income Medicare Beneficiaries. Washington, D.C.

Gruber, J., et. al., (1999). Physician fees and procedure intensity. *Journal of Health Economics* 18, 473–90.

Holloway, M. (2000). *Expanding Health Insurance for Children.* Robert Wood Johnson Foundation.

Kaiser Commission on Medicaid and the Uninsured (1999). *Health Coverage for Low-Income Children.*

Kaiser Commission on Medicaid and the Uninsured (2000). *Medicaid Enrollment in 50 States.*

Kaiser Family Foundation, (2000). *Uninsured in America,* 2nd ed., Menlo Park.

Klarman, H. (1974). Major public initiatives in health care. In E. Ginzberg and R. Solow (eds.), *The Great Society.* New York: Basic Books.

Levitt, K.R., Lazenby, H., Broden B. (1998). National health spending trends in 1996. *Health Affairs* 17 (1), 35–51.

Marmor, T. (2000). *The Politics of Medicare,* 2nd ed. New York: Aldine de Gruyter.

Merrell, K., Colby, D.C. and Hogan, C. (1997). Medicare beneficiaries covered by medicaid buy-in agreements. *Health Affairs* (16) (1), 175–184.

Moon, M., Brennan, N. and Segal, M. (1998).

Options for aiding low-income Medicare beneficiaries. *Inquiry* 35, 346–56.

Morone, J. (1990). American political culture and the search for lessons from abroad. *Journal of Health Politics, Policy and Law* 15 (1), 128–43.

Nemore, P.B. (1999). *State Medicaid Buy-In Programs: Variations in Policy and Practice.* The Henry J. Kaiser Family Foundation.

O'Brien, M.J., Archdeacon, M., Barrett, M., Crow, 5., Janicki, 5, Rousseau, D, William C. (2000). *State experiences with access issues under children's health insurance expansions.* The Commonwealth Fund.

Rowland, D. Salganicoff, A., Keenan, P. (1999). The key to the door: Medicaid's role in improving health care for women and children. *Annual Review of Public Health* 20, 403–26.

Selden, T., Banthin J. Cohen J. (1998). Medicaid's problem children: Eligible but not enrolled. *Health Affairs* 17 (3), 192–200.

Serafini, M.W. (2000). Prescription drugs: The state experience. *National Journal* October 7.

Shaner, H., (1999). *Dual Eligible Outreach and Enrollment: A View from the States.* Health Care Financing Administration.

Storing, H. (ed.). (1985). *The Anti-Federalist.* Chicago: University of Chicago Press.

World Health Organization (2000). *World Health Report, 2000: World Health Systems—Improving Performance,* Chap. 2.

9

Health-Care Justice and Agency

Patricia S. Mann

> Justice requires that we treat those who are alike—in relevant ways—equally; and those who are different—in relevant ways—differently, in proportion to their difference.
>
> Aristotle, *Nicomachean Ethics*

> A requirement for democratic peace . . . Basic health care assured for all citizens.
>
> Rawls, *The Law of Peoples*

> The adult who lacks the means of having medical treatment for an ailment from which she suffers . . . may also be denied the freedom to do various things—for herself and for others—that she may wish to do as a responsible human being . . . Responsibility requires freedom.
>
> Amartya Sen, *Development as Freedom*

The failure of the United States to provide basic health-care coverage for a growing number of its citizens is one of those startling public facts—along with our huge prison population, and our continued use of capital punishment—that leads international commentators to shake their heads and puzzle over an American barbarian streak. Moreover, within U.S. society, there is a large gap between how this issue is understood by actual policymakers, and how it is understood by philosophers analyzing issues of just distribution.

For many political philosophers, including John Rawls, Ronald Dworkin, and Amartya Sen, it is a simple matter to show that distributive justice requires universal health-care coverage in a society with the material and technological resources of the United States. Indeed, all other affluent democratic societies today provide such coverage. Yet despite media attention to the suffering of the millions of children and adults who lack adequate access to basic

medical and dental treatment, universal coverage does not appear to be on the immediate political agenda in this country. Why not? If, as a problem of distributive justice, universal health care is a "no-brainer," then what other vectors of analysis are necessary to portray it as the difficult political decision it is today in the United States?

THE HEALTH-CARE ENIGMA

In this chapter, I want to investigate this gap between our political ideals and our current political practices. The existence of this gap becomes even more puzzling when we take into account the fact that we are deviating from a standard of domestic policy established by other industrialized nations since World War II. We have been global leaders historically in many areas of social justice policy, from land ownership to universal education, and our leadership in areas such as women's rights in employment and sports today is an important basis for democratic pride.[1] How does America, as the largest, richest democracy, accept the degrading physical suffering, combined with the assault on dignity, involved in the fact that 44 million people do not have health coverage?[2]

Amartya Sen, in *Development as Freedom* (2000), draws attention to an interesting difference between attitudes toward individual and social responsibilities in the United States and Europe. After noting the large number of people lacking health care in the United States, Sen states: "A comparable situation in Europe, where medical coverage is seen as a basic right of the citizen irrespective of means and independent of preexisting conditions, would very likely be politically intolerable . . . On the other hand, the double-digit unemployment rates that are currently tolerated in Europe would very likely be political dynamite in America, since unemployment rates of that magnitude would make a mockery of people's ability to help themselves"(Sen, 2000, p. 99). Sen never analyzes this difference in political attitudes, but he suggests an explanation for apparent American heartlessness with respect to health-care coverage when he states that Americans would never accept the high unemployment rates of Europe because they "would make a mockery of people's ability to help themselves." In this chapter, I will suggest that an ethic of self-sufficiency or, more formally stated, a narrative of autonomous economic and political agency does much to explain our failure to enact a national health-care program.

Historian Joyce Appleby supports this notion of a peculiarly American narrative of autonomous individual agency. In her recent book, *Inheriting the Revolution: The First Generation of Americans*, Appleby (2000) explains the origins of such a discourse in terms of the demands and opportunities for individual initiative and commercial enterprise in eighteenth-century America. According to Appleby, this first generation after the Revolution created a "social framework we are still living with," constructing the peculiar national identity of autonomous and enterprising individuals that has come to characterize Americans.[3] According to this familiar narrative, each American has the opportunity to succeed if he or she really makes the effort, and each of us is responsible for making this effort. A political corollary of this ideal of autonomous individualism is that it is unjust to tax the property of those who are enterprising and successful in order to support those who do not make a sufficient effort to become economically independent. Insofar as individual economic autonomy remains a dominant, idealized feature of our American national identity, redistributive social policies are likely to be represented as unjust.

Although the economic and political context of American society has changed dramatically over the past 200 years, the power of this ideology of individual autonomy, according to Appleby, is such that it has remained difficult for subsequent generations to set forth alternative identities and meanings of America. Compounding the problem is the fact that political philosophers do not typically confront ideologically specific components of our national identity. Because political philosophers presume to address universal selves rather than embedded American individuals, theories of distributive justice fail to engage Americans as situated moral and political agents.[4]

Of course, it has been possible to make arguments asserting that justice demands redistributive taxation in particular contexts. Welfare legislation was originally supported in the early twentieth century as an aid to widows and children, who were not presumed to be autonomous economic agents. (Skocpol, 1991). The defeat of welfare policies in the late 1990s is related to our radically changed view of women as economic and political individuals having equal capacity and responsibility to participate alongside men in the workplace.

Because of the tension between the underlying national narrative of autonomous economic agency, and contrary narratives of social injustices that demand a political response, it is possible to identify a pattern of national indecisiveness and vacillation in responding to problems of justice in our society. Consider antipoverty policy over the last 40 years: During a time of national prosperity in the 1960s, we responded to evidence of widespread hunger and poverty with legislation greatly expanding the provision of welfare to those in need. Yet opposition to these welfare entitlements grew as conservative politicians insisted upon promoting our national identity of individual economic self-sufficiency. Ironically, the civil rights movement and the women's movement, in asserting the full citizenship of minorities and women, provided ideological support for applying the identity of autonomous individuals to these two groups. Federal welfare programs were drastically reduced in the late 1990s. The argument was not that poverty had been eradicated—indeed, a new and growing problem of homelessness had manifested itself. The argument was simply that adults should be required to work in order to maintain themselves and their children, and that welfare creates a harmful cycle of dependency.[5]

One of the cruel features of the current Workfare era is that in localities like New York City, administrators are making it harder for the poor to get food stamps and Medicaid, two federal entitlement programs supposedly exempt from work requirements. "The city's approach seems to view any safety-net assistance, even food for pregnant women, as encouraging dependency."[6] Although no one actually argues that children should be autonomous, we have no adequate conceptual framework to critically evaluate personal and social responsibility toward children.

An ideology of autonomous and enterprising individual agency places major constraints upon political initiatives addressing forms of structural injustice in contemporary U.S. society. It distorts our political

perspective on a number of contemporary issues, especially those in which there is a need to rethink traditional forms of individual and social responsibility.[7] The currently fraught issue of health care is one of those issues, and it provides a good occasion for critically grappling with this national narrative of individual self-sufficiency, showing its crucial limitations. In this chapter, I will explain how an alternative theory of engaged individual agency better enables us to address changing structures of individual and social obligation in health policy.

RONALD DWORKIN'S APPROACH

Political philosophers today are rarely interested in discussing the gap between our political ideals and our political practices. John Rawls's theory of justice, for example, is concerned with establishing the ideal conditions under which individuals would contract for a just distribution of social goods, and in outlining the distributional principles of such a society. Those who work in a Rawlsian mode may deem certain technical questions about what counts as just distribution of a good, such as health care, philosophically interesting. However, it is up to politicians to work out the legislative means to accomplish this just distribution. While Marxist philosophers such as Rodney Peffer (1990) have suggested that such legislation is highly unlikely within capitalism, Rawls explicitly dismisses such suggestions.[8] For Rawls it is enough that distributive justice is hypothetically possible under liberal democracy, and he reserves all judgment as to the practical likelihood that the political will or means will be found.

In his recent book, *Sovereign Virtue*, Ronald Dworkin (2000) criticizes what he calls Rawls's "detached" conception of democracy, and indeed, stands out among legal and political philosophers today in his efforts to address the gap between our political ideals of distributive justice, and our liberal democratic political practices.

Dworkin offers moral as well as political arguments for policies aimed at moving closer to a defensible distribution of basic goods such as health care within the United States. Unlike a Marxist theorist such as Peffer, Dworkin does not explain this gap in terms of a capitalist political economy. Instead, he explains it in terms of the moral and political principles that inform our individual and collective sense of agency (Dworkin, 2000, pp. 186–90, 232).

By contrast with the Rawlsian theory of justice that cannot be articulated apart from its ideal methodological starting point of an original position, Dworkin proposes a theory of "ethical individualism" that addresses us as individuals in the flux of daily life. He insists that we acknowledge a basic "real world" problem for any theory of distributive justice today: We live in affluent societies in which the majority of people accept a high degree of inequality, and indeed, seem to prefer it over policies that would address this inequality.

The challenge for Dworkin's theory of ethical individualism is to justify forms of redistribution necessary to ameliorate distributive injustices today. Dworkin cites two principles as fundamental to his theory of ethical individualism: (1) The principle of "equal importance," according to which "it is important, from an objective point of view, that human lives be successful rather than wasted, and this is equally important, from an objective point of view, for each human life", and (2) the principle of "special responsibility," according to which "though we must all recognize the equal objective importance of the success of a human life, one person has a special and final responsibility for that success—the person whose life it is" (Dworkin, 2000, p. 5). Like Rawls, Dworkin is concerned with remedying basic injustices of people's starting positions, unchosen aspects of their lives that disadvantage them. In an ideal world, people would start out with equal resources. However, Dworkin goes beyond Rawls in worrying about how to justify a redistributive policy in the context of our actual political situation. Our politicians will never make policy from behind a Rawlsian veil of ignorance, so Dworkin attempts to provide a narrative of moral and political agency that addresses each of us directly, in whatever our social position. Rawls's two principles articulate the ideal basis for a politically just distribution of goods.[9] Dworkin's two principles, by contrast, attempt to provide a framework for re-thinking the relationship between our moral and political obligation to others (his first principle) and to ourselves (his second principle). His goal is to combine a liberal notion of personal responsibility with a collective sense of social responsibility for just treatment of others, arriving at what he terms an "integrated liberal" moral perspective (Dworkin, 2000, p. 233).

Dworkin's general idea is that certain constraints on individual freedom of choice may be justified in order to ameliorate societywide distributive injustices, while other constraints on freedom of choice may not be justified. Constraints on freedom of choice that remove advantages of economic power that a person would not have in a more just system of distribution are justifiable. By contrast, it would not be acceptable to remove an individual's liberty of speech or of sexual activity because this would diminish an individual's freedom from what it would be under any defensible system of just distribution. This latter sort of restriction would victimize individuals, while merely constraining an individual's use of excessive economic power would not (Dworkin, 2000, p. 180). Some liberties allowed under our system are more important to individual freedom than others. Dworkin makes the case, as a twenty-first century liberal, that economic redistribution undertaken in order to ameliorate great economic injustices does not jeopardize fundamental liberties (pp. 175–80).

Within liberal theory, individual persons are usually assumed to be the "unit of agency," and Dworkin retains this assumption, while arguing for a more nuanced vision of our individual political agency, such that our political identity may affect our sense of moral agency. According to the communitarian philosopher Michael Sandel (1998), individuals are metaphysically embedded within a larger community; our individual actions are not comprehensible except in the context of the community as a collective unit of agency.[10] Dworkin believes that such a broad theory of metaphysical embeddedness threatens basic liberal beliefs about individual autonomy; yet he suggests that there are specific situations in which a practical vision of political integration is appropriate and morally significant. Just as individual members of an orchestra readily distinguish between their own individual interests and the interests of the orchestra which they participate in, Dworkin argues that many or most individuals see themselves both as private agents and as members of a larger political community whose interests they participate in. Our liberal ideals of tolerance, and our respect for different individual preferences with regards to various living styles, sexualities, and beliefs, rely upon preserving a sense of the private, individuated aspect of our lives. And yet, as integrated members of a political community, Dworkin argues, we feel our lives diminished insofar as we live in an unjust community. Indeed, Dworkin maintains, "An integrated citizen accepts that the value of his own life depends on the success of his community in treating everyone with equal concern" (Dworkin, 2000, p. 233).

HEALTH CARE AND THE INTEGRATED LIBERAL TODAY

According to Ronald Dworkin, if you are an integrated liberal acting according to the two principles of ethical individualism, you will recognize that your life will go better in a just society. You will act on the basis of both your sense of responsibility for yourself, and on the basis of your sense that others should have basic forms of equality. In a society where basic health care is not available to 44 million people, it may seem obvious that ethical individuals will act politically to end this form of inequality, which Dworkin indignantly terms a "national disgrace."

Moreover, statistical evidence compiled by government agencies demonstrate that our current system of profit-driven HMOs is extremely inefficient relative to alternatives. According to statistical projections done by the Congressional Budget Office and the Government Accounting Office, a single-payer nationalized system would save the United States more than 10% of all health costs annually just by reducing paperwork. This would amount to $225 billion by 2004, providing enough money to cover all the uninsured, provide better health care for the underinsured, and improve the quality of health care for all. The Canadian health-care system, as well as various European programs, concretely demonstrate the possibility for combining greater efficiency and equity through tax-funded, single-payer health-care delivery systems.[11]

Even Americans with "good" medical coverage are experiencing the frustrations of increasingly coercive micro-management by the large HMOs attempting to maintain their profit margins. Media coverage of the windfall profits of pharmaceutical companies and the suffering of the growing numbers of people who lack access to adequate medical care has been extensive. Yet there is no national discussion of alternatives to a profit-driven system. National health care is not visible as even a blip on our political horizon.

Insofar as European and Canadian health-care systems offer more equitable and efficient models of care, why are Americans not clamoring for a single-payer national health insurance system on both moral and pragmatic grounds? I can only conclude that our sense of moral and political reality is clouded by an American identity of economic self-sufficiency, the enduring eighteenth-century ideology of enterprising and autonomous agency identified by historian Joyce Appleby. It encourages Americans to rationalize the injustices of our health-care system, as well as to be fearful of available alternatives. However, there are reasons to believe that this national identity is evolving in ways that will undermine this mythology of individual self-sufficiency, enabling Americans to evaluate health-care options more realistically at some future point.

By emphasizing responsibility aspects of individual agency, Ronald Dworkin's two principles of ethical individualism help to reveal problems with our current ideals of individual self-sufficiency rather than to provide a new schema capable of resolving current problems of justice.

Consider Dworkin's First Principle of Ethical Individualism, the *Equal Importance Principle*. As Amartya Sen (1995, p. ix) has explained, most people are committed to equality as a political ideal, but there is a big question about what we mean by equality and equal treatment. If you subscribe to the ideology of autonomous economic individualism, you may conclude that everyone has an equal opportunity to succeed in America, and that our responsibility to others is satisfied by participating in the system already in place. In other words, our responsibilities to others are fulfilled by doing our best within this system to reach our own ends.

Consider Dworkin's Second Principle, the *Special Responsibility Principle*, according to which each adult is responsible for securing the basic welfare of himself or herself, above all. This principle corresponds fully with an ideology of enterprising personal autonomy. Basic welfare has always included food, shelter, education, and health care. Thus, the integrated liberal may feel uncomfortable when hearing that 44 million people in this rich country do not have access to health care, but he or she will not have a moral or political justification for demanding that our system change to provide care for everyone.

An individual might be committed to both of Dworkin's principles without acknowledging health-care injustices in our

society. His theory of ethical individualism alludes to problematic issues of responsibility today, but it does not provide a framework for responding to them. Insofar as many Americans consider health-care coverage just deserts for their enterprising individual agency, they may be distressed that not everyone is sufficiently enterprising to deserve health coverage; but despite Dworkin's support for a redistributive solution, it is not required by his theory of ethical individualism.

Moreover, the very idea of participating in a tax-funded national health-care community is contrary to an ethic of enterprising autonomy in at least two ways. First, insofar as individual autonomy is understood as self-sufficiency, membership in a national health-care community implies interdependencies that deny or compromise one's self-sufficiency. Second, insofar as individual autonomy is understood as self-determination, Americans are fearful that without market competition they will not have the freedom to choose their doctors and their treatments. Of course, corporate medical interests encourage these fears.

THE SHIFTING SANDS OF CONTEMPORARY AGENCY

Two related social changes may help transform this ideology of enterprising autonomy. First, I suggest we think of our historical moment as a period of fundamental "social unmooring." One of the consequences of this period of social turmoil is that our narratives of individual selfhood and agency are changing. An earlier period of social unmooring occurred in Europe at the end of feudalism, when the hierarchical and prescribed relationships of entire communities came to an end as individuals were cast off the landed estates of feudal lords. European society was reorganized around industrial workplaces and competitive market relationships between male workers. Only the patriarchal family retained its organic, hierarchical, and involuntary structure.[12]

Rene Descartes and Thomas Hobbes responded to this dramatic social moment by finally overthrowing the classical paradigms of Plato and Aristotle and by theorizing a rational, autonomous, desiring individual self. Modern society as we know it, liberal democracy as well as capitalism, developed upon these particular social and theoretical foundations. If Appleby is correct, this narrative of independent, self-made individualism develops in post-Revolutionary America far beyond its European prototype in response to unprecedented economic and political opportunities.

We are experiencing a second period of social unmooring today, as women's new economic and reproductive agency brings an end to the prescribed and hierarchical relationships of patriarchal families. Traditional kinship practices organized around women's maternal role are rapidly vanishing as countries struggle against overpopulation and promote women's use of contraception. And as their kinship roles decline, women are a growing presence within the global workforce. In a process that I term "the social enfranchisement of women," women come to have not merely the right, but also the responsibility to participate within the public workforce and to choose when and if they will have children.[13]

In this context, lifetime familial commitments become unnecessary and problematic. We make and unmake family units in response to a logic of individual choice that has long structured public interactions. There is a radical sense in which individualism now goes all the way down, into the most personal aspects of our lives. Metaphorically, but also quite literally, women and children, and men as well, are unmoored today from the lifetime family unit that has historically provided individuals with their most basic interpersonal foundations.

Life is chaotic to a degree perhaps rivaling that at the end of feudalism, whose intense dynamics Thomas Hobbes so memorably evoked. But Hobbesian man had a familial community to retreat to, while in today's chaos there is often no secure familial harbor. Even the most self-sufficient modern men took familial foundations for granted, and as these begin to fail, such individuals find themselves negotiating new social connections. Moreover, insofar as they recognize the significance of the loss of these previous familial foundations, men may finally acknowledge that their autonomy itself has been grounded in and promoted by supportive kinship relationships. That is, men's experience of liberal autonomy, paradoxically, may decline when they are freed from their familial moorings.

A second form of social transformation is occurring today and may also lead to a displacement of the American mantra of enterprising autonomy. In this case, it is not the social structure, but the meaning and motivation that people accord their actions, or their agency, that is changing.

I have been interested in this issue of agency, or the meaning and motivation individuals ascribe to their actions, for at least 25 years. Ever since as a teenager musing about my goal of becoming an aggressive trial lawyer, I kept wondering how it was possible for me to have such a goal (or for all my female friends to have such goals) while knowing that our mothers and their mothers, and their mothers . . . had not been active participants in the public sphere, and for the most part did not even imagine the possibility of such participation. Clearly, society was changing, but what explained the willingness of our mothers to accept their consignment to the private, subordinate, dependent realm of a patriarchal system if in truth they had the capacities to act in the public realm alongside men?

According to the accepted Hobbesian/Cartesian inspired image of men as desiring, rational agents, women of previous generations simply did not possess a modern form of individual agency. However, when social conditions changed sufficiently in the 1970s in the United States, vast numbers of women—many of them our mothers—overnight it seemed, found themselves entering the public workforce and behaving quite capably alongside men as desiring, rational agents. In retrospect, it seems likely that these women did not acquire the capacity for agency overnight. Instead, it seems that our modern theories had not been sufficiently complex to articulate the dimensions of agency women had exhibited in the context of their familial roles as wives and mothers.

In my book, *Micro-Politics: Agency in a Postfeminist Era*, I proposed a three-dimensional theory of agency within which the desiring rationality associated with liberal citizenship is only one of the basic dimensions of individual action. *A full understanding of anyone's actions involves inquiring not merely about one's desires, but also one's sense of responsibility, as well as one's expectations of recognition and reward in taking a particular action* (Mann, 1994, p. 14). According to this multidimensional theory of agency, our individuality can only be understood in the context of our social engagement.

This three-dimensional theory of agency reveals social hierarchies between individuals insofar as societies have distributed the dimensions of agency among individuals according to particular social patterns. In modern society, the agency of various subordinate groups—not just women, but also workers, servants, and slaves—has been seen primarily in terms of the dimension of responsibility. Correspondingly, modern societies have emphasized the desires and given the most important forms of recognition and reward to a privileged group of men. I posited that we could chart changing power relations in terms of changing distributions of the three dimensions of agency. I predicted that the empowerment of women would be reflected by greater concern for their desires, as well as by their growing expectations of recognition and reward.

Twenty years later, we do have greater concern for the desires of women, and women have greater expectations of recognition and reward. However, as women have gained greater social participation and status, the dimension of responsibility

often remains primary when women articulate their sense of power and authority. Indeed, women now experience intense daily conflicts and uncertainties with respect to their competing public and private responsibilities. Insofar as women experience their agency in terms of competing responsibilities to self and others, women may be more prepared to comprehend our current health-care dilemma as one of reforming a distorted system of public and private responsibilities.

It is not that women do not value their autonomy. Having been denied autonomy for so long, it is an important goal for many women. However, we must distinguish between two sorts of autonomy. Autonomy, as freedom from patriarchal constraints, as freedom to determine one's own life plans, is fundamental to women's emancipation. Alternatively, the mantra of enterprising agency has historically idealized autonomy as self-sufficiency. Women are not as likely to embrace this latter notion of autonomy. First, this ideal was always more of an illusion than a reality; autonomous men relied upon the daily familial labors of a wife without acknowledging their real dependency upon their wives. Having performed this role for men, women are not as likely to fall prey to illusions of their own self-sufficiency. We know our lives would run more smoothly if we had wives.

Second, I have suggested that women's sense of empowered agency remains a responsibility-dominated agency, rather than becoming a desire-dominated agency comparable to that of modern men. If even very powerful and successful women tend to understand their agency in terms of the demanding, significant responsibilities they have taken on, then it would seem that women's empowerment has not resulted in liberal selfhood in the traditional American mode. Rather, it has led them to see themselves as the engaged social selves of a system that values social solidarity, perhaps more in the mold of European welfare democracy.

It is not that women as a group are currently identifiable for their radical critiques of American society. Women may be as vulnerable as men are to neo-liberal arguments that there is no serious alternative to privatization and market competition in health care. I am simply arguing that as more and more women gain positions of power and authority in our American system, the mantra of enterprising autonomy should prove less of an impediment to progressive moral and political analysis. The different underlying quality of women's agency at this point in history—I do believe men's agency will also become responsibility-dominated eventually—may be significant. It should make women more capable of recognizing the moral and pragmatic arguments for a national health-care system funded by taxation.

FURTHER IMPLICATIONS OF A THREE-DIMENSIONAL THEORY OF AGENCY

Contemporary philosophers rarely discuss contextual features of our individual agency.[14] Because of our idealization of individual enterprising autonomy as a basic perspective of liberal individualism, we rarely notice the complex social nexus within which individual actions occur. Yet ours is an era of fundamental social transformations. I believe we require a theoretical framework that better represents the multiple, ineradicably social dimensions of individual action if we are to fully analyze contemporary problems and the possibilities for resolving them.

Modern ethics has emphasized responsibilities to oneself (and loved ones as familial extensions of oneself), while ignoring larger, social-responsibility dimensions of individual agency. However, the realities of modern medicine create a pressing demand for rethinking our assumptions about how our responsibilities for ourselves and for others are connected. We require an understanding of ourselves as individuals that allows for our individual autonomy, understood as freedom for creative self-development and freedom from unrea-

sonable social constraints. Yet as Amartya Sen suggests, these sorts of individual freedom are entirely compatible with acknowledging various forms of dependency upon others, as well as various forms of responsibilities toward others.[15] Our eighteenth-century ideal of enterprising autonomy can only be salvaged if we acknowledge the emergence of a dynamic continuum between responsibilities to self and others in the world of the twenty-first century.

A three-dimensional theory of engaged autonomy highlights obligations to others, as well as recognition by others as basic dimensions of individual agency. Neither of these two features of agency were visible as social variables in the liberal model of desiring autonomous individual agency. However, to evaluate and rectify injustices in our health-care system we need to go beyond the fact that each individual desires to remain healthy. My three-dimensional theory encourages us to rethink the quality of our health-care obligations. It also encourages us to reflect upon our individual participation in societal problems of recognition and reward.

A three-dimensional agency analysis enables us to recognize the social nexus within which our actions occur, making it possible to continue to see ourselves as enterprising and relatively autonomous individual agents while also acknowledging our dependency upon a larger community. Autonomous individuals have always had familial relationships within which their responsibility for themselves was continuous with responsibility and dependency relationships with others. Contemporary social issues, from environmental concerns to child care to assisted suicide and other end-of-life issues, will only be resolved if we can abandon a false ideal of individual self-sufficiency and view them in terms of complicated responsibility and dependency relationships.[16]

For example, the relevance of economic distinctions between *private* goods, like clothes and cars, and *public goods*, like defense, mail service, environmental protection, and health care, may become visible in the twenty-first century once we acknowledge that individual autonomy does not preclude specific forms of social interdependency. The market mechanism is geared to private goods, and as many economists have explained, it does not function efficiently in relation to public goods.[17] A three-dimensional theory of individual agency encourages Americans to evolve beyond a market-dominated sense of entrepreneurial freedom. Acknowledging membership in a national health-care community, or in an international environmental and economic community, would seem an increasingly necessary basis for a secure sense of self-determination and freedom in our daily lives.[18]

A three-dimensional theory of agency also enables us to respond to health-care injustices involving the dimension of recognition. A number of studies have recently shown that women and minorities presenting the same medical symptoms are less likely than white men to be referred for heart bypass surgery or other advanced forms of treatment.[19] No one believes that doctors intend to treat patients in racially or sexually biased ways. But they do. Socrates, of course, defined wisdom as knowing what you do not know. In medicine, the ideology of enterprising autonomy, along with the ideology of scientific objectivity, makes it difficult for individual physicians to acknowledge the degree to which their own medical skills are embedded in learned patterns of differential treatment.

Racial and sexual biases are a major factor in unjust distribution of medical treatment. These biases are not addressed by an analysis that simply prescribes that individuals should be treated equally, if that means being given equal rights to visit a doctor.[20] The medical profession will only become capable of changing biased treatment patterns insofar as individual doctors recognize that they are not autonomous medical agents, but socially embedded selves who make predictable and corrigible forms of medical errors. A three-dimensional theory of agency can acknowledge the desire of physicians to treat patients fairly, while also holding them responsible for changing racially and sexually biased forms of medical recognition that are demonstrably at odds with these desires.

A three-dimensional theory of agency allows us to acknowledge our social embeddedness without compromising our sense of individual agency. Instead, it clarifies how our individual agency is enriched by, and indeed requires, three-dimensional relationships with others. We can still think of ourselves as relatively autonomous actors in various economic and political contexts. Most importantly, we can articulate responsibility and recognition relationships that are currently problematic, and attempt to renegotiate them.

CONCLUSION

There is evidence that a growing majority of people in the United States are dissatisfied with health-care policies and are prepared for a change. The percentage of gross domestic product (GDP) spent on health care rises as contact time with physicians declines, hospital care deteriorates, rights of patients and doctors to make decisions over basic care is usurped by insurance bureaucrats, and growing numbers of people lack health-care coverage altogether. Yet despite persuasive statistical projections indicating that we could achieve greater efficiency as well as equity by changing to a national health-care program there is no national outcry demanding national health care, and not even a serious debate about the issue.[21] I have maintained that a political discourse of enterprising freedom and autonomy has a lot to do with the failure of the populace to demand national health care.

Unsurprisingly, given the tremendous lobbying power of insurance, pharmaceutical, and other corporate medical interests, neither one of our two major political parties is suggesting that we move to a national single-payer health-care system.

Only a powerful public movement demanding such a change could motivate serious political support for national health care. Political conservatives have successfully used the discourse of enterprising and autonomous individual agency to erode public support for policies aimed at achieving greater justice in the United States Along with insurance, pharmaceutical, and other medical corporate interests they have successfully wielded this narrative to make support for nationalized, single-payer health care seem un-American.

A three-dimensional theory of agency relations exposes the fallacies and hypocrisies in this corporate narrative of individual freedom. If Americans accept a more complicated identity as engaged individuals whose individual agency is multidimensional and socially embedded, our sense of individual agency will not seem compromised by a national health-care program. We will become capable of evaluating the efficiency and equity of such a program more objectively. Conservative idealizations of individual self-sufficiency will appear anachronistic.

Ronald Dworkin is right to deny arguments that nationalized health care is a socialist program violating important economic liberties (2000, p. 319) And he is correct in emphasizing that health-care injustices be seen as continuous with our concerns as integrated moral and political agents. But a commitment to equality does not provide an adequate critique of our private health-care system; integrated individuals will comprehend the need for a national program only if they recognize that responsibility to oneself exists on a continuum with one's responsibility and dependency upon others. This evolving continuum of personal and interpersonal responsibility can only become evident insofar as we gain a historical perspective on our national identity as enterprising and autonomous agents. We may continue to see ourselves as enterprising and relatively autonomous individual agents. However, to be morally and politically responsible agents in relation to health care we need to admit our very real embeddedness within a larger community. Only then will we be capable of recognizing the complexity of our relationships and of negotiating a set of responsibilities required by justice. We are individuals whose freedom and equality depend upon our engagement in a just community.

NOTES

1. Amartya Sen points out that famines, which had occurred quite regularly in India prior to independence, ceased to occur in India after 1946, when India became a democratic nation and elected leaders took the necessary steps to avert famines whenever they threatened. Indeed, Sen reports that a famine has never occurred in a democratic nation, while they continue to occur quite regularly in nondemocratic ones. See Sen, *Development as Freedom*, particularly chap. 7.

2. See Farmer, "On Suffering and Structural Violence: A View from Below."

3. Appleby documents the highly self-conscious formation of this national consciousness, emphasizing the risks and failures as well as the rewards of this new entrepreneurial mode of life. "In embracing the virtues of personal autonomy and individual responsibility, they rallied around qualities with wide appeal across the spectrum of classes, faiths, families, and even races. The range of human potentialities engaged by this model of excellence was narrow, but widely shared" (Appleby, 2000, p. 259)

4. See Margaret Archer, *Realist Social Theory: The Morphogenetic Approach*. Archer's analytical dualism is directly relevant here. This American identity is part of the ideological context of American politics. Philosophers address us universally and atomistically, overlooking the relevant existence of, in Archer's terms, "pre-existing structures," be they ideological or sociopolitical structures. This aspect of identity is not so self-conscious as the laissez-faire egalitarianism of political conservatives. It is a taken-for-granted feature of individual identity in situ in America, and as such informs our sense of individual and social responsibility and fairness. It is a basic, easily recognized feature of American political discourse. Amartya Sen, an economist, Joyce Appleby, a historian, recognize its significance. Philosophers, for the most part, do not.

5. For an historical overview of the changing

meanings of "dependency," see Fraser and Gordon, "A Genealogy of 'Dependency': Tracing a Keyword of the U.S. Welfare State."

6. *New York Times*, editorial, July 31, 2000; see also "Bingo, Blood and Burial Plots in the Quest for Food Stamps," *New York Times*, August 12, 2000.

7. See Patricia Mann, (1998), "Meanings of Death," for a discussion of the problematic effects of this ideal of autonomous agency on the assisted suicide debate.

8. See Peffer, *Marxism, Morality, and Social Justice*, p. 14. See also Rawls, *Political Liberalism*, p. 7.

9. See John Rawls, *A Theory of Justice* (Cambridge: Harvard University Press, 1971), pp. 60–75.

10. See Sandel, *Liberalism and the Limits of Justice*, pp. 62–65, 179–83.

11. See Physicians for a National Health Program website: David Himmelstein and Steffie Woolhandler, "Single Payer Fact Sheet," citing the General Accounting Office's projection of administrative savings of 10% a year in 1994; citing the Congressional Budget Office projecting a $225 billion savings by 2004 despite expansion of comprehensive health care to all Americans. See also, "Why the U.S. Needs a Single Payer Health System." Citing as their sources the *New England Journal of Medicine* and *JAMA*, Himmelstein and Wollhandler argue that Canada spends $1,000 less per capita on health care, while offering more care and greater choice for patients. About 96% of people and 85% of doctors prefer their system to ours. There is almost no wait for most kinds of care. "An oft-cited survey that alleged huge waiting lists counted every patient with a future appointment as 'in a queue.' . . . More legitimate research shows that the average waiting time for knee replacement in Ontario is 8 weeks, as compared to 3 weeks in the U.S."

12. See Patricia Mann, (1994), *Micro-Politics: Agency in a Postfeminist Era*, particularly the Introduction and chap. 4, for an analysis of this process of social unmooring.

13. Ibid., pp. 21–23, 35–36, 163.

14. Pierre Bourdieu is an important exception. According to his theory of individual and collective social practices, a discourse of enterprising autonomy could be seen as a component of a homogenizing American "habitus," a generative system of structured and structuring dispositions, produced by history and oriented toward practical functions. See Bourdieu's *The Logic of Practice*, pp. 52–55.

15. Sen's capability notion of freedom and equality offers a positive alternative to the economic autonomy ideal. It complements my three-dimensional analysis of individual agency,

making any absolute notion of autonomy appear foolish, while allowing for a relative notion of autonomy as part of what we mean by freedom and equality. See Sen, 2000, pp. 283–84, particularly.

16. See Mann, (1998), "Meanings of Death," in *Physician Assisted Suicide: Expanding the Debate*, for my analysis of how the debate over assisted suicide would be transformed by an explicitly social framework of analysis, and specifically by a three-dimensional theory of agency.

17. Accoding to Sen (*Development or Freedom*, p. 325, n.38–40), the literature on this topic is vast. He cites Paul Samuelson's "The Pure Theory of Public Expenditure," *Review of Economics and Statistics* 36 (1954), and "Diagrammatic Exposition of a Pure Theory of Public Expenditure," *Review of Economic and Statistics* 37 (1955) as classic analyses of "market failure." He also cites Kenneth Arrow, "The Organization of Economic Activity: Issues Pertinent to the Choice of Market versus Non-market Allocation," in *Collected Papers of K.J. Arrow*, vol. 2 (Cambridge, MA: Harvard University Press, 1983). Andreas Papandreou, *Externality and Institutions* (Oxford: Clarendon Press, 1994), is cited as offering a good overview of the currently vast literature on public goods and the "need for institutional enhancement beyond reliance on traditional markets."

18. See Amartya Sen's insightful analysis of this issue in *Development as Freedom*. See particularly chap. 12, pp. 283–84; and chap. 5, pp. 128–29.

19. See *New York Times*, February 25, 1999, citing an article in the *New England Journal of Medicine*: "A new study of 720 physicians found that with all symptoms being equal, doctors were 60% as likely to order cardiac catheterization for women and blacks as for men and whites. For black women, the doctors were 40% as likely to order catheterization, considered the gold standard diagnostic test for heart disease. 'Most likely this is an underestimate of what's occurring,' Dr. Kevin Schulman of Georgetown University Medical Center said, because the doctors knew their decisions were being recorded, but not why."

20. Amartya Sen's "capabilities approach" to freedom and development assessment enables us to discuss such forms of differential treatment. But it remains an outcomes test, focusing on the goal of achieving equal functioning and capabilities for minorities and women. It does not assess the social relationships that must change for this to be effected. See Sen's *Inequalities Reexamined* and *Development as Freedom*.

21. See Marcia Angell, (2000), "Patients' Rights Bills and Other Futile Gestures." As the

outgoing editor of the *New England Journal of Medicine*, Angell critically reviews proposals for reforming the current system and dismisses them. She explains the structural problems with a system in which employers and investor-owned managed-care companies presume to represent the interests of workers and doctors. She repeats a call she made in 1993 for a universal single-payer system, basically an extension of Medicare to everyone, emphasizing its greater efficiency and equity.

See also Physicians for a National Health Program website: David Himmelstein and Steffie Woolhandler, "Why the U.S. Needs a Single Payer Health System."

REFERENCES

Angell, M. (2000). Patients' rights bills and other futile gestures. *New England Journal of Medicine* 342, 22–xx.

Appleby, J. (2000). *Inheriting the Revolution: The First Generation of Americans.* Cambridge, MA: Harvard University Press.

Archer, M. (1995). *Realist Social Theory: The Morphogenetic Approach.* Cambridge: Cambridge University Press.

Aristotle ([fourth century B.C.] (1941). *Nicomachean Ethics.* R. McKeon. (ed.), In *The Basic Works of Aristotle.* New York: Random House.

Battin, M. Rhodes, R., and Silvers, A. (eds.). (1998). *Physician Assisted Suicide: Expanding the Debate.* New York: Routledge.

Bourdieu, P. (1990). *The Logic of Practice.* Stanford, CA: Stanford University Press.

Dworkin, R. (2000). *Sovereign Virtue: The Theory and Practice of Equality.* Cambridge, MA: Harvard University Press.

Farmer, P. (1997). On suffering and structural violence: A view from below. In A. Kleinman, V. Das, and M. Lock (eds.), *Social Suffering.* Berkeley: University of California Press.

Fraser, N. and Gordon, L. (1997). A genealogy of "dependency": Tracing a keyword of the U.S. welfare state. In N. Fraser, (ed.), *Justice Interruptus: Critical Reflections on the 'Postsocialist' Condition.* New York: Routledge.

Himmelstein, D. and Wollhandler, S. (2000a). Single Payer Factsheet. Physicians for National Health Program (PNHP) website.

Himmelstein, D. and Wollhandler, S. (2000b). Why the U.S. Needs a Single Payer Health System. Physicians for National Health Program (PNHP) website.

Mann, P. (1994). *Micro-Politics: Agency in a Postfeminist Era.* Minneapolis: University of Minnesota Press.

Mann, P. (1998). Meanings of death. In M. Battin, R. Rhodes, and Anita Silvers (eds.), *Physician Assisted Suicide: Expanding the Debate.* New York: Routledge.

Peffer, R. (1990). *Marxism, Morality, and Social Justice.* Princeton, NJ: Princeton University Press.

Rawls, J. (1971). *A Theory of Justice.* Cambridge, MA: Harvard University Press.

Rawls, J. (1993). *Political Liberalism.* New York: Columbia University Press.

Rawls, J. (1999). *The Law of Peoples.* Cambridge, MA: Harvard University Press.

Sandel, M. (1998). *Liberalism and the Limits of Justice.* Cambridge: Cambridge University Press.

Sen, A. (1995). *Inequalities Reexamined.* Cambridge, MA: Harvard University Press.

Sen, A. (2000). *Development as Freedom.* New York: Anchor Books.

Skocpol, T. (1991). *Protecting Soldiers and Mothers: The Politics of Social Provision in the U.S., 1870–1920.* Cambridge, MA: Harvard University Press.

10

Treatment According to Need:
Justice and the British National Health Service

Roger Crisp

The British National Health Service (NHS) was founded in July 1948 on the basis of three principles: universality, comprehensiveness, and free access (Webster, 1998, p. 22). That is, it was to provide health care to all, regardless of age, class, sex, religion, or geography; the care it provided was to be complete, rather than, for example, only a basic package of care; and there was to be no cost to the patient for the treatment provided. These three principles were seen as expressions of the more fundamental principle that treatment should be supplied according to need (and not, say, according to ability to pay).

At first, it was thought that the NHS might be so beneficial to the country's economy that it would constitute an overall saving, and that it would be little used once the population had been raised to a certain level of health. Almost immediately these hopes proved ill founded. In the first nine months of the NHS's existence, real cost outran the estimated amount of just under £200 million by over £75 million (Ross,

1952, p. 15). Not only had demand been underestimated, but also the potential for development in medical science. Over the next few decades, scientists made huge advances, offering treatments hitherto unavailable, which were often of great benefit to the patient while of great cost to the NHS budget. It soon became clear that, though formally each individual might be entitled to make a demand on the NHS, the principle of free access had to be limited. To restrict usage, prescription costs and other charges were introduced. And in more recent times, the principle of comprehensiveness also has been explicitly constrained. In 1991, for example, the North East Thames health region stated that patients would not be treated for certain conditions, including the removal of nonmalignant lumps (Ham, 1992, pp. 244–5). And yet it is still widely believed that the NHS has, in essence, remained true to its founding principle of treatment according to need (see, e.g., Webster, 1998, p. 215). Indeed, the latest proposals for governmental reform of the NHS open with the suggestion that: "[The] founding principles of providing access to care to all on the basis of need, not ability to pay, remain as important today as in 1948" (Preface, *NHS Plan*, 2000).

As soon as it becomes obvious that the NHS is unable to meet all the health-care needs of all the population, one must see the principle of treatment according to need as a principle concerning the just allocation of scarce resources (i.e., of rationing). In this chapter, I intend to examine the notion of treatment according to need so as to examine whether the NHS has indeed respected its founding principle.

WHAT IS A NEED?

Before we consider what it is to treat "according to" need, we should first discuss the notion of need itself. What is a need? There are several important points to make here.

First, the phrase "P needs N" is elliptical. The need-relation is triadic, involving not only a needing subject and a needed object, but also a purpose. Needing subjects do not, of course, have to be human beings. Cars need oil, for example; but they need oil so as to function properly, that is, efficiently, effectively, and without breaking down. Nor are all needs tied to functionings. If I am to attend the dinner this evening, then I need a dinner jacket.

Secondly and relatedly, need-satisfaction understood independently of its purpose cannot ground any reasons for action, moral or otherwise. My car may well need oil, but if I know that it will shortly be scrapped, and will never be driven again, it would be absurd to think that its need for oil provides me with any reason to provide it with some. Surely, however, this cannot be the case with serious human needs, such as the need of some person in severe pain for a painkiller? Here, however, it is again not the need-satisfaction that provides the reason, but the purpose—in this case, the avoidance of severe pain. What is needed

is always needed as a means—instrumental or constitutive—to some end, and it is only the ends that can plausibly ground reasons.

Thirdly, in the case of human needs, any reason to meet them must rest, at least partly, on the advancement of well-being. This is true even in trivial cases. If you have a reason to lend me your dinner jacket, because I need one for the dinner, that is because attending the dinner is something that I want to do, something that I will enjoy. And advancing my enjoyment is advancing my well-being, or at least a constituent of it.

THE NEED FOR HEALTH CARE

Now let us consider the need for health care. On one view, human beings have certain so-called basic needs—for basic food, basic shelter, and basic health, for example—and these basic needs can be understood as independent of, and as making claims independent of, wants, desires, or preferences (for discussion, cf. Daniels, 1985, pp. 13–14; Wiggins, 1987, pp. 15–16). If we apply this notion to health, it might be argued that the needs to be met by the NHS are basic needs, that is, needs for basic health care: relief from severe suffering, for example, or life-saving surgery. This was certainly not the view of the founders of the NHS, as the principle of comprehensiveness makes explicit. Nor can it be seen as a plausible interpretation of present practice: The NHS continues to provide sticking plasters for sore fingers, for example. But we shall return to the question of comprehensiveness later.

So we must at least begin with a less restricted conception of a health-care need. Let us say that "A needs treatment T" is elliptical for "A's health is such that, if she does not receive treatment T, her life will go less well for her." This definition builds the notion of treatment into that of a health-care need, on the one hand, to allow for less important health-care needs, and, on the other, to prevent needs—of whatever stringency—for non–health-related objects coming within the purview of the Health Service.

If a need, whether health-related or not, must ultimately be grounded on the advancement of well-being if it is going to give us reasons for action, does this mean that we must supply an account of well-being if we are to interpret the notion of treatment according to need? Strictly, yes, because strength of reason will be tied, in important part at least, to advancement of well-being, and how much certain treatments advance well-being depends on the theory of well-being at stake.

There is, standardly, said to be a trio of main theories of well-being (see Parfit, 1984, App. I). (There are problems with the distinctions drawn between members of this trio, but it will serve our present purposes well enough.) These are:

1. *Hedonism*: Well-being consists in pleasurable experiences, and the pleasurableness of these experiences is what makes them good.
2. *Desire accounts*: Well-being consists in the fulfilment of desires or preferences.
3. *Objective list accounts*: Well-being consists in the instantiation in a being's life of certain objective values, such as accomplishment, personal relationships, or understanding.

Now consider a case in which a decision must be taken whether to provide a lifesaving treatment to one of two individuals: *Happy*, or *Sad*. Happy is a very bubbly person, who vastly enjoys her life. She lives for everyday pleasures, but manages to achieve a large number of them across a wide range. Sad, on the other hand, is morose, anxious, and always unhappy. But she paints, almost compulsively, the most wonderful pictures. According to hedonism, Happy's need for the treatment is far greater than Sad's: After all, Sad will gain nothing from continuing to live. On the objective list account, however, it may well be that, because of the centrality of accomplishment to well-being, Sad has the

stronger claim on the basis of need. Indeed, if trivial pleasure is either absent from or given low priority on the list, it may well be that, according to this theory, Happy has little reason to go on living.

Examples could, of course, be constructed to demonstrate that desire accounts may also differ in their implications from either hedonism or objective list accounts. Now, given these differences, can we really proceed with our argument without deciding between the theories? In fact, we can, since the cases on which the theories differ are highly unusual. The theories will largely agree, that is to say, on how well people are doing. This is because most people enjoy and desire the items that are found on plausible objective lists (and surely any such list must itself include pleasure, and on its corresponding list of what makes life go worse for a person include pain?). Most accomplished painters, for example, greatly enjoy painting, and they strongly desire to continue to engage in that activity. Further, because of the scale of health-care provision at the national level, generalizations about the effects of various conditions are unavoidable if resources are to be rationally distributed. (More on this last point in my conclusion.)

TREATMENT ACCORDING TO NEED

Given that rationing of care is inevitable in the NHS, which interpretation of its governing principle provides the most morally plausible implications for distribution of health care in conditions of scarcity?

On one view, our aim should be equality of need-satisfaction across society as a whole. Indeed, it might be claimed, the founding idea of the NHS was equality: No citizen was to count more than any other.

There is a serious problem with any such account of egalitarianism, brought out well in recent work by Derek Parfit and Larry Temkin (Temkin, 1993; Parfit, 1998). Egalitarianism runs into what Parfit has called "the levelling-down objection." Consider a case in which you are confronted by two patients. Patient P is in fairly great need; that is to say, she has some fairly serious health problems, for which treatment is available. Patient Q, however, is in greater need—that is, she is more ill. There are three options open to you: you can treat P, and remove her need entirely; you can treat Q, and satisfy her need to some extent, though she will be left still considerably worse off than P; or you can "treat" both P and Q in such a way that both will be left much worse off, but will be in equal and very great need.

The problem with the principle that we should aim at equality of need-satisfaction is that it appears to speak in favor of the last option, which many will find not only ethically unacceptable, but also absurd. How can there be anything to be said for acting in such a case so as only to harm and to do no good to either patient?

One response here is that the case for equal need-satisfaction is grounded on the value of fairness (Broome, p. 1991, p. 193; Temkin, 1993, p. 13). It is unfair that Q is in greater need than P (through, we are assuming throughout, no fault of her own). If both are at the same level of need, then there is no unfairness. I have two doubts about this conception of fairness. The first concerns its source. Something very like this conception of fairness is one of the first morally loaded notions used by children, and the difficulty for its defender is to disentangle it from unjustified resentment at the good fortune of others—that is, envy. Complaints based on envy will be appropriate in exactly those cases in which complaints based on this egalitarian conception of fairness arise, and I submit that this is more than a coincidence. The egalitarian conception of fairness is merely envy transmuted into a moral principle.

But, it may be suggested, surely relative positions should concern us in distributions of health care, or of any other good? Do we not believe that, in the case above, the fact that P and Q are at different levels of

need makes a difference to their moral claim on any available treatment? Well, of course we do. But it must be the case that the relevance most people will attach to this difference in position is different from that attached to it by the egalitarian. For most people will suggest that Q should be treated.

It is highly tempting, in other words, to claim that—if we leave aside questions of responsibility of a patient for her condition—those with the greater need should be given priority over those with lesser need: I shall call this the "absolute priority view" (the term "priority view" is taken from Parfit, 1998). First, this seems to provide a plausible account of what is required in certain simple situations, such as that of P and Q above. The notion that the person in greater need should be given priority, and receive the treatment, seems much more attractive than several other options: tossing a coin, splitting the drug equally between the two patients, or selling it to the highest bidder. Secondly, this interpretation of the principle captures what some see as a central aspect of the most plausible view of ethics: individuality. Consider Thomas Nagel's view that, in seeking the most plausible principle of distribution, we are looking for a kind of "unanimity" in assessing outcomes:

The essence of such a criterion is to try in a moral assessment to include each person's point of view separately, so as to achieve a result which is in a significant sense acceptable to each person involved or affected. Where there is conflict of interests, no result can be completely acceptable to everyone. But it is possible to assess each result from each point of view to try to find the one that is least unacceptable to the person to whom it is most unacceptable. This means that any other alternative will be more unacceptable to someone than this alternative is to anyone. The preferred alternative is in that sense the least unacceptable, considered from each person's point of view separately. A radically egalitarian policy of giving absolute priority to the worst off, regardless of numbers, would result from always choosing the least unacceptable alternative, in this sense. (Nagel, 1979, p. 123)

This conception of ethics, according to which principles must be acceptable to each person affected, taken one by one, and not based on the aggregation of goods across individuals and the idea of benefiting groups, has been taken further in T.M. Scanlon's version of contractualism (see Scanlon, 1998, chaps. 4 and 5).

However plausible this conception of ethics is in itself, it has some very unattractive implications. Consider a case in which you can either treat a single person, who is in great need (let us say, for the sake of argument, at need-level 10, though there is no intention of this number's representing anything precisely), or treat a group of 1,000 people at a lower need level: 8. In the first case, you will benefit the patient by "one point" (so the individual, if treated, will be at level 9); if you treat the members of the group, however, each of them will benefit greatly, and end up at level 1. The view we are considering speaks in favor of treating the single individual— and it will have the same implication however many are in the group, and however much they can be benefited. Because this view is "innumerate," as Nagel puts it, and a "maximin" principle (see Rawls, 1972, pp. 152–56), it will allow the smallest amount of need-satisfaction for the smallest number of neediest to trump the largest amount of need-satisfaction to any but the neediest, even the next neediest.

What appears to be required, then, is a principle that allows us to give some priority to people the more needy they are, but in giving priority to take into account the amount of need-satisfaction at stake, and the number of people whose needs will be satisfied. So understood, the priority view is essentially a nonlexical weighting principle: Satisfying needs matters more the worse off the needy people are, the more of those people there are, and the greater the level of need-satisfaction that can be achieved.

This principle—call it the "weighted-need principle"—permits us to satisfy the needs of the less needy, if the level of need-satisfaction one can achieve for them is significantly greater than that possible for the more needy, or if the less needy are greater in number. Judgment will be required, of course, to decide in any particular case how the variables of existing need, available increases in need-satisfaction, and number of individuals weigh one against another. But I now want to suggest that whatever weights are attached to these factors the weighted-need principle allows too much in certain cases. Consider the following example, in which "extra moral weight" is attached to using medical care to decrease a person's neediness according to how needy he or she is. The central idea is that the moral value of decreases of a single unit can be "multiplied" to give an overall moral value, the multiplier being proportionally greater the greater the neediness of the individual helped. We have to imagine that 0 need is the level of perfect health and 100 is the level of maximum need.

Improvement in Level of Need	Multiplier	Overall Moral Value
100→99	100	100
99→98	99	99
98→97	98	98
. . . .		
3→2	3	3
2→1	2	2
1→0	1	1

If, for example, I can decrease the level of need of R, who is at 100, to 99; or decrease the level of S, who is at 99, to 97; or decrease the level of T, who is at 3, to 0, the overall moral value of each treatment is:

R: 100 = 100
S: 99 + 98 = 197
T: 3 + 2 + 1 = 6

Attention to degree of need-satisfaction, then, requires me to treat S. But if we imagine that there is a second person in R's position, whom I may also treat along with R, the value of this option will be 200, and hence the more valuable of the three options available. In this case, the number of needy outweighs the importance of the amount of need-satisfaction available to any particular individual.

The multipliers I have set here are quite arbitrary. One might, for example, use a much larger multiplier at higher need levels (so, for example, bringing someone from 100 to 99 might be multiplied by 1,000). But I now want to demonstrate that a serious problem arises for the weighted-need principle whatever the multiplier used. Imagine a case in which you can decrease the level of need of 100 people, who are maximally needy and hence at level 100, by 100. That is, you can make entirely healthy 100 people who are suffering terribly, and as sick as they could be. Alternatively, you can provide a high-quality skin cream to a million otherwise healthy individuals, to bring their level of need down from 1 to 0. That is, you can make entirely healthy people who are pretty well already as healthy as they could be.

The value of treating the thousand is:

$$(100 + 99 + 98 \ldots + 3 + 2 + 1)$$
$$\times \ 100 = 550{,}000$$

The value of treating the million is:

$$1 \times 1{,}000{,}000 = 1{,}000{,}000$$

In other words, the weighted-need principle, though it may avoid requiring us to help the smallest number of neediest in the smallest possible way instead of helping the largest number of those only slightly less needy in the largest possible way, does require us to treat the very minor ailments of the already almost entirely healthy instead of giving hugely significant forms of treatment to the very sickest individuals. Its readiness to aggregate need-satisfaction across individuals all the way up results in

a failure to give the appropriate moral significance to levels of existing need, increases in need-satisfaction, and numbers of needy. This result seems to me perhaps even less attractive than the implications of the original, individualistic, absolute priority view, which at least always distributes health care to the most needy.

It might now be suggested that we try to block the aggregations that lead to these unacceptable outcomes by putting restrictions on aggregations when gaps between levels of existing need are large. Now it depends, of course, what is meant by large, but let us assume that a gap of 10 is large. Then a restriction on aggregation would prevent, for example, our bringing 10 million individuals down from a level of 15 to a level of, say, 10, instead of bringing one individual down from a level of 25 to a level of, say, 20. This modification is too extreme: From giving insufficient weight to distribution, and too much to aggregation, we have moved to the opposite position, attaching far too much significance to distribution and no serious weight to aggregation. (This, you will recall, was exactly the problem with the absolute priority view discussed above.) At less severe levels of need, aggregation seems quite appropriate.

What is required is a principle that allows us to give priority to those who are in serious need, but otherwise maximizes need-satisfaction overall, taking into account the factors of existing need, available levels of need-satisfaction through treatment, and number of beneficiaries. Let me call this the threshold principle (TP):

(TP) Priority is to be given to satisfying the needs of those above a threshold of health need. Above the threshold, satisfying needs matters more the needier the individuals in question, the more of them there are, and the greater the available level of need-satisfaction through treatment. Below the threshold, or in cases concerning only trivial decreases in need above the threshold, need-satisfaction overall is to be maximized.

In effect, TP reintroduces the idea of basic needs for health care, although it does of course allow for needs all the way up (that is, not all needs are basic). Individuals whose health-care needs are basic have a special claim on health-care resources, and they can justifiably complain if serious improvements to their health are ignored in favor of treating those below the threshold. In effect, this is a way of spelling out the notion of "sufficiency" as a principle of justice in allocation of health care: When you are healthy enough, you have less claim on resources than those who have not reached the level of sufficiency (see Frankfurt, 1988). Where the threshold falls, of course, is the key question any proponent of this view must answer. Much work has been done on clinical priority setting in the UK over the last 20 years (see, e.g., New, 1997a), but a lot more remains to be done. Let me for the sake of illustration suggest that the following conditions bring a person above the threshold:

Conditions causing severe pain over a sig-nficant period (e.g., certain cancers)
Conditions seriously affecting mobility, and other central physical capacities (e.g., Parkinson's disease)
Conditions that seriously impair mental functioning (e.g., severe schizophrenia)

And the following conditions are clearly insufficient to take a person above the threshold (in the UK, such conditions are frequently treated by primary health care practiioners):

Mild skin complaints
Sore throats
Mild hay fever

Thus, to take an example, if we are to treat people according to need, on the most plausible understanding of that notion as a conception of justice, in a situation of scarce health resources, nontrivial medical benefits should be supplied to those in severe pain over a significant period, rather than, say, lozenges for those with sore throats, however few those in pain are, and however many there are with sore throats. Now it may well be that considerations of, for example, utility, or efficiency, would outweigh the principle of treatment according to need in cases such as those we have mentioned. But we should be clear about the implication here: Treating people on the basis of efficiency is not treating people in accordance with their need.

THE NEW NHS AND TREATMENT ACCORDING TO NEED

How close does the NHS, in its current incarnation, come to adherence to its founding principle, that patients should be treated according to need? It comes closer than it might, but there is substantial room for improvement.

The main problem, from the perspective of treatment according to need, is that no serious attention has been paid to the question of what package of health care the NHS as a whole is intended to provide. There have been developments at local levels in the NHS: One-quarter of health authorities in 1996 and 1997, for example, included explicit statements in their purchasing plans that they would not contract for certain services, such as the removal of tattoos (Redmayne, 1996). But explicit rationing by condition appears absent from the proposals in *The NHS Plan* of 2000. There are several possible reasons for this. First, explicit discussions of priority-setting by condition, as in New Zealand, the Netherlands, and Oregon, have not been entirely successful. Secondly, such explicit priority-setting, even if allowance is made for clinical judgment and unusual cases, is not only highly controversial at the margins, but also makes patent exactly where the NHS stops. At present, the limits of NHS funding are hidden behind a woolly commitment to comprehensiveness and rationing by waiting lists, budgetary limits, and other contingencies. Finally, and relatedly, governmental priority-setting by condition would amount to giving up on one of the principles on which the NHS was founded: comprehensiveness. Indeed, comprehensiveness is stated in the NHS Plan as the second core principle, after treatment according to need: "The NHS will provide a comprehensive range of services" (Preface, *NHS Plan*, 2000).

But that the NHS cannot be comprehensive was not only one of the things that became clear after the euphoria surrounding its foundation in 1948 had died down, but in fact implicitly denied even in the very nature of the NHS as it was then conceived. Even in 1948, the founders of the NHS would have been well aware that providing each citizen with his or her own personal doctor, available on call 24 hours a day, would have met certain health-care needs that otherwise would go unmet. But of course such a program was inconceivable. A case could be made for a certain range of treatments and services, and above these a line would be drawn: The NHS was not, at its very inception, comprehensive. The necessity for further explicit priority-setting has emerged as demand for that range has exceeded supply, and the range itself has increased hugely with changing health needs and availability of new treatments.

The NHS Plan includes a discussion of alternative conceptions of the NHS (*NHS Plan*, 2000, chap. 3: "Options for Funding Health Care"): private insurance; charges; social insurance; rationing the service down to a fixed core. That rationing should be discussed in this chapter is odd, since it is not relevant to funding; likewise it is strange that, in section 3.4, it is stated that each proposal has been "examined against two key criteria"—efficiency and equity—and that in the discussion of rationing alone no mention is made of these criteria. There are nevertheless some objections offered to the proposal.

The first is that "advocates of this position usually have great difficulty specifying what they would rule out. The sort of services that commonly feature . . . account for less than 0.5% of the NHS budget" (section 3.29). There are several responses to

this objection. First, that a position is difficult to state is, in itself, no objection to that position. Secondly, to make the proposal more practically significant will require slimming down the core service considerably; but, as we have seen, this is required if treatment is to be delivered according to need within a limited budget. Thirdly, as I have just demonstrated, the notion of comprehensiveness is an unattainable ideal. Lines have been and will continue to be drawn, and certain health-care needs are above those lines. The rational approach must be to consider whether the lines as they are currently drawn—largely as a result of historical, political, and social contingencies—are reasonable. It may be, of course, that on reflection they will indeed be seen to be reasonable, in which case what the NHS currently supplies would be its "core service." The NHS Plan fails to consider rationing seriously because it fails to recognize that the proposal that the boundaries of NHS treatment be considered is not equivalent to the proposal that certain less important services be cut.

The second objection to the proposal is that "different patients under different circumstances often derive differing benefits from the same treatment" (section 3.30). Now this is of course the case, and I said a little about this question above, in my discussion of the relation of needs and well-being. But this fact is a problem for any cash-limited health-care system, not only for a rationed system. The NHS will not be able, and has never been able, to meet all health-care needs of all UK citizens. The present system of rationing by waiting lists makes no room for the fact that different patients derive different benefits from the same treatment.

Further, as should be fairly obvious, generalizations about the benefits to be gained from various treatments can easily and plausibly be made, and indeed some of the central proposals in the Plan rest on such generalizations: More funding is to be given for treatments related to cancer, coronary heart disease, and mental health. But it is clear that some of the patients who will benefit from these new treatments will benefit less than certain other patients, with other conditions, who remain untreated. Consider, for example, someone who because of some illness has only a few agonizing months to live, suffers a heart attack, and whose life is prolonged for those few months because of the increased funding, as opposed to someone with very many fulfilling years left who dies after a road accident because of the unavailability of an intensive care bed.

What sort of further generalizations *might* be made? (I say "might" because much further thought and research would be required: My proposal is merely that this thinking be carried out.) Consider cataract extraction. Cataract extractions cost significantly less than £1,000 each, but the NHS might expect to perform over 150,000 per year (*Financial Times;* www.surgicare.co.uk). Now some of these patients are almost certainly in dire need of care, but in a not insignificant number of cases the patients will be able to see quite well. It is at least arguable, then, that funding should be shifted to some degree from cataract removal to, for example, psychiatric care for late adolescents with a severe psychosis, which at present is very underfunded, on the ground that the impact of their condition upon their well-being brings them well above the threshold of basic need, whereas certain cataracts do not bring patients above the threshold. As it happens, many who require cataract surgery could afford to pay for it; but that is merely a fortunate coincidence. Even if they could not, the claim of the psychotic adolescents could be said to be greater.

Other treatments that might not be included in the package are, in addition to the standard instances (cosmetic surgery, varicose vein removal, wisdom teeth extraction, and sterilization or vasectomy reversal), treatments for several gynecological and urological conditions, contra-

ception, and life-prolonging treatment for those with a very low quality of life. But let me stress again that these are merely off-the-cuff suggestions that might begin a debate or a research program. And note too that this chapter concerns the principle of treatment according to need. There may well be other very strong reasons for public funding of, say, contraception. In particular, there may be reasons based on the advancement of well-being overall, but it is important to remember that these reasons will then have to be weighed against those resting on the principle of treatment according to need.

Finally, it is worth noting that because a patient's condition can be described in various ways, the concerns about a package's ruling out a treatment that will, unusually, provide a major benefit to a certain patient are largely misplaced (see New, 1997b, pp. 83–84). Consider the commonly cited case of someone who is suffering extreme psychological distress from a tattoo. It might be thought that if tattoo removal is not part of the NHS package, this patient must remain untreated. But that is a mistake: Serious psychological distress is something for which treatment would almost certainly be provided within the package.

What appears to be the third objection to rationing to a core service is hard to interpret, so let me state it in full:

The NHS is not a system under which each patient only gets a fixed "ration" of healthcare, regardless of their personal need and circumstances. The fact that a patient has previously been treated for one condition will not of itself prevent her or him from being treated for subsequent conditions. If, however, "rationing" merely means that it has never and will never in possible in practice to provide all healthcare theoretically possible, then it is true of every health care system in the world. (section 3.31)

The first part of this point seems a wilful misinterpretation of a proposal that has been clearly stated a few paragraphs above in the document. The notion of rationing to a core service is quite different from that of rationing individuals to a certain share of health care. The second part is no better. Those proposing rationing to a core service are obviously not claiming merely that there are limits to health care, but that these limits should be imposed in a particular way. And the recognition of limits, as I have shown, is in itself inconsistent with any claim to comprehensiveness.

The final paragraph in the section discussing rationing to a core service is a little worrying. It states that: "Under the NHS, treatment is based on peoples' ability to benefit . . . [National Service Frameworks, etc.] will help the NHS to focus its growing resources on those interventions and treatments that will best improve peoples' health" (section 3.32). On one reading, this is a proposal to give up the founding principle of the NHS, and no longer to treat individuals according to their need, but to maximize the well-being of the population overall. And even if this is said to be treating according to need, it will result in the minor interests of the many trumping the significant interests of the few. On another and perhaps more plausible reading, the proposal is that priority setting in the NHS continue to be the result of largely uncontrollable contingencies on an undiscussed and unplanned package of health care. Treatment according to need surely demands more than that.[1]

NOTES

1. I wish to thank participants in the 1999 Mt. Sinai–Oxford Consortium on Medical Ethics, and especially my co-presenter, Catherine Paxton, and the editors for helpful comments on previous versions of this chapter.

REFERENCES

Broome, J. (1991). *Weighing Goods.* Oxford: Blackwell.

Daniels, N. (1985). *Just Health Care.* Cambridge: Cambridge University Press.

Financial Times, January 5, 2000.

Frankfurt, H. (1988). Equality as a moral ideal. In H. Frankfurt (ed.), *The Importance of What We Care About.* Cambridge: Cambridge University Press.

Ham, C. (1992). *Health Policy in Britain,* 3rd ed. Basingstoke and London: Macmillan.

Nagel, T. (1979). Equality. In T. Nagel (ed.), *Mortal Questions.* Cambridge: Cambridge University Press.

New, B. (ed.) (1997a). *Rationing: Talk and Action in Health Care.* London: BMJ Publishing Group and King's Fund.

New, B. (1997 b). Defining a package of health-care services the NHS is responsible for: The case for. In B. New, *Rationing: Talk and Action in Health Care.* London: BMJ Publishing Group and King's Fund.

NHS Plan, The (2000). Norwich: Stationery Office.

Parfit, D. (1984). *Reasons and Persons.* Oxford: Clarendon Press.

Parfit, D. (1998). Equality and priority. In A. Mason (ed.), *Ideals of Equality.* Oxford: Blackwell.

Rawls, J. (1972). *A Theory of Justice.* Oxford: Oxford University Press.

Redmayne, S. (1996). *Small Steps, Big Goals: Purchasing Policies in the NHS.* Birmingham, UK: NAHAT.

Ross, J.S. (1952). *The National Health Service in Great Britain.* London: Oxford University Press.

Scanlon, T.M. (1998). *What We Owe to Each Other.* Cambridge, MA: Belknap Press.

Temkin, L. (1993). *Inequality.* New York: Oxford University Press.

Webster, C. (1998). *The National Health Service: A Political History.* Oxford: Oxford University Press.

Wiggins, D. (1987). *Needs, Values, Truth.* Oxford: Blackwell.

11

Rationing Decisions: Integrating Cost-Effectiveness with Other Values

Tony Hope, John Reynolds, and Siân Griffiths

Health-care systems throughout the world face the problem of how the resources available should best be allocated. No system has sufficient funds to provide the best possible treatment for all patients in all situations. On average, three new pharmaceutical products are licensed each month in the United Kingdom. Almost all have some benefit over existing drugs. Many are expensive. When is the extra benefit worth the extra cost? Both managed-care systems in the United States and publicly funded systems such as the British National Health Service (NHS) face this fundamental issue.

Philosophers and economists have struggled with the question of which principles should determine the allocation of health-care resources. Various approaches have been proposed such as welfare theory (Williams, 1996; Edgar et al., 1998), needs theory (Daniels 1980, 1985), and the use of a lottery (Harris, 1985). Each theory faces difficulties, and none can be applied unambiguously to many of the allocation decisions that have to be made. Perhaps be-

cause of these apparent limitations to the various theories, recent philosophical attention has turned to the process by which allocation decisions are made, in contrast to the reasons for those decisions (Daniels and Sabin, 1997; Daniels, 2000). The hope may be that if we can specify the conditions required for a just decision-making process, then we can sidestep the difficulties in determining the principles that should be applied to individual decisions.

Daniels and his colleagues have provided the most sustained theoretical analysis of the conditions required for a just decision-making process. Singer, Martin, and their colleagues are carrying out empirical research on such a process in practice in the context of the Canadian health-care system (Martin and Singer, 2000).

According to Daniels and Sabin, one feature of a just decision-making process is a "relevance condition"—that is, that a decision must rest on evidence, reasons, and principles that all fair-minded people can agree are relevant (Daniels and Sabin,

1997). Daniels has analyzed the concept of "accountability for reasonableness." One of the four conditions he identifies in order to implement such accountability is "reasonableness." He writes that "the rationales for coverage decisions should aim to provide a *reasonable* construal of how the organization should provide 'value for money' in meeting the varied health needs of a defined population under reasonable resource constraints. Specifically, a construal will be 'reasonable' if it appeals to reasons and principles that are accepted as relevant by people who are disposed to finding terms of co-operation that are mutually justifiable" (Daniels, 2000, p. 92). The Oxfordshire Health Authority in the United Kingdom has developed a procedure for making some resource allocation decisions that meet this criterion on reasonableness (Hope et al., 1998; Griffiths et al., 2000).

A central feature of both the process described by Singer and colleagues in Canada, and the one adopted by Oxfordshire Health Authority (and indeed by other U.K. health authorities), is that a group of people come to a decision about a specific allocation issue on the basis of evidence and after deliberation. This feature is likely to be a part of any process that meets Daniels's criteria. From our experience in Oxfordshire this core decision-making group faces two types of difficulty. The first is that evidence about the effect of spending resources in one way rather than another is often poor. This is particularly the case for the more "macro-level" decisions, such as whether to divert resources from a small local hospital to a large city hospital, or vice versa. We will not discuss this issue any further. Instead, we will focus on the second difficulty: Even when the evidence concerning both the cost and the effect of a health-care intervention is good, the members of the group frequently face problematic ethical choices. The group struggles with questions about what are the right principles to apply to the specific allocation decisions that need to be made. Thus, a fo-

cus on the process by which allocation decisions should be made leads back to questions about what are the right principles and theories on which to base such decisions. We cannot avoid questions of principle by a focus on process. However, the experience gained from developing better processes has, we believe, clarified some of the key ethical issues that require further philosophical analysis.

In this chapter we consider one type of decision that health-care systems face: whether to spend resources on a new, expensive, therapy. We will assume, as is often the case, that particularly with new drug treatments, there are good data on the cost and the effect of the therapy. We will describe a four-step method that can be applied by a decision-making group, which, we believe, meets Daniels' and Sabin's criterion for a "relevance condition" and addresses how Daniels' criterion of reasonableness can be tackled in practice. We then identify six specific ethical issues that the decision-making group is likely to face. These complement the allocation problems outlined by Martin and Singer (2000). One strength, we believe, of the method we present is that it allows the integration of values taken from welfare theories of resource allocation with values taken from needs theories. This method highlights those issues of value concerning the allocation of resources that must be faced by decision makers, and that will repay philosophical analysis.

In the United Kingdom, major decisions about what to fund, or what not to fund, fall squarely on the shoulders of health authorities, who are charged with purchasing health care on behalf of the population they serve. Health authorities are likely to continue to play this central role despite current NHS reforms (see Chapter 10). Oxfordshire Health Authority set up a "Priorities Forum" in order to advise it on resource allocation decisions. In the appendix we describe the origin, structure, and work of this forum. The question we will consider is how should such a forum approach the question of whether or not to fund a new treatment, or other health-care intervention. We will argue that the starting point for considering this issue should be a measure of cost-effectiveness, such as the quality-adjusted life-year (QALY).

The essence of a QALY is that it takes a year of healthy life expectancy to be worth 1, but regards a year of unhealthy life expectancy as worth less than 1. Its precise value is lower the worse the quality of life of the unhealthy person (which is what the quality adjusted part is all about) (Williams, 1996). The general idea behind the QALY approach is that a beneficial health-care activity is one that generates a positive number of QALYs, and that an efficient health-care activity is one where the cost per QALY is as low as it can be. A high priority health-care activity is one where the cost per QALY is low, and a low priority activity is one where cost per QALY is high.

We describe an approach to decision making that allows values that are not part of cost-effectiveness analysis to be taken into account in a semi-quantitative way. We hope that this approach contributes to both the theoretical and practical development of a reasonable attitude to resource allocation that goes "beyond . . . cost-effective analysis" (Martin and Singer, 2000, p. 143) and beyond the phase of simple solutions (Holm, 1998; Klein, 1998).

COST-EFFECTIVENESS SHOULD BE THE STARTING POINT FOR RATIONING DECISIONS

Many criticisms have been leveled at the use of QALYs, or other measures of cost-effectiveness, as the criterion to be used for deciding issues of resource allocation (Harris, 1985, 1987, 1988; Broome, 1988). Quite different approaches to resource allocation have been developed (Daniels, 1985; Harris, 1985). However, it is our view that the starting point for deciding an issue, such as whether a new and expensive cancer drug should be funded for a particular group of patients, has to be some form of cost-effective analysis. Lottery theory (Harris, 1985) provides a method (whether or not it is the morally right method) for deciding which patient should be given the only organ available for transplant. That method is to choose by lottery. However, it does not provide a clear method for deciding whether or not a new and expensive cancer treatment should or should not be funded as it is quite unclear what outcomes should be put into the lottery.

"Needs theory" (Daniels, 1980, 1985; Doyal and Gough, 1984) has more general application than lottery theory. It suggests there are some treatments that amount to fulfilling a need, whereas other treatments, while being of benefit, do not address a need. It suggests that needs should be met before other benefits even if this leads to less welfare overall. However, it cannot be applied directly to the question of whether or not to fund the new cancer drug. This is partly because of the difficulty in deciding whether the relative benefit of the new drug compared with current treatment amounts to satisfying a need. What increase in five-year survival rates, for example, would constitute a need rather than a mere benefit? But it is also because there is no way of taking cost into account. Even if it were agreed that relevant patients "needed" this new drug, a health funder could not afford to pay an unlimited amount for it.

Many people consider that any method of cost-effective analysis, such as QALYs, leads to the ethically wrong distribution of resources. How then can we have a method for deciding the allocation of resources that makes use of cost-effectiveness data while allowing other values to be taken into account?

COMBINING COST-EFFECTIVENESS ANALYSIS WITH OTHER VALUES: A FOUR-STEP METHOD

The task facing the decision-making group in considering whether a particular health-care intervention should be provided can be summarized as answering the following questions.

- Is there evidence that the intervention is effective?
- How good is this evidence?
- What is the cost of bringing about the effect?
- What is the value of this effect (using "value" in the sense described in the appendix).
- Is it worth paying the cost, given the value of the effect, and in light of what the particular health authority can afford to pay?

In theory these questions can be asked without any formal cost-effectiveness data. The group of people around the table can be given a clear account of the effect that the intervention brings about; the group of patients for whom the treatment is effective; the chance of the treatment working; and the cost (expressed, for example, as cost per patient, or per patient who benefits). The group could then make a judgment as to whether, given what the authority can normally pay, this particular intervention should or should not be provided. In practice, however, this judgment would be very hard to make without some common currency by which to judge this intervention against others that are, or are not, provided. Without a "common currency" it would be difficult to ensure consistency between decisions, or to provide clear justification for the decisions taken. It would also be difficult to ensure that the decisions adequately take into account the amount of money that is available. The QALYs, or in the case of treatments that are primarily life-extending, cost per life-year extended, provide common currency.

The Oxfordshire Health Authority can currently afford to pay about £15,000 per QALY for new treatments, although in the longer run this will be dependent on the number of patients who receive treatment. This figure provides guidance to the Priorities Forum when considering whether to purchase a new treatment or other intervention. A practical approach to addressing the above questions is to apply the following four-step method.

1. To start with evidence as to how much the treatment costs per life-year extended (or per QALY).
2. To compare this cost with the "guide cost"—the amount, on average, that the funding body can pay (i.e., about £15,000 in the case of Oxfordshire Health Authority).
3. If the proposed treatment is less than this amount then the presumption is in favor of providing the treatment, and there would need to be a reason not to provide it. If the proposed treatment is more than this amount then the presumption is that it should not be provided, and there would need to be a reason to provide it (see below).
4. If the proposed treatment costs more that the "guide cost" then two questions arise: (a) are there grounds for paying more than the usual amount (per QALY or life-year extended); and, if there are, (b) do those grounds justify paying that much more (i.e., however much more it is)?

This approach is flexible. It ensures that the decision-making group takes into account the key factors of cost and effectiveness, while also allowing other values to be considered. The group can recommend interventions that would not be supported by the QALY calculation if it believes that there are further grounds—for example, those espoused by needs theories—that justify straying from the QALY calculation. This approach requires the group to make a judgment as to how much weight should be given to these further grounds in terms of how much more than the "guide cost" is justified.

Six Key Ethical Issues

We will now consider six situations that arise in practice and that raise the question of whether more (or less) should be spent per QALY than the "guide cost."

Should treatments for the young have a different priority from treatments for the old?

Life-years, and quality adjusted life-years treat years at different ages as of equal value. If a treatment has an effect on quality or length of life for the two years from ages 25 to 27 years, this is given identical value as the same effect over the two years from ages 80 to 82 years, or from ages 2 to 4 years.

Some philosophers have argued that it is wrong to treat years at different ages as of equal value (Daniels, 1985; Lockwood, 1988). At least in the case of life-extending treatments there is more value if the life extension is from age 30 to 35, than if it is from 70 to 75. Lockwood observed: "To treat the older person, letting the younger person die, would thus be inherently inequitable in terms of years of life lived: the younger person would get no more years than the relatively few he has already had, whereas the older person, who has already had more than the younger person, will get several years more (Lockwood, 1988, p. 50). Daniels (1985) comes to a similar conclusion, applying a variant of Rawls's veil of ignorance (Rawls, 1972). If, behind the veil, we were choosing a type of health insurance scheme for our entire lives—from cradle to grave—Daniels argues that it would be rational for us to give relatively greater priority to a treatment to extend our life at the age of 30 years than to a treatment to extend life at the age of 70 years.

The issues that come to the Priorities Forum are never of the form of a choice between two individuals of different ages. However, different health-care interventions often primarily affect people of different ages, because they relate either to a disease or a service that affects one age group rather than another. The question that arises, therefore, is whether the "guide cost" in terms of cost per QALY should be different for different age groups. Should a funding authority be prepared to spend more per QALY for diseases of childhood? This would not be on the grounds that the benefits of the health-care intervention in childhood will be enjoyed for longer as that factor is already taken into account in the QALY calculation. The grounds would be, at least for life-extending treatments, that a youthful year has more value than an aged year.

Our purpose, in this chapter, is not to argue in favor of one position or another. It is to suggest that it is possible, within the framework we describe, to adjust the "guide cost per QALY" for different ages. It is interesting to note, in this context, that disability-adjusted life-years (DALYs), which have been developed to measure the "burden of disease" for different diseases worldwide, have explicitly given a different value to life at different ages—valuing young adulthood more than either old age or childhood (Murray, 1994; Anand and Hanson, 1997; Murray and Acharya, 1997).

Should identifiable patients be favored over nonidentifiable patients? The rule of rescue

Consider two different types of treatment. The first is a drug that will change the chance of death by a small amount in a large number of people. For example, out of every 2000 people in the group, if A is not given then 100 people will die over the next few years. If A is given then only 99 will die. Drug A is cheap.

The second drug, drug B, is effective for an otherwise life-threatening condition. Those with this condition face a greater than 90% chance of death over the next year if not given B. If given B then there is a good chance of cure—say greater than 90%. Drug B is expensive.

The question is, should we be prepared to spend more per life-year extended on drug B than we would on drug A? The first type of treatment is typical of many preventive health-care strategies. One example is cholesterol-lowering drugs. The Oxfordshire Health Authority tends to spend less per life year extended on treatments of this kind than on treatments that extend the lives of identifiable people. This is not simply an issue of saving a current life versus saving a future life. Even if there is some justification for some discounting of future lives, as some economic models hold, this would only justify a relatively small extra cost per identifiable life saved. Furthermore, the difference between saving the identifiable life and preventing the loss of the unidentifiable life is not fundamentally about whether one is in the present and one is in the future. Some preventive treatments—for example, drugs reducing the risk of death following a heart attack—prevent unidentifiable deaths over the next few days and months. Conversely, some treatments given to identifiable people may save lives sometime in the future.

There is a widely held view that we should put more into saving the life of an identifiable person than into saving lives of "statistical people." This is sometimes called "the rule of rescue" (Hadorn, 1991). The QALY calculation does not support this rule of rescue. A decision-making group must decide whether the money available should be used to maximize the life years extended overall or whether more money, for a given outcome such as life year extended, should be spent on those treatments that will extend the lives of identifiable people. A health-care funding organization is not in a position to pay an unlimited amount even for extending the lives of identifiable people. But it can certainly pay a different price. For example, a funder that is working with a "guide cost" of £15,000 per QALY might decide to provide cholesterol-lowering drugs up to £10,000 per QALY but be prepared to pay £50,000 per QALY for a treatment for extending the lives of identifiable people. It might not be prepared to pay £300,000,

however, for the latter type of treatment. One of us (Hope, 2001) has argued against the "rule of rescue" as applied to such decisions. However, the point we want to emphasize is that the process described in this chapter is sufficiently flexible to allow more to be spent on treating identifiable patients than on "statistical" people.

Should palliative care be given higher priority than would result from the QALY calculation?

Good palliative care for those near the end of life might come out as expensive under the QALY calculation because the patients do not live very long. However, many people believe that palliative care for those near the end of life should have a higher priority than might result from the QALY calculation. The QALY calculations, and similar cost-effective analyses, give equal weight to each time slice. One issue, which we have raised above, is whether a time slice at the age of 40 years should count for the same as an identical time slice at the age of 80 years. The issue of palliative care raises the question of whether a time slice is altered, not by the person's age, but by the relationship to the person's death. A life, on this view, is not simply the sum of each time slice. The way in which a novel ends can have special significance. In an analogous way, how a life ends may have particular significance. The quality of care and patients' experiences for the last period of their lives should, on this view, be accorded more weight than other periods in life. A further reason for according a high priority to palliative care is that the ending of a person's life is of particular importance to those individuals who are close to the dying person.

If palliative care is valued for these reasons they can be taken into account by the health funder in paying more per QALY than the guide cost. This does not open the door to paying an unlimited amount. The question is how much more should the funder be prepared to pay for good palliative care than the QALY calculation would support.

Should higher priority be given to those who are particularly badly off with regard to their health?

One implication of Daniels's (1985) approach to justice is that higher priority than most cost-effectiveness analyses allow should be accorded to those who are particularly badly off. Consider two treatments for different conditions. One raises the quality of life of the patients from 0.2 to 0.5. The other treats a different group of patients and raises the quality of life from 0.6 to 1.0. Both treatments cost the same per patient treated. Thus, the second treatment is better value according to the QALY calculation. If the use of resources is to be prioritized on the basis of QALYs, then the second treatment should have priority over the first. However, it might be argued that the first treatment should have higher priority. This is because the first treatment helps those who are worse off even though it leads overall to a smaller increase in quality of life.

Although this criticism of QALYs has considerable weight, it would be reckless of a funding authority to put considerations of cost-effectiveness to one side. This would result in spending enormous resources on the treatment of very sick patients, with little health gain. On the model described in this chapter, a funder could be prepared to pay more per QALY than the guide price for those who are particularly badly off without paying an unlimited amount more.

This issue has been relevant to a number of decisions faced by Oxfordshire Health Authority, such as whether the authority should pay for very expensive drugs that improve the symptoms of multiple sclerosis or Alzheimer's disease. Beta-interferon is a drug that provides some improvement for some sufferers of multiple sclerosis (MS). It does not increase life expectancy but it does tend to reduce the frequency of relapses. Varying cost-effectiveness analyses suggest a cost per QALY of about £800,000 with a range from £74,500 to over £35 million—showing just how problematic such analyses can be (Nicholson and Milne, 1999). Even at best this is five times the authority's "guide cost." Should Oxfordshire Health Authority pay more than its guide cost for beta-interferon on the grounds that those with MS are in greater need than most patients? If it should, should it pay five times the guide cost?

Should higher priority be given if there is no alternative treatment?

Consider the following hypothetical, but realistic, situation. Several current treatments exist for cancer A. None are curative, but the current best treatment very significantly improves five-year survival compared with no treatment. A new treatment for cancer A is developed. It gives better five-year survival than the current best treatment but is somewhat more expensive. It costs £20,000 per life-year extended. Cancer B is a cancer for which there is no treatment other than palliative care. A new drug is developed that offers, for the first time, an improved five-year survival. The cost per life-year extended is £40,000. Should we pay more than the guide cost in the case of the treatment of cancer B, on the grounds that this is the only effective treatment, while not paying for the new and more cost-effective drug for cancer A? Sufferers of cancer A, it might be argued, already have access to a reasonable treatment, although not the best.

How is "double jeopardy" to be dealt with?

Harris pointed to the issue of double jeopardy as a problem with the QALY approach (Harris, 1987, 1995; see also Singer et al., 1995). This arises when a person has a chronic condition that lowers quality of life—for example, bad arthritis. If that person then has another condition, which may or may not be life-threatening, the treatment of that second condition may turn out to be more expensive, and therefore of lower priority, because of the first condition. Thus, a life-extending treatment will produce fewer QALYs for the same number of years of life extension in the person with arthritis because the arthritis lowers the quality of life. Similarly, a quality-enhancing treatment may not produce so much increase in quality of life because the increase in quality has a ceiling placed on it by the arthritis.

Consider another example: the question of dental treatment for people with severe learning disability. The cost of dentistry can be greater in this group because of lack of cooperation with the treatments. It is possible, at least in theory, that a dentistry service that was available (within the "guide cost") for most people would cost more than the guide cost for people with learning disability, who, because of behavioral difficulties, required a special service. If this did arise, one way in which it could be handled is by deciding whether to buy the service with reference to the cost for the population in general. If the service turned out to be cost-effective for the population as a whole then it could be made available for all regardless of any other condition that might affect the individual cost. This might lead to the health authority paying more than its guide price for a subgroup of people. It remains an ethical issue as to whether it is right for more to be paid for this subgroup. The point, however, that we wish to emphasize is that the problem of "double jeopardy" does not often arise, and when it does it can probably be dealt with through the method outlined above.

RESOURCE ALLOCATION IN THE REAL WORLD

We have focused, in this chapter, on the ethical framework that informs a process of decision making for the allocation of health resources. There are other factors, of course, that are outside this framework and that a decision-making process has to take into account. These other factors include political concerns: local factors such as issues dealing with community hospital pro-

vision, and national factors. The British NHS has recently set up the National Institute of Clinical Excellence (NICE) [available online at www.nice.org.uk], which considers the evidence for effectiveness of some, but by no means all, new treatments. It is yet to be seen how the individual health authorities respond when NICE judges an expensive treatment to be effective, with the implication that it should be provided by the NHS, but a health authority considers it too expensive, and that overall, given the other demands on its budget, it is not cost-effective.

CONCLUSIONS

We have argued that the question of how scarce health-care resources should be allocated cannot be solved by specifying the criteria for a just process, important though this is. Such a process will involve a group of people who need guidance from philosophical analysis in coming to decisions. Based on our experience with a process for making allocation decisions within the British National Health Service, we propose a framework for decision making that allows cost-effectiveness to be combined with other values. We identify six specific ethical issues that any group empowered to make allocation decisions will need to tackle.

APPENDIX

The Oxfordshire Priorities Forum

The Oxfordshire Health Authority is responsible for the health care of everyone who lives in the County of Oxfordshire: a total of about 600,000 people. The city of Oxford is the largest city or town in the county, with a population of about 120,000. The county, is predominantly rural. The Health Authority receives a budget from the government—as part of the NHS–and has the responsibility of using this money to purchase the health care for the population it serves. The Health Authority pays for almost all the hospital care that is provided by the NHS and the cost of drug treatment provided both by hospitals and in primary care. The government also provides some money directly to primary care so that some services and drugs can be purchased on behalf of patients by primary care doctors independently of the Health Authority. In practice, however, primary care physicians usually follow the decisions made by the authority, particularly with regard to rationing decisions.

The process that has been developed for deciding on priority setting and rationing focuses on the Priorities Forum (Hope et al., 1998). This forum is a subcommittee of the Oxfordshire Health Authority and reports its advice to the public meetings of the authority. Strictly speaking, the Priorities Forum is advisory and it is the board of the Health Authority that makes the final decisions. In practice, the board normally follows the forum's advice. The forum brings together primary care physicians from across the county, medical directors of the local hospital trusts, Health Authority staff (both medical personnel and others, such as the finance director), hospital doctors and nurses, and nonexecutive lay members of the Health Authority. Members of the local community health council, which is the body that represents patients' interests within the NHS, attend as observers. They did not wish to participate as voting members so as to remain independent of the decisions taken, as these decisions involve choosing between the interests of different patient groups.

During the early years of the forum's existence it became clear that some of its decisions were inconsistent with previous decisions. Furthermore, although the Priorities Forum provided a process for making decisions, the grounds on which these were made were not always apparent. The forum decided, therefore, that it should articulate an "ethical framework" with three main aims:

1. To help in the structuring of discussions and ensure that key points were properly considered.

2. To help ensure consistency of the decision making, both from one meeting to another, and with respect to decisions concerning different clinical settings.

3. To enable the Priorities Forum to articulate the reasons for its decisions. This is crucial both for an appeals procedure and to enable the forum's methods of working to be open and transparent. This framework has guided the forum's work for three years. As originally articulated it has proved to be insufficiently detailed, particularly in describing how the values of cost-effectiveness and equity should be combined, and in clarifying how equity is to be understood.

The Ethical Framework

The original ethical framework was structured around three main components: evidence for effectiveness; equity; and patient choice.

Evidence of effectiveness

The framework distinguishes effectiveness, value, impact, and efficiency. The main purpose in making these distinctions is to help the Priorities Forum distinguish between factual statements and value judgments.

"Effectiveness" is the extent to which a treatment (or other health-care intervention) achieves a desired effect (for example, the proportion of patients who would be expected to show the effect). Effectiveness is a matter of fact, although the evidence may be incomplete and some judgment may need to be made as to the likely effectiveness of an intervention based on the evidence available.

"Value" is a judgment as to the value of the effect in the relevant patient group, relative to the value of other treatments. A treatment that saves the life of young adults and restores them to full fitness is of high value. A treatment that removes a slight blemish from an unexposed part of the body would normally be of low value.

"Impact" is the value of an intervention weighted for the degree of effectiveness.

"Efficiency" is the impact per unit cost.

The evidence of effectiveness for a particular intervention can fall broadly into one of three categories:

1. There is good evidence that the treatment is not effective.
2. There is good evidence that the treatment is effective.
3. The evidence either way is not good.

It is clear that treatments in the first category should not be funded. Few new drug treatments fall into this category as the licensing system will normally ensure that only effective treatments are licensed. For treatments that fall into the second category the Priorities Forum has to consider the value, impact, and efficiency of the treatment. Treatments that are in the third category are, typically, established treatments that are currently being carried out but which have never been subjected to a proper trial of effectiveness. In judging the quality of the evidence, the Priorities Forum will often benefit from the advice of those expert in the area. When seeking advice, the Forum requires, from the adviser, a full declaration of interests. Forum members have to come to a decision about the quality of evidence, and to weigh this with the value of the intervention. This is, inescapably, a matter of judgment.

Equity

The basic principle of equity is that people in similar situations should be treated similarly. For this reason it is important that there is consistency in the way in which decisions are reached, at different times and in different settings. The principle of equity also requires that no distinction exists in treatment on grounds that are irrelevant to priority for health care. The ethical framework identifies a number of such grounds as irrelevant. These include race, social position, financial status, religion, and place of abode (within the area covered by the local health authority). These basic constraints around equity do not get us very far. The original ethical framework was not explicit about the more contentious aspects of equity. It accepted that the cost-effectiveness of a treatment (or other health-care intervention) as measured, for example, by quality-adjusted life-years (QALYs) (Williams, 1996; Edgar et al., 1998) was important. But it also stated that other considerations should be taken into account. For example, the maximization of welfare (which is the focus of the QALY approach) takes no account of how the welfare is distributed between different people. Equity would seem to require giving some priority to those most in need even if this does not produce the greatest level of welfare overall. The framework did not give much guidance to the Priorities Forum on how it should deal with the different values encapsulated in different theories of resource allocation.

Patient choice

Respecting patient autonomy and choice is a value that the Priorities Forum considers to be important, and it is highlighted by being the third main consideration in the ethical framework. However, it has not proved to be a very useful value in the context of the decisions that the forum has to make. The value of patient choice does have three implications for the work of the Priorities Forum.

1. In assessing research on the effectiveness of a treatment, it is important that the outcome measures used in the research include those that matter to patients.
2. Within those treatments (or other health-care interventions) that are provided, patients should be able to make their own choices as to what they want.
3. Each patient is unique. Good-quality evidence about the effectiveness of an intervention normally addresses outcomes in a large group of people. There may be a good reason to believe that a particular patient stands to gain significantly more from the intervention than most of those who formed the study group in the relevant research. This may justify a particular patient receiving treatment not normally provided.

However, in terms of the decisions that are made at the level of the Health Authority, these considerations are rarely crucial. Normally, the Priorities Forum is making decisions about which treatments should, and which should not, be purchased. The treatments that are not purchased are typically of benefit, but the cost of gaining that benefit is considered to be too great given what the authority can afford. Thus, in practice, the decisions that are made have the effect of limiting treatment opportunities for one group of patients for the sake of other patients. It would normally be inequitable, in the eyes of the forum, to make an exception to a decision not to purchase a particular intervention simply because a patient wishes to have that intervention. One patient's choice may result in another patient's lack of choice.

Types of Decisions the Priorities Forum Has to Make

The Priorities Forum is called on to make a number of different decisions:

1. Whether to normally fund a new treatment or investigation. The most common new treatment is a drug treatment. However, other novel treatments or management methods are also considered.
2. Whether to fund, or cut, a service (such as a small local hospital, or a school health program).
3. Whether the current funding for one area of medicine is equitable compared with another area. For example, are the services available for someone with life-threatening renal disease equitable compared with the services for life-threatening ovarian cancer?
4. Whether a particular medical intervention (for example, some kinds of assisted reproduction) should have a claim on the health budget at all.
5. The Priorities Forum considers a few cases involving individual patients. For example, most patients with a severe eating disorder are treated locally under

a contract between the Health Authority and the local psychiatric hospital trust. Occasionally a patient will ask to be treated at a highly specialized national center for eating disorders on the grounds that the local facilities are not providing effective therapy. Most individual requests are dealt with by the Health Authority staff, but cases raising unusual issues are considered by the Priorities Forum. In such cases the forum has to consider whether the extra resources that would be needed to provide this particular patient with the specialized treatment should be made available and whether it is fair to do so taking into consideration other patients with a similar condition, and other patients more generally.

REFERENCES

Anand, S. and Hanson, K. (1997). Disability-adjusted life years: A critical review. *Journal of Health Economics* 16, 685–702.

Broome, J. (1988). Good, fairness and QALYs. In J.M. Bell and S. Mendus (eds.), *Philosophy and Medical Welfare*. Cambridge: Cambridge University Press.

Daniels, N. (1980). Health care needs and distributive justice. *Philosophy and Public Affairs* 10, 147–76.

Daniels, N. (1985). *Just Health Care—Studies in Philosophy and Health Policy*. Cambridge: Cambridge University Press.

Daniels, N. (2000). Accountability for reasonableness in private and public health insurance. In A. Coulter and C. Ham (eds.), *The Global Challenge of Health Care Rationing*. Buckingham, UK: Open University Press, pp. 89–106.

Daniels, N. and Sabin, J. (1997). Limits to health care: Fair procedures, democratic deliberation and the legitimacy problem for insurers. *Philosophy and Public Affairs*. 26, 303–50.

Doyal, L. and Gough, I. (1984). A theory of human needs. *Critical Social Policy* 4, 6–38.

Edgar, A., Salek, S., Shickle, D., and Cohen, D. (1998). *The Ethical QALY—Ethical Issues in Healthcare Resource Allocations*. Haslemere, UK: Euromed Communications.

Griffiths, S., Reynolds, J. and Hope, T. (2000). Priority setting in practice. In A. Coulter and C. Ham (eds.), *The Global Challenge of Health Care Rationing*. Buckingham, UK: Open University Press, pp. 203–13.

Hadorn, D. (1991). Setting health care priorities in Oregon. Cost-effectiveness meets the rule of rescue. *JAMA* 265, 2218–25.

Harris, J. (1985). *The Value of Life: An Introduction to Medical Ethics.* London: Routledge.

Harris, J. (1987). QALYfying the value of human life. *Journal of Medical Ethics* 13, 117–23.

Harris, J. (1988). More and better justice. In J.M. Bell and S. Mendus (eds.), *Philosophy and Medical Welfare.* Cambridge: Cambridge University Press.

Harris, J. (1995). Double jeopardy and the veil of ignorance—A reply. *Journal of Medical Ethics* 21, 151–57.

Holm, S. (1998). Goodbye to the simple solutions: The second phase of priority setting in health care. *British Medical Journal* 317, 1000–1002.

Hope, T., Hicks, N., Reynolds, D.J.M., Crisp, R. and Griffiths, S. (1998). Rationing in the Health Authority. *British Medical Journal* 317, 1067–69.

Hope, T. (2001). Rationing and life-saving treatment: Should identifiable patients have higher priority? *Journal of Medical Ethics* 27, 179–185.

Klein, R. (1998). Puzzling out priorities. *British Medical Journal* 317, 959–60.

Lockwood, M. (1988). Quality of life and resource association. In J.M. Bell and S. Mendus (eds.), *Philosophy and Medical Welfare.* Cambridge: Cambridge University Press.

Martin, D.K., and Singer, P.A. (2000). Priority setting and health technology assessment: Beyond evidence-based medicine and cost-effectiveness analysis. In A. Coulter and C. Ham (eds.), *The Global Challenge of Health Care Rationing.* Buckingham, UK: Open University Press, pp. 135–45.

Murray, C.J.L. (1994). Quantifying the burden of disease: The technical basis for disability-adjusted life-years. *Bulletin of World Health Organisation* 72, 429–45.

Murray, C.J.L. and Acharya, A.K. (1997). Understanding QALYs. *Journal of Health Economics* 16, 703–30.

Nicholson, T. and Milne, R. (1999). Beta-interferons (1a and 1b) in relapsing-remitting and secondary progressive multiple sclerosis. Southampton, UK: Wessex Institute for Health, Research and Development; 1999 June. Development and Evaluation Committee Report no. 98.

Rawls, J. (1972). *A Theory of Justice.* Oxford: Oxford University Press.

Singer, P. McKie, J., Kuhse, H. and Richardson, J. (1995). Double jeopardy and the use of QALYs in health care allocation. *Journal of Medical Ethics* 21, 144–50.

Williams, A. (1996). QALYs and ethics—a health economist's view. *Society for the Science of Medicine* 43, 1795–1804.

12

Resources and Rights: Court Decisions in the United Kingdom

Richard H. S. Tur

This chapter is about the judicial review of resource-allocation decisions by what I shall call "primary institutions." Such primary institutions include public authorities responsible for health care, for welfare, and for education. Among "some very obvious generalizations—indeed truisms—concerning human nature and the world," Hart[1] included "limited resources." Primary institutions inevitably encounter this truth, sometimes in heart-rending and tragic circumstances. Understandably, their resource-allocation decisions can cause acute disappointment, and sometimes they are challenged in the courts by way of application for judicial review. This chapter seeks to explore and learn from the styles of reasoning deployed by judges in exercising their review function with respect to resource-allocation decisions of primary institutions.

These concerns grow in part out of current debate in Britain not only as to the future, if any, of the welfare state in general and the National Health Service (NHS) in

particular, but also as to the legitimacy of judicial review, which appears to some people to lack sufficient, if any, democratic warrant but which has nonetheless become well established as a central feature in the relationship between the citizen and the state in modern Britain. The growth in public law in the last third of the twentieth century is indeed remarkable.[2] By the time of this writing it had become a commonplace that the British welfare state was seriously underresourced[3] by the national government, which claimed electoral warrant for and curried electoral favor with their low-taxation policies. Accordingly, it appears that by the late 1990s in Britain, judicial review had become increasingly a means for asserting health and welfare claims against primary institutions, seriously starved of resources and stretched still further by the increasing costs of a widening range of expensive drugs[4] and medical procedures.[5] Long-term health care had a cumulative effect on resources, and for some the policy of "care in the community" meant the closure of their only and permanent home, whereas for others the closure of such institutions had become an economic necessity.[6]

These debates were sometimes played out in the courts. More often than not the judicial debates turned upon classical rule-based reasoning by way of interpretation of statutes that appeared to impose obligations on primary institutions struggling to discharge them for want of resources. Given that successive governments showed no readiness openly to repeal such duty-imposing statutes, attempts were made, sometimes successfully, to reconstruct the statutory schemes as merely empowering rather than requiring provision of health care and welfare services.[7] Such reconstruction allows the legislation to remain on the statute book and thereby saves the government any political embarrassment associated with repeal or amendment while liberating the primary institutions from any duty to expend resources, thereby permitting government to adhere to a policy of low taxation. Robust judicial interpretation reaffirming the existence of statutory duties maintains pressure on primary institutions and through them on government to deliver the necessary resources by increased taxation if necessary. However, early in the new millennium there have been government promises of significant new resources for the NHS over the next 10 years. Even if these promises are honored in full, resource-allocation questions will inevitably require answers from primary institutions.

Sometimes judges have reached beyond rule-based reasoning toward reasoning based on secular rights. Thus, in one case[8] where the primary institution had decided on economic grounds to close a long-term residential facility, in addition to other independently convincing arguments, the court expressly invoked Article 8(1) of the European Convention of Human Rights, which enshrines the right that everyone has to respect for their private and family life and their home. Miss Coughlan had been grievously injured in a road traffic accident in 1971. She is tetraplegic; doubly incontinent, requiring regular catheterization; partially paralyzed in the respiratory tract, with consequent difficulty in breathing; and subject not only to the attendant problems of immobility but to recurrent headaches caused by an associated neurological condition. She had been promised a "home for life" and the extent to which the public cost was going to be reduced by moving her was not dramatic. She regarded the loss of her accommodation as "life-threatening," but even if that was thought "unreal" the court recognized that the enforced move could not be other than "emotionally devastating and seriously anti-therapeutic." The trade-off for the economies included a clear breach of a plain promise and the loss of her only home and a purpose-built environment, which meant more to her than a home does to most people. The court readily concluded that by closing the residential facility the primary institution had reached a decision that could not be justified given the substantial interference with human rights.

In another and tragic case "Child B" was denied further medical treatment for acute myeloid leukemia, in circumstances giving rise to allegations that the primary institution had reached its negative decision exclusively on resource-allocation grounds. The ensuing public debate and judicial hearings showed the primary institution's position to be somewhat more complex, but insofar as the case focused attention on the resources issue, the difference in reasoning between Mr. Justice Laws (as he then was) in the Divisional Court and Sir Thomas Bingham MR in the Court of Appeal is important and instructive.

One significant implication is that medical and management decisions may, perhaps must, be distinguished. In practice, medical and management decisions may shade imperceptibly into each other, but in principle medical decisions may be subject to "relaxed" scrutiny because they involve professional medical judgment, whereas management decisions may be subject to

more "rigorous" scrutiny because such decisions are inherently more susceptible to
infection by irrelevant considerations. This
further distinction, between levels of judicial scrutiny (or review), is more familiar
to American than to British lawyers, but it
is essential to a proper understanding of
the role of rights in public law adjudication, and is increasingly important in British courts especially as influenced by the
European Convention of Human Rights
under the rather opaque heading of "proportionality." Such rights-based reasoning
is flexible and scalar in that it contemplates
degrees of justification depending on the
weight of the individual right, the importance of the state interest, and the appropriateness or fit of the means adopted. In
such a decisional matrix, resources may be
relevant to a degree which is dependent on
context. By comparison, rule-based reasoning is rigid and polar. In English public law
a decision by a primary institution can be
quashed if it took irrelevant considerations
into account or if it failed to take relevant
considerations into account. This has led to
framing the resource-allocation question in
the context of judicial review as asking
whether resources are irrelevant or relevant. And the answer to that question in
turn means that resources have either no
weight or weigh so very heavily as to be
near-conclusive.

Mr. Justice Laws thought that "fundamental rights . . . [have] . . . a secure home
in the common law" and that even a
"modest chance . . . of longer survival had
to be unimaginably precious." I call this
"rights-based" reasoning. Human rights,
including the right to life, are so deep and
fundamental as to require very weighty reasons indeed to be overridden. In the opinion of Mr. Justice Laws the primary institution had simply not adequately explained
or justified the funding priorities that had
led to its decision not to provide further
treatment for "Child B." Accordingly, he
quashed that decision and required the
health authority to reconsider, but he re-

fused to make an order requiring the health
authority to fund the treatment.

In contrast, Sir Thomas Bingham in the
Court of Appeal treated medical and management decisions as cut from the same
cloth and, just as it is not and cannot be
part of a court's function to make medical
judgments, so neither is a court in a position to decide on the correctness of the difficult and agonizing judgments that had to
be made by primary institutions as to how
a limited budget was best allocated to the
best advantage of the maximum number of
patients. Clinical decisions must therefore
always be taken by primary institutions
with due regard to the resources available,
and the courts should be slow to intervene.
With respect, I submit that there was no
attempt by Mr. Justice Laws simply to assess substantively the correctness of either
medical or managerial decisions concerning
"Child B." Rather, he took the view that
the right put at risk by these decisions was
so significant that a compelling justification
was necessary in law and that the primary
institution had not, in his judgment, produced sufficient justification. Far from attempting to substitute his own decision—
for example, by requiring the primary institution to fund the treatment—Mr. Justice Laws simply referred the matter back
to the primary institution for reconsideration. Accordingly, the two judges differed
not so much as to the relevance of resources but as to the point at which limited
resources ceases to be a sufficient justification for infringing a right as fundamental
as the right to life.

To facilitate exploration of styles of judicial reasoning, I adopt and explain a tripartite historical analysis of phases of judicial reasoning in British courts: (1)
natural law; (2) legal positivism; (3) secular
human rights. My interest is ultimately to
explore whether what I call "secular rights-
based judicial reasoning," which I claim to
be a current, or emergent, strand in English
courts generally, and increasingly visible in
public law adjudication, is at all apt in as-

sessing the quality and merits of answers to difficult questions about allocation of resources reached by primary institutions and whether such reasoning can ever legitimate decisions contrary to government policy or the "plain meaning" of enacted legislation. The discussion is informed by several recent high-profile and controversial decisions of the appellate courts in the English legal system. Although the cases analyzed are from one jurisdiction and the context of the problem addressed is given by the institutional and economic arrangement peculiar to Britain, I hope that the analysis will nonetheless generate insights of some general philosophical interest and validity.

The "mighty problem"[9] of judicial review is the problem of legitimacy: On what basis, if at all, can such judicial intervention be justified? The problem is exacerbated by populist conceptions of democracy, which find unelected judges overriding the clearly stated intentions of a duly elected legislature odd and open to question. Indeed, some legal theorists take the view that in an ideal legal system the judiciary would be constrained by relatively specific rules and not qualified to overrule otherwise valid legislation either by invocation of general principles of common law or principles of civil liberties and human rights.[10]

Natural law thinking is the first of three distinctive historical and theoretical answers to the mighty question. Here the core notion is the pre-eminence of "God's law." In the seventeenth century the common law was understood as the perfection of right reason itself[11] and that which was not consonant with Holy Scripture in the law of England was not the law of England.[12] Nothing that is not reason or religion is law. On such a view there is ready-made justification for restricting the scope or even nullifying statutes made by the legislature, should the need arise, because any statute inconsistent with right reason or religion is simply invalid.[13] Judicial review of primary legislation is an integral and non-problematic component of this system of thought, and something like this grounded the American constitutional tradition.

Natural law also grounds two great principles of natural justice: (1) *nemo judex in rem suam*—not to be judge in one's own cause; and (2) *audi alteram partem*—to hear both sides. Compliance with these principles is widely—and rightly—regarded as basic to the fairness of decision making. But although these principles have endured they cannot of themselves guide the resource-allocation decisions of primary institutions or adequately equip the judiciary to review such decisions. Furthermore, the metaphysical and epistemological burdens of moving beyond these core procedural principles toward substantive principles of (distributive) justice and fairness are signigicant, and the fruits of such intellectual labors would be highly controversial. In any event, as a historically and sociologically valid system of thought, natural law was replaced over time by legal positivism.

The core notion of *legal positivism* is that law is an artefact of human will. As this plays out in English constitutional and legal history it leads to the pre-eminence of "man's law" and hence to "parliamentary sovereignty"—the doctrine that all that a court can do with an act of Parliament is apply it—and the denial of judicial review of primary legislation. The natural law system of thought was only gradually replaced by the legal positivist approach, but sometime in the nineteenth century and no later than 1871 the transition was complete. In that year the courts held that Parliament could even pass a law making one judge in one's own cause, although absent clear words to that effect the courts would assume that the intention of Parliament was not to do so.[14] In judicial review of secondary legislation and administrative decision making, this system of thought grounds the doctrine of *ultra vires*—that is, the principle that only rules or decisions authorized by primary legislation are *intra vires* or within the powers of the subordinate rule or decision maker and anything else may be set aside by the court. The major difficulty with this position is that as long as a government takes care to ensure that its subordinate rule and decision-making agencies have been clearly granted the powers exercised, there is little, or nothing, that the courts can do to protect the citizen from the state. Nevertheless, British judges deployed considerable ingenuity and imagination—mostly by way of canons of statutory interpretation—to reach beyond the formal question of *vires* toward substantive principles of (distributive) justice and fairness.

The history of judicial review in Britain has given special weight to rule-based reasoning and, until the final third of the twentieth century, judicial quietism prevailed. The *locus classicus* is *Associated Provincial Picture Houses Ltd* v. *Wednesbury Corporation*[15] The local authority had the power to grant licences for the opening of cinemas subject to such conditions as the authority "thought fit." The authority, when granting a Sunday licence, imposed a condition that no child under 15 be admitted. The question for the court was whether there are any limits on the exercise of discretion. The court took the view that there are limits, including unreasonableness, bad faith, dishonesty, taking account of irrelevant considerations, not taking account of relevant considerations, disregard of proper procedure, and so on. As to "unreasonableness," the test propounded in that case was whether the authority had acted so unreasonably that no reasonable authority could have reached the decision. This was glossed by Lord Diplock in a later case[16] as limiting judicial intervention to a decision "so outrageous in its defiance of logic or of accepted moral standards that no sensible person who had applied his mind to the question to be decided could have arrived at it."

The strengths and weaknesses of this approach are obvious. It preserves the integrity of the decision of the primary institution. Only where the decision of the primary institution is unlawful, procedurally flawed, or completely mad can the courts legitimately intervene. But the disadvantage of this is that instances exist where the exercise of a discretion, though lawful, procedurally correct, and not completely mad, nonetheless generates legitimate criticism and tempts activist judges to intervene. Thus, in a recent case Lord Justice Mummery observed, "In examining the decision-making with an over-critical eye, there is a danger that a legitimate exercise in review of legality becomes an impermissible appeal on the merits and that imperfections in the process are equated with irrationality in the result."[17] There is, in short, a tendency for the review court to reach to the merits of the decision of the primary institution. A like tendency, no less controversial, is seen in the move in American constitutional adjudication from procedural due process to substantive due process.[18]

In Britain, there has been significant movement since the landmark decision a half century ago, and we are now well beyond "the crude bludgeon" of *Wednesbury*. Reviewing the cases suggests a development from self-imposed judicial restraint to a form of qualified activism, and a sea-change in justificatory judicial rhetoric and, in particular, a move from rule-based to rights-based reasoning. In 1948, and for quite some time after, only a wholly mad decision could be quashed; if a decision survived all other tests it was very unlikely to be quashed as "unreasonable." However, cases in the 1960s and 1970s show the courts inching beyond *Wednesbury*, albeit by stealth, and primary decisions slightly less than wholly mad may sometimes be quashed as "unreasonable." Somewhere hereabouts *ultra vires* reasoning begins to be perceived and described by commentators and occasionally by judges as "unreal" and merely "a fig leaf."

In the 1970s and 1980s the common law was afforced by back-door absorption as persuasive of ideas and reasoning based on the European Convention of Human Rights, and some tentative use of ideas such "proportionality" and "co-sovereignty" suggest that novel ideas were being grafted on and starting some kind of sea-change in the idiom of legal justification. Hereabouts, some believe, lies the corpse of the doctrine of parliamentary sovereignty, though, rather like Bentham, it has been stuffed and is wheeled around by some minders as if still alive and kicking.

In the 1990s, courts and the legislature sought were boldly to "bring home" rights, culminating in the passage into law of the Human Rights Act in 1998 and fully in effect toward the end of 2000. This made explicit the sea-change, although the enabling human rights (and devolution) legislation still pays lip service to the continuing sovereignty of Parliament and still presupposes the unitary state. Under the Act, primary (Westminster) legislation cannot be disapplied by the courts even if adjudged to be contrary to European Convention rights, but primary decisions can be quashed even though procedurally impeccable and comfortably *intra vires* if substantively defective as measured against a cluster of secular human rights, at least where no compelling justification has been provided by the primary institution under review. This suggests that the reasoning of Sir John Laws in *ex parte B*, invoking human rights as a ground for inviting a primary institution to reconsider was approximately five years ahead of its time.

Hereabouts notions of legal pluralism may quietly begin to take root and local legal norms may sometimes be subject to qualification by global principles of human rights. Change is increasingly necessary, therefore, in legal theory, and the concept of law and the "hard" outlines of classical legal positivism are softened.[19] The point here is not whether these diluted positivist theories work as philosophical constructs but how they reflect the *Zeitgeist*. Hegel observed that "when philosophy paints its grey on grey, then has a shape of life grown old . . . the owl of Minerva spreads its wings only with the falling of the dusk."[20] The suggestion is that classical legal positivism has grown old. However, that may reflect my conceit that I am writing about an epoch-making movement in the history of my subject. But Hegel warned against such self-importance: "The materials are patent to every writer: each is likely enough to believe himself capable of arranging and manipulating them; and we may expect that each will insist upon his own spirit as that of the age in question."[21] Perhaps the perception of an emergent new form of legal life is fanciful and prediction hazardous. Nonetheless, the future may involve "chartering" the Human Rights Act 1998 (as in Canada), so as to subject even primary (Westminster) legislation to judicial (secular human rights) review.

As to *secular human rights* reasoning, two dicta of Lord Bridge are important in understanding its nature. First, in an asylum-seeker's case he said,

I approach the question raised by the challenge to the Secretary of State's decision on the basis of the law stated earlier in this opinion, *viz.* that the resolution of any issue of fact and the exercise of any discretion in relation to an application for asylum as a refugee lie exclusively within the jurisdiction of the Secretary of State subject only to the court's power of review. The limitations on the scope of that power are well known and need not be restated here. Within those limitations the court must, I think, be entitled to subject an administrative decision to the more rigorous examination, to ensure that it is in no way flawed, according to the gravity of the issue which the decision determines. The most fundamental of all human rights is the individual's right to life, and when an administrative decision under challenge is said to be one which may put the applicant's life at risk, the basis of the decision must surely call for the most anxious scrutiny.[22]

Second, in a later case concerning the power of government ministers to direct broadcasters to refrain from airing direct speech by persons representing terrorist groups, he said,

I do not accept that . . . the courts are powerless to prevent the exercise by the executive of administrative discretions, even when conferred, as in the instant case, in terms which are on their face unlimited, in a way which infringes fundamental human rights. . . . [W]e are . . . perfectly entitled to start from the premise that any restriction of the right to freedom of expression requires to be justified and that nothing less than an important competing public interest will be sufficient to justify it.[23]

In these two passages, Lord Bridge anticipates increasing use by British judges of the European Convention of Human Rights as a basis for their reasoning and as a justification for their decisions. That use has been given increased impetus by the Human Rights Act 1998, which does not yet fully incorporate the European Convention into domestic law but certainly more directly integrates it than hitherto.[24] Although these are controversial issues, one can only expect the use of rights-based reasoning to increase both generally and in respect of the allocation of health care and welfare resources.

In *R v. Gloucestershire County Council and another ex parte Barry*,[25] the English House of Lords considered services for and assessment of the needs of sick and disabled persons and faced the question of whether a primary institution can, in assessing and reassessing needs, take into account the effect on its resources. Michael Barry, 79 years of age and severely disabled, lived alone in his own home and had no contact with his family. In 1992 his local authority assessed his needs as requiring home care help twice a week for shopping, collecting his pension, laundry and cleaning, and meals on wheels four days a week. Under section 2(1) of the Chronically Sick and Disabled Persons Act 1970, if a local authority was satisfied that it was necessary to make arrangements in order to meet the needs of a chronically sick or disabled person it was the "duty of that authority to make those arrangements." In September 1994 the local authority informed Michael Barry that it would no longer be able to

provide services to meet his full needs as assessed and that the cleaning and laundry services would be withdrawn because it had suffered a cut of £2.5 million in the funds allocated by the central government. The Court of Appeal accepted, by two judges to one, that a person's needs depended on the nature and extent of his disability and could not be affected by, or depend on, the local authority's ability to meet them. However, by a majority of three to two, the House of Lords reversed, holding that for the purposes of section 2(1) of the 1970 *as is or* Disabled Persons Act 1970 Act, a chronically sick or disabled person's "needs" were to be assessed by taking into account the cost of providing the benefit and the impact that that cost would have on its resources, which in turn would depend on the authority's financial position. In short, a chronically sick or disabled person's need for services could not sensibly be assessed without having some regard to the cost of providing them. This important decision affirms the style of argument adopted and the conclusion reached by the Court of Appeal in Child B's case to the effect that, in assessing medical needs, due regard must be taken of the resources available.

By contrast, in a later case, *R v. East Sussex County Council, ex parte Tandy*,[26] the House of Lords held unanimously that the resources available were irrelevant in the determination of educational needs. Beth Tandy was born in February 1982 and was thus a child of compulsory school age until February 1998. She had suffered from myalgic encephalomyelitis since the age of seven, in consequence of which she found it very difficult and at times impossible to attend school. From May 1992 onwards her local education authority had provided five hours per week home tuition for her under section 298 of the Education Act of 1993 (now re-enacted in section 19 of the Education Act 1996). Under section 298 each local education authority was required to make arrangements for the provision of suitable full-time or part-time education at school or otherwise than at school for those children of compulsory school age who, by reason of, *inter alia,* illness, might not otherwise receive suitable education.

In October 1996 the education authority gave notice that, for financial reasons, the maximum number of hours of home tuition provided under section 298 would be reduced from five hours per week to three. On judicial review of that decision, the judge held that the education authority had taken into account an irrelevant factor (i.e., the shortage of resources) when deciding to reduce the number of hours of home tuition, that the decision was made in pursuit of an ulterior purpose, namely the reduction of expenditure, and that it was irrational. The Court of Appeal, however, reversed this decision by a majority on the ground that it was legitimate for the education authority to take into account the shortage of resources. In unanimously reversing the Court of Appeal, the House of Lords held that on a true construction of section 298 of the Education Act 1993, there was no reason to treat the resources of a local education authority as a relevant factor in determining what constituted "suitable education." However, if there was more that one way of providing "suitable education," the education authority would be entitled to have regard to its resources in choosing between different ways of making such provision. It followed that the decision of the education authority to reduce the hours of home tuition provided to Beth Tandy for financial reasons was unlawful. Lord Browne-Wilkinson stressed that "the courts should be slow to downgrade such duties into what are, in effect, mere discretions."

This is perceived as a preferable outcome to that in Michael Barry's case, which was only distinguished and not overruled, but any rejoicing should be tempered by the realization that nearly all such cases have turned primarily on questions of statutory interpretation. The question is whether Parliament intended to impose and did impose a duty rather than a power. In a sense, Beth Tandy's case affirms "rights," but only in a very narrow sense, as the correlative of a legal duty. Therefore, this decision, like that in Michael Barry's case, better fits the *legal positivism* paradigm than the model of *secular human rights.* There is something philosophically displeasing about embedding questions of "need" in questions of resources. In the British context it is particularly questionable that primary institutions should be able to convert duties into powers by tolling the bell of scarce resources, not least because this allows the central government to maintain the popular policy of low taxation without being associated with the unpopular consequences of denying health care, welfare provision, and education to the needy. In the history of British legal and political debate, members of the judiciary have usually been perceived as hostile toward the welfare state, but on the basis of Beth Tandy's case, the judges emerge as its defenders.

But the style of reasoning whereby the judges defend the welfare state is highly unsatisfactory. On *Tandy* reasoning, even the most trivial duty trumps even the most compelling power, and a primary institution ought to fulfil all its duties in preference to exercising any of its powers; Suppose an authority [A] has (say) five duties (a, b, c, d, and e) and (say) three powers (x, y, and z). Suppose too, albeit implausibly, that all five duties and all three powers cost exactly the same, say, 1,000 Euros each to deliver. Consider the following two hypothetical resource situations: (1) A has 7,000 Euros and (2) A has 4,000 Euros. On the first hypothesis, A has sufficient resources to discharge all duties and some powers; *Tandy* says fulfill all these duties but it offers no guidance as to prioritizing powers. On the second hypothesis, A has not even enough resources to fulfill all duties, but *Tandy* provides no guidance as to prioritizing duties.

Furthermore, the *Tandy* presupposition means that even if A prioritizes its duties and powers for good and sufficient reasons, say, as follows: *a, z, e, y, d, c, x, b*; *A* must nonetheless allow lesser duties to trump greater powers. Of course, the idea that a power may be more important than a duty might appear counterintuitive, but where, as in Child B's case, the power relates to life and death it may well be rational and desirable to exercise the power even at the cost of not fulfilling some duty. In other words, mapping legal powers and duties against secular human rights may produce a prioritizing that does not subordinate all powers to all duties. To accept *Tandy* as rational, one would have to claim that Parliament always perfectly matched the power/duty distinction to minor and major goods. But such matching may not even have been in the draftsman's contemplation—*a fortiori* given that different powers and duties may be vested at different times under different statutes in the same authority, leaving the authority to prioritize among powers and duties that the draftsman and the parliamentarians may not even have juxtaposed in their thinking.

The idea that Parliament intended *A* to fulfil duty *b* (imposed, say, by a statute in 1981) rather than exercise power *y* (vested, say, by a statute in 1995) is unreal. The reality may be that *b* and *y* were never weighed against each other in the thinking of those participating in the legislative process. Further, if the matter had been contemplated by a legislature already attuned to *Tandy* reasoning the 1995 statute might have imposed *y* as a duty in order to prevent it being subordinated to *b*. But even then, a legislature already attuned to *Tandy* reasoning could not, as long as that case holds sway, prioritize *y* over *b* because *Tandy* supposes that all duties are equal, whereas it may be that some duties are more compelling than others. What we need are principles allowing for reasoned choices between competing duties and for preferring a compelling power to a less compelling duty. Perhaps mapping duties and powers against human rights could achieve this. I do not believe that statutory interpretation can achieve it, least of all a closed-code, literalist mode of statutory interpretation as is encountered in *Tandy* and in *Barry*.

Moreover, statutory interpretation is uncertain, unreliable, and potentially unprincipled. For example, the eight appellate judges who considered the relevance of resources in Michael Barry's case divided four-four. Section 3 of the Human Rights Act 1998 will, when it is fully in force, require judges in Britain not to apply statutes exclusively in terms of their literal meeting but as far as possible in a manner consistent with the European Convention of Human Rights. I suspect that this will take us away from the literalism of *legal positivism* and move us toward rights-based reasoning. It may be that there is insufficient guidance in Bills, Charters and Conventions of Rights, but the alternative method for determining questions of the allocation of health-care resources, as I understand it, namely the notion of the quality-adjusted life-year (QALY) seems far too computational. That, I believe, revisits in a new guise the philosophical chestnut of utilitarianism versus rights to which I now turn.

The metaphor of "trumps" for rights "in the strong sense"[27] is commonplace. On this view even the smallest individual right overrides even the largest collective interest. But, as a matter of historical and sociological fact, collective interests sometimes override individual rights, especially if these interests are regarded as "compelling." Assuming that at least some of these instances are morally defensible, the conceptual primacy of rights over interests is difficult to sustain. However, various moves can be made at this point to preserve the primacy of rights. First, interests could be reinterpreted as rights so that the question is reformulated as a competition between two rights of which one may have more weight, just as a low trump card loses the trick to a higher card. But if such reinterpretation of interests is alway possible, the problem of the relationship of rights and interests is not so much explained as explained away. And if some interests prove resistant to reinterpretation, the move saves only some appearances and is not a complete answer.

Second, some theorists take refuge in the limiting case of moral catastrophe, in which all intellectual bets are off.[28] An illustrative argument here is that if sleep deprivation will certainly cause the suspect to reveal where the bombs are hidden surely the compelling interest in saving many lives should be resistant to the suspect's right not to be tortured and accordingly the right should not trump the interest.[29] But even if one accepts this limiting move at face value—though it is worrisome that the right should be most easily dispensed with when it is needed most—this move does not save the appearances because, in fact, there are many cases where the cost of compliance with a right is high but not catastrophic, and yet the collective interest justifiably prevails over the individual right.

Third, one might abandon the concept of rights altogether. An extreme act-utilitarian decides all cases directly by reference to the principle of utility. There is no need or place for rights. A crude rule-utilitarian adopts a two-tier decision-making process such that decisions are justified by rules and rules justified by the principle of utility. Even if—in a hard case—it should happen that faithful application of the justified rule generates an outcome inconsistent with what direct application of the principle would require, the rule-determined outcome prevails. Again, there is no need or place for rights. A more sophisticated rule-utilitarian decisional matrix accommodates "rights" as a side constraint or filter that precludes certain types of decisions even if generated by faithful application of the justified rule. In such cases "the evil of observing the rule might surpass the evil of breaking it."[30] A weakness of this rule-utilitarian accommodation of rights is that rights must be understood as commensurable with interests—otherwise how could one know that the evil of compliance surpasses that of deviance—which presup-

poses that all rights are consequentialist and none are deontological. But if all rights are treated as consequentialist then this sophisticated rule-utilitarian approach actually obliterates the concept of a right while retaining the language of rights to refer to a certain cluster of privileged consequences. This approach proves on analysis to be exclusively consequential and, like its utilitarian cousins, has no need or place for rights, properly so-called. Although some so-called rights are perhaps susceptible of reduction to consequences without remainder, others seem somehow deeper or more fundamental and, therefore, resistant to recasting as consequentialist. For Hart, if there are any natural rights, "freedom" is one, and Dworkin emphasizes the "same" or "equal concern and respect."[31] Other deontological candidates include human dignity and privacy. Such deontological rights are found enshrined in constitutional documents such as the American Bill of Rights, the Canadian Charter, and the European Convention. But important as they undoubtedly are, even these entrenched categorical rights are susceptible of override by compelling state interests. It follows that the assimilation of rights to trumps is descriptively inaccurate and potentially misleading.

Schauer,[32] like Hart,[33] proposes the different and more appealing metaphor of rights as shields or suits of armor. He observes that there is a difference between the "violation" and the "infringement" of a right. Violation is conceptually tied to remorse and compensation, whereas infringement is not. On this approach a right to X is a right not to have X infringed without a justification of a special strength, and it is a commonplace of constitutional adjudication that there is a sliding scale of justification from "rational" to "compelling" depending on context. Rights can best be understood as shields against governmental interference. This is an important function because governments and their administrative agencies are all too prone to maximize efficiency at the expense of individual liberty and welfare. The shield protects the citizen from unnecessary interference with liberty and welfare and seeks to ensure that any interference is the minimum necessary to achieve the legitimate or compelling state interest.

Frederick Schauer suggests that the concept of a shield is a "useful tool" for explaining both the resistance of rights to interests and the overriding of even categorical rights by sufficiently compelling interests. Whereas a medieval suit of armor might well protect against slings and arrows, it is ineffective against bombs or scud missiles. What one gets with a right is a level of protection but not a guarantee of invincibility. Having a right requires a higher level of justification from government and its agencies. The precise level of justification is dependent on the context, the nature of the individual right at risk, and the nature of the collective interest in play. Taking all these considerations properly into account calls for reasonableness, proportionality, and sound judgment. As Sir Thomas Bingham MR put it, "The more substantial the interference with human rights, the more the court will require by way of justification before it is satisfied that the decision is reasonable"[34] or, as the Court of Appeal subsequently added in *Coughlan*, "fair."[35]

Finally, a cautionary note: The three styles of reasoning stand not in a relationship of supersession but of transcendence, such that the later style includes and goes beyond the earlier one. Thus, secular rights reasoning does not cancel or prevent continued use of rule-based reasoning. There will be cases in which a rights dimension is minimal or nonexistent, and in any event courts may prefer traditional forms of argument wherever possible. Even now one encounters judicial exasperation with "unfocused recourse to . . . [the Strasbourg] jurisdiction, whether before or after the absorption of part of the Convention into the law of England and Wales, [which] is not helpful to the Court. Indeed, it is positively unhelpful . . ."[36] It is no part of the thesis advanced in this chapter that rights-based reasoning is or should be the sole or chief mode of reasoning about resource allocation by primary institutions. However, the metaphor of a shield is a "useful tool" and the ideas that (a) having a right requires higher levels of justification from decision makers and that (b) the more important or fundamental the right, the greater the need for justification, illustrate a specific form of reasoning that may sometimes assist primary institutions faced with difficult and agonizing decisions in the allocation of scarce resources.

NOTES

1. H.L.A. Hart, *The Concept of Law*, 2nd edition. Oxford: Clarendon Press, 1994, pp. 193–200.

2. P. P. Craig, *Administrative Law*, 4th edition London: Sweet & Maxwell, 1999, chap. 2.

3. "It was common knowledge that health authorities were pressed to make ends meet; that they could not provide the payment for nurses, the treatment, the equipment, the research or the buildings that they would like." *R v. Cambridge District Health Authority, ex parte B* [1995] 1 WLR 898, 906 per Sir Thomas Bingham MR. The *London Times* reported on July 13, 200, that "80,000 cancer patients have been denied vital drugs because the NHS cannot afford them, doctors said yesterday. A coalition of cancer specialists reporting on the extent of underfunding for cancer treatments said that another £207 million was needed to give patients the care they required. This would more than double the Government's spending on the drugs, which are often denied to patients depending on whether their local health authorities will pay for them."

4. *R v. North Derby HA ex parte Fisher* (1997) 38 BMLR 76 (beta-interferon); *R v. Secretary of State for Health, ex parte Pfizer Ltd* [1999] Lloyd's Med Rep 289 (viagra). Concern has been expressed about the "tens of millions of pounds" annually that viagra might well cost the National Health Service given figures of 1.8 million who suffer total and eight million who suffer partial erectile dysfunction, and the *Sunday Times* on September 27, 1998, reported with a sense of outrage that "Homosexuals to get Viagra on the NHS."

5. *R v. Cambridge District Health Authority, ex parte B, The Times*, March 15, 1995 (Mr. Justice Laws);[1995] 1 WLR 898 (Court of Ap-

peal): chemotherapy and a second bone marrow transplant; *R v. North West Lancashire Health Authority, ex parte A and others* [1999] Lloyd's Rep Med 399: gender reassignment surgery.

6. *R v. North and East Devon Health Authority, ex parte Coughlan* [2000] 2 WLR 622; a similar case is pending at the time of this writing concerning Orchard Hill Center in Surrey, which provides a home for 110 adults with profound mental and physical handicaps; some of them have lived there for more than 20 years. The patients reside in 15 bungalows on the site, where there is a full range of therapeutic services, including an education center, hydrotherapy pool and a garden, all aimed at giving the patients as good a quality of life as possible. Last year Merton Sutton and Wandsworth Health Authority decided to close the center and send patients to homes in the community, stating that this fitted in with government policy on care in the community. Apparently the site might be sold to developers for about £20,000,000. An application for judicial review of the decision to close the center has now been brought by three parents on behalf of their children who live at Orchard Hill. Media reports suggest that leave was granted on July 31, 2000.

7. *R v. Gloucester CC ex parte Barry* [1996] 4 All ER 421 (Court of Appeal); [1997] AC 584 (House of Lords); *R v. East Sussex CC, ex parte Tandy* [1998] 2 All ER 769.

8. *R v. North and East Devon Health Authority, ex parte Coughlan* [2000] 2 WLR 622, 657–58.

9. M. Cappelletti, "The Law-Making Power of the Judge and Its Limits: A Comparative Analysis" (1981) 8 *Monash Univ. L. Rev.* 15; M. Cappelletti, "The 'Mighty Problem' of Judicial Review and the Contribution of Comparative Analysis" (1980) 53 *Southern Cal L Rev.* 409.

10. Tom D. Campbell, *The Legal Theory of Ethical Positivism.* Aldershot, UK: Dartmouth Publishing, 1996, pp. 116, 161.

11. Sir Edward Coke, *First Institute* (1628), p. 1: "Reason is the life of the law; nay, the common law itself is nothing else but reason. . . . The law, which is perfection of reason. . . ."

12. *R v. Love* (1653) 5 S T 43, 172 per Keble J, "Whatsoever is not consonant to Scripture in the Law of England, is not the Law of England."

13. *Dr Bonham's Case* (1610) 8 Coke's Reports 114, 118: ". . . it appears in our books, that in many cases the common law will control Acts of Parliament and sometime adjudge them to be utterly void: for when an Act of Parliament is against common right or reason, or repugnant, or impossible to be performed, the common law will control it and adjudge such an Act to be void."

14. *Lee v. Bude and Torrington Junction Rly* (1871) LR 6 CP 576.

15. [1948] 1 KB 223.

16. *Council of Civil Service Unions v. Minister for the Civil Service* [1985] AC 374, 410.

17. *R v. East Sussex County Council, ex parte Tandy* [1997] 3 WLR 884.

18. *DeShaney v. Winnebago County Dept of Social Services* 489 US 189 (1989); Eugene W. Hickok and Gary L. McDowell, *Justice vs. Law: Courts and Politics in American Society.* New York: The Free Press, 1993.

19. On "presumptive positivism," see Frederick Schauer, *Playing by the Rules.* Oxford: Clarendon Press, 1992, pp. 196–206, and Frederick Schauer, "The Jurisprudence of Reasons" (1987) 85 *Michigan L. Rev.* 847–70; on "inclusive positivism, see W. J. Waluchow, *Inclusive Legal Positivism.* Oxford: Clarendon Press, 1994; on "soft positivism," see H.L.A Hart, *op cit,* pp. 250–54.

20. T. M. Knox, *Hegel's Philosophy of Right.* Oxford: Oxford University Press, 1976, p. 13.

21. G.W.F Hegel, *The Philosophy of History.* New York: Dover Publications, 1956, p. 7.

22. *R v. Home Secretary, ex parte Bugdaycay* [1987] AC 514, 531.

23. *R v. Home Secretary, ex parte Brind* [1991] 1 AC 696, 748–9.

24. At the time of this writing the Human Rights Act 1998 was not yet in effect in England and Wales but already its anticipatory impact on judicial decision making is evident as shown, for example, by *R v. DPP, ex parte Kebilene and Others; R v. DPP, ex parte Rechachi* [1999] 4 All ER 801 (Queen's Bench Division); [1999] 3 WLR 972 (House of Lords).

25. [1997] AC 584.

26. [1998] 2 All ER 884.

27. Ronald Dworkin, *Taking Rights Seriously.* London: Duckworth, 1981, p. 269: "If someone has a right to do something, then it is wrong for the government to deny it to him even though it would be in the general interest to do so."

28. Ronald Dworkin, *op cit,* p. 191.

29. *See Ireland v. United Kingdom* (1978) 2 E.H.R.R. 25. Some rights are subject to derogation under Article 15 of the European Convention of Human Rights, but neither the right to life (Article 2) nor the freedom from torture (Article 3) is included in the list.

30. John Austin, *The Province of Jurisprudence Determined.* London: Weidenfeld & Nicholson, 1955, p. 53.

31. H.L.A Hart, "Are There Any Natural Rights?" (1955) 64 *Philosophical Rev.*, 175–91; Dworkin, *op cit,* pp. 199, 273.

32. Frederick Schauer, "A Comment on the Structure of Rights" (1993) 27 *Georgia L. Rev.*

415–34. I gratefully acknowledge that my own analysis has been much assisted by this excellent article.

33. H.L.A Hart, "Between Utility and Rights," 79 *Columbia L. Rev.*, 828–46, at 845.

34. *R v. Ministry of Defence, ex parte Smith* [1996] QB 517, 554E.

35. *R v. North and East Devon Health Authority, ex parte Coughlan* [2000] 2 WLR 622, 658.

36. *R v. North West Lancashire Health Authority, ex parte A and others* [1999] Lloyd's Rep Med 399, per Auld LJ. Both Buxton and May LJJ offered similar observations.

13

Justice and the Social Reality of Health: The Case of Australia

Mark Sheehan and Peter Sheehan

Nothing is more fundamental than the span of life and the health that permits life to be lived to the full. In many of the world's poorer countries, life is short and lived in wretched conditions, plagued by avoidable disease. This is undoubtedly the greatest injustice of our time. Yet even in the most developed nations, health outcomes and the life chances to which they give rise are unequally distributed by social class and income level. The great injustice of the unequal distribution of health outcomes is not just a phenomenon of the poorer countries; it reaches right into the heart of the developed world.

By contrast to this harsh reality, one central foundation of a just society is widely held to be an equal distribution of health outcomes across social classes and income groups. If both the span of life and the health quality of life are unequally distributed, then many other inequities must inevitably follow. This requirement can be expressed in terms of Amartya Sen's "ca-

pabilities approach": Justice requires equal access to basic capabilities to be and to do, and this in turn requires equal access to health outcomes. But a similar requirement in respect of health is shared by, and can be expressed in terms of, other theories of justice.

Many contemporary approaches to justice, including the *capabilities approach,* are set within an individualistic framework. In one sense at least, justice is indeed an individual matter. That is, justice requires that each *individual* have equal access to basic capabilities and to the level of health that makes such capabilities possible. Beyond this point, there has been intense debate in the philosophical literature over whether justice can be adequately described and supported in an individualistic framework, with Sandel's (1982) well-known criticism of Rawls (1971, 1975) being a case in point. Equally, it has been fiercely debated for over two centuries whether just outcomes can be achieved by programs that, in giving priority to the liberties and rights of individuals, rely mainly on market-based instruments.

A central theme of this chapter is the social reality of health. By this we mean that a person's health cannot be understood in purely individual terms, but is the outcome of complex social *and* individual factors. A person's health and life expectancy are strongly influenced by inherited biological characteristics and patterns of behavior, as well as by current social circumstances, activities, and expectations. As J. M. Najman and G. Davey Smith (2000) put it, "The human body is the physical manifestation of an individual's history of socially determined experiences and exposures" (p. 3). Our argument, along with our discussion of aspects of the Australian health system, is based on this concept.

There is now overwhelming evidence that, in the developed countries including Australia, massive inequalities exist in health outcomes by income and social class. The evidence is of three types of effect. First, life expectancy and freedom from disease are positively related to income and social class, so that the poor (and/or those of lower socioeconomic status) tend to have higher disease and mortality rates. But, second, disease and mortality rates also tend to be higher, for a given level of average income, in communities that are more unequal—unequal communities have lower health outcomes than do more equal ones, for a given level of income. Third, particular groups, such as indigenous Australians or African Americans, also have particularly adverse health outcomes. These disturbing facts are powerful evidence for, and can only really be explained in terms of, the social reality of health. Thus, the fact that 40% of indigenous Australians die before age 45, whereas only 8% of nonindigenous Australians die before reaching this age, is the starkest possible expression of this reality.

The social reality of health has many implications beyond the scope of this chapter, such as for the theory of justice and for philosophical issues about the practice of medicine. It can also contribute to the explanation of the fact that some highly funded national health systems may have much worse outcomes, both in terms of equity and of overall health levels, than some lower-cost systems. Thus, for example, the United States spends about 65% more on health as a share of gross domestic product (GDP) than does Australia, but it still has age-adjusted death rates nearly 40% higher than in Australia. Indeed, despite its failures and of the many serious challenges, Australia's health system achieves better overall health outcomes with less inequality than do systems in many other countries, at about the average cost for developed countries. Hence, Australia's attempts to deal with these challenges may be worth examining.

Both the social reality of health and the character of health services as a knowledge-based industry imply that the social optimum cannot be achieved in health by market-based policies alone. Thus, in examining the Australian case we look at the major policy initiative directed at the goal of universal provision, the Medicare system of universal health funding. We also briefly examine issues associated with the health of indigenous peoples in Australia.

The Australian experience shows mixed lessons. On the one hand, the record of Medicare and its successors shows that policy initiatives can be effective in achieving the three goals of improved outcomes, equity, and cost-effectiveness. In particular, it shows the special value, in terms of both equity and efficiency, of health programs with universal coverage. But structural initiatives of this type have always been controversial, reflecting the continuing clashes both of philosophy and self-interest that bedevil health reform around the world. Public systems have also been under severe pressure in recent years, as governments search for ways of containing costs while responding to rapid changes in health technologies. On the other hand, Australia's dismal failure to achieve acceptable health outcomes for indigenous peoples, despite some efforts, shows how unprepared governments are to respond in an effective, strategic manner to even the sharpest manifestations of the social reality of health.

PERSISTENT INEQUALITY IN HEALTH OUTCOMES

Despite a widely proclaimed commitment to justice, large inequalities in health outcomes by income levels and social class persist in all developed nations, including Australia. These inequalities appear to be particularly marked in the English-speaking countries, and they embody the three main effects distinguished above. In this section we briefly review the evidence about these three effects, with special reference to Australia and to the English speaking nations more generally.

Income Level, Social Class, and Unequal Health Outcomes

Documentation of social inequalities in health has a long tradition in a number of countries, especially Britain. Evidence of these unequal outcomes was an important element in the *Beveridge Report* of 1942, which led to setting up the welfare state in the United Kingdom. The report of the Working Group on Inequalities in Health (the *Black Report*) in 1980 was an early example of a systematic, official review of these inequalities and of policies that might address them (Townsend et al., 1988). This was followed by the report of the Health Education Council, *The Health Divide*, of 1987 (Townsend et al., 1988) and the more recent *Independent Inquiry into Inequalities in Health* of 1998 (Acheson, 1998), to which the government of the UK responded with a comprehensive program of measures in its 1999 statement titled *Reducing Health Inequalities: An Action Report* (UK Department of Health, 1999).

Because health, whether good or bad, is such a diverse and complex state, inequalities in health related to income or class are inherently difficult to measure. One approach is to study the incidence of different diseases by income level, but because there are so many diseases, it is difficult to draw a sharp overall conclusion. Thus, the two most widely used methods are the study of death rates and of self-reported assessments of health. Self-reported assessments raise issues about the influence of subjective and cultural factors, and the possible variation of these factors across countries. Although these issues are of considerable interest, especially given our theme of the social reality of health, they take us beyond the scope of this chapter. Hence, we briefly review the evidence on mortality rates.

In respect of mortality rates, Najman and Davey Smith (2000) summarize the position succinctly:

Class-related inequalities in mortality rates are observed in almost every country for which data are available. These inequalities in mortality are observed for causes of death that make up well over three-quarters of all deaths. . . . These inequalities are found for all age groups from infancy to childhood, adolescence, adulthood and old age. The magnitude of these inequalities varies from country to country, as well as over time in particular countries. (p. 3)

Unfortunately, no simple set of comparative data is available to allow us to readily illustrate these facts.

Some indication of the magnitude of these inequalities in England and Wales can be gleaned from Table 13–1, compiled from the 1998 UK report. Between 1970 and 1972, mortality rates for unskilled men aged 20 to 64 years were about 80% higher than for professional men, and about 70% higher than for men in managerial and technical occupations. Between 1970 and 1972 and 1991 and 1993, mortality rates in the two higher social classes fell by over 40%, whereas they fell by only 10% for unskilled men. Thus, between 1991 and 1993, mortality rates for unskilled men were nearly three times those for men in professional, managerial, and technical occupations. These data need to be treated with some caution, in particular

Table 13–1. Mortality Rates by Social Class, England and Wales, Men Aged 20 to 64 Years, Selected Periods

| Social Class | Death Rates per 100,000 Population | | | Relative Death Rates | |
| | (1970–72) | (1979–83) | (1991–93) | (1970–72) | (1991–93) |
				(Professional = 1)	
Professional	500	373	280	1.00	1.00
Managerial/Technical	526	425	300	1.05	1.07
Skilled (nonmanual)	637	522	426	1.27	1.52
Skilled (manual)	683	580	493	1.37	1.76
Partly skilled	721	639	492	1.44	1.76
Unskilled	897	910	806	1.79	2.88

Source: Acheson (1998), Table 2.

because some part of the differences described may be due to the changing composition of the social classes within the 20–64-year-age group. Yet they do illustrate two widespread facts. One is that the prospect of premature death is closely related to social class or income. The other is that the benefits, in terms of lower death rates, arising from advances in health and medical practice over the past few decades have had limited impact among many less privileged groups with in society.

More recently, increasing attention has been given to a new technique (disease-adjusted years of life, or DALYs) developed by the Harvard School of Public Health in conjunction with the World Health Organization for the Global Burden of Disease Study (Murray and Lopez, 1996). This approach aims to estimate and add together the years of healthy life lost through death and through living with disease, impairment, and disability, thus providing a powerful tool with which to study the distribution of the burden of disease and ill-health. While several studies are proceeding, few completed studies for individual developed countries are yet available. However, some preliminary results from the U.S. Burden of Injury and Disease Study (Murray et al., 1998) have highlighted the massive variations in mortality rates by county, race, and income in the United States.

Australia is one of the few countries for which a substantial burden of injury and disease study using these techniques has been completed (Mathers et al., 1999). In terms of socioeconomic incidence, their estimates are based on a classification of local government areas by an index of socioeconomic disadvantage, and analyses of the burden of injury and disease across areas classified in these terms. As shown in Table 13–2, this burden is 30% to 40% higher, for all three measures, for regions in the lowest socioeconomic quintile relative to those in the highest quintile, and it is more marked for men than for women. This and other evidence indicates that, while not nearly as pronounced as in the United States, social inequalities in health outcomes are persistent in Australia.

Income Inequality and Unequal Health Outcomes

Thus far we have documented a relationship between income level or social position and health outcomes. But it has also become clear from recent studies that there is an additional effect, over and above the income level effect: The level of inequality within a community has a separate, negative effect on the health levels of a community. For technical reasons, most of the studies that show this effect use a measure of inequality in terms of income rather than social class or status. But, given the pervasive correlation between income and

Table 13–2. Differentials in the Age Standardized Burden of Injury and Disease, Top and Bottom Socioeconomic Quintiles, Australia, 1996

	Ratio of Bottom-to-Top Quintile		
	Men	Women	Persons
Age-standardized death rates	1.41	1.26	1.35
Disease free years of life lost	1.32	1.29	1.30
Disease-adjusted life-years lost (DALY)	1.37	1.27	1.32

Source: Mathers, Vos, and Stevenson (1999).

social position in the countries being studied, there is little doubt that these results can also be interpreted in terms of social inequality more broadly defined.

An important recent study here is by Lynch et al. (1998), who investigated income inequality and mortality in 283 metropolitan areas in the United States, and again found evidence of a positive association between per capita income and mortality. But they also found that "metropolitan areas which had higher income inequality had significantly greater age-adjusted total mortality than those with low inequality, regardless of which measure of inequality was used" (pp. 1077–78). For example, dividing the 283 cities up into quartiles by per capita income, for each quartile they found higher mortality rates in more unequal cities. Comparing the two extremes—cities with high inequality and low per capita income and cities with low inequality and high per capita income—they found that the death rate per 100,000 population was 139.8 deaths higher in the former cities than the latter. Such differences are very large:

To place the magnitude of this difference in some perspective, an appropriate comparison would be that this mortality difference exceeds the combined loss of life from lung cancer, diabetes, motor vehicle crashes, HIV infection, suicide and homicide in 1995. (Lynch et al., 1998, p. 1079)

They also found that the per capita income effect was weaker than the income inequality effect.

This finding of a strong effect of the degree of inequality on health outcomes, separate from and in addition to the effect for income or social position, is replicated in many others studies for a number of countries, such as Davey Smith et al. (1998), Stanistreet et al. (1999), and Wolfson et al. (2000).

The Position of Disadvantaged Groups

Thus, there appear to be two ways in which social position affects health outcomes. First, the social position of individuals is correlated with their health outcomes and, second, the degree of social inequality in a community is negatively correlated with the average health outcomes of that community, after correcting for the average level of income of the community. But there are also massive variations in health outcomes relative to national norms for specific social groups in many nations, of such a magnitude that they cannot be explained in terms of these two effects (measured in terms of national averages) alone. The two cases that we highlight here are African Americans and the indigenous peoples of Australia, again using mortality data.

Table 13–3 summarizes some representative data for African-American and white

Table 13–3. Mortality Among African-American and White Men, United States, 1980 and 1990 (men aged 15 to 64 years only)

	Percent of Families Below Poverty Level (%)	Death Rate (per 100,000 population)	Excess Death Rate	Age-Adjusted Rate Ratio
African-American males				
1980	26.5	809	332	1.70
1990	26.3	791	374	1.90
White males				
1980	7.0	477		1.00
1990	7.0	417		1.00

Source: Geronimus, (1999), Table 2, p. 27.

Table 13–4. Deaths by Age, Indigenous, and Nonindigenous Australians

Age of Death	Proportion of Population (%)		Cumulative Proportion of Population (%)	
	Indigenous	Nonindigenous	Indigenous	Nonindigenous
Under age 25	16	3.1	16.0	3.1
25–44 years	24.4	4.9	40.4	8.0
45–64 years	32.2	13.8	72.6	21.8
65–74 years	14.1	21.6	86.7	43.4
75 years and over	13.4	56.7	100	100

Source: Australian Bureau of Statistics, Cat. No. 3315 (2000), Table 4.4.

males in the United States in 1980 and 1990. By 1990, death rates for African-American men (791 per 100,000) were nearly double those for white men nationally, with an excess death rate of 374 per 100,000. This comparison is not significantly affected by age distribution, and the relative position of African-American men deteriorated between 1980 and 1990. What is more, these national differences mask even more profound variations in particular regions and communities. Geronimus and his colleagues (Geronimus, 1999) studied all African-American and white men aged 15 to 64 years, in 12 regionally diverse, impoverished areas in the United States. They found that, particularly in urban communities, African-American men face extremely high death rates, and the situation deteriorated markedly over the 1990s. In Harlem and the South Side of Chicago, two-thirds of 15-year-old males cannot expect to survive to 65 years, a rate less than half that of white males nationwide. Circulatory disease is the great killer, and HIV and homicide are much less important in explaining the difference than is widely believed.

Striking as the African American story is, these differences are modest compared to those between indigenous and nonindigenous Australians. In the eighteenth and early nineteenth centuries, a substantial majority of the aboriginal population of Australia died from European diseases before even coming into contact with a white person. In the ensuing two centuries, the remaining communities have suffered grievously from a mixture of direct oppression, neglect, and misguided policies. One result of this is the continuing serious situation in aboriginal health, summarized in terms of mortality rates in Table 13–4. Death rates for indigenous Australians up to the age of 44 years are about five times those of the nonindigenous population, and over 40% of indigenous Australians die before the age of 45. Nearly three-quarters of indigenous Australians will die before age 65, by comparison with just over one-fifth for the rest of the population. Thus, mortality rates for the whole of the indigenous population of Australia (which accounts for about 2% of the total) are worse than for African-American men in the impoverished urban regions of the United States.

JUSTICE AND THE SOCIAL REALITY OF HEALTH

Amartya Sen has suggested that most theories of justice can be analyzed in terms of two aspects, the selection of *relevant personal features* and the choice of *combining characteristics* (Sen, 1992). Relevant personal features are to be distributed justly, and the combining characteristics represent the way those features are to be distributed. Examples of relevant personal features cited by Sen include liberties and primary goods (Rawls), rights (Nozick), resources (Dworkin) and individual utilities. Formulae for combining these features include simple summation, sum-maximization, utility-based maximin, and equality. For example, Rawls' theory of justice requires primary goods to be equally distributed and social and economic inequalities to be justified only in terms of providing the greatest benefit to the least advantaged members of society (Rawls, 1982).

Whereas Rawls' work has been most influential in the theory of justice, the utilitarian answer has been dominant in economics, with utility interpreted mainly as preference satisfaction. Powerful economic theories were built on the calculus of utility, defined in terms of ordered sets of preferences. The most dominant and persistent has been the pure competition model of Arrow and Debreu (Debreu 1959). Although Rawls (1971) disputed the utilitarian case and the welfare view (Cohen, 1990), arguing that neither "offensive tastes" nor "expensive tastes" imposed an obligation in justice, his objections had little impact on prevailing economic theories.

Sen's "capabilities view" has recently become influential in both philosophy and economics and may be particularly relevant to the issue of health care. Sen focuses the discussion of equity and justice on what individuals are able to do and to be (Sen, 1980, 1985, 1993). As Nussbaum has put it, "instead of asking about people's satisfactions, or about how much in the way of resources they are able to command, we ask, instead, about what they are actually able to do or to be" (Nussbaum, 2000, p. 12).

The most basic concept in this approach involves "functionings," the various things that an individual manages to do or to be in living a life. Some functionings are elementary, such as being nourished or being in good health, while others might be quite complex. Many different types of functioning will be possible for a given individual, and he or she must choose one at some point. Thus, the person's actual functionings through life will represent choices from a broader set of possibilities. Someone's functionings are what the person actually does and is, while the capabilities are the broader set of what the person was able to choose to do and to be.

On this view, a just society is defined in terms of the capabilities that it makes available to the individuals within it. For example, it might be argued that equality in some "basic" capabilities is a fundamental condition of justice and of an egalitarian society (Sen, 1992). However basic capabilities may be defined, it is clear that life, health, and physical well-being underpin a wide range of other capabilities. Most valuable human functionings, and a corresponding level of capability, require physical and mental health. That is, if one individual suffers diseases more often and more severely than another, then the set of possible functionings from which the former will be able to choose will necessarily be more constrained than that of the latter, other things being equal. An individual who lacks health has limited access, limited choice, and limited use of whatever package of goods is being distributed.

In this sense, at least, justice is clearly an individual matter. Justice requires that each person have equal access to basic capabilities and to the level of health that makes them possible. The distribution of these capabilities within families and communities—for example, between women and men—is a matter of great concern for justice (Nussbaum, 2000). It is not enough, for instance, for resources and life chances to be equally distributed among families, if within those families the men largely appropriate those resources and life chances. For justice to be fully achieved in a society, each individual person must receive justice.

It does not follow from this point that the way to think about, and to achieve, justice is through an individualistic theory. But Rawls's theory of justice, neoclassical economic theory, and the capabilities approach are each firmly set within an individualistic framework of analysis. To use Sen's classification, the relevant personal features to be distributed are those of discrete individuals, and the combining characteristics involve uniting those features in ways that respect their discreteness. But the viability of this individualistic approach has been widely disputed in ways that are particularly relevant to the case of health.

For example, at the heart of Sandel's criticism of Rawls is his attack on the concept of the person (the "deontological self") implicit in individualistic theory. In Sandel's view, this concept of the self—independent from our attachments, never identified by our aims, and always able to stand back and reassess—is inconsistent with key features of our moral being (Sandel, 1982). Rather, the central attachments that we have and the allegiances that we share are often constitutive of who we are. A person without such attachments is not an ideal moral agent, perhaps not a moral agent at all. To take an example presumably congenial to Sandel's view, the basic attachments and allegiances of the Yorta Yorta indigenous people of the Murray-Goulbourn region of Australia are not particular values, which they could stand back from, assess, and perhaps revise. They are fundamental to who these people are, having been forged over the many millennia of their history and shaping not only their goals and choices but how they think of themselves and their world.

It is again another question whether just outcomes can be achieved by programs that rely almost exclusively on market-based instruments, motivated in part by theories that give priority to the liberties and rights of individuals. Even if justice could be adequately described as a function over discrete individuals, it does not follow that justice can be achieved by such methods. The calculus of discrete individuals might prevail in the theory of justice, yet the causes of persisting injustice might still be found in powerful social forces and the self-reinforcing paths to which they give rise. There may well be a large gap between the theoretical tasks that philosophers set themselves and the problems confronting policymakers.

It is characteristic of individualistic, at-omistic philosophies—whether in philosophy, economics, or politics—to treat each person as a discreet entity and to analyze their welfare in individual terms. A person's health is normally taken to be a classic case of an individual matter. Whether a person is healthy or sick here and now is a purely atomistic fact, to be determined independently of his or her goals, values, or social context. Although history is relevant to both diagnosis and treatment, this is the individual medical history of the particular patient. Thus, medical treatment, health economics, and public policy development, drawing on an ancient philosophical tradition, each take the discrete individual as the unit of analysis, to be dealt with independently of his or her personal or social context and history.

But the three facts we have documented briefly above about persistent inequalities is health outcomes call this approach into question. Each of these three facts are indicative of the intimate, self-reinforcing relationship between the social history of a group and the physical health of its members. They seem to imply that, contrary to prevailing ideologies, a person's health is not simply an atomistic, individualistic fact, but is intimately bound to the past history and present experiences and practices of the communities with which the person is involved.

Consistent with this, recent research reported in the medical literature has broken down the sharp distinction between the physical and the social dimensions of health (Davey Smith 1996; Kuh and Ben-Schlomo 1997; Najman and Davey Smith, 2000). In this interpretation, "the human body is the physical manifestation of an individual's history of socially determined experiences and exposures" (Najman and Davey Smith, 2000, p. 3). Both a person's health and his or her life expectancy are in part shaped by historically determined biological characteristics, as well as by inherited patterns of behavior and by current social circumstances, activities, and expectations. This is not, of course, to propound a theory of the social determinism of individual health. But it is to recognize the intimate connections between health and social history and experience, as a basis for explaining the persistent inequalities in health outcomes documented above. These intimate connections we refer to as the *social reality of health*. The social reality of health stands as a negative claim, guarding against purely individualistic assumptions about the influences on a person's health. In much the same way that Sandel challenged Rawls's conception of the self by denying that the self should be seen as separable from its attachments and allegiances, the social reality of health forces us to see social and cultural circumstances as crucial for an adequate understanding of an individual's health.

In our view, recognition of the social reality of health is likely to have important implications for the theory of justice and for philosophical issues concerning the practice of medicine, as well as for health policy. Further analyses of both this concept and of the philosophical issues it raises are beyond the scope of this chapter. But it does provide the framework in which we interpret the Australian experience.

RESPONDING TO THE SOCIAL REALITY OF HEALTH: ASPECTS OF THE AUSTRALIAN EXPERIENCE

National Systems and the Social Reality of Health

National health systems in the developed countries differ widely in both their cost and social effectiveness. However, one of the paradoxes of the study of these systems is that they also differ radically in cost-effectiveness. That is, there appears to be great diversity across national systems in the extent of effective health care achieved for a given level of cost. This diversity, which in our view is closely linked to the extent of policy recognition of the social reality of health, can be illustrated by the fact that the U.S. health system costs nearly 14% of GDP, by far the highest level of any country, but it delivers both overall health and equity outcomes below those of many other, cheaper systems.

In our present context, the comparison of the United States and Australia in these regards is of interest. In 1997 the overall cost of the Australian health system was 8.4% of GDP, only about 60% of the cost of the American system. But, as we have seen, the level of inequality in health outcomes was much higher in the United States, while the overall level of health outcomes is lower. This latter point is evident from age-specific mortality data and other information. For example, age-specific mortality rates, for ages up to 64 years, are on average more than 40% higher in the United States than in Australia. A similar conclusion holds also for the comparison between the United States and Sweden, which has a health system that costs about the same as Australia but has even lower mortality rates up to age 45 years.

Many factors influence the comparative effectiveness and efficiency of national health systems, but it seems beyond doubt that high on the list must be institutional and policy structures, and how well these structures address the social reality of health. As the authors of the U.S. Burden of Disease and Injury Study concluded:

In a country with the highest per capita expenditure on health care in the world, the extraordinary variation at the county level by race forces one to take a broad view of the determinants of health outcomes (Schwartz, et al. 1990). Viewing the much smaller variation in life expectancy in other high income countries, it is tempting to assume that the organisation of the US medical care system and perhaps more importantly the US public health system are the critical factors. (Murray et al. 1998, p. 11)

Thus, how well the institutions of a national health system are attuned to address the social reality of health is likely to be a key determinant of the performance of that system.

The Evolution of the Australian Health System

The Australian health system can only be properly understood in terms of the historical evolution of a complex, path-dependent social system. In the late nineteenth century, Australian hospitals were dangerous places, medical services were largely provided to the well-to-do in their own homes, and the poor relied on religious and charitable institutions for medical care. From that starting point a healthcare system with the following features evolved by the mid 1940s: (1) the provision of free or heavily subsidized services by public hospitals, which were charitable institutions increasingly supported by state governments; (2) an extensive private-friendly social system, which pooled financial risks among members and their dependents, and (3) a three-tiered price discrimination system operated by the medical profession, with different prices charged for the poor, the lower paid working class, and the middle class (Scotton and Macdonald, 1993).

This system, such as it was, had come under increasing pressure during the 1930s, and clearly it was not viable for an expanding country in the postwar period. Thus, the intense debates in the decade after World War II, and the changes to which they gave rise, were pivotal in forming Australia's contemporary health system. The other decisive period was 1972 to 1975, when the Whitlam government attempted to establish a universal health insurance system; such efforts were reshaped in the aftermath of that government's dissolution by the Governor General in November 1975.

Prior to 1946, the Commonwealth government had virtually no role in health, but the national referendum in 1946 gave the Commonwealth an array of powers over social security and health. The two central health issues debated prior to and immediately after this referendum were a national pharmaceutical scheme and a national health insurance scheme. The Pharmaceutical Benefits Act of 1947 was soon passed to establish a national scheme, but a national insurance program did not survive the debates and the changes of government in the late 1940s. In the upshot a new version of the three-tiered funding system was put in place. This provided for free services for pensioners and for subsidised voluntary health insurance through the private health funds, while leaving individuals free to opt out entirely and to determine their own arrangements through the market if they wished.

As the result, the health system administered for many years by the conservative Menzies government involved three main elements: (1) a highly regulated pharmaceutical scheme, providing access to drugs to all at low cost; (2) free hospital and medical care for pensioners, and (3) a heavily subsidised voluntary health insurance scheme available to all others, although a significant proportion of the nonpensioner population were not covered by insurance.

This system was generally well accepted by the public, with about 70% of the population taking out health insurance by 1960, and it was, in many respects, effective. However, deficiencies of the voluntary insurance system increasingly emerged over time and became a key factor in the 1972 federal election. We trace the subsequent evolution of key elements of a new system below.

Universal Access to Services: Medibank and Medicare

The deficiencies of the system of voluntary health insurance were largely hidden from view during the period of prosperity and public quiescence during the 1950s and 1960s, but these were brought to light by pioneering academic research toward the end of the latter decade. In essence, it was a heavily subsidized private system lacking any real elements of competition, with heavy monopoly power exercised by the medical profession and the health funds, and with an increasingly regressive social impact over time.

On the finance side, the proportion of the population that was uninsured did not fall below 17% at any stage, and many of the uninsured were low-income individuals and families. For uninsured low-income people, the burden of meeting medical and hospital bills from their own resources was often crippling. As costs rose, with medical fees determined by the medical profession, health insurance fees rose also, making it harder for lower-income groups to afford insurance. What is more, health insurance fees were flat rate, tax-deductible charges, with a lower after-tax cost to those on higher marginal tax rates. They were, however, community rated—a single rate applied for everyone, rather than fees being rated by risk status—which limited their impact on individuals more at risk. On the supply side, the proportion of beds in public hospitals used by private patients doubled from about 25% in 1954 to about 50% by 1975, so that they increasingly became vehicles for servicing higher income groups.

The basic elements of the alternative proposal, developed by two Melbourne University economists[1] and first proposed publicly by the Labor Party leader Gough Whitlam (then in opposition) in 1968, were simple: (1) free standard treatment, including medical care, in public hospitals for all Australians, with doctors reimbursed at sessional rates for services provided in public hospitals; (2) free medical treatment for all Australians by general practitioners and specialists, at fees to doctors set at 85% of a schedule of rates; (3) the program to be substantial funded by a new income-related tax, and otherwise from consolidated revenue; (4) the program to be overseen by a new Health Insurance Commission, with an overall management responsibility for the health system; and (5) continued freedom for individuals to insure privately, or to pay individually, for additional care over and above that provided by the universal system. While this proposal was never implemented in its entirety, it was substantially put in place, and its various versions

have provided the foundation of the operation of the Australian health system for nearly 30 years. It remains the most substantial reform ever undertaken in the Australian health system to address, in a systemic way, the social reality of health.

The vicissitudes of the universal insurance proposal, which have been heavily determined by the changes in the balance of political power in Australia, can only be reviewed briefly here. The central issues have related to the familiar debate between universal access and controls on service provider incomes on the one hand and freedom of choice for patients and doctors and the role of the private health funds on the other.

The Whitlam government established the Health Insurance Commission to implement the proposal in 1974, and the new scheme was termed "Medibank." But critical elements of the proposal, and especially the Medibank levy, were rejected by the Australian Parliament in 1974. A scheme funded from existing revenue sources was put in place before the Whitlam government was sacked in November 1975. In 1976 the Fraser government restructured the scheme, introducing a Medibank levy of 2.5% of taxable incomes, together with a crucial provision that individuals with hospital and medical insurance with a private fund could opt out and be exempt from the levy. This meant the maintenance of a two-tier system, with a public scheme funded by the levy and a private scheme funded by insurance contributions. The Health Insurance Commission became one of the leading insurers.

The reelection of a Labor government, this time led by Bob Hawke, in 1983 brought further changes. A new version of the basic scheme was introduced, now called *Medicare*, and the opting out provisions were removed. Individuals could still privately insure for additional hospital or medical services, but they were not freed from the Medicare levy as a result of doing so. This led, inter alia, to a steady reduction in the proportion of the population taking out private insurance (65.8% in March 1983 to 30.3% in March 1999), and to greatly increased pressure on public hospitals. As a result, with the election of the conservative Howard government in 1996, the wheel took another turn. In particular, the government introduced in 1999 a nonmeans-tested 30% rebate for contributions to private health insurance, at a full year cost of $1.7 billion, and moved to allow the health funds to charge individual risk premiums rather than be confined to a single community-rating schedule.

The Australian debate remains dominated by the balance between public and private, and hence the degree to which individuals with financial resources and market power can use those assets to obtain privileged outcomes. But the fact remains that the public hospital system, together with low-cost access to basic hospital and medical services for all, has provided an overall level of equity and effectiveness in health care comparable to international best practice. There is no doubt that the system can be much improved, but it does continue to provide high-quality care at an affordable cost to the community at large.

Aboriginal Health Programs

The striking exception to Australia's record of relative equity and efficiency in health care is the health of indigenous Australians. Indeed, issues of aboriginal health have been strikingly absent from many policy discussions, including those that explicitly target the health needs of the more disadvantaged groups within society. The implicit assumption seems to have been that broadly based health policies directed at social equity would meet the needs of all individual groups. Thus, for example, it is only in recent times that a serious assessment has been made of total spending on aboriginal health (Deeble et al., 1998), and the results of that assessment were surprising. Despite the depth of their health needs, total per capita expenditure on the health of aboriginal and Torres Strait Islander people is only marginally higher than that

for Australians as a whole—2% of the population accounted for 2.2% of total health expenditure.

As noted earlier, Australia's indigenous peoples illustrate the social reality of health in its sharpest manifestation. Their health is intertwined in complex ways with history, poverty, current lifestyle, educational levels, and deep-seated factors that have to do with community cultures and their preservation and adaptation. While the policy challenge is undoubtedly intensely difficult, Australia's dismal failure to achieve acceptable health outcomes for the indigenous population shows how unprepared governments are to respond in an effective, strategic manner to these profound challenges.

Acknowledgments

The authors are especially grateful for the expert assistance of Margarita Kumnick in the preparation of this chapter. Peter Sheehan is also grateful to the Australian Research Council and to the Henderson Foundation for support related to the topic of this chapter.

NOTES

1. Indeed, the development, implementation, and success of a system of universal health insurance in Australia is a classic case of effective applied academic research. In a series of joint and individual papers published between 1967 and 1969, two young researchers (Dick Scotton and John Deeble) at the Institute of Applied Economic and Social Research at the University of Melbourne developed a penetrating critique of the voluntary health insurance system. Asked in June 1967 by the leader of the then opposition Labor Party, Gough Whitlam, to produce a detailed alternative policy, by May 1968 they had developed a detailed plan for a compulsory insurance system (Scotton and Deeble, 1968). After seven years of bitter debate, a limited version of this proposal was implemented by the Whitlam government on July 1, 1975, as Medibank, and Scotton became chairman of the new Health Insurance Commission. In 1976, after the sacking of Whitlam in November 1975, Scotton and Deeble's revised proposals, designed to address the new government's financial parameters while preserving as much as possible of the original intent, formed the basis

of Medibank Mark II implemented in late 1976. For further details, see Scotton and Macdonald (1993).

REFERENCES

Acheson, D. (1998). *Independent Inquiry into Inequalities in Health Report*. London: The Stationery Office.

Australian Bureau of Statistics (ABS) (2000). *Mortality of Aboriginal and Torres Strait Islander Australians*. Occasional Paper, Cat. No. 3315.0, Canberra.

Australian Institute of Health and Welfare (2000). *Australia's Health 2000*, AIHW, Canberra.

Cohen, G. (1990). Equality of what? On welfare, goods and capabilities. In M. Nussbaum and A. Sen (eds.), *The Quality of Life*. Oxford: Clarendon Press. 9–29.

Cunningham, J. and Paradies, Y. (1997). *Mortality of Aboriginal and Torres Strait Islander Australians*. Occasional Paper, Cat. No. 3315.0, Australian Bureau of Statistics, Canberra.

Davey Smith, G. (1996). Income inequality and mortality: Why are they related? *British Medical Journal* 312, 987–98.

Davey Smith, G., Hart, C., Watt, G., Hole, D. and Hawthorne, V. (1998). Individual social class, area-based deprivation, cardiovascular disease risk factors and mortality: The renfrew and Paisley Study. *Epidemial Community Health* 52, 399–405.

Deeble, J., Mathers, C., Smith, L., Goss, J., Webb, R. and Smith, V. (1998). *Expenditures on Health Services for Aboriginal and Torres Strait Islander People*. Australian Institute of Health and Welfare and NCEPH, Canberra.

Debreu, G. (1959). *The Theory of Value*. New York: John Wiley.

Geronimus, A. (1999). Economic inequality and social differentials in mortality. *Federal Reserve Board of New York Economic Policy Review*, September, pp. 23–36.

Kuh, D. and Ben-Shlomo, Y. (1997). *A Lifecourse Approach to Chronical Disease Epidemiology*. Oxford: Oxford Medical Publications.

Lynch, J., Caplan, G., Pamuk, E., Cohen, R., Heck, C., Balfour, J. and Yen, I. (1998). Income inequality and mortality in metropolitan areas of the United States. *American Journal of Health* 88 (7), 1074–80.

Mathers, C., Vos, T. and Stevenson, C. (1999). *The Burden of Disease and Injury in Australia*. Australian Institute of Health, Cat. no. PHE 17, Canberra.

Mooney, G., Jan, S., and Wiseman, V. (1998). Economic issues in Aboriginal health care. In G. Mooney and R. Scotton (eds.), *Economics and Australian Health Policy*. Sydney: Allen and Unwin.

Murray, C. and Lopez, A. (1996). *The Global Burden of Disease*. Cambridge, Mass: Harvard University Press.

Murray, C., Michaud, C., McKenna, M. and Marks, J. (1998). *US Patterns of Mortality by County and Race: 1965–1994*. Cambridge, MA: Harvard Center for Population and Development Studies. (http://www.hsph.harvard.edu/organizations/bdu/papers/usbodi/index.html).

Najman, J.M. and Davey Smith, G. (2000). The embodiment of class-related and health inequalities. Editorial, *Australian and New Zealand Journal of Public Health*, 24 (1).

Nussbaum, M. (2000). *Women and Human Development: The Capabilities Approach*. Cambridge: Cambridge University Press.

OECD (1998). *OECD Health Data 1999*. Paris.

Rawls, J. (1971). *Theory of Justice*. Cambridge, Mass Harvard University Press.

Rawls, J. (1975). Fairness to goodness. *Philosophical Review* 84, 536–54.

Rawls, J. (1982). Social unity and primary goods. In A. Sen and B. Williams (eds.), *Utilitarianism and Beyond*. Cambridge: Cambridge University Press.

Sandel, M. (1982). *Liberalism and the Limits of Justice*. Cambridge: Cambridge University Press.

Schwartz, E., Kofie, V., Rivo, M. and Tuckson, R. (1990). Black/white Comparisons of deaths preventable by medical intervention: United States and District of Columbia 1980–1986. *International Journal of Epidemiology* 19, (3), 591–97.

Scotton, R.B. (1999). *Managed competition: The policy context*. Melbourne Institute Working Paper No. 15/99. University of Melbourne, Melbourne, Australia.

Scotton, R.B. and Deeble, J. (1968). Compulsory health insurance for Australia. *Australian Economic Review*. Fourth Quarter, Institute of Applied Economic and Social Research, Melbourne.

Scotton, R.B. and Macdonald, C.R. (1993). *The Making of Medibank*. Australian Studies in Health Service Administration Series, No. 76. University of New South Wales, Sydney.

Sen, A. (1980). Equality of what?. S. McMurrin (ed.), *Tanner Lectures on Human Values*. Cambridge: Cambridge University Press.

Sen, A. (1985). *Commodities and Capabilities*. Amsterdam: North-Holland.

Sen, A. (1992). *Inequality Reexamined*. Oxford: Clarendon Press.

Sen, A. (1993). Capability and well-being. In M. Nussbaum and A. Sen (eds.), *The Quality of Life*. Oxford: Clarendon Press.

Stanistreet, D., Scott Samuel, A. and Bellis, M. (1999). Income inequality and mortality in England. *Journal of Public Health Medicine* 21 (2), 205–7.

Townsend, P., Davidson, N. and Whitehead, M. (1988). *Inequalities in Health: The Black Report and the Health Divide*. London: Penguin Books.

UK Department of Health (1999). *Reducing Health Inequalities: An Action Report*. London: Department of Health.

Wolfson, M., Kaplan, G., Lynch, J., Ross, N. and Backlund, E. (2000). Relation between income inequality and mortality: Empirical demonstration. *Western Journal of Medicine* 172, 22–24.

14

Justice for All? The Scandinavian Approach

Tuija Takala

Philosophically speaking, we can identify at least five major theories of justice, each of which can be interpreted in different ways (Gillon, 1986). Many varieties of the concept of justice are also specified in the opening chapters of this book. In this chapter I take justice in health care to mean the national system's ability to respond equally to the medical *needs* of the entire population. I argue that, in this sense, the Scandinavian health-care policies meet the requirements of justice, at least in spirit. The strong commitments to solidarity, equity, and universality make these systems just. Empirical studies have shown that even the macroeconomic changes of the 1980s and 1990s did not shake this core ideology of the Nordic welfare states (Kautto et al., 1999; Nordlund, 2000). The financial difficulties encountered did, however, present new challenges to the ability of the Scandinavian health-care systems to meet the requirements of justice.

Ideological objections to tax-paid health services are mainly based on neoliberal thinking. In addition, increased emphasis on patient rights—especially the right to choose one's doctor, treatment, and place of care—has revealed inherent tensions in the model. In this chapter I examine the ideological basis of the Scandinavian health-care systems and outline their struggles to uphold the ideals of solidarity, equity, and universality.

IS THERE A SCANDINAVIAN APPROACH?

There are three preliminary matters of dispute that I should address before going to the actual theme of this chapter. First, what are the Scandinavian countries? Second, are there good grounds for assuming that a "Scandinavian approach" exists? And third, further clarification of the definition of justice in health care is needed.

In this chapter the Scandinavian countries, also referred to as the "Nordic" countries, are taken to include Denmark, Finland, Norway, and Sweden. This is a compromise often utilized in studies conducted on the welfare policies of the Northern European nations. According to *Merriam-Webster's Collegiate Dictionary* (1997), "Scandinavia" is either Denmark, Norway, and Sweden, or it can be taken also to include Finland and Iceland. But, for a discussion of similar social policies in sufficiently similar cultural and political environments, Iceland, with a population only a fraction of the other Scandinavian nations, is often dismissed as unsuitable for comparative analyses. (The populations of the Scandinavian countries in 1998 were: Denmark, 5,270,000; Finland, 5,154,000; Iceland, 276,000; Norway, 4,419,000; and Sweden, 8,875,000.) The relevant features of Finland, in contrast, are similar enough to the other Scandinavian countries so that its inclusion is likely to enrich the analysis.

The assumption that there exists a health-care system, or more generally a social policy, typical to the Nordic countries, unified to the degree that it can be studied as a whole, has been challenged (e.g., Alban and Christiansen, 1995). Yet most still hold that the overall similarity of the Scandinavian welfare policies is analytically too important a tool to be discarded, regardless of the divergence on particular issues (e.g., Kautto et al., 1999). In the following discussion I recognize the differences, but hold to the conviction that the health-care systems of Denmark, Finland, Norway, and Sweden reflect ideals that can be labeled as the "Scandinavian approach." The means, goals, values, and outcomes are roughly the same, and the similarities of many cultural and historical features of these countries make them comparable, even if a comprehensive list of what is included in this model cannot be explicated.

Justice in health care can, according to Saltman (1997), mean different things, depending whether the focus is on processes, outcomes, or a mix of the two. If the focus is on the process, the idea of a "fair equal opportunity," a fair process, is stressed. If justice is measured in outcomes equality, the emphasis is on ensuring that needed care of an appropriate standard is available to everyone—not just to the industrious and talented (Saltman, 1997). It can be argued that there has been a shift from the latter toward the former in the Scandinavian health-care systems within the past decades.

WHAT IS THE SCANDINAVIAN MODEL?

Three central ideological features characterize at least the rhetoric of the Scandinavian model: universality, solidarity and equity (Erikson et al., 1987; Holm et al., 1999). Like justice, these concepts have many meanings. Solidarity can be explained as analogous to "brotherhood" or "neighborhood" (Ashcroft et al., 2000). It carries the idea that "we are in this together, and we have to take care of each other." To make this a bit more complicated, there are two main roots to solidarity. One can be said to have arisen from the universalistic, rights based Anglo-Saxon world, and the other from the more community-centered Continental tradition. And in many respects, the Nordic countries represent a collision point of these two traditions. It can be argued, though, that solidarity, in both of these forms, adds to justice a shared goal and a feeling of interconnectedness (Houtepen and ter Meulen, 2000). Like solidarity, equity and universality can be understood as further aspects of justice. The basis of the Scandinavian health-care ideology is to provide health-care services equally and universally to all residents, and, in the spirit of solidarity, to devote special consideration to the needs of the weakest (Holm et al., 1999).

In practice, the reliance on universality, solidarity, and equity means that health care is mainly funded by tax revenues, most hospitals are publicly funded, and the system is organized to ensure that all residents have access to health services regardless of where they live or what their economic status is. One of the peculiarities of Scandinavian health care is that the rich as well as the poor have traditionally made use of the publicly funded services. In the Scandinavian countries the term "welfare state," therefore, refers to a system of entitlement to health services based on one's permanent residence in a particular country. This use of the term should be distinguished from another interpretation of a "welfare state," which is better characterized with the label "poor law model," where people are entitled to certain goods based on certain social criteria, such as poverty. It is noteworthy, however, that in Scandinavia the right to health care is not a legal right (or a claim right)—that is, people do not have an absolute right to health care. They only have a right to their just share of the limited resources at hand. Governments have the duty to provide high-quality services for all, but the scarcity of resources may restrict the available services.

Primary care is cost-free for children (in Finland under age 15, in Norway under age 7, and in Sweden under 20 years of age). In Denmark all general practitioner (GP) services for all age groups are free, with the exception of vaccination for travel to foreign countries. In the other Scandinavian nations an out-of-pocket co-payment is required for primary care. In Finland the fee is approximately $20 for as many visits as needed within a 12-month period, or $10 for one appointment (this cannot be charged more than three times a year). In Finland, Norway, and Sweden some additional payments are charged for certain diagnostic procedures. In Denmark, as in other Scandinavian countries, co-payments are charged for pharmaceuticals and for consultations with specialists. Dental care is also, to a degree, financed by co-payments. In Finland, dental care is, in theory, free for everyone born after 1955.

All the Scandinavian countries have 24-hour emergency units in hospitals for acute medical needs. Again, in Denmark these services, like other hospital services, are free, but in Finland and Sweden a co-payment of approximately $20 is required.

For longer hospitalization, the fee is approximately $25 each day, including the required examinations, procedures, and medication. The needed care is provided even if the patient has no money at all. Fees are usually collected after discharge, and the system is flexible to the degree that should all else fail, social services will be there to assist any patient who is unable to pay. For long-term special care, the Scandinavian countries set limits to the overall amount one is expected to pay for health services within a year. For example, in Finland the maximum is about $700.

Public health care in Scandinavia is mainly funded by tax revenues, and most health services are provided in the public health system. Public expenditure as a percentage of the total expenditure on health is 84.3% in Denmark, 73.7% in Finland, 82.0% in Norway, and 78.0% in Sweden, yet the percentage of gross national product (GNP) spent on health-care services is relatively low. By the end of the 1990s the percentage of GNP spent on health care was 8.0% in Denmark, it was 7.6% in Finland, 6.5% in Norway, and 9.2% in Sweden. (World Health Organization [WHO], 2000). The relatively small percentage of GNP spent on health care is partly due to the relatively large allocation of funds to the social services that are also provided by the Scandinavian governments. Social services provide for a range of things that people need which are not quite medical care, such as some services for the elderly. When we compare the portion of GNP spent on health care in different countries, we have to make sure we are comparing similar services. It should also be noted that co-payments required for certain health-care services may ultimately come from the social services.

PROBLEMS IN THE 1980s AND 1990s

The *World Health Report 2000* was not very flattering to us Scandinavians who, to this day, believe that our health-care systems are among the best in the world. In the overall ratings of health-care systems worldwide, Norway ranked 11th, followed by Sweden 22nd, Finland 31st, and Denmark 34th (WHO, 2000). The rankings and relative differences can be explained in part by the variables used. But the rankings also show that the ideals of the Scandinavian system fall short of realization. For instance, Finland's biggest problems are the expansion of the private sector in health care, the fact that life expectancy for men is considerably lower than that of women, and the variations in morbidity among social groups (Keskimäki, 1997; Ministry of Social Affairs and Health, Finland, 1999). These problems reflect, in part, our genetic heritage, especially the prevalence of cardiovascular disease, which tends to shorten the lives of men rather than those of women. Whether this particular matter should cast doubt upon the justice of our health-care system can surely be disputed. The other matters are more problematic.

In the beginning of the 1980s the Nordic welfare model experienced its "Golden era." The economies were growing and the resources to meet the needs of all were in hand. For Finland and Sweden a severe recession began at the start of the 1990s, and both countries have not yet fully recovered from it. Oil reserves helped to pull Norway out of its recession and its bank crisis. And even though the macroeconomy of Denmark has been struggling since the 1970s, Denmark has managed to fulfill its health-related tasks as a welfare state. The economic difficulties, however, took their toll on the health-care systems of the Scandinavian nations. Costs had to be cut. The general trend has been to move patients from inpatient care to outpatient care simply to reduce the number of hospital beds. The long-term economy of this is not, however, evident (Kautto et al., 1999). Other methods used to save money have included the enlargement of health-care municipalities and the centralization of special-care units. Although these moves have been statistically efficient, they have also resulted in inequalities of access to health services, as those living near mainly urban, special-care units have easier access to those services than do the residents of rural areas.

The new challenges to the health-care systems are intensified by the accompanying difficulties of unemployment, disability pensions, and early retirement. Many of these have been caused, more or less directly, by the economic difficulties of the past decades. Also, the aging of the population, partly due to successful health policies, adds to these problems. And because health care is financed by tax revenue, as the relative number of taxpayers goes down, the problem of scarce funds for social services and health care seems inescapable.

Cutbacks in the public health sector during the years of recession made room for private health care. Especially in Finland and Sweden, the proportion of private, self-paid services has expanded at the expense of the public sector. With rapid advances in medical technologies from the 1990s onward—which created new and often expensive methods of diagnosis and treatment—equal access to state-of-the-art health care has been challenged. Those better-off can buy the services they need from the private sector, where treatments are available to anyone who can pay for them, whereas those who depend on the public system are forced to queue for special care. Everyone still has the right to whatever health care is needed, but only within the limits of available resources. And in the age of scarcity, not all needs can be met. To the extent that justice in health care means equal access to health services according to medical need, the existence of a private sector of any size undermines the provision of justice. The conclusion that can be drawn from this inequality in access to care is problematic. "If it cannot be given to all, none shall have it" is not an obvious solution.

An additional problem is that employment in the public sector has become increasingly unrewarding for both doctors and nurses. Attempts to reduce costs have led to personnel cuts in hospitals and other medical care units. This means that public health professionals have to work under stress and deal with more patients than they can properly handle and at salaries that are not competitive with those paid in the private sector. The result may be that some of those who can (the best or the greediest?) move to the private sector. This relocation of personnel can mean that patients within the public system will not receive the care that they should, either due to the lack of professional skill or because of the exhaustion of the staff. Some seem to believe, however, that this trend will not bring about the fall of the Scandinavian health-care model, as the market competition between virtually free public health care and expensive private health care does not work in favor of private enterprises (Holm et al., 1999). At present, with relatively small disparities in income among individuals in the Nordic countries, this is probably true. But the fairly even income distribution might someday change. Gains from stock market investments and the development of new technologies have already created a new class of wealthy people. Should the income gaps become wider, it will, arguably, strengthen the private health-care sector, which, in turn, will ultimately weaken the public sector. If this possibility is not recognized and addressed it might become a reality.

FUTURE CHALLENGES

The Finnish Ministry of Social Affairs and Health (1999) has listed future challenges that our health-care system is likely to face. These include most of the already mentioned concerns: loss of public funds, unemployment, large municipalities, aging of the population, advances in medical technology, and the rights of patients to influence their treatment. These problems are with us already.

An important, but not yet tackled, feature is the growing value given to an individual's rights to choose her doctor, and the means and the place of her treatment. Finland was one of the first countries in the world to implement a patient rights act (1993), and slowly, toward the very end of the twentieth century, patients in Scandinavia started to become clients and active participants instead of passive receivers of health-care services. This change in attitude is at odds with the inherent structure of the Scandinavian health system, which is, and has been from the beginning (to some degree), paternalistic. The GP (general practitioner) system of Denmark and Norway can be seen as an expression of the built-in paternalism of the Scandinavian health-care system. In Denmark every resident has a duty to register with a GP, through whom all further medical needs are addressed. In 2000, Norway introduced a similar model.

The reason for the paternalism in the Scandinavian model is historical. The birth of a welfare state is often linked with the national need to ensure primarily that men and women are fit to undertake industrial work or to fight in actual, or feared, wars and not so much with individuals' need for well-being as such (Ashcroft et al., 2000). The Nordic countries are no exception. To recover from the world wars it was in the interests of these countries to have a working health-care system: It takes healthy people to rebuild a country. That partly explains why the Scandinavian health-care model has been thus far more interested in the outcomes than in the justness of the processes and why its strength, in terms of efficiency, has been in numbers. The idea has been that "the system takes care of medical needs as defined by the system"— people do not use the system to satisfy their medical needs.

By the beginning of the 1990s the political and ideological climate had in many ways changed. Globalization, individualization, expansion of higher education, and new ways of earning money gave birth to a new generation of Scandinavians who would no longer accept the postwar health-care system. They knew their rights and did not tolerate being treated as unintelligent subjects of the health-care services. Medical paternalism was no longer accepted.

Also, economic difficulties, followed by cuts in health services, had driven the Scandinavian systems away from their traditional focus on equality of outcome and toward procedural justice, "fair equal opportunity." A convenient way to make the necessary cuts is to ensure that medical services are still, in theory, available for all, in the spirit of "fair equal opportunity," although they are not overtly advertised to those who do not claim them as their due. This entails, further, that those who know the system and are capable of utilizing its full potential are likely to get better treatment than the less savvy. For instance, it is the right of a patient to get a second opinion if she so wishes, but in most cases she needs to ask for it first. The patient's ability (mental, physical, educational, linguistic, social) to demand what is rightfully her due as a resident of a particular Nordic country has an effect on how the health-care system works for that person (Holm et al., 1999).

Furthermore, the number of nights spent in hospitals, or the number of vaccinations given, in this or that municipality, does not prove that the medical needs of individual patients have been met. Keskimäki's study (1997) of inpatient care in Finland shows that even if statistics lead us to believe that health-care services are provided according to need, closer examination reveals that the needs of those better-off are more likely to be satisfied than those of the less well-off. This is partly due to the abilities needed to actually secure one's entitlements.

The transition from equity in outcomes to fair processes is the result of two completely different developments, one ideological, another material. Ideologically, political pressures have weakened the inherent paternalism of these models and moved them toward the procedural idea of justice. Materially, the public image of the financially challenged system has been defended by placing emphasis on equal opportunities rather than on actual outcomes.

The problem with the introduction of the right-to-choose principle into the Scandinavian welfare model is that as long as public funds in health care are scarce, the private sector can better live up to the expectations created by the principle. A further problem arises, as I have argued above, from the introduction of individual choice to the essentially paternalistic system. The idea that choices have high value in the provision of health care is somehow at odds with the ideology of the welfare state. No nation has sufficient wealth to satisfy all its citizens' health-related needs as defined by the citizens themselves. Only needs defined by public health authorities can be met by the resources allocated to public health care, even in the most dedicated welfare states.

SOME INTRINSIC TENSIONS IN THE WELFARE MODEL

The justice found in the Scandinavian health-care systems is usually considered a reflection of their strong commitment to the equality of citizens expressed in terms of equal access to health-care services according to medical need. Although this commitment can be essential to justice (e.g., Caplan et. al., 1999), it nonetheless creates problems. In an influential book, Michael Walzer has argued that the grounds for distribution should vary according to the goods distributed. According to Walzer, justice in health care requires that the distribution be based on medical need and not on ability to pay (Walzer, 1983). This is also the position of many World Health Organization (WHO) policies, which, among other things, stress the importance of equal access based on medical need. Similarly, the Finnish Ministry of Social Affairs and Health has set as its future goal that "all the residents of Finland are equally entitled to top-quality services regardless of their place of residence or economical status" (Ministry of Social Affairs and Health, 1999).

The problem is that not all medical needs can be met, at least through public funding. In such circumstances, justice, if it is simply taken to mean equal access to equal services in the spirit of the WHO policies, would require that everyone should be equally deprived of the most expensive medical services. What this would entail in practice seems impossible to formulate. The idea of rationing has been employed to answer the question. But if rationing is practiced on the basis of age, life expectancy, or the like, justice—to each according to medical need—ceases. And the same is true if some expensive treatments are made altogether unavailable. It is, then, not to *each* according to need, but to some according to need, while *some* needs are not met.

There are two lines of argument against the welfarist health-care systems of our time, one ideological, the other practical. According to the neoliberals or libertarians, the welfare model lacks justification. It is quite nice if people get the health care they need, but the problem is how to fund it. Why should all pay for the health care of some? Why should anyone pay for someone else's misfortune? It is not other people's fault in any way (Nozick, 1974). This line of reasoning has not been very popular in the Scandinavian countries where solidarity and equity are deep and shared commitments. It is, in fact, "politically incorrect" to propose such libertarian ideas.

Sticking to what is politically correct, however, gives rise to the other problem. Everyone knows that there is not enough money to sustain the ideal of health care for all. Yet hardly anyone seems prepared to say what exactly should be done to cut costs, as any explicit rationing would go against the sacred ideals of equity, solidarity, and universality. The result is that the cuts are "hidden" in the system as queues for special care and difficulties in getting needed care. It might be prudent, and fair,

to recognize the scarcity of resources as a fact and to start building a just system from there. In this way we could at least have justice in terms of equal access within the public system, even if the existence of the private sector would disturb the fairness of health-care provision overall.

SCANDINAVIAN WELFARE STATES IN THE TWENTY-FIRST CENTURY

The Scandinavian welfare states seem to have survived the economic challenges of the 1980s and the 1990s without any drastic policy changes either in the field of health care or in other areas (Kautto et al., 1999; Nordlund, 2000). Some cuts have been made to both health care and social services, but the outcome seems to be more satisfactory than some social scientists first assumed. Kautto et al. (1999) speculate that the limited effect of the reduction in services might be the result of the system's ability to adapt to changing circumstances, or an indication that the economic and political changes have not been so dramatic after all, or evidence that the Nordic way of thinking is somehow so firmly rooted in its institutions and culture that politics and economics cannot easily upset it.

If equal access to top-quality health services is the goal that we all agree on, we must decide what to sacrifice in order to achieve it. Should we ban private health-care provision, limit freedom, and risk our health-care professionals fleeing abroad? Or should we cut other government programs so as to ensure the government's ability to respond to the basic welfare needs of its residents? Or should we increase co-payments as a means to maintain the high quality of public health care (Holm et al., 1999) and possibly undermine equal access?

Apart from the old problems of resource allocation, Scandinavian countries are now facing two new challenges—the rise of a private health-care sector, and the introduction into the system of individual choice as a central value. The private sector does not have to be a threat to the equity of the system, provided that the quality and accessibility of care in the public sector can be maintained or increased from current levels. What is needed to accomplish this is ultimately an empirical question. The value of choice, in contrast, is an admonition of another kind. It challenges the very core of welfare policies. Therefore, it is not only a question of how to cope with what seems to be a lack of material and financial resources, but also a question of what the welfare state should do, and what we want it to do in the twenty-first century in terms of health-care policies.

Acknowledgments

My thanks go to Dr. Sakari Karjalainen (Secretary General, Research Council for Health, Academy of Finland) and to Rosamond Rhodes for their insightful comments.

REFERENCES

Alban, A. and Christiansen, T. (eds.). (1995). *The Nordic Lights: New Initiatives in Health Care Systems*. Odense, Denmark: Odense University Press.

Ashcroft, R.E., Campbell, A. V., and Jones, S. (2000). Solidarity, society and the welfare state in the United Kingdom. *Health Care Analysis* 8: 377–94.

Caplan, L.R., Light, D. W., and Daniels, N. (1999). Benchmarks of fairness: A moral framework for assessing equity. *International Journal of Health Services* 29: 853–69.

Erikson, R., Hansen, E. J., Ringen, S. and Uusitalo, H. (eds.). (1987). *The Scandinavian Model: Welfare States and Welfare Research*. Armonk, NY: M.E. Sharpe.

Gillon, R. (1986). *Philosophical Medical Ethics*. Chichester: John Wiley.

Holm, S., Liss, P.-E. and Norheim, O. F. (1999). Access to health care in Scandinavian countries: Ethical aspects. *Health Care Analysis* 7: 321–30.

Houtepen, R. and ter Meulen, R. (2000). New types of solidarity in the European welfare state. *Health Care Analysis* 8: 329–40.

Kautto, M., Heikkilä, M., Hvinden, B., Marklund, S. and Ploug, N. (eds.). (1999). *Nordic Social Policy: Changing Welfare States*. London and New York: Routledge.

Keskimäki, I. (1997). *Social Equity in the Use of Hospital Inpatient Care in Finland*. Stakes Research Reports 84. Jyväskylä, Finland: Gummerus.

Merriam Webster's Collegiate Dictionary, 10th ed. (1997). Springfield, MA: Merriam-Webster.

Ministry of Social Affairs and Health, Finland. (1999). *Guidelines on Health Care in Finland*. Helsinki, Finland.

Nordlund, A. (2000). Social policy in harsh times. Social security in Denmark, Finland, Norway and Sweden during the 1980s and 1990s. *International Journal of Social Welfare* 9: 31–42.

Nozick, R. (1974). *Anarchy, State, and Utopia*. Oxford and Cambridge: Basil Blackwell.

Patient rights act ("Laki potilaan asemasta ja oikeuksista"). (1993). *Statutes of Finland* 782/92.

Saltman, R. B. (1997). Equity and distributive justice in European health care reform. *International Journal of Health Services* 27: 443–53.

Walzer, M. (1983). *Spheres of Justice*. Oxford: Basil Blackwell.

World Health Organization (WHO). (2000). *World Health Report 2000*.

15

Ethics, Politics, and Priorities in the Italian Health-Care System

Giovanna Ruberto

> A rational man acting in the real world may be defined as one
> who decides where he will strike a balance between what he
> desires and what can be done. It is only in imaginary world
> that we can do whatever we wish.
> Walter Lippermann, *The Public Philosophy*

The constitutions of all Western countries revised after World War II incorporated a new focus on citizens' rights: the right to personal liberty, to health, to well-being, and so forth. In fact, equal and free access to health care and to education are now seen as fundamental rights throughout Western Europe. They are considered to be as basic as the right to freedom of speech, and they are seen as necessary constituents of and means to freedom.

In the Constitution of Italy, individuals' right to health care is specifically decreed in Article 32 where the government pledges free health care to all, including the indigent. Legislation related to the health-care system was revised in 1978 by Law 883 and also by subsequent legislative decrees. As recently as 1998, Law 40 was passed, which clearly asserts that all foreign citizens, even illegal immigrants, have an equal right of access to health care. The sum total of this legislation makes health care a fundamental right for everyone in Italy. Access to the health-care system is free for everyone living in or simply visiting the nation.

The Italian National Health System (NHS)is financed by the general tax revenue and an additional health-care tax. Expenditures of the NHS are based on a budget that is voted every year by Parliament. The annual appropriation for the NHS is approximately 7% of the Italian gross domestic product (GDP). Wealthy people pay more taxes, but all people receive the same comprehensive health-care assistance without regard to income or tax contribution. Health care is provided through a structured network of territorial agencies, each financed by a state budget. These agencies purchase treatments or social services from public health facilities and occasionally from private hospitals when a specific treatment is needed and the patient cannot wait for it from the usual public sources. The National Health Care Plan, which sets the standards for medical care and social services, is formulated by the Ministry of

Health in collaboration with regional health councillors. In sum, the state takes responsibility for the health care of all people through a regionally organized system that is completely patient-oriented. In Italy, there is no private health insurance system, and even supplemental health insurance is very uncommon because, in effect, no one needs it. Private donations are only used in a supplementary way to support research and sometimes to purchase new equipment.

Traditionally in Italy, public services are better than private services. Medicine is no exception. The Italian public health hospital system offers more comprehensive treatment options than do private hospitals, and the quality of the services is also better than what is available through the private sector. Like the British National Health Service, the Italian National Health System provides uniform and universal coverage. This means that everyone has free access to hospital care (e.g., medical, surgical), to sophisticated therapies (e.g., transplantation, genetic counseling), to preventive medicine (e.g., vaccination), and to continuing care from family physicians.

In 2000 the World Health Organization (WHO) published *World Health Report 2000*, its evaluation of the performance of health-care systems in 190 countries around the globe according to how well they met three goals: (*1*) attainment of health for the population, (*2*) responsiveness, and (*3*) fair financing. Western European countries achieved the highest rankings on the list. Italy was ranked second only to France as having the best health-care system in the world.

Despite our extraordinarily high ranking on performance in health-care delivery, some of the problems inherent in our system were not reflected in the WHO assessment. The level of our assistance has grown nationally, but allocation and development is organized regionally. The consequence of this regional design is that there are some regional differences in health care. Most of the hospitals, and specifically most of the

excellent hospitals, are located in the northern part of the Italy (Lombardia, Emilia-Romagna, Toscana). Nevertheless, because we have the freedom to travel and receive health care anywhere in the country, a kind of health migration has developed to allow people to utilize the highest quality of medical care and the most effective diagnosis and treatment. For example, the hospital where I work is in Pavia. More than 40% of its patients come from outside the city and the region.

While Italy has thus far been able to offer its people exemplary health care, the rising costs are putting the system in jeopardy. To continue to provide its excellent level of comprehensive health-care assistance, the nation will have to adopt a number of measures to contain costs. We have heard the call for moving away from the traditional public management of the system and for the introduction of strong professional private sector management styles. We have also heard the demand for a clear definition of explicit objectives for our National Health System as a prelude to rationing. And we have heard the demand for family doctors to take on a crucial role in filtering access to care and controlling the use of expensive prescription drugs. Setting priorities for a health-care system encompasses three main issues:

- the allocation of resources (the portion of resources to be spent on health care and how these resources should be divided among the various types of services)
- optimal production (how health care can be efficiently put together in both ethical and economic terms)
- distribution (how health care should be distributed among the people).

Yet, in our recent efforts in allocating health-care resources we encounter a number of problems (*Hastings Center Report*, 1996).[1]

Recent goals and reforms in the health-care system are economically unsustainable. They tend to generate unaffordable medicine, which in itself is going to be the most unacceptable problem in the future. Bloated expectations tend to widen the inequitable gap between the rich and the poor in the same country and between developed and developing countries.

The situation is also clinically confusing. It is hard to find a good balance between care and cure, between conquering disease and improving the quality of life, between reducing mortality and morbidity, and between investing social resources in health care and the actual improvement in the health of the population. In reality, the enormous investment of resources directed toward achieving good health has undeniably increased the average life span and improved the quality of life in general. Nevertheless, we must acknowledge that people die from medical conditions associated with their way of life or social status even in countries that spend more than others on their health-care system. This should make us seriously ponder how we spend the resources we have before deciding how much of them to spend.

Recent efforts to resolve the problem have been socially frustrating, fostering false and unrealistic hopes in the public and creating expectations of wonders from modern medical technology that cannot be met or that can only be met at an unaffordable and exorbitant cost. It is worth noting, for example, that great hopes have been invested in gene therapies that are still ineffective. Consider also how we fool ourselves into believing that we have found the cure for cancer every time new and more costly drugs are developed. In reality, our form of medicine is still essentially diagnostic, it primarily treats symptoms and is less than modestly curative. Many previously acute diseases can now be maintained in the chronic phase. We can cure only very few. This situation raises another problem, namely the cost of chronic treatment for an increased number of people who live with disease for a significant number of years.

Regional reforms lack coherent direction and purpose. They respond to pressures from special-interest groups (multinational pharmaceutical companies, the academic world, etc.) with unrelated objectives or in the name of market freedom. These piecemeal changes accept no direction, no vision of worthy goals oriented toward the needs and desires of people, and no meaningful picture of medicine's contribution to the individual's well-being.

The aging population is yet another complicating factor. It is a real problem now and it is expected to become an even greater problem in the future. The number of people over the age of 65 is constantly increasing. It is obvious that this is an important achievement, but it is equally obvious that we must begin to consider the age factor as an increasingly important variable in the public health-care system.

Many factors are responsible for increasing the average life span: greater attention is given to prevention, improved living conditions (e.g., hygiene, nutrition) and increased ability to maintain people with diseases in the chronic phase when only a few years ago these same diseases ended with death in the acute phase (e.g., renal failure, cardiovascular diseases, neurodegenerative diseases, cancer). As a consequence, we find ourselves confronting patients who cannot be considered healthy and who need costly medications and/or surgical procedures for many years. Many new medical technologies now in the research and development phase will further extend the lives of the elderly and, at the same time, raise the cost of caring for them. Every developed nation is going to face a significant increase in the number of people over the age of 85. This problem will be intensified by further technological developments, which will not only allow us to treat the elderly more effectively, but also increase the cost of their care, both in long-term care facilities and in the home-care setting.

We are also going to face a greater public demand for good medical care. Publicized research results create expectations that are typically followed by people clamoring for the newest technology. Researchers and the media have fed the hunger for results and nourished the belief that medicine can cure every illness, or at least provide treatment. We have also communicated the idea that money can allow you to avoid disease and its fatality.

All these factors together, an increased life span, more "state of the art" medical procedures, and higher expectations have made it necessary for us to reexamine the dimensions our public health-care budget and to scrutinize our values and our conception justice. If, for example, we decided to treat only the sick with acute conditions, neglecting those with chronic conditions, we could be valuing productivity and efficiency because by favoring the patients who can be cured, the cost-benefit ratio becomes more efficient. Doing the contrary, as Callahan (1987, 1998) polemically and paradoxically suggests, treating only chronically ill patients who cannot be successfully cured, results in increased costs for less benefit. The values that support this type of choice are solidarity and the dignity of the person. We need to forge a strong bond among bioethics, health-care economics, and politics so as to decide together what is the common good. To make the choices that cannot be avoided, we must find a consensus on where to start rationing and from which criteria.

The history of the Italian health-care system reveals that Italy chose to let supply direct demand. For example, The National Health Care Plan, which represents the government's health-care objectives at the practical level, has the task of determining "the level of health care services which in any case must be guaranteed to all its citizens." In fact, this strong commitment to universe access to health-care keeps the cost-benefit concept from rendering the aims of the health care system meaningless. The National Health Care Plan is committed to defend and promote the dignity of the people, especially those who are most fragile. As with most Scandinavian and southern European countries, Italy has also chosen to guarantee access to the health care system to everyone by utilizing tax revenues as the main financing source. Public funding of medicine is widely accepted because it guarantees a fair distribution of resources and allows everyone to utilize the system.

Nevertheless, Italian health professionals are aware that as medical procedures become more complex and costly, we will be obligated to establish criteria for withholding treatment. We will have to develop a system that will not only protect those utilizing the system but that also reflects solidarity by not excluding or selecting individuals based on their social condition, culture, income, physical or psychological weaknesses. The development of health-care policy should be based on the concept of a renewed agreement among citizens, health care workers, and elected officials.

All questions do not have an immediate or a single answer. Starting with the premise that the present standard of universal access to health-care services must continue, we can imagine the first step in limiting health care. For example, we can start from an issue that is rarely mentioned in resource-allocation discussions, which is serious consideration of the role of medical education. We teach our students to be hi-tech doctors, forgetting about the primacy of the doctor–patient relationship. Today, the ability to take a patient's medical history, to examine the patient, and to listen to the patient are replaced by an emphasis on hi-tech diagnostic tests and analyses. In a certain sense, we teach as if making a diagnosis based on the results of hi-tech equipment (CT scan, MRI, etc.) is more objective than basing diagnosis on the signs and symptoms of an illness. Most freshly trained doctors do not know how to interpret the sounds they hear with their stethoscope, yet they know details about every single laboratory test that has just been discovered. This excessive reliance on technology also reflects deterioration of the doctor–patient relationship. Today the doctor's fear of legal action is constantly present and prompts the call for tests and analyses just to avoid being accused of malpractice. Recuperating trust in the doctor–patient relationship can help family practi-

Table 15–1. Alternative Strategies for Cost-Containment in the Pharmaceutical Sector in the EU Member States

Strategies Regarding the Supply	
Fixed estimated budgets for doctors	Family practitioners in the UK
Estimated cost guidelines for doctors	Germany
Fixed estimated budgets for medications	Germany, Italy
Training	France
Evaluating economic feasibility	UK
Checking prescriptions	Almost every country except the UK
Disease management	France, UK
Positive and/or negative lists	Every country
Limit the number of products	Denmark, the Netherlands, Norway
Create a market for generic drugs	Almost every country except France
Strategies Regarding the Demand	
Sharing the costs	Almost every country except the Netherlands
Health-education programs	The Netherlands, UK, Italy
Strategies Aimed at the Market as a Whole	
Keeping prices low	France, Italy, Sweden, Norway
Regulating profits	UK
Referencing prices	Denmark, Germany, the Netherlands
Expected earnings or fixed estimated budgets for industry	France, Spain
Taxes on promotional expenses	France, Spain, Sweden
Creating a market for generic drugs	Almost every country

Source: E. Mossialos and B. Abel-Smith, Cost-containment in the pharmaceutical sector in the EU Member States. London: London School of Economics, 1996.

tioners to treat their patients better without wasting resources. The problem of allocating scarce medical resources makes rethinking and reviewing the framework that sustains the doctor–patient relationship crucially important. The context of rationing provides pressing reasons for restoring dignity to the doctor who must cease to be a mere provider of medical services and must reclaim responsibility to the patient who must not regard medicine as a store where one gets whatever health care one desires.

Another aspect of the current view that we can correct is tied to the idea that medicine should only treat or cure. We invest enormous resources to study new diagnostic procedures, to provide more sophisticated transplants, to develop more costly drug therapies, and to perform extravagant procedures for assisted reproduction, yet little is spent on prevention. Patients, doctors, and elected officials must unite around the concept of "shared responsibil-

ity." The government has to guarantee fair and equal access to medical treatment. The doctor has to utilize the knowledge and skills of medicine to treat and cure patients without wasting resources. The citizen has to learn and practice a way of life that keeps diseases at bay or that limits their impact and progress. Diet, lifestyle, and physical exercise are fundamental components in maintaining well-being. Smoking is unhealthy, and so is being overweight and leading a sedentary lifestyle. In fact, the government is now focused on these strategies to contain the cost of the medication expenses. (See Table 15–1.) We also need to take care of the environment in which we live. Consider the cost of diseases related to environmental pollution (e.g., the treatment of asthma or allergies).

Furthermore, we need a strong cultural effort to encourage people to accept the idea of limits and the inevitability of suffering and sickness as they once did. If a child is hyperactive today, he is quickly medicated. If one feels unhappy or depressed for a very serious personal problem, she takes a pill.

Health-care workers, patients, and citizens are aware that we are at a medical frontier. We are about to reach goals in understanding biological processes and curing diseases that were, until recently, unimaginable. This knowledge should not become the privilege of a few at the expense of the health of the majority. Fair allocation of these resources is what we should all want. We therefore need to consider seriously about quickly building a value system for just allocation before economic needs dictate the allocation policies and before we lose the heritage that the European health-care systems have constructed and strengthened over the last 20 years.

Acknowledgment

I want to thank Caterina Campani, who helped with the final version of the chapter.

NOTE

1. The *Hastings Center Report* provides a systematic overview of the health-care problem. The expert panel classified the reasons for reestablishing the priorities of health care into four categories.

REFERENCES

Callahan, D. (1987). *Setting Limits: Medical Goals in an Aging Society*.
Callahan, D. (1998). *False Hopes*. New York: N.Y. Simon & Schuster by D. Callahan 1987 Simon & Schuster.
Hastings Center Report (1996). The goals of medicine: Setting new priorities. Special Supplement, November, pp. S1–S27.

16

Philosophical Reflections on Clinical Trials in Developing Countries

Baruch A. Brody

Ever since the publication of the results of the AIDS Clinical Trial Group (ACTG) 076 (Connor et al., 1994), it has been known that an extensive regimen of zidovudine provided to the mother and to the fetus can drastically reduce (25.5% to 8.3%) the vertical transmission of HIV, the virus that causes AIDS. Unfortunately, the regimen in question is quite expensive and beyond the means of most developing countries, some of which are the countries most in need of effective techniques for reducing vertical transmission of HIV. This realization led to a series of important clinical trials designed to test the effectiveness of less extensive and less expensive regimens of antiretroviral drugs. These trials were conducted by researchers from developed countries in the developing countries that were in need of these less expensive regimens.

These new trials have been very successful. The Thai CDC trial (Shaffer et al., 1999) showed a 50% reduction (18.9% to 9.4%) in transmission from a much shorter antepartum regimen of zidovudine combined with a more modest intrapartum regimen. The PETRA trial (DeCock et al., 2000) showed that zidovudine and lamivudine provided in modest intrapartum and postpartum regimens also significantly reduced transmission, whether or not they were provided antepartum, although there was a trend to more reduction of transmission if they were provided in a short antepartum regimen (16.5% to 7.8%) than if they were not (16.5% to 10.8%). Most crucially, there was no reduction (16.5% to 15.7%) if they were not provided postpartum. Finally, a single dose of nevirapine provided intrapartum and postpartum was shown in HIVNET 012 (Guay et al., 2000) to significantly reduce transmission (21.3% to 11.9%). In all cases except HIVNET 012, the control group received only a placebo. In HIVNET 012, the control group received a modest regimen of intrapartum and postpartum zidovudine. It is crucial to keep in mind that all these results relate to short-term benefits. Whether or not those benefits can be sustained over time, especially in a breast-feeding population, remains to be seen.

As a result of these trials, developing countries with some significant financial capabilities have the opportunity to drastically reduce vertical transmission by proven less expensive regimens. This constitutes an important contribution of these trials. Unfortunately, however, the poorest of the developing countries (including some in which these trials have been run) may not be able to afford even these shorter regimens unless the drugs in question are priced far less expensively for those countries. Efforts have begun to make that possible (Brown, 2000).

Many critics of these trials have argued that they were unethical. Some have attempted to explain how the information might have been obtained in other more ethical trials while others have not. The focus in this chapter is not on that question. Instead, I want to address the arguments offered in support of the claim that these trials were unethical. I see the critics as advancing three very different criticisms, which they do not carefully distinguish. The first criticism is that an injustice was done to the control group in each of these trials (with perhaps the exception of HIV-NET 012) as the subjects in the control group only received a placebo and were denied proven effective therapy. The second criticism is that participants in the trial were coerced into participating and did not give voluntary consent, because they had no real choice about participating as antiretroviral therapy was otherwise unavailable to them. The third criticism is that the countries in question were exploited by investigators from the developed nations because they were testing the effectiveness of regimens that would not be available after the trial to the citizens of the countries in which the trials were conducted.

The goal of this chapter is not just to deal with these three criticisms as they apply to the vertical HIV transmission trials. It also is an attempt to develop understandings of justice in research, coercive offers,

and exploitation that can be applied to the analysis of other clinical trials in developing countries.

THE JUSTICE OF THE USE OF THE PLACEBO CONTROL GROUP

The scientific importance of the use of concurrent placebo control groups is well illustrated by the PETRA trial. If there had been no such control group and the various regimens had been compared to the historical control group in ACTG 076, then the intrapartum-only arm would have been judged a success, for its transmission rate was only 15.7% as compared to the 25.5% HIV transmission rate in the control group in ACTG 076. But it actually was no better than the placebo control group in PETRA (16.5%). When the rate of HIV transmission varies from one setting to another, historical control groups cannot be used. Despite this scientific value, the critics have argued that it was wrong to use a placebo control arm because the patients in that arm were being denied a proven therapy (the 076 regimen) and were being offered nothing in its place. (Lurie and Wolfe, 1997) The critics claim that this was unjust according to the standard for justice in research articulated in the then-current (and since essentially reaffirmed) version of the Declaration of Helsinki: "In any medical study, every patient, including those of a control group, if any, should be assured of the best proven diagnostic and therapeutic method" (World Medical Association, 1975).

Defenders of these trials quite properly note that none of the participants in these trials would otherwise have received any antiretroviral therapy, so nothing was being denied them that they would otherwise have received. How then, ask the defenders, have members of the control group been treated unjustly? This led to a proposed, but subsequently rejected, revision of the Declaration of Helsinki, which read: "In any biomedical research protocol every patient–subject, including those of a control group, if any, should be assured that he or she will not be denied access to the best proven diagnostic, prophylactic, or therapeutic method that would otherwise be available to him or her" (Proposed revision, 1999). The point of this revision was to maintain that the justice or injustice of what is done to the control group depends on what members of that group *would* have received had the trial not been conducted.

Though the reality of what members of the control group would have received is obviously relevant, I am not satisfied that this proposed revision has properly taken that into account. Would it be just, for example, to use such a placebo control group in a trial in a developed country where the antiretroviral therapy is widely available except to members of some persecuted minority from whom the control group is drawn? They *would* not have received the treatment had the trial not been conducted, although they *should* have received it given the resources available in the developed country; their use in a placebo control group is therefore not justified. The proposed revision was too descriptive, and not sufficiently normative.

A recent workshop has proposed instead that "study participants should be assured the highest standard of care practically attainable in the country in which the trial is being carried out" (Perinatal HIV, 1999). This seems better. After all, it was certainly practical to provide the treatment in question to members of the persecuted minority, even though that would not have occurred because of discrimination in the country. Thus, the use of members of the persecuted minority from the developed country in a placebo control group would not be justified under the workshop standard. Nevertheless, that standard may require too much. Suppose that the treatment is practically attainable in the developing country but only by inappropriately cutting corners on other forms of health care that might have a higher priority in that country. Then, under the workshop standard, the

study participants in the control group must receive the treatment in question, but that seems inappropriate in light of the realities of health-care resources available in the country.

I would suggest, therefore, that the normative nature of the standard should be made explicit. It would then read that all participants in the study, including those in the control group, should not be denied any treatment *that should otherwise be available to him or her in light of the practical realities of health-care resources available in the country in question*. The question for institutional review boards overseeing proposals for such research is then precisely the question of justice. In the case of the persecuted minority in the developed country, subjects in the control group must receive the treatment, and not a placebo, because that treatment should otherwise be available to them in light of the realities of health-care resources in the country. In the case of inappropriately cutting corners to make the treatment available in the developing country, members of the control group need not receive the treatment, and may only receive a placebo, because the treatment should not otherwise be available to them in light of the practical realities of available health-care resources. Perhaps the information in Table 16–1 will be helpful in summarizing the results of this analysis.

On such an account, the trials in question were probably not unjust, although there is some debate about the THAI CDC trial in light of resources that appropriately became available in Thailand during the interval between its being planned and its being implemented (Phanuphak, 1998). Such trials will be harder to justify in the future given the availability today of proven but much less expensive therapies that arguably are appropriately attainable even in some of the poorest countries. It is of interest to note that HIVNET 012 was not a placebo control trial. But it was a superiority trial, and active controlled trials are less problematic scientifically when they are

Table 16–1. Research Standards

	Desired Conclusion	Then Current Declaration of Helsinki	Rejected Revised Version of Declaration of Helsinki	Workshop Standard	Brody Normative Proposal
Persecuted Minority in Developed Country	Not permissible to use them in placebo control group	Not permissible	Permissible	Not permissible	Not permissible
Treatment Attainable in Developing Country only by Inappropriate Cutting of Corners	Permissible to use placebo control group	Not permissible	Permissible	Not permissible	Permissible

superiority trials. That may well be the way future transmission trials will be run.

Two final questions need to be addressed about the standard I have proposed. The first relates to different standards of justice in different countries. The second relates to the justice of the international economic order.

The standard of justice for the use of a placebo control group is a single standard meant to apply to all questions about clinical trials employing such control groups. Because it makes reference to the practical realities of the health-care resources available in the country in question, its implications will vary from one nation to another, but this does not change the fact that this is a single standard. The single standard that friends should help each other accomplish their major goals may have very different implications for how different friends are treated, as different friends have different goals, but it remains a uniform standard across friends. Thus, critics of the vertical HIV transmission trials who say that the trials employed different standards of justice in different countries simply misunderstand the difference between standards and their applications.

Some may also object that, by referring to the practical realities of health-care resources available in the country in question, the proposed standard too easily accepts the realities of the current international economic order, with its wide disparities of available resources in different countries. This chapter is not the place to address the broad and crucial issue of justice in the international economic order. All I can say is that I agree that justice requires the elimination of the extreme disparities, although I am far from being clear what degree of disparities remain acceptable. If one grants that this is so, then it might be suggested that the standard should be modified to read "... *should not be denied any treatment that should otherwise be available to him or her in light of the practical realities of health-care resources that would be available in the country in question if the unjust disparities in the international economic order were eliminated.*" Such a suggestion would have profound implications for clinical trial design, although the exact nature of those implications would, of course, depend upon what remaining disparities were still just.

However, I would reject this suggestion

on the grounds that it requires too much from clinical trials, which are not the appropriate means for addressing all issues of injustice. We need to have both global principles of justice, including ones addressing disparities in the distribution of resources internationally, and activity-specific principles of justice, which place significant demands on those who engage in particular activities without demanding that their activities presuppose the total realization of our global conceptions of justice. In formulating my standard, I demanded that researchers, in their use of placebo control groups, do not take advantage of discrimination in a country's health-care system or of a failure of the country's system to provide needed treatments that are appropriately attainable. That seems to me sufficient for an activity-specific principle, in part because it seems realistically attainable by those engaged in the activity. I recognize that others may deny this distinction among principles of justice or may demand more than I would for this particular type of activity-specific principle.

COERCIVE OFFERS

It has been suggested by other critics that participants in these trials were coerced into participating because of their desperation. "The very desperation of women with no alternatives to protect their children from HIV infection can be extremely coercive," argue one set of critics (Tafese and Murphy, 1998). One of the requirements of an ethical trial is that participants voluntarily agree to participate, and how can their agreement to participate be voluntary if it was coerced?

This line of thinking is analogous to the qualms that many have about paying research subjects substantial sums of money for their participation in the research. Such inducements are often rejected on the grounds that they are coercive, because they are too good to refuse. The International Conference on Harmonization Guidelines for Good Clinical Practice is

one of many standards that incorporate this approach when it stipulates that the "[Institutional Review Board/Institutional Review Committee] should review both the amount and method of payment to subjects to assure that neither present problems of coercion or undue influences on the research subject" (ICH, 1996).

Normally, coercion involves a threat to put someone below his or her baseline, either by actively worsening the person's condition or by interfering with an expected improvement in the condition, unless the individual cooperate with the demands of the person issuing the threat (Nozick, 1969). As the researchers were neither going to actively worsen the condition of those who chose not to participate nor going to interfere with any expected improvement in their condition, they were clearly not threatening them. Further evidence that offering the treatment in these cases should not count as coercion comes from the reflection that threats are unwelcome to the parties being threatened, but there is no reason to suppose that the potential subjects in these trials saw the request to participate as something unwelcome. Even the critics recognize this. The potential subjects were being offered an opportunity that might improve their situation. This was an offer "too good to refuse," not a threat. The critics are arguing, however, that such offers can also be coercive.

Should we expand the concept of coercion to include these very favorable offers? Several reasons exist for thinking that we should not. These offers are opportunity expanding, and opportunity expansion seems to be related more to the enhancement of freedom than to the limitation of freedom involved in coercion. Moreover, the individuals in question want to receive these offers, and this makes the offers very different from coercive threats, which the recipients usually do not want to receive (Wilkinson, 1997). It is important, of course, that participants understand that what they are being offered is *a chance* to receive a treatment that *may* reduce HIV transmission (as this is a randomized placebo controlled trial of a new regimen). Ensuring that participants do understand this is essential for the consent to be an *informed* consent. But as long as care is taken to ensure that this information is conveyed in a culturally sensitive fashion, and that it is understood, then there seems to be little reason to be concerned about coercion simply because a good opportunity is being offered to those individuals with few opportunities.

Sometimes, important issues are intuitively sensed and then misdescribed. This may be one of those cases. The critics who have raised the issue of coercive offers begin with the intuition that there is a problem related to the desperation of the potential subjects. They then (mistakenly, I have argued) describe that problem as a problem about coercion. But I can suggest two alternative hypotheses about what is problematic. One is that the desperation puts the potential subjects at risk of being exploited. This is supported by the notion that we might be less troubled about the trials if the subjects were offered far better conditions for participating in the trial (say, state-of-the-art therapy for them and/or their child for their lifetime). But these far better conditions would make the offer to participate even harder to refuse, so if the problem raised by their desperation really was a problem about coercion, the problem in the trials with those better terms should be worse, not better. If, however, the problem is a worry about exploitation, then such a better offer would be less troubling. I will explore the issue of exploitation in the next section of this chapter.

The other suggestion is that the desperation may result in people discounting long-term harms from participation, because the very substantial short-term benefits may cloud their judgment. This is suggested by some of the language used by the critics, such as subjects being "seduced" into participation. This may indeed be a ground for concern in some cases, but it is difficult to see how it would apply to

the vertical HIV transmission trials, as it is unclear what these long-term harms could be, given the minimal toxicities found in ACTG 076. For these vertical transmission trials, it is appropriate to conclude that the concerns about coercion were unfounded and that the only concern raised by the desperation of the subjects is the concern about exploitation. I turn, therefore, to that concern.

EXPLOITATION OF SUBJECTS

The final criticism of the trials has raised concerns that these trials are exploitative of developing countries and their citizens because the interventions in question, even if proven successful, will not be available in these countries. To quote one of the critics: "To use a population as research subjects because of its poverty and its inability to obtain care, and then to not use that knowledge for the direct benefit of that population, is the very definition of exploitation. This exploitation is made worse by the fact that richer nations will unquestionably benefit from this research . . . [they] will begin to use these lower doses, thereby receiving economic benefit" (Glantz and Grodin, 1998).

There are really two claims being advanced in that statement. The second claim, that the developed countries ran these trials to discover cheaper ways of treating their own citizens, is very implausible as pregnant women in developed nations are increasingly receiving even more expensive cocktails of drugs both to treat the women and to reduce HIV transmission. But that, of course, is only a side issue. The crucial issue is whether the trials exploit the developing countries.

There seems to be a growing consensus that the trials are exploitative unless certain conditions about future availability in the country in question are met. The Council of International Organizations of Medical Societies (CIOMS) is the source of this movement, as it declared in its 1992 guidelines that "as a general rule, the initiating agency should insure that, at the completion of successful testing, any products developed will be made reasonably available to residents of the host community or country" (CIOMS, 1992). A slightly weaker version of this requirement was adopted by a recent workshop, which concluded that "studies are only appropriate if there is a reasonable likelihood that the populations in which they are carried out stand to benefit from successful results" (Perinatal HIV 1999).

This growing consensus is part of what lies behind the effort to secure these benefits by negotiating more favorable prices for the use of the tested drugs in developing countries. It seems highly desirable that this goal be achieved. But I want to suggest that it should be viewed as an aspiration, rather than a requirement, and that different and more modest requirements be met to avoid charges of exploitation.

A good analysis of exploitation is that it is a wrong done to individuals who do not receive a fair share of the benefits produced by an activity in which they voluntarily take part, even if they receive some benefit (Wertheimer, 1996). This is why a mutually beneficial voluntary activity, one from which both parties will be better off, can still be exploitative when one of the parties uses its greater bargaining power to harvest most of the benefits and the other party agrees because it needs whatever modest benefit it will receive.

This is a good analysis of exploitation, precisely because it enables us to distinguish exploitation from other moral issues. One is the issue of wrongfully harming others. Sometimes, people suggest that there can be nothing wrong with a mutually beneficial activity precisely because everyone benefits. The above analysis of exploitation is a good analysis precisely because it enables us to see that someone can be wronged by being treated unfairly even when the person has benefited in the process. A second is the issue of coercion. Sometimes, people suggest that there can be nothing wrong with a mutually beneficial activity

into which all parties have entered voluntarily precisely because everyone has voluntarily entered into the activity. The above analysis of exploitation is a good analysis of exploitation precisely because it enables us to see that someone can be wronged by being treated unfairly even when the individual has voluntarily agreed to enter into the activity. In short, the above analysis enables us to focus on what is crucial to the issue of exploitation, the issue of the fairness of the distribution of benefits.

As we apply this concept to the trials in question, we need to ask who needs to be protected from being exploited by the trials in question. It would seem that, first and foremost, it is the research subjects. Are they getting a fair share of the benefits from the trial? This is a particularly troubling question when we consider those in the control group, whose major benefit from participation may have been an unrealized possibility of getting treated. We may judge that this possibility, even though unrealized, is a sufficient benefit so that they were not treated unfairly. But if we judge that the subjects, especially those who were in the control group, have not received enough, then *they* must receive more. An obvious suggestion is that *they* (either just the subjects in the control group or all the subjects, depending upon whom we deem has not received a fair share of the benefits) be guaranteed access to any regimen proved efficacious in any future pregnancies (or perhaps even that they be granted access to antiretroviral therapy for their own benefit). This would be analogous to familiar concepts of subjects receiving continued access to treatment after their participation in a trial is completed. Such additional benefits to *them* may be necessary if we are to more fairly distribute the benefits of the activity among the participants in the activity; conversely, it is unclear why making the drugs generally available in the country in question is necessary for a fair distribution of the benefits among the participants. Those who have proposed the more general requirement seem to have confused laudable aspirations, or the demands of global justice (if, indeed, it demands that these drugs be available—see our discussion above), with what is required to eliminate the exploitation of the subjects.

It might be objected that others in the less developed country, aside from the subjects who have been involved in the activity, must be protected from exploitation. These others may include health-care workers or, it might be suggested, the health-care infrastructure of the country. The former suggestion is easier to deal with. As long as health-care workers have been appropriately compensated for their activities, what reason is there to suppose that they have been exploited? The latter suggestion is more complex and deserves further discussion.

One possible impact of running the trials in a developing country is that its meager health-care infrastructure resources are diverted to running the trial, instead of to helping other patients with their medical problems. Those other patients would be harmed (not exploited) by the trial, and that must be avoided. Let us suppose, then, that this possible harm has been avoided by an augmentation of the health-care infrastructure through an infusion of resources provided by the sponsors of the trial. Then there would be no one outside of the trial who is harmed because the health-care infrastructure's ability to treat other patients has not been diminished. Often, in fact, the augmentation of the infrastructure (including training of personnel and developing facilities) remains as a residual benefit of the trial. (Leaving such residual benefits is something else to which we should aspire, although this may not be required by the concept of exploitation.) Who then has been exploited? It cannot be these other potential patients because they are not participants in the activity, only (perhaps) unwitting beneficiaries. But if neither the other participants nor the health-care workers are exploited, then it is not clear

that talk about exploitation of the country's health-care infrastructure is morally meaningful.

Let me repeat that I certainly support every reasonable effort to increase access to treatments that will reduce vertical HIV transmission in developing countries. I also support leaving residual augmentations of the country's health-care infrastructure after running trials in developing countries. But imposing the types of communitywide requirements for access and for infrastructure improvement that have been suggested, but not necessarily justified if the above analysis is correct, may prevent important trials from being run because of the potential expense. Such proposals should be treated as moral aspirations. Exploitation should be avoided by focusing on what is owed to those who have participated in the trials. It is they, after all, who are primarily at risk for being exploited.

There is one final observation I want to make about the issue of exploitation. Suppose that there was a case in which someone proposed running a placebo controlled clinical trial in a developing country, but that the subjects in the trial, especially those in the control group, could not receive sufficient additional benefits to meet the challenge that they were being exploited. (Perhaps because there will be no access in that country after the trial to the treatment in question.) Suppose, moreover, that all subjects have participated voluntarily and have benefited from that participation, even though they have not benefited enough. Is the wrong of exploitation a sufficient reason for the trial not to be run? What is the moral force of the wrong of exploitation? This question has been raised by others (Radin, 1996) in discussing other wrongs that are not harms, and it deserves more attention in the case of exploitation than it has received until now.

CONCLUSION

These reflections are important for what they teach us about research in developing countries in general, and not just about research on vertical HIV transmission. Three lessons have emerged. The standard for when a placebo control group is justified is a normative standard (what they should have received if they were not in the trial) rather than a descriptive standard (what they would have received if they were not in the trial). Coercion is not a serious concern in trials simply because attractive offers are made to the subjects. Legitimate concerns about exploiting subjects should be addressed by ensuring their future treatment, rather than by asking what will happen in their community at large.

Acknowledgment

This chapter is an expanded version of a paper I gave at the 2000 International Long-Term Clinical Trials Meeting in London entitled, "Ethical Issues in Clinical Trials in Developing Countries." That paper is forthcoming in *Statistics in Medicine*. This chapter expands upon the clinical and ethical analysis of the earlier effort and offers a more philosophical defense of the conclusions of that earlier work.

REFERENCES

Brown, P. (2000). Cheaper AIDS drugs due for third world. *Nature* 405, 263.

CIOMS (1992). *International Ethical Guidelines for Biomedical Research Involving Subjects*. CIOMS p. 68.

Connor, E.M., Sperling, R.S., Gelber, R., et al. (1994). Reduction of maternal–infant transmission of human immunodeficiency virus type 1 with zidovudine treatment. *New England Journal of Medicine* 331, 1173–80.

DeCock, K., Fowler, M., Mercier, E., et al. (2000). Prevention of mother-to-child HIV transmission in resource poor countries. *JAMA* 283, 1175–82.

Glantz, L. and Grodin, M. Letter (1998). *New England Journal of Medicine* 338, 839.

Guay, L.A., Musoke, P., Fleming, T., et al. (2000). Intrapartum and neonatal single-dose nevirapine compared with zidovudine for prevention of mother-to-child transmission of HIV-1 in Kampala, Uganda. *Lancet* 354, 795–802.

ICH (1996). *Guideline for Good Clinical Practice*, IFPMA, Geneva. Guideline 3.1.8.

Lurie, P. and Wolfe, S.M. (1997). Unethical trials of interventions to reduce perinatal transmission of the human immunodeficiency virus in developing countries. *New England Journal of Medicine* 337, 853–56.

Nozick, R. (1969). Coercion. In S. Morgenbesser (ed.), *Philosophy, Science, and Method*. New York: St. Martin's, Press.

Perinatal HIV Intervention Research in Developing Countries Workshop Participants (1999). Science ethics and the future of research into maternal–infant transmission of HIV-1. *Lancet* 353, 832–35.

Phanuphak, P. (1998). Ethical issues in studies in Thailand of the vertical transmission of HIV. *New England Journal of Medicine*, 338, 834–35.

Proposed revision of the Declaration of Helsinki (1999). *Bull Med Ethics* 18–21.

Radin, M. (1996). *Contested Commodities*. Cambridge, MA: Harvard University Press.

Shaffer, N., Chuachoowong, R., Mock, P.A., et al. (1999). Short-course zidovudine for perinatal HIV-1 transmission in Bankong, Thailand: A randomised controlled trial. *Lancet* 353, 773–80.

Tafesse, E. and Murphy, T. (1998). Letter. *New England Journal of Medicine* 338, 838.

Wertheimer, A. (1996). *Exploitation*. Princeton, NJ: Princeton University Press.

Wilkinson, M. and Moore, A. (1997). Inducement in research. *Bioethics* 11, 373–89.

World Medical Association (1975). Declaration of Helsinki–Principle II.3.

III

SPECIAL NEEDS OF SOCIAL GROUPS

Groups of people with special needs present a variety of challenges for medical justice. Discussions in other sections of this volume illuminate several such issues. Individuals who need extremely expensive care may be as deserving of successful medical intervention as other people are, but the price of treating them may cut into the amount of ordinary care available to everyone else. Individuals who need resources in short supply, such as a human organ for transplant or a drug that has not completed testing phases, compete for treatment, raising questions about the justice of selecting a few recipients while rejecting other, equally needy people. Individuals who need unusual kinds of care may find themselves unable to obtain it because providers offer only those interventions that command large markets, or are otherwise established, popular, or profitable. Discussions of values and principles that may govern such hard cases are found in earlier parts of the book.

In Part III, we look at people whose social status is at least as special as their medical conditions. All are associated with groups that at some point in recent history have been identified as "weak" or vulnerable classes. This means that the group's members have been characterized as less competent or productive than the desirable norm for citizens, and thus have been at higher than usual risk of suffering from discrimination or other forms of injustice. As such, they warrant special protective measures within the health-care system, either for their own sake because of their fragility, or for society's sake in order to enhance their potential to be contributing citizens.

The contributors to this section of the book all explore dimensions of the relationship between generalized cultural stigma or social marginalization and access to medical care. The chapters present different ways in which social devaluation is tied to special claims upon justice within the health-care system. Taken together, they reveal a spectrum of connections between the social injustice that damages our everyday civic and commercial interactions with one another and inequalities and failures in our medical system.

We begin in Chapter 17 with a group whose special need is for an intangible: namely, trust. Given their history of mistreatment by medical professionals, Howard McGary contends, African Americans have a reasonably heightened distrust of the current health-care system. For example, a comparison between the infamous Tuskegee Syphilis Study of half a century ago and contemporary public health programs directed at HIV/AIDS infection in the African-American community finds disquieting similarities. Calling upon arguments advanced by Julia Driver and John Rawls, McGary concludes that mitigating such distrust is a matter of social justice incumbent on public policy. As trust is a central element of effective relations between patients and health-care professionals, African Americans will not have equitable access to health care until trust is established. McGary goes on to identify aspects of the current health system that continue to undermine African-Americans' trust in it and to consider whether health-care professionals have yet formed a resolve to repair the distrust.

Social transformation is also the goal of Rosemarie Tong and Nancy Williams. They seek gender justice in the health-care system. Justice theory in health care should focus on vulnerability, especially on the recognition of women who are disadvantaged because they care for vulnerable people who cannot care for themselves. Some important feminist approaches to equality—for instance, the difference approach, the dominance approach, and the diversity approach—continue to center on independent, self-interested, rational agents. In reality, however, we are interdependent. That this is so means that some community members must assume care of others. "If society cared about its 'carers' as much as it expects its carers to care about society," Tong and Williams point out, women's health would be less compromised, for there would be "less wear and tear on their bodies and psyches." To achieve this level of equality of health, we must support the work of caregivers by directing more resources to support long-term care for the chronically ill.

Anita Silvers's theme is whether the system of allocating rehabilitative care to disabled patients can preserve impartiality without obscuring their personal characteristics and values. She asks whether bedside justice is well served by adopting species-typical functioning as the standard for rehabilitation patients' goals. In answering this question, Silvers develops an approach she calls "multifunctionalism," which should command as much recognition and respect as its analogue, multiculturalism.

Most analyses of achieving social justice in and through medicine focus on acute care of physical illness or injury. It is not clear whether psychiatric illness is well represented by the models assumed in such discussions. Michael Teitelman has his doubts. At the very least, health-care insurance does not offer individuals with mental pathologies that can be mitigated or cured the same benefits provided for people whose physical pathologies can be remedied. This deficiency exists in both private and public coverage. Teitelman attributes such disadvantageous treatment to the social stigmas imposed on the mentally ill.

Perhaps compassion can overcome stigma. But, Teitelman notes, like mental disease, "dental disease does not have outcomes that evoke compassion." Like mental disease, there is no empathic pressure to provide broad and equitable access to treatment of dental disease. Compassion alone cannot be the answer. We must pursue cultural transformations that both acknowledge the reality of the full spectrum of human suffering and support efficacious medical interventions in relieving it.

There are reasons beyond stigmatization for the disregard of certain social groups within the health-care system. Even though our children are our future, Loretta M. Kopelman points out in Chapter 21, they are not provided with the basic health care that adults enjoy. Kopelman demonstrates our duties in this regard, explains why we fail to fulfill these duties, and considers what is needed programmatically to build support for improving children's health.

Kopelman's concern is with the health-care needs of those at or near the start of life. Leslie Pickering Francis writes about the elderly, who are near the end of life. Some of the most respected commentators on health-care justice, such as Daniel Callahan and Norman Daniels, hold that people who belong to the social group labeled "the elderly" should be assigned less priority to access health-care resources. Francis observes that Callahan and Daniels proceed as if the question can be resolved by ideal theory. Their paradigmatic elderly individual is a person who does not enter old age already damaged by prior injustices in the health-care system and by general social injustice. A fairer approach, Francis proposes, is to turn from ideal theory to partial compliance theory, which assumes that decisions about rationing and other public policy issues apply to a world in which some members of large populations such as "the elderly" already bear the marks of a history of inequitable treatment. Francis therefore lays out the constraints that partial compliance theories of justice are likely to impose on health-care rationing as it affects elderly people.

James Lindemann Nelson calls attention to "specific and serious kinds of vulnerabilties" that families develop when total responsibility for ill or disabled family members falls completely on them. Families in this position risk being exploited and becoming dysfunctional because they are drafted into substituting their labor for professional caregivers. Nelson argues that communities have a duty of distributive justice to deploy resources for the support of families with such special needs. This obligation is at least as strong as the requirement for providing health care, and it is even more justified because family members who provide home care for their relatives do a service for the entire community.

Advancing to a similar conclusion, Eva Feder Kittay speaks about the importance, for justice, of increasing both respect and material resources for individuals who occupy caregiving roles, whether they do so professionally or out of love for and obligation to a family member. She accentuates the connectedness that is crucial for all people, whether or not they are disabled. Those in a position of vulnerability need to trust others, and when others are vulnerable to us, we need to know how to be worthy of their trust. We often find ourselves in transition from one role to another, especially as we wend our way through stations of life. Of course, some individuals are continuously rather than intermittently dependent, and there also are people who are extraordinarily detached from all others. We need to develop institutions and ethical strategies that are pertinent to all these extreme conditions, and also to the very wide variety of situations that are more common.

Finally, in Chapter 25 Patricia Smith picks up and deals systematically with questions about financial resources. These questions are raised either explicitly or implicitly in many of the earlier essays in Part III, for populations subjected to general social injustice often are less affluent than are members of favored groups. Smith shows us how intimately poverty, ill health, and lack of health care are connected. Poor health both results from, and exacerbates, poverty. This state of affairs is not only inhumane and unjust; it is also inefficient. As Michael Teitelman finds compassion to be an inadequate antidote to the inadequacy of health care for the mentally ill—a socially devalued group— so Smith argues that charity is an ineffective route for securing health care for the poor. The fundamental problem, she believes, lies in our having made health into a commodity and consequently having set a high price on the means of maintaining it. "Medicine should be dedicated to health without qualification," Smith urges. Neither poverty, nor age, race, gender, nor type of disability should disqualify individuals from equitable access to effective means of caring for their health and the health of their families.

17

Racial Groups, Distrust, and the Distribution of Health Care

Howard McGary

Philosophers have divided the study of ethics into three branches: *descriptive ethics, meta-ethics,* and *normative ethics.* People who do descriptive ethics are interested in providing a correct description of the ethical norms and values in a given society. However, there is no attempt to analyze or evaluate these norms and values.

Philosophers doing meta-ethics analyze or explain the meaning of ethical concepts. They analyze words like *right, wrong, good, bad,* and *ought,* and they attempt to explain how or if ethics differs from other human endeavors such as art, mathematics, and science. Philosophers who do meta-ethics attempt to give us insight into the nature of moral reasoning.

Philosophers who examine normative ethics attempt to justify principles that can be used to make judgments about what is actually right or wrong, good or bad, and morally obligatory. *Applied ethics* is located within this branch of ethical inquiry. People studying applied ethics attempt to apply the results of their normative inquir-ies directly to specific questions in various professions. Or they use a process of *reflective equilibrium* to go back and forth between their intuitions about what is moral and the accepted standards in the given professions.

In the last 30 years, some professional philosophers have trained their critical gazes on a host of ethical issues and problems in a variety of professions. These professions include business, education, journalism, the law, medicine, the military, politics, and science. Their goal is to help these professionals come to careful conclusions about their ethical responsibilities.

A profession that has received a great deal of attention by philosophers is medicine. The issues range from abortion to euthanasia and from genetic engineering to debates over what counts as morally appropriate systems for the delivery of health care. There is some controversy about how effective philosophers or ethicists can be in altering the attitude and behaviors of medical professionals. Some critics question whether there is any real impact when it comes to medical practice.

In this chapter I shall examine an important but neglected topic in medical ethics. In a recent article in the *Mount Sinai Journal of Medicine,* I argued that the medical distrust that African Americans exhibit toward the health-care system is not unreasonable and that addressing this distrust is a matter of social justice (McGary, 1999). Nonetheless, physicians are reluctant to confront this distrust in their medical practice. Thus, the primary aim of this chapter will be to argue that medicine should address African-American distrust. Before I examine this issue, however, I shall present my reasons for believing that African-American distrust of the health-care system is real and also a matter of social justice.

DISTRIBUTIVE JUSTICE AND HEALTH CARE

In the United States, health care, food, and housing are considered to be primary goods (Rawls, 1971, p. 62). According to John Rawls, one of the leading political philosophers of the twentieth century, primary goods are things that every rational person is presumed to want (1971, pp. 90–95). These goods have value to a rational person no matter what his plan of life might be. Rawls goes on to argue in books such as *A Theory of Justice* (1971) and *Political Liberalism* (1992) that these goods are subject to the constraints of justice and they have a bearing on a rational person's self-concept. The cornerstone of Rawls's account of social justice is his belief that the least-advantaged members of society, as measured by their possession of the primary goods, should be the gauge by which we assess the justness of the basic structure of society (1971, pp. 76–80).

Given Rawls's focus on the least-advantaged members of society, he endorses taxing those who are better off in order to make the least-advantaged better off than they would be under any alternative arrangement. However, Rawls's critics from the political right contend that egalitarian/welfarist conceptions of justice violate the individual's right to liberty (Nozick, 1974, chap. 7). Rawls's critics on the left claim his commitment to equality is not strong enough (Nielsen, 1985). They argue that the needs of many, especially the poor, will always go wanting in a capitalist mode of production.

As we can see, there are various ways of conceptualizing the demands of justice. Studies have shown that many African Americans distrust the health care system (Baker, 1999). Does this distrust raise specific issues of social justice or should it be viewed as an instance where people are unreasonably failing to take advantage of existing opportunities? I argue that the response to this distrust is an issue of social justice and that the state does have an obligation to eliminate or mitigate this distrust. In this chapter, I will not explore the more general question about what is the correct account of distributive justice; instead, I shall address the ways race should or should not affect the delivery of health-care benefits in a system that is just.

Scholars who have been concerned with the justice of health care delivery have asked some pertinent questions, such as: What is the nature of a right to health care? Who has the responsibility for financing health care? What should be the priorities in the allocation of health-care resources? (Mappes and Zembaty, 1981, chap. 11). These are all difficult and important questions. How we answer them will have a direct bearing on the quality of our lives. This is true in a racially homogeneous society, but they become even more complex in a racially heterogeneous society with a long history of racial oppression.

No matter which account of distributive justice we embrace, when we say that an institution or practice is unjust we believe that this fact gives us a compelling reason for altering or abandoning it. Because justice is considered to be the first virtue of social institutions, injustice demands action. The action can, and often does, de-

mand state intervention. In capitalist societies like the United States with a
Constitution that vest rights in individuals
and gives great weight to individual liberty,
there is a separation of the right from the
good. Individuals are allowed to pursue
their own conceptions of the good provided they respect the rights of others.

There is a widespread view that justice
demands that we respect the rights of individuals. This is true whether we interpret
rights in consequentialist or deontological
terms (Sen, 1988). On both accounts, injustice or rights violations provide us with
a strong motive for change, a reason for
feeling sympathetic to the victims of injustice, and a basis for claiming that the victims deserve to be compensated for violations of their rights.

HEALTH CARE AND RACISM

Discussions about what should be done in
the aftermath of slavery and a system of
legal racial discrimination have invoked
strong reactions. Some people argue that
state-sanctioned racism is a thing of the
past, and that racial minorities should forget about the past and work to take full
advantage of present opportunities (Steele,
1990). Others argue that the vestiges of a
system of legal discrimination still exist,
and racial minorities will not be able to develop their skills and reach their full potential until society takes steps to break down
the barriers that have been erected by a
long history of racism (West, 1992). The
position that one takes in this debate will
bear directly on where one stands regarding the relevance of race in the distribution
of health care.

For those who believe we ought to put
the past behind us, it is hard to imagine
why a person's race should be seen as morally and socially relevant in the delivery of
health care. For people who view things in
terms of a current time-slice, our horrible
racial history does not justify giving health-
care resources in order to remedy past racial discrimination.

In this postmodern age, some scholars

have argued that we need to totally rethink
the whole concept of race. For them it is
wrong to think of races as natural kinds or
as groups that can be defined in biological
and genetic terms. Some of these commentators even conclude that racial classifications are fictional entities that cause more
harm than good in our legal, moral, and
social deliberations. They believe that we
would be better served by doing away with
the concept of race altogether. We cannot
make race relevant without engaging in unjust discrimination or racism. On their
view, a just society must be completely
blind to race.

But is it overly optimistic to believe that
a society can achieve a just distribution of
health-care benefits without recognizing
people as members of racial groups? Some
scholars have maintained that race is a
meaningless concept that should not have
any significance (Soo Jin et al., 2001). They
argue that as long as we give it significance
(no matter how pure our motives) this will
only encourage and sustain racist ways of
thinking. According to these authors, eliminating documented health disparities
found within the U.S. population is a laudable goal, but they warn us that we face
the following dilemma when we use race to
try to understand the sources of these disparities (Soo Jin, et al., 2001, p. 33). Either
health disparities are the result of unequal
distribution of resources or they are the result of inherited characteristics of individuals defined as ethnically or racially different (Soo-Jin et al., 2001, p. 34). The
authors warn us that how we conceptualize
race when we address this dilemma will
have serious moral consequences. They argue against the use of the concept of race
as a legitimate scientific variable.

These researchers are reluctant to asso-
ciate particular diseases with so-called racial groups. Because they conceptualize
race as a social rather than a biological
kind, they believe that we encounter conceptual and moral problems by trying to
locate identity in genes. They reject naïve
genetic determinism that not only reinforces the belief that discrete human races

exist but also directs attention away from the complex environmental, political, and social factors that contribute to an inequitable distribution of illness.

In contrast, some scholars who deny that races are natural biological kinds go on to claim that races are social constructions that do have a reality. For them, this reality should be taken into account in moral, legal, and social discussions. Those who argue that our history of racism has had an impact on present health care believe that the society must address past racial injustices as a matter of social justice. They view the present situation of racial differences in life expectancy and racial differences in medical treatment as clear consequences of past racist practices that were in many instances condoned by the government. For these scholars, race-based compensatory health-care programs may be necessary to bring about social justice.

The long period of American slavery, Jim Crow segregation, and the use of African Americans in morally questionable medical research differentiates the experiences of African Americans in unique ways from other groups. This history is the primary reason why people who are concerned about the justness of health care believe that we cannot create a just health care system without taking into account the unique history of African Americans.

There is also a third group that, like the second group above, believes a just society must acknowledge race, but it does not have to compensate the descendants of members of racially oppressed groups. According to their view, the good or just society has good forward-looking reasons for taking the steps necessary to make society more egalitarian and open to all. These individuals are not concerned about identifying wrongdoers and providing compensation to those who have been aggrieved. They argue that there are good consequentialist reasons for providing additional resources to persons in certain racial groups (Wasserstrom, 1980).

Even if we could show that race is irrelevant in our personal private relations, it would be hasty to assume that this is also true about public relations. Having said this, many people are still reluctant to conclude that someone's race should matter when it comes to the distribution of health-care benefits.

When asked to reflect on how health care should be distributed, most people claim that medical need should be the primary consideration, although, after further consideration, they will usually conclude that things like the ability to pay might also be a relevant factor. If medical need and ability to pay are relevant considerations in the delivery of health care, then one might conclude that a person's race is relevant because it has an important bearing on who is medically needy and who can afford to pay for medical services. People who argue in this way usually point to the general disparities of health and wealth that exist in American society between African Americans and whites to maintain that race is relevant (Baker, 1999, pp. 212–17). They produce evidence to show that these disparities are widespread, and are especially prevalent in the field of medicine.

But even with this said, others are still reluctant to use race as a characteristic because of the history of how racial identities have been used in the United States to subjugate members of certain groups. There is a long history in America of picking people out by skin coloring for unequal treatment (Baker, 1999, pp. 217–21). African Americans have been the prime victims of unjust discrimination. This discrimination was once so pervasive that it was (and some would say still is) an integral component in the design of American institutions. But will we ever be able to put racism behind us if we do not give moral and legal significance to races?

AFRICAN AMERICANS, DISTRUST, AND HEALTH CARE

Let us turn to the issue of African-American distrust of the health-care system. Is the distrust by African Americans rationally grounded? And if the distrust is unreasonable, does this mean that a just society is under no obligation to address it?

Let me begin with the second question. The mere fact that many African Americans distrust the health-care system does not mean that the system is unfair to them. Nor does it directly follow that the system ought to be altered or abandoned. It depends upon why they distrust the system. If the distrust is based upon misconceptions, then one may initially believe there is no need to change the system.

But this initial reaction may be mistaken. Just because a system is fair does not mean that it can be readily be seen as such. A part of what we mean by a good health-care system is that it is perceived so by those who use it. This is one reason why systems analysts are concerned to produce systems that are simple and readily accessible to the general public. Being a fair system may not be good enough. It may also be necessary for the system to be viewed by the general public as fair.

To be responsible to the needs of the entire community, the health-care system may have an obligation to address even the erroneous perceptions of the system by African Americans. Even if the system is just, and the distrust is not well founded, the long and troubled relationship between African Americans and various components of the health care system may explain the distrust if not justify it. Given our history, perhaps an equitable system should be willing to make reasonable efforts to dispel feelings of distrust. As Aristotle said, the equitable person is not a stickler for justice, especially when doing so does not serve the wider demands of morality (Aristotle [384–322 B.C.], p. 1987).

But what should count as reasonable efforts in such a situation? In my view, two factors would have to be considered. One of them is how much this distrust impacts the delivery of quality health care to African Americans. Another important factor is to what extent do the costs associated with eliminating this unfounded distrust divert funds from medical concerns that may be more pressing. An equitable health-care system must be willing to address these factors in a candid and public way. Doing so will make it clear to all involved that the system is concerned about the interests of the entire community, and that it is sensitive to the historical context that gives rise to this distrust.

From a moral point of view, why should a just society cater to the false perceptions of a large segment of the African-American population? One might argue that an action that is not in itself immoral can be described as morally faulty if it closely resembles an immoral act (Driver, 1992). Immanuel Kant's arguments against the mistreatment of animals are often cited as such an instance. Kant claims that we have duties not to be cruel to animals because this type of cruelty will undermine the genuine duties that we owe to all persons (Kant [1775], 1963). Although treating animals in a cruel manner does not violate Kant's categorical imperative, such treatment damages our benevolent feelings and makes us prone to be cruel to people. Resemblance is taken to be a morally relevant feature of our actions because it can corrupt the actor and it can also mislead others in ways that lead to their moral corruption.

Does the resemblance argument have any application to the debate over minority distrust and the delivery of health care? Perhaps it does. If efforts by public health officials to reduce the risks of AIDS in predominantly African-American communities resemble the strategies that were used in the now infamous Tuskegee Syphilis Study (Jones, 1993), then one might argue that through resemblance such acts, although not in themselves morally wrong, may be faulty because of their tendency to corrupt the actors or those who witness such acts. The Tuskegee Study was a research project that has become symbolic of deception and abuse by the medical establishment of the African-American community. The researchers used culturally sensitive techniques on the grassroots level to ensure the

involvement and participation of the subjects. In the 40-year Tuskegee Study, 399
black men with syphilis and 201 controls
were involved. The unwitting participants
were not exposed to syphilis by the researchers. But even after the discovery of
penicillin, the men in the study with syphilis were not informed about their condition nor were they treated. In order to keep
the participants ignorant, there was an extensive collaboration among a variety of
government agencies, private institutions,
and community-based organizations.

If public health programs resemble, in
form but not in content, the practices in the
Tuskegee Study, then this might give many
people in poor black communities pause.
Sensitive public health officials have attempted to design programs to address the
distrust in these communities. However,
strategies like hiring grassroots people from
the community can backfire and further
contribute to the distrust (Thomas, 1991).
Such efforts often resemble the Tuskegee
Study.

Julia Driver has argued that one of the
basic reasons for thinking that acts that resemble immoral acts are faulty is that we
may be unsure about the moral status of
these acts (Driver, 1992, p. 337). Because
we are unsure, we tend to play it safe and
regard these actions as morally faulty. Can
we justify calling health and public health
programs in black communities morally
objectionable when they appear objectionable to members of these communities?
Some would argue against such a characterization. They might contend that to do
so would be unreasonable. Are they
correct?

Whether they are correct depends upon
how confident we are about the safety and
fairness of these programs. As the probability approaches 1.0, we are inclined to reject the misgivings of African Americans.
But when the evidence is less persuasive,
given the past abuses of African Americans,
such programs will require greater evidence
of propriety than would be required for
people who do not have such a history.

What will count as reasonable will depend
upon past experiences, the extent of the
possible harm, and the resources that are
available to cope with untoward eventualities. This, of course, is not to deny that the
probabilities should rationally dictate
whether African Americans should be involved with such programs. My point is
simply: Human beings more often than we
might think do not do what the probabilities dictate they ought to do. We have seen
that African Americans avoid the health-
care system because of their distrust.

Driver also argues that there are sometimes good consequentialist reasons for refraining from doing something that is not
in itself wrong. She cites the case of a
woman who pays for a vase that she knew
that she did not break to prevent any of
the negative consequences that might result
from misunderstandings concerning the
breaking of the vase (Driver, 1992, p. 341).
In a like manner, a public health-care system may expend funds to forestall the unjustified misgivings that may result from
misunderstandings regarding legitimate efforts to reduce the risk of communicable
diseases. Even though there may be some
bad consequences connected with pander-
ing to people's false perceptions, the good
consequences outweigh the bad.

There may be a more compelling argument for using government resources to
mitigate the bad consequences created by
an understandable, but unreasonable distrust of the health-care system. In *Political
Liberalism*, John Rawls has argued that
stability is an important component of a
just society. According to Rawls (1992,
p. 143):

[t]he problem of stability is not that of bringing
others who reject a conception to share it, or to
act in accordance with it, by workable sanc-
tions, if necessary, as if the task were to find
ways to impose the conception once we are convinced it is sound. Rather, justice as fairness is
not reasonable in the first place unless in a suitable way it can win its support by addressing
each citizen's reason, as explained within its
own framework.

Rawls recognizes that, for a society to be correctly described as just, citizens and public officials must comply with the rules laid down by the basic institutions of society. This compliance must be sustained over a period of time, and those who are expected to comply with it must feel they have a reasonable basis for doing so. For Rawls, it would not be permissible to coerce, pressure, or trick citizens into this compliance.

Stability must be achieved by addressing each citizen's reasons. If stability is an important requirement of the just society, then a society in which a significant number of people believe that they are being treated unjustly will be unstable. Even if the society is just, it has an obligation to reasonably demonstrate to all of its citizens that it is indeed just and trustworthy.

Many African Americans believe the health-care system in the United States is not designed in accordance with principles that are fair and just. If stability is important, and I believe it is, then a just society should be willing to expend the resources to demonstrate the justness of the system. This is especially important where there has been a history of isolating a segment of society by race and then treating this segment in unfair ways. Because African Americans have experienced such a history, it is only reasonable that they would be skeptical about the kind of treatment they might be accorded.

While this skepticism can be overcome, it is naive to think that special efforts will not be required to do so. Although I do not want to encourage wild conspiracy theories about government-sanctioned programs of black genocide, we must not be cavalier about the possibility that African Americans may be the victims of racist injustice. We have made great strides in race relations in this country, but there is still much work to be done. Because of this unfinished work, a just society must be willing to make special efforts to ensure that African Americans can have confidence that the basic institutions of their society will provide them with fair access to health care, respect their rights, and treat them with dignity.

IS DISTRUST A PROBLEM?

Does this mean that we should alter our health-care system? I think so. But if changes are to be effective, we need to realize that the systemic distrust that African Americans feel is not limited to health care. It is a part of a more general distrust for public and private institutions that have a racist history (Herk and Hochschild, 1990). Past policies and practices have certainly played a role in engendering this distrust. No one can seriously dispute the host of serious injustices that have been committed against African Americans by the criminal justice and health-care systems. Although racial discrimination has been reduced, critics complain of a crippling "victim's mentality" that prevents many black Americans from taking full advantage of existing opportunities (Steele, 1990) and that encourages them to blame their personal failings on racism.

According to the philosopher Laurence Thomas, we must exhibit a minimal amount of trust when it comes to strangers without having overwhelming evidence that they are trustworthy (L. Thomas, 1989, pp. 176–86). But can we afford to trust strangers in cases where life and death are at risk? When we are vulnerable to significant bodily or economic harm, should rational people require strong evidence of the trustworthiness of the person or institution upon which they are relying? Do African Americans have good reason to distrust the health-care system?

The continued existence of antiblack racism, as documented by scholars like Andrew Hacker in his book *Two Nations: Black and White, Separate, Hostile, Unequal* (Hacker, 1992), undermines the belief that African Americans are treated fairly by institutions controlled by whites. Hacker assumes that all racism must be eliminated before African Americans can drop their skeptical attitudes. But as our experiences with school desegregation cases shows us, the elimination of intentional racism is not enough (Hacker, 1992). De facto racial discrimination can be just as debilitating as de jure discrimination. As we are well aware, efforts to eliminate de facto segregation in the schools, and in other walks of life, have met with strong opposition. Many African Americans view this opposition as evidence of the lack of goodwill toward their plight. To the extent that they are right, there is a rational basis to be skeptical about how they will fare when they seek health care.

But even if African Americans are justified in thinking that their race could adversely affect the quality of health care they will receive, this would not show they are being treated unjustly unless the system does not attempt to eliminate their distrust. It is not enough to make health-care programs available to African-American communities. Additional efforts and resources should be made available to these communities to overcome the skepticism that many members have toward these programs.

The 40-year Tuskegee Study is unambiguously a case where people's rights were violated, but it is also a case that gives even the most secure African Americans pause about what their government might do in the name of maximizing the common good (Thomas, 1991). The Tuskegee Study and the disproportionate impact that AIDS is having on the black community help fuel conspiracy theories about black genocide. These theories, in turn, breed distrust in a population that is poor and resentful in the wake of persistent inequality. Given that the present political and social reality was created in large part by the past unjust actions of the government, state action is necessary to alter this reality. Whether one uses the language of rights or the vocabulary of the common good, special governmental efforts are required if public health programs are to overcome distrust that took years to construct. We should not be surprised to find that engendering trust in such a system will not be achieved overnight.

There is also widespread distrust about public health programs to combat contagious diseases and also about the quality of primary health care that poor African Americans receive. Given the changes that have occurred in black communities in the wake of racial integration and a growing black underclass, we still find few black health professionals to serve a population with serious health-care needs. These factors combine to cause African Americans to receive inadequate health care.

Trust in a doctor/patient relationship is an important ingredient in receiving good medical care. It is especially important for members of the black underclass to have trusting relationships with people who provide their care (Thurston, 1996). It is not that the doctors are unwilling to develop these relationships, but because patients do not see the same physician on a consistent basis, the familiarity that is necessary to build the bonds between doctors and patients are often lacking. Old family doctors knew that the human side of medicine is important. The lack of familiarity, and thus a lack of trust, unfortunately leads many poor African Americans to avoid seeking health care until they absolutely have no other choice.

Distrust, and the harm that results because of it, cannot be addressed without making fundamental changes in the way our society conceptualizes obligations and priorities. We cannot make changes without reaching some public consensus about how to eliminate the remaining vestiges of a system of racial discrimination. A consensus about the requirements of justice is probably the best that we can do in a democratic society that is defined by racial and cultural pluralism and a belief that each citizen is entitled to shape one's own conception of the good life.

WAYS TO OVERCOME THE DISTRUST

Let us assume, for the sake of argument, that I have established a prima facie case for the claim that a just society should take steps to eliminate the well-founded distrust that many black Americans have toward the health-care establishment. How can this be achieved? Should affirmative action be used to recruit and train African American medical students who may be more aware of the plight of black Americans? This seems like a sensible proposal. However, some conservative writers have raised objections to the idea that a person's race is an indicator of who would be better at serving the needs of a particular community.

Nevertheless, it is doubtful that the number of African-American physicians can be increased enough to have much of an impact on the distrust problem unless we employ very aggressive affirmative action measures. Instead, I wish to examine some of the problems that we face in trying to convince physicians who are not African Americans that this is a problem that they can and should address.

Morally responsible physicians believe they have the best interests of their patients as their primary concern. And many believe that their good intentions, commitment to sound medical practices, and adherence to the law is sufficient for safeguarding the interests and well-being of their patients. So, unfortunately, they doubt whether reflecting on minority distrust of the health-care system will enhance their behaviors as physicians. There are a number of reasons why physicians might adopt this attitude.

Reason One

Many physicians believe that there are some clear-cut things that are right and wrong and good or bad, but that when it comes to many ethical disputes there is no clear-cut position that reasonable people can all agree upon. About these controversial issues, they embrace a kind of ethical relativism. They doubt whether we can reach some reasonable overlapping consensus about certain ethical concerns. For example, they might argue about the morality of abortion (Thomson, 1998).

This objection may be valid in the case of abortion, but I doubt that it can be used to support failing to address the issue of minority distrust of the health-care system. There are no troublesome premises of a metaphysical or moral sort in the argument in favor of taking African-American distrust seriously. Reasonable consensus can be found on this question. Therefore, it would not be reasonable for a morally decent physician to ignore distrust on this ground.

Reason Two

Physicians are viewed as very intelligent and caring people. In fact, to be admitted to medical school students must give evidence that they possess both characteristics in some abundance. We are reluctant to view caring and intelligent people as harboring racial biases. However, this assumption is wrong. Doctors suffer from the same biases and prejudices that are found in the general population.

In her book *Vulnerable Populations and Medicare Services: Why Do Disparities Exist?*, Marian E. Gornick uses Medicare data to demonstrate the racial disparities that exist in Medicare utilization and treatment between elderly people of color and elderly white Medicare patients (Gornick, 2000). By focusing on Medicare recipients, Gornick is able to eliminate class and income factors that complicate making comparisons between blacks and whites in the general population.

Gornick's study shows that black Medicare patients are not given the same quality of care as their white counterparts. She indicates that they are subjected more often than white patients to radical debilitating surgical procedures and that they are less likely to be given the most advanced medical procedures. Physicians unwittingly bring their biases and prejudices to bear when treating black patients. They often assume that blacks are less able to understand certain courses of treatment or that blacks do not have the patience and perseverance that white patients have. This causes doctors to mistakenly believe that there is a rational basis for recommending certain treatments to their white, but not to their black, patients.

Once this information is brought to the attention of doctors, can we rely on them to change their conduct, or will a watchdog agency have to monitor and coerce physicians to do the right thing? History has shown that even when de jure racial discrimination is brought to the attention of the offending parties and laws and rules are changed to correct the bias, de facto racial discrimination still exists. I do not see why things would be different in this case. Without some authority using its power to bring about changes, I doubt that things will be different.

In the present conservative political climate where there is an emphasis on deregulation, there is not much political capital that can be brought to bear through regulations designed to eliminate racial discrimination in the delivery of health care. Doctors already feel that they are overburdened with paperwork from insurance companies and government agencies. It is doubtful that the American Medical Association (AMA) would support moving in this direction even if state and federal legislators were amenable.

Reason Three

Because doctors are experts in one area (medicine), they often mistakenly believe that their expertise carries over into other areas. This belief often generates a harmful paternalistic attitude that often prevents doctors from doing the kind of assessment of their medical decisions and practices that is necessary to ensure that their patients are receiving good medical care and are treated with the respect and dignity they deserve.

During the time of slavery there was a dominant conception of male blacks as childlike figures labeled "Sambos" and, in the case of female slaves, selfless caregivers called "mammies" (McGary and Lawson, 1992, Introduction, chaps. 2 and 3). These stereotypical images of blacks persist today in American culture. As I have argued elsewhere, paternalistic motives often put behavior that we consider morally unacceptable in a more positive light. The person who acts in a way that is harmful to another for paternalistic reasons is seen as misguided rather than evil, for the individual's motive is to do good and not to cause harm or suffering. There is a tendency to believe that such people should be educated rather than punished. This view is very Kantian (Kant 1775 1963). It assumes that people's motives are primary in determining the moral worth of their conduct. People who adopt a more consequentialist perspective put greater weight on outcomes. They might judge that harmful acts even done out of paternalistic motives should be censured and punished.

Even though Americans care about outcomes, we still believe that why a person does what she does (motive) is an important part of any moral assessment of the person and the behavior. Ample evidence shows there is still a widespread belief in the culture that blacks are less intelligent than whites, whether this position is justified by appealing to genes or social conditioning. With either rationale the result is that blacks are stereotyped as less intelligent.

Saddled with this stereotype of blacks, it is no wonder that many doctors prescribe different courses of treatment for their white and black patients (Gornick, 2000, p. 43). Of course, any stereotype or racial generalization can be theoretically overcome in a given case by contrary evidence. However, erasing or repairing stereotypes also requires some substantial personal experience. Because many black patients do not see the same doctor on a regular basis, the sustained interaction that is necessary to overcome the stereotype does not exist in many cases.

Reason Four

The final excuse that many doctors give for failing to address the problem of minority distrust of the health-care system is that they just do not have the time to do so. They do not deny that this is an important problem, but they question the priority that should be given to it. They believe that there are more pressing concerns that require their attention. From their point of view, resources and time are better expended helping patients who are not so distrustful of the system.

This is not an unreasonable stance for doctors to take. Physicians very often engage in cost-benefit analyses to determine which of the courses of action available to them will produce the greatest good. I do not question their method. I have reservations about whether they will indeed achieve greater good by not addressing the distrust that we find in many African American communities.

CONCLUSION

We should be careful to distinguish the nature of the distrust that doctors are being asked to address. Some people within black communities are so distrustful that they only see doctors in cases of medical emergencies; others may practice preventative care, but they do not have complete confidence that their physicians have their best interests at heart. Many patients believe that doctors are more concerned with their own material interests than with the welfare of black patients. As a consequence, black patients do not take full advantage of the medical expertise and resources that are available.

As I have argued above, all of this distrust is not unfounded. Most people act upon generalizations in all aspects of their lives. This is certainly true when it comes to our health. If African Americans discover that a significant percentage of their racial group are being exploited or misused in certain institutional settings, then they will be distrustful or extremely cautious when it comes to their dealings with these institutions. This is also true for whites, but I believe it has greater pertinence for Afri-

can Americans given the history of anti-black racism in this country.

It is very difficult for people from different races to build the bonds that will allow them to trust one another. The doctor–patient relationship is also susceptible to these difficulties (L.M. Thomas, 1999). People are able to trust those of different races by getting to know them. This can only happen through greater association with people we perceive to be different. Overcoming prejudices and stereotypes is something that can only be achieved when the parties involved have open, frank, and sustained interactions with one another. In most medical settings today this sustained interaction is hard to come by.

It would be nice to think we can overcome racial misunderstandings by simply pointing out the ways that these misunderstandings occur. However, this way of viewing the problem gives too much weight to rationality and not enough attention to the role that our emotions play in how we conduct our lives. Even when we know that something is the reasonable thing to do, our emotions often stand in the way of doing what we know to be best. Race relations in the United States invoke strong emotions in the parties involved. Understanding and addressing these emotions can only occur where there is meaningful and sustained interaction.

It is doubtful that medical practices today lend themselves to many sustained and meaningful interaction between white doctors and their black patients. This is especially true where the class and cultural backgrounds of the parties involved are also very different. The establishment of such interactions should be high on the priority list of health-care providers and therefore merit the expenditure of resources. In the end, these resources would help doctors detect and ward off illnesses that require even greater expenditures. It is shortsighted for health providers to save now, but spend vast sums of money later, when they have to deal with the medical consequences of patient distrust.

The problem of minority distrust of the health-care system is a serious but solvable problem. I have tried to suggest how it might be solved without turning to affirmative action in medical school admissions. Kenneth DeVille (1999) has given us good reasons for thinking that affirmative action is a viable option for overcoming distrust. However, I am not sure that in the present climate there is enough resolve to allow us to use affirmative action for this purpose. Therefore, my intent here is to suggest alternatives. I only hope my remarks will encourage others to give this issue the frank and public discussion that it deserves.

REFERENCES

Aristotle [384-322 B.C.] (1987). *Nicomachean Ethics*, 5th ed. Book V. Translated by M. Ostwald. New York: Macmillan.

Baker, R. (1999). Minority distrust of medicine: A historical perspective. *Mount Sinai Journal of Medicine* 66, 212–22.

DeVille, K. (1999). Trust, patient well-being and affirmative action in medical school admissions. *Mount Sinai Journal of Medicine*, 66, 247–56.

Driver, J. (1992). Caesar's wife: On the moral significance of appearing good. *The Journal of Philosophy* 89, 331–43.

Gornick, M.E. (2000). *Vulnerable Populations and Medicare Services: Why Do Disparities Exist?* New York: The Century Foundation.

Hacker, A. (1992). *Two Nations: Black and White, Separate, Hostile, Unequal.* New York: Scribner's.

Herk, M. and Hochschild, J. (1990). Yes, but . . . : Principles and caveats in American racial attitudes. In J.W. Chapman and A. Wertheimer, *Majorities and Minorities.* New York: New York University Press, pp. 308–35.

Hochschild, J.L. (1985). *Thirty Years After Brown.* Washington, DC: Joint Center for Political Studies.

Jones, J.H. (1993). *Bad Blood: The Tuskegee Syphilis Experiment.* New York: Free Press.

Kant, I. [1775] (1963). *Lectures on Ethic.* Translated by L. Infield. Indianapolis, IN: Hackett.

Mappes, T.A. and Zembaty, J.S. (1981). *Biomedical Ethics.* New York: McGraw-Hill.

McGary, H. (1999). Distrust, social justice, and health care. *Mount Sinai Journal of Medicine* 66, 236–40.

McGary, H. and Lawson, B.E. (1992). *Between Slavery and Freedom: Philosophy and American Slavery.* Bloomington: Indiana University Press.

Nielsen, K. (1985). *Equality and Liberty: A Defense of Radical Egalitarianism.* Totowa, NJ: Rowman and Allanheld.

Nozick, R. (1974). *Anarchy, State and Utopia.* New York: Basic Books.

Rawls, J. (1971). *A Theory of Justice.* Cambridge, MA: Harvard University Press, p. 62.

Rawls, J. (1992). *Political Liberalism.* New York: Columbia University Press.

Sen, A.K. (1988). Rights and agency. In S. Scheffler (ed.) *Consequentialism and Its Critics.* Oxford: Oxford University Press, pp. 187–23.

Soo-Jin, L.S., Mountain, J. and Koenig, B.A. (2001). The meanings of "race" in the new genomics: Implications for health disparities research. *Yale Journal of Health Policy, Law, and Ethics* 1, 33–76.

Steele, S. (1990). *The Content of Our Characters.* New York: Saint Martin's Press.

Thomas, L. (1989). *Living Morally: A Psychology of Moral Character.* Philadelphia: Temple University Press.

Thomas, L.M. (1999). Trusting under pressure. *Mount Sinai Journal of Medicine* xx, 66(4), 223–28.

Thomas, S.B. (1991). The Tuskegee syphilis study, 1932 to 1972: Implications for HIV education and AIDS-risk reduction programs in the black community. *American Journal of Public Health* 81, 1498–1504.

Thomson, J.J. (1998). A defense of abortion. In L.P. Pojman and F.J. Beckwith (eds.), *The Abortion Controversy: 25 Years After Roe v. Wade.* Belmont, CA: Wadsworth, pp. 117–31.

Thurston, J. (1996). Death of compassion: *The Endangered Doctor–Patient Relationship.* Waco, TX: WRS Publishers.

West, C. (1992). *Race Matters.* New York: Beacon Press.

Wasserstrom, R. (1980). Racism and sexism. In R.W. Wasserstrom, *Philosophy and Social Issues.* West Lafayette, IN: University of Notre Dame Press.

18

Gender Justice in the Health-Care System: Past Experiences, Present Realities, and Future Hopes

Rosemarie Tong and Nancy Williams

Increasingly, society recognizes that gender, race, ethnicity, nationality, and class affect people's health. Although feminists are concerned about all disparities in people's health status and access to health care, they are, of course, primarily concerned about *gender* disparities. Specifically, they seek to determine whether health-related gender disparities are simply a matter of happenstance and states of affair beyond anyone's control, or whether they are instead the result of discrimination against women.

When feminists express concerns about health-related gender disparities, they raise considerations about justice and gender that traditional philosophers have either not raised or raised somewhat weakly (Okin, 1989). Among these new gender-sensitive justice perspectives is Eva Kittay's "dependency" approach. In her book *Love's Labor: Essays on Women, Equality, and Dependency*, Kittay discusses the popularly accepted view that equality for women consists in women being given the same opportunities to enjoy "the resources and privileges now concentrated in the hands of men" (Kittay, 1999, p. 8). Like many contemporary feminists, Kittay rejects the "sameness" interpretation of equality on the grounds that the "reference class" for women's aspiration (that is, men) is a class whose self-definition, behaviors, values, and virtues have caused a great amount of injustice. Thus, for women to want to be like men is for women to ask for something that it would be better for them not to desire.

Having expressed her primary reason for rejecting a "sameness" approach to gender justice, Kittay proceeds to discuss in some detail the three standard feminist alternatives to it: (*1*) the difference approach, (*2*) the dominance approach, and (*3*) the diversity approach. According to *difference* feminists, women do not have to become like men in order to become men's equals. On the contrary, gender-equality depends on society recognizing that women's differences from men are absolutely essential to society's well-being. Because life would indeed be "nasty, brutish and short" without women's caregiving touch, it is incumbent upon society to esteem "womanly" values at least as highly as it esteems "manly" values.

Although *dominance* feminists agree that the human community is in great need of nurturant people, they nonetheless observe that the tendency to view *women* as society's primary caregivers contributes to women's subordination to men. Exhausted by their self-imposed as well as socially required labors of love, women have relatively little, if any, energy left to pursue their own interests. Thus, dominance feminists maintain that equality for women consists neither in women becoming the same as men nor in women maintaining their difference from men. Rather, it consists in women liberating themselves from men. To achieve equality with men, women need to identify and explore those attitudes, ideologies, norms, systems, and structures that keep women the "second sex."

A final feminist critique of the sameness approach to gender equality is the "diversity" critique. According to *diversity* feminists, the equality problem for women is a matter of eliminating disparities not only between men and women but also between different kinds of women. Equality is a moving target that shifts its meaning depending on the context in which it is sought. The price of achieving equality with one reference group in one dimension of human existence might be the loss of equality with another reference group in another area of life.

In this chapter we explain the ways in which the sameness, difference, dominance, and diversity perspectives function in analyses of gender-based disparities in health status and health care. We also discuss how Kittay's own alternative to the sameness view of equality, the dependency view, might bring us closer to eliminating these disparities. As we see it, gender justice in the health arena will continue to elude us unless understandings of equality based on

individuals' purported independence are replaced by understandings of equality based on individuals' interdependency.

THE SAMENESS APPROACH TO ACHIEVING GENDER JUSTICE IN THE WORLD OF HEALTH CARE

In general, "sameness" feminists claim that two types of gender-based assumptions or "lenses" have made the world of health care a realm in which women are treated as less than men's equals. One of these lenses is so-called male bias, which "refers to the 'observer bias' present in scientific inquiry when scientist-observers adopt male perspectives" (Mastroianni et al., 1994, p. 111). The other one is the so-called male norm, which "refers to the tendency to perceive men's identity and experience as the characterization or standard of what it is to be a person and to portray female differences, where they occur, as deviant" (Mastroianni et al., 1994, p. 111).

Sameness feminists believe that male bias and the male norm explain why many physicians (especially male physicians) tend to treat female patients with less respect and consideration than male patients. Although considerable efforts have been expended to make physicians more aware of their gender biases (Weisman, 1998), female patients continue to report difficulties in communicating with their physicians. For example, in a 1997 *New York Times*/CBS News poll, 59% of 1,453 women interviewed said their own physicians talked down to them half or most of the time, irrespective of the women's level of education (Elder, 1997, p. 8). In addition, 47% of these women said they perceived physicians in general as taking men's complaints far more seriously than women's. Among the most highly educated of the women polled, this perception jumped to 63%. Moreover, because of their less-than-ideal relationships with their own physicians, a majority of all the women surveyed said they sought most of their medical information from television, newspapers, and magazines, with the most educated of them relying on medical websites for their health-care and health status information (Elder, 1997, p. 8).

According to lawyer–bioethicist Rebecca Dresser, American society still tends to view women as less in control of their emotions (fears, anxieties, phobias) than men and, therefore, as worse decision makers than men (Dresser, 1992) Thus, it is not surprising that despite increased efforts to respect all patients' autonomy, paternalism is not dead in the health-care establishment. In fact, the kind of paternalism that aims to protect *women* from making poor judgments about what is in their and their children's (and even fetuses') best interests shows no signs of significant weakening. Many physicians still feel free to make decisions for female patients that they would be loath to make for male patients who supposedly do know what is best for themselves (Miles and August, 1990, p. 87).

The desire among physicians to protect women is apparently shared by research scientists. Traditionally, researchers have defended their exclusion of women from clinical drug and treatment trials primarily on the ground that women of childbearing age need to be protected from harm to their reproductive systems. Sameness feminists object to this exclusion of women. They note that not all women of childbearing age can have or want to have children (Council on Graduate Medical Education, 1995); moreover, men of childbearing age are routinely included in clinical studies of drugs and treatments that might harm *their* reproductive systems. This state of affairs is unfair to women, according to sameness feminists. On the basis of all-male or nearly all-male studies, drugs and therapies are developed and used on women, despite the fact that many diseases have different frequencies, symptoms, and/or complications in women than in men.

Theorizing that as soon as there are as many female as male physicians and researchers, women's and men's health status and health-care needs will be equally well

met, sameness feminists have sought to increase women's access to medical schools and doctoral programs in the natural sciences. But even though women have gone from 17,300 (6% of all physicians) in the 1960s to 104,200 (17% of all physicians) in the 1990s (*American Medical News*, 1992, p. 19), female physicians continue to cluster in the relatively low-paying and low-status areas of medicine such as pediatrics, psychiatry, dermatology, preventive medicine, pathology, and obstetrics/gynecology (Klass, 1988, p. 35), whereas men continue to dominate in such lucrative and prestigious specialties as organ transplantation, neurology, and vascular surgery (Pool, 1990).

The situation for women is much the same in the sciences. Women now constitute 35% of PhD's in the life sciences (Pool, 1990), yet female scientists are not as honored, privileged, and well-financed as are male scientists, largely because of their lack of "connections" to those who make granting and funding decisions (Angier, 1992, p. B8). Indeed, the situation for female scientists has not changed much from 1989 when only 14% of the National Institutes of Health (NIH) research projects were directed by women (Council on Graduate Medical Education, 1995). Thus, sameness feminists continue to espouse affirmative-action initiatives aimed at not only increasing the number of women in previously male-dominated professions but also their rank and salary in them.

THE DIFFERENCE APPROACH TO ACHIEVING GENDER JUSTICE IN THE WORLD OF HEALTH CARE

"Difference" feminists claim that the crucial mistake of sameness feminists is their failure to realize that gender disparities in health status and health care will not disappear just because more women become physicians, health-care professionals, or scientists. In the estimation of difference feminists, women often emerge from medical school and graduate school thoroughly infected by the male norm and male bias, and they are overly eager "to prove they can be just as *good* as any male physician" (Dresser, 1992, p. 28). Only if women practice medicine and do research *as women*, that is, from a gynocentric perspective, will the health-care and science establishments become more humane environments in which patients' psychic, spiritual, and emotional needs are taken as seriously as their somatic and medical needs (Angier, 1992, p. B8).

Difference feminists are strong advocates for the creation of a women's health specialty and of women's health centers. In the early 1990s, Dr. Karen Johnson proposed the creation of a woman's *total* health specialty capable of meeting all of women's basic health care needs: nonreproductive as well as reproductive (Davis, 1993). In support of Johnson's recommendation, difference feminists noted that throughout history women have sought all-female environments in which to address their most serious health-care concerns. Maternity hospitals thrived in the 1800s; family planning centers grew in the early 1900s; and birth control, abortion, and birthing centers appeared in the 1970s (Weisman, 1998). Thus, in the estimation of difference feminists, new-millennium, one-stop women's health-care centers staffed primarily by female health-care practitioners (Gross, 1997) are just the latest additions to a long tradition of all-female health-care environments.

Predictably, sameness feminists have opposed both a women's health specialty and one-stop women's health centers. For example, Dr. Michelle Harrison, a sameness feminist, insists that women are better served when women's similarities to men are emphasized. Her main concern is that with the creation of a women's health specialty, the already established specialties may pay even less attention to women than they do now. Rather than being viewed and used as a resource that other specialties should tap for valuable information about women's health, a women's health specialty

might instead be viewed as a "ghetto" for women and minority physicians and research scientists: an underpaid, low-prestige, domestic specialty for "do-gooders" (Harrison, 1992, p. 169). Similarly, instead of being presented to female patients as high-quality, state-of-the-art, efficient medical complexes, women's health centers might instead be marketed to women as "the medical version of the Kaffee Klatsch, Tupperware party or consciousness-raising group of old" (Gross, 1997).

THE DOMINANCE APPROACH TO ACHIEVING GENDER JUSTICE IN THE WORLD OF HEALTH CARE

As "dominance" feminists see it, neither a sameness nor a difference approach is likely to yield a just health care system for women. Not only does a sameness approach use men as women's measure, so too does a difference approach (Littleton, 1987). Sameness feminists fail to see that in wanting women to be like men, they purchase for women precisely those "male" attitudes, behaviors, and values that have resulted in women's subordination to men. Similarly, in defining women as men's opposite, difference feminists celebrate a set of traditional "feminine" virtues and values (interdependence, community, sharing, emotion, body, trust, absence of hierarchy, nature, innocence, process, joy, peace and life) (Jaggar, 1992) that, though distinct from traditional "masculine" virtues and values (independence, autonomy, intellect, will, hierarchy, domination, transcendence, product, war and death) (Jaggar, 1992), result in women's caring too much for others and not enough for themselves. Justice for women will not be achieved in the realm of health care, according to dominance feminists, unless women stop looking to men and concentrate instead on exploding the kind of power structures that have made women the "second sex." In particular, feminists need to focus less on the people who have most of the power (physicians, high-status health-care professionals, and research scientists), and more on the people who are the most vulnerable: that is, the patients (Fee, 1983, p. 24).

Among the interesting points that dominance feminists make is that women probably had more control over their health care during the eighteenth and nineteenth centuries than they do now. Before scientific biomedicine became capable of effecting dramatic cures for diseases, women were, literally, the doctors in the house. They developed an amazing panoply of relatively effective home remedies for common, chronic ailments. In addition, they routinely served as midwives, relying upon their own experiences to assist other women through what was, at the time, the perilous course of giving birth (Speert, 1980).

Midwives' and women's general control over reproductive matters was not to remain unchallenged, however. As scientific biomedicine, often referred to as "regular" or "allopathic" medicine, began to grow in power and prestige, its practitioners, most of whom were men, claimed they could offer women better pregnancy services than midwives could. Although it was initially difficult for the regulars/allopaths to convince American women to use their services, they gained inroads into the realm of obstetrics/gynecology subsequent to their increased use of painkillers and forceps, two innovations that helped them to ease the birth process for women and to reduce infant mortality (Weisman, 1998, pp. 40–41).

Not only did regulars/allopaths gradually take over midwives' role, they made it extremely difficult for women to join their ranks, going so far as to exclude all women from membership in the newly established American Medical Association (1847). Nevertheless, despite the fact that women had to jump very high hurdles to gain admission to medical schools, a small but extremely able and articulate group managed

to do so. Not surprisingly, these female physicians became leaders in the early-nineteenth century Popular Health Movement, one of the aims of which was to reduce the large number of children that women typically had (Bogdan, 1990). They urged "respectable" women (that is, women who supposedly had no interest in sex except for procreative purposes) to practice "voluntary motherhood" (i.e., birth control) by simply saying "no" to their husbands requests for sex (Weisman, 1998, p. 44).

But "respectable" nineteenth-century women probably did more than just say "no" to their husbands' sexual advances. Most likely they used the contraceptives and abortifacients then available (douching preparations, vaginal sponges, condoms and the like) (Brodie, 1996). In the estimation of dominance feminists, women's increasing willingness and ability to control their reproductive and sexual rhythms set the stage for major post–Civil War efforts to limit women's reproductive choices. The war had left the American male population decimated, and society wanted women to resume their reproductive role full force. "Involuntary motherhood" once again began to displace "voluntary motherhood."

Speculating that not only women's growing inability to produce large numbers of children but also women's increasing "restlessness" were manifestations of "imbalances" in women's reproductive system, regulars/allopaths sought to restore women's wombs to "health." They claimed that concentrated study, focused reading, and creative writing drew too much of women's blood to their brains, depriving their reproductive organs of proper nourishment. Worried that "brain work" was the worst thing possible for women's reproductive health, physicians routinely prescribed "rest-cures" (long periods of bed rest devoid of intellectual activity) as proper treatment for women's menstrual problems, failed pregnancies, and infertility (Speert, 1980).

Reflecting on the development of scientific biomedicine in the United States and elsewhere, dominance feminists conclude that the health-care establishment has done at least as much harm as good to women in the past and still does so today. Specifically, they claim that women often require more health care than do men not so much because they are actually more ill than men, but because medical entrepreneurs deliberately create pseudo-medical "needs" for women. At a time when health-care costs are escalating and third-party payers are growing ever more stingy, dominance feminists fear that an increasing number of health-care administrators and professionals are aiming to capitalize on female baby boomers, the generation of women now hitting their fifties and whose average life expectancy is 79 (National Center for Health Statistics, 1996).

Currently, scores of products, both conventional and alternative, are being developed to meet aging women's supposed need to stay young and healthy. For example, hormone replacement therapy (HRT) is regularly touted as a panacea for women's wrinkles, hot and flushed bodies, weak bones, sexual dysfunctions, and memory gaps. Moreover, infertility services are increasingly offered to post-menopausal women (or nearly post-menopausal women) who are told it is never too late to try for a perfect baby. In addition, cosmetic surgery is, more often than not, being presented as an opportunity that any woman who "cares about herself" ought to seize lest she become an unsightly mess. Finally, drugs are pushed everywhere as the magic cure not only for true depressions but for everyday "blues." For all these reasons and more, dominance feminists increasingly express the concern that all too much of what passes for "medicine" may simply be a prescription for women's enslavement to ever more unrealistic standards for physical and psychological "health." Women, they say, would be better were they to rely less on the "experts" and more on themselves.

THE DIVERSITY APPROACH TO ACHIEVING GENDER JUSTICE IN THE WORLD OF HEALTH CARE

Although dominance feminists initially confined their discussions to gender inequities, they gradually came to the conclusion that women's oppression is a complex phenomenon consisting of several interconnecting parts. Redescribing themselves as diversity feminists, this group of feminists agreed with Charlotte Bunch that "domination on the basis of race, class, religion, sexual preference, economics, or nationality cannot be seen as a *mere additive* to the oppression of women by gender" (Bunch, 1985, emphasis ours). Thus, as diversity feminists see it, depending on facts about herself over and beyond her "femaleness," one woman will receive better health care than another woman will. For example, if a woman has "made it" in this society, she will go to the kind of women's health center that caters to middle-aged and upper-middle-class women, employed and insured, white and well educated. There she will be served by physicians, most of whom will fit her same privileged profile, in a "spa"-like environment where she will be treated to "boutique health care" (Gross, 1997).

At the opposite end of the spectrum, the woman who has not made it in this society will go to another kind of women's health center called the "Medicaid clinic." To be sure, the typical Medicaid clinic does not bill itself as a women's health center, but its clientele is certainly mostly female. Depending on the level of state and federal support available, a woman who depends on Medicaid funds for her care will be provided with a more or less basic package of services delivered by a hurried and harried staff.

Diversity feminists note that differentials in the kind of health care unprivileged women as opposed to privileged women typically receive are especially obvious with respect to currently available reproductive and genetic technologies. For example, in the United States, permissive sterilization, contraception, and abortion policies have worked only to certain women's advantage. A situation illustrating this point is the now defunct "rule of 120." Widely followed by obstetrician-gynecologists for their healthy, white, middle-class patients up through the 1960s, this rule recommended sterilization for a woman only if her age times the number of her living children equaled 120 or more. Angered by physicians' attempts to control their reproductive destinies, these advantaged women pressed for permissive sterilization policies. It never occurred to them that the same obstetrician-gynecologists who were reluctant to sterilize "good stock" were often quite willing to sterilize "inferior stock" (e.g., women of color, especially indigent ones). Indeed, in some Southern states, sterilizations of indigent black women were so common that they were irreverently referred to as "Mississippi appendectomies" (Rodriguez-Trias, 1982, p. 150).

More recently, it has become clear that expensive fertility treatments involving in vitro fertilization and extensive genetic services are available only to women who can pay for them out of pocket. As a result, poor women do not have the same opportunities to procreate as do rich women; and they do not generally receive the kind of prenatal testing and counseling they need in order to make a good decision about the best way to handle the news that their fetus has a genetic disease or defect (Mehlman and Botkin, 1998, pp. 55–87).

To be sure, this state of affairs is not unique to the United States. According to diversity feminists, it is a situation familiar to women all over the world, particularly women in many developing nations. Depending on a society's population size, available health-care services, and beliefs about the value of women, it will use reproductive and genetic technologies for or against women's best interests (Petchesky and Judd, 1998, p. 298). Sadly enough, in all too many countries, scant attention is paid to the ways in which reproductive and genetic "health care" policies contribute to the breakdown not only of women's bodies but also their psyches.

THE DEPENDENCY APPROACH TO GENDER JUSTICE IN THE WORLD OF HEALTH CARE

Clearly, sameness, difference, dominance, and diversity feminists have made significant contributions to improving women's health status and health care. But, in our estimation, they have not focused nearly enough on health issues related to older women. The health of elderly women is generally worse than the health of elderly men, primarily because women live longer than men; and the longer one lives, the more one is afflicted by chronic conditions and disabilities. Aging women's health is also worse than aging men's health because more older women than older men are poor, and the poorer one is, the less likely one is to have access to adequate health care. Although women constitute 58% of the over-65 population, they constitute 75% of the impoverished elderly, and this percentage is growing (Baird, 1998, p. 167). The reasons for women's relative poverty are many, but in general they are related to women's lower income throughout their lifetime, increased poverty from widowhood, and longer life span that depletes savings (Rowland and Lyons, 1996). Thus, elderly women rely on Medicare and Medicaid more than elderly men do.

In 1996, Medicare covered 38.2 million people; of them, 22 million were women, but only 16 million were men. Medicare covers hospitalization and, for additional money, physician bills. Medicare does not cover long-term care or prescription drugs, a fact that distresses all elderly people, but particularly elderly women who constitute nearly 80% of the population in long-term care facilities. Because Medicare does not cover long-term care but Medicaid does, and because most nursing-home residents do not have private health-care insurance that covers long-term care (which, by the way, typically costs $49,820 per annum in 2000 and is expected to rise to $89,220 per annum in 2009!), most nursing-home residents have to "spend down" their personal assets until they become poor enough to qualify for Medicaid (Moon, 1993). Unfortunately, because Medicaid reimburses physicians at very *low* rates, many physicians refuse to accept Medicaid patients. Thus, it is not surprising that many nursing-home residents rarely see a physician. Their care is provided mainly by nurses and nurse ancilliaries. Unfortunately, most nursing homes are so understaffed that 34% of them fail to provide patients with at least two hours of daily care from nurse's aides, and 31% of them fail to provide patients with at least 12 minutes of daily care from a registered nurse. As a result, a very high number of nursing home patients suffer from dry skin, bedsores, malnutrition and excessive weight loss. There are simply not enough hands available to clean and feed patients, let alone to comfort and provide solace to them (Pear, 2000). As sad as this state of affairs is, even sadder is the fact that many nursing-home residents have little contact with family members or old friends. Women in nursing homes tend to be even lonelier than the men there, if only because there are far more widows than widowers over the age of 85.

Clearly, there is something morally unsettling about the fact that those who did most of society's "caring" work when they were younger and healthier tend to get less good health care in old age than those who did far less "caring" throughout their lives. Most of the care needed by the elderly is provided by family members, approximately three-quarters of whom are women. Many women in this position do not shoulder this responsibility, which typically lasts for about two decades, without some reservations and even reluctance. Often they do so because it is either they who do it or no one (AARP, 1989).

Given the fact that caring for an elderly parent or a family member with disabilities at home is usually a very demanding and time-consuming task, many female caregivers find they must give up or substantially reduce work outside of home, and/or pass up any career advancement that conflicts with their attempts to care for their loved one(s). Moreover, if a woman is married, she will probably proceed from taking care of her parents to taking care of her elderly husband at home for as long as possible. When the time comes for the wife to move her husband into a nursing home, it will not be long before the bills wipe out whatever financial assets the couple have. The "good news" about this state of affairs is that the husband will probably not be a Medicaid patient for too long because male life-expectancy projections are such that he is likely to die shortly after he qualifies for Medicaid. Over and beyond the death of her husband, the "bad news" for the wife is that when the time comes for her to move into a nursing home, she will probably not only be a widow but also a very poor and lonely one.

As a Medicaid patient, she will be tended primarily by health-care auxiliaries, most of them women, who will, on the average, eventually meet with the same fate (Fee, 1983, p. 31). Wages and benefits for unskilled health-care workers are meager, particularly if they work as part-time help. Some of these employees perform their jobs grudgingly and/or perfunctorily, but most of them give their work a whole-hearted effort, frequently doing far more than the letter of the law requires of them to do.

To be sure, this situation, which, as we have previously indicated, strikes us as unfair, could be rectified either by getting women to die earlier or by encouraging women not to care for others. Neither of these "solutions" to the problem we have identified has much appeal. Instead, of great interest to us are some of Eva Kittay's suggestions for making the world we live in, including the realm of health care, more just.

According to Kittay, the traditional idea

of equality presumes that all people are in-dependent, symmetrically situated, and wanting the kind of life privileged white men have traditionally had. The problem with this conception of equality is, in Kit-tay's estimation, not only that people are more or less dependent on each other and asymmetrically situated, but also that the kind of life privileged white men and those like them have is made possible by those who do "dependency work" for them. Ac-cording to Kittay, this type of work, tra-ditionally done by *all* women, is increas-ingly done by marginal women as the gaps between privileged and disadvantaged women widens (Kittay, 1999).

Kittay defines a "dependency" worker as someone whose labor enhances the power and activity of another—for example, the woman who has taken care of Kittay's se-verely developmentally disabled daughter, Sasha, for 23 years has enhanced Kittay's ability to pursue successfully the lifestyle of a high-status academic (Kittay, 1999). Sig-nificantly, Kittay wishes to temporarily ex-clude two groups of people from the cate-gory of dependency workers; namely, (1) wives of *healthy* husbands who could do much of the work their wives do for them themselves; and (2) high-status profession-als (lawyers, physicians, teachers) who are amply rewarded for the services they pro-vide to others. When Kittay talks about de-pendency workers she has in mind, first and foremost, the kind of people we de-scribed above: women who formally or in-formally care for vulnerable people who cannot take care of themselves, and who suffer negative personal and/or profes-sional consequences as a result of the work they do. Kittay claims that if we desire a better theory of equality than we have had in the past, we must focus on securing full citizenship for dependency workers. They, rather than the traditional subjects of jus-tice theory—independent, self-interested, rational agents—should be the major focus of our attempts to eliminate injustice (Kit-tay, 1999, p. 38).

Kittay claims that the first goal of public

policy should be "to empower the depen-dency worker with respect to her own in-terests and, whenever possible, to decrease the dependency of the dependent as well" (Kittay, 1999, p. 37). Possible ways to in-crease the power and autonomy of depen-dency workers are to pay them higher sal-aries; expand legislation such as the Medical and Family Leave Act so that it protects the jobs of all workers with care-giving responsibilities; and provide more community-based and workplace care cen-ters for children and for frail elders. Kittay stresses that, in a just society, all mothers, for example, would have the wherewithal to preserve the lives of their children, to foster their growth, and to help them be-come contributing members of a society to which they feel connected (Kittay, 1999, p. 154).

CONCLUSION

Kittay's views on justice would, in our es-timation, go a long way toward eliminating remaining gender disparities in health care. If society cared about its "carers" as much as it expects its carers to care about society, then women would reach old age with ade-quate monies, with less wear and tear on their bodies and psyches, and with more people eager to care for them. As Kittay and we see it, care or dependency work is essential for society's survival. Someone has to do this work if we are to remain a hu-mane society.

To be sure, men need to assume more of the burden of care than they have in the past. But just in case it turns out, as Kittay speculates, that the expectation that women will do dependency work is some-how "integral to our understanding of sex-uality, to the shaping of emotional re-sponse, and to the creation of personality" (Kittay, 1999, p. 188), the safest way for people who care about women's well-being to proceed is simply to provide dependency workers with the material and spiritual re-sources that permit a person to lead a fully human life. A good place to begin is with the creation of a public health-care policy that provides all citizens with health-care coverage: a package of basic health-care services that preeminently includes ample coverage for some of the most vulnerable sections of the population: namely, those who need several years of good long-term care and those who suffer from permanent disabilities and/or chronic illnesses.

Considerations about sameness, difference, dominance, and diversity have done much to eliminate disparities between men and women; but it is considerations about dependency that are most likely to complete this essential task. Unless we abandon the traditional conception of equality, the ethics of justice that bolsters it and the ontology of the separate and independent self that masterminds it, and substitute for it a new concept of equality supported by an ontology of interconnectedness and an ethics of care, dependency workers will remain at the bottom of society and women will continue to be treated less well than most men. As Kittay stresses, we are not so much independent equals as dependent nonequals. Thus, any theory of justice that fails to see the way the world actually is will disserve everyone, but particularly those who not only recognize the fragility of human beings, but also take it upon themselves to weave the relational webs that sustain society as we know it.

REFERENCES

AARP (1989). *Working Caregivers Report: National Survey of Caregivers Final Report.* March. Washington, DC. American Association of Retired Persons. American Medical News (1992):

Angier, N. (1992). Bedside manners improve as more women enter medicine. *New York Times,* June 21, p. B8.

Baird, K. (1998). *Gender Justice and the Health Care System.* New York: Garland Publishing.

Bogdan, J. (1990). Childbirth in America, 1650 to 1990. In R.D. Apple, (ed.), *Women, Health, and Medicine in America: A Historical Handbook.* New Brunswick, NJ: Rutgers University Press, chap. 4.

Brodie, M. (1996). Americans' political participation in the 1993–94 national health care reform debate. *Journal of Health Politics, Policy and Law* 21, 99–128.

Bunch, C. (1985). U.N. World Conference in Nairobi. *Ms.* magazine, June, p. 82.

Council on Graduate Medical Education (1995). *Fifth Report: Women and Medicine.* Rockville, MD: U.S. Department of Health and Human Services.

Davis, F. (1993). Who should doctor women? *Working Woman,* March, pp. 81–86.

Dresser, R. (1992). Wanted—Single, white male for medical research. *Hastings Center Report* January/February, pp. 24–29.

Elder, J. (1997). Poll finds women are the health savvier sex and the warrior. *New York Times,* June 22.

Fee, E. (1983). Women and health care: A comparison of theories. In E. Fee (ed.), *The Politics of Sex in Medicine.* Farmingdale, N.Y.: Baywood Publishing.

Gross, J. (1997). Is there a doctor in the house? Whatever kind you need. *New York Times,* Sunday, June 22, p. 15.

Harrison, M. (1992). Should women's health be a separate medical specialty? *Glamour* magazine, p. 169.

Jaggar, A. (1992). Feminist ethics. In L. Becker and C. Becker (eds.), *Encyclopedia of Ethics.* New York: Garland, pp. 363–64.

Kittay, E. (1999). *Love's Labor: Essays on Women, Equality, and Dependency.* New York: Routledge.

Klass, P. (1988). Are women better doctors? *New York Times Magazine,* April 10, pp. 35–97.

Littleton, C. (1987). Sexual equality reconsidered. *California Law Review* 75, (4), 1279–1337.

Mastroianni, A., Fader, R. and Federman, D. (1994). *Women and Health Research. Ethical and Legal issues of Including Women in Clinical Studies.* National Academy Press: Washington, D.C.

Mehlman, M.J. and Botkin, J.R. (1998). *Access to the Genome: The Change to Equality.* Washington, DC: Georgetown University Press.

Miles, S. and August, A. (1990). Courts, gender, and the right to die. *Law, Medicine and Healthcare* 18 (1–2), p. 87.

Moon, L. (1993). *Medicine Now and in the Future.* Washington, DC: Urban Institute.

National Center for Health Statistics (NCHS) (1996a). *Health United States, 1995–1996.* Hyattsville, MD: Public Health Service.

Okin, S.M. (1989). *Justice, Gender, and the Family.* New York: Basic Books.

Pear, R. (2000). U.S. recommending strict new

roles at nursing homes. *New York Times*, July 23, pp. 1, 15.

Petchesky, R. and Judd, K. (1998). *Negotiating Reproductive Rights: Women's Perspectives Across Countries and Cultures*. London: Zed Books.

Pool, R. (1990). Who will do science in the 1990s? *News & Comment*, April 27, pp. 433–35

Rodriguez-Trias, H. (1982). Sterilization abuse. In Hubbard, R., Henifin, M.S., and Fried B. (eds.), *Biological Woman: The Convenient Myth*. Cambridge, MA: Scheneman.

Rowland, D. and Lyons, B. (1996). Medicare, medicaid, and the elderly poor. *Health Care Financing Review* 18(2), 61–85.

Speert, H. (1980). *Obstetrics and Gynecology in America: A History*. Chicago: American College of Obstetricians and Gynecologists

Weisman, C.S. (1998). *Women's Health Care: Activist Traditions and Institutional Change*. Baltimore: Johns Hopkins University Press.

19

Bedside Justice and Disability: Personalizing Judgment, Preserving Impartiality

Anita Silvers

Commenting on changes in the culture of health care, Eric J. Cassell observed: "Although [I] could rise in outrage at the idea of the concept of justice at the bedside in 1981, less than twenty years later it has a secure place at the head of the patient's bed" (Cassell, 2000, p. 21).

Over the decades to which Cassell refers, an abundance of conversation has professed that health is good for justice, and justice is good for health. As a result, it hardly seems strange to think of justice as being an appropriate and important component of decisions that determine patient care. Nevertheless, the conduct of justice in the sick room remains troubling.

BEDSIDE JUSTICE

Justice's role at the bedside, Cassell (2000) says, is "to insure that the patient gets a fair share (but not more) of the medical resources and that the social system gets its money's worth" (p. 21). But is justice, when conducted as usual, sufficient for

these guarantees? A troublesome discrepancy appears as we consider whether procedures central to judgments about justice suit the delivery of health care. The traditional approach to dispensing justice is (figuratively) to don a blindfold. But it is not at all reassuring to envision the dispensing of medical treatment in a blindfold, even a figurative one.

Consequently, in this chapter, I begin an exploration of the propriety of regarding, rather than blinding ourselves to, patients' individual characters and personal values in deciding what is no more nor less than each patient's fair share of medical services. Should we weigh patients' nonbiological differences for purposes of just allocation of medical attention and materials? May we do so and yet achieve the impartiality ordinarily demanded by justice? Here, I will consider whether certain medical resource distribution decisions, made with the goal of normalizing patients' functioning, ought to be influenced by patients' personal values in regard to modes of functioning, and by the character traits and ideas about the good that underlie people's individual preferences for different goals. Is such personalization compatible with a just allocation system? And whose preferences about modes and levels of functioning justly take precedence in determining what medical services a patient should get—the patient's? the medical professional's? the dominant social group's?

For purposes of this discussion, I will assume a society that tolerates different ideas of the good. Various paths traveled to different goals may equally be of social benefit and therefore deserving of support from collective resources. As multiculturalism recognizes that the practices and convictions of various cultures are equally valuable, I will argue, multifunctionalism similarly acknowledges the equivalent value of various modes of performing such important human functions as mobilizing, socializing, acquiring information and communicating it. Appreciating multifunctionalism is as important for healthcare justice, I will suggest, as appreciating multiculturalism is for justice in other areas of social policy.

Brief though the discussion will be, it should throw some light on how to endow justice with a bedside manner that has a personal touch. It thus will afford a bit of insight into designing health-care distribution systems capable of inspiring patients' confidence in the system's justice. To gain perspective, we will consider alternative approaches to allocating fair shares of medical resources under the constraint that Cassell applies to distributive justice, namely that "the social system gets its money's worth."

Depersonalizing Medical Decisions

Impartiality is a mark of justice. Our usual understanding is that justice abstracts from, and is expected to be blind to, personal traits that make some recipients more satisfying or attractive or otherwise pleasurable to serve than others. Initially, this standard appears not only appropriate to, but also advisable for, medicine. Arguably, medical allocation decisions would verge on injustice were we deliberately to give charming, appealing or admirable patients, or those who share our values, priority in obtaining treatment, especially if having traits like these becomes the reason one patient rather than another receives the means for being cured.

Some biological characteristics are no more relevant to the justice of providing a person with health care than are the individual's character and other personality traits. Being in danger of having one's flourishing health compromised, or of losing the use of a superlatively functioning part of one's body, should afford an individual no priority for preventative or reparative medical care over others, with the same medical needs, who have flabby bodies or are in imperfect health. Nor should patients' skin, eye, or hair color procure priority for them (unless such a trait supports a diagnosis warranting urgent intervention, as, for instance, a patient's having red hair might support scheduling a dermatological examination because of the association of red hair with an elevated risk of skin cancer) (Satz and Silvers, 2000).

Clearly, not every feature of a person's biological condition justly influences the allocation of potentially successful medical treatment. Even some conditions associated with the biological anomalies we consider to be impairments should not do so. For instance, United States disability discrimination law prohibits viewing Down syndrome as categorically precluding eligibility for organ transplantation, except where a particular patient's level of Down-associated circulatory or cognitive dysfunction may contraindicate the success of a transplant (Cole, 1996).

It usually is considered wrong to allow a patient's character and personal values to influence whether he or she receives medical resources. We are not comfortable with the thought that being virtuous should gain priority for individuals in securing scarce pharmaceuticals or organs for transplantation. Arguably, some aspects of a patient's character do bear on allocation decisions. But Moss and Siegler have pointed out that even these tend to be "medicalized" and thereby depersonalized and objectified. For example, as Moss and Siegler (1991) show, distaste for permitting individuals whom we hold responsible for their own physical deterioration to have access to replacement organs is camouflaged by contentions about their heightened risk of replacement organ failure. In a similar process of medicalizing value judgments, the global devaluation of persons with anomalous cognitive traits due to Down syndrome has prompted unsubstantiated clinical decisions that those with Down syndrome cannot be compliant with a post-transplant regimen. In general, this process camouflages personal bias against patients by disguising medical professionals' reluctance to engage with them individually as judgments about the riskiness of treating members of their group.

Depersonalizing judgment does not guarantee that it is unbiased. When health-care allocation schemes deprive people with Down syndrome and other disabilities of equitable health-care opportunity, they typically do so by devising impersonal measures that become proxies for personal traits. When not protected by strong disability discrimination statutes, people with Down syndrome often have been denied life-saving treatment available to other citizens, but not with direct reference to a personal trait. Instead, the policies that deprive them apply depersonalized quality-of-life or disability-adjusted measures (Glatzer, 1999).[1] These quality of life measures usually stipulate that, in general, living with a disability makes people deficient in personal success. They do so by defining species-atypical biological limitations as equivalent to reduced ratings on their scales of the value of life. They thereby deflect medical decision making from attend-ing to the real textures and values of each patient's life.

JUSTICE AND HEALTH

Justice Is Good for Health

Can justice be good for our health if judgments about justice depersonalize patients? Answering requires considering why bioethicists and other health-policy scholars often seem to view health and justice as symbiotic. Literature describing correlations between health and justice is plentiful and need not be reported except in general outline here. The point of the brief review that follows is to see why some bioethicists believe that securing social justice will make us healthier.

Injustice is manifested in the denial of important goods such as health and education to those who deserve and need them. Thus, without committing to any specific theory of justice, we can expect that more citizens in just societies will have access to the material resources needed to achieve and sustain good health, and to the educational resources needed to understand the importance of maintaining health, than in unjust societies.

Further, a just society is organized to promote the good of citizens collectively, whereas an unjust society ignores the good of the many and serves only the few. We thus can anticipate that just societies are likely to pursue broad public health initiatives for their citizens, seeking to improve conditions for all types of citizens, whereas unjust societies focus on health issues of importance to the most influential citizens, if they cultivate public health at all. Similarly, just societies will promote health-care research equity. For example, in a just society the principles regulating drug development and testing will ensure that therapies benefit women as positively as men, and that remedies for illnesses prevalent in minority or powerless populations are sought as energetically as for the illnesses of large or influential populations.

In sum, we can postulate that larger proportions of the citizenry of just societies will live in conditions that improve health than will the citizenry of unjust societies. Parenthetically, although more citizens will be healthier in just societies than in unjust ones, just societies will not necessarily manifest higher aggregated levels of health than unjust ones. In a just society, broad-based access to health support likely will maintain at-risk individuals whose lives would be lost in an unjust society. To illustrate, a society where the concern to improve everyone's health creates programs that prevent polluted urban air may maintain the lives of more sufferers of serious respiratory disorders than a society in which only the powerful have access to clean air. A society where dialysis is available without regard to age or cause of kidney failure is likely to maintain the lives of more elderly diabetics than one that denies this lifesaving treatment to whatever groups cannot meet the eligibility qualifications to have more years of life. And a society where fragile neonates are treated regardless of their prospects of disability is likely to increase the proportion of disabled children in its population.

Once we understand this, we can see that to affirm that justice is good for health does not entail any claim about the superiority of aggregated health in just societies or about the propriety of using aggregated health as a measure of social justice. The standard of justice in health care is not "the nation's health," although a depressed level of aggregated health may be a sign of neglect of the welfare of many citizens. Equitable personal healthiness, at levels appropriate to facilitate different individuals' securing of their own variety of goods, is what we should expect of a just system.

Health Is Good for Justice: Equalizing Welfare

As justice is good for health, health also is good for justice. The idea here is that health is necessary to each citizen's pursuit of welfare. Thus, whether justice is thought of in terms of equality of outcomes, or in terms of equality of opportunity to realize desirable outcomes, being reasonably healthy enables individuals to benefit from justice. Equally healthy citizens are equally well-positioned, at least in this respect, to benefit from justice.

Those who take the view that justice must offer more than opportunity urge that something more than leveling the playing field must be done. Individuals with health problems must be made capable of leaving the starting gate in pursuit of opportunity, even if doing so requires an unevenness in how health services are allocated. If individuals' poor health impedes their pursuit of opportunity, just societies should allocate more health-care resources than is common to them to help overcome their disadvantage. For example, Amartya Sen famously argues that it is not unfair to allocate unequally large amounts of resources to those special individuals who need to repair or compensate for certain kinds of deficiencies so that they can acquire the basic capabilities the rest of the population enjoys. (Sen, 1980, 1992, 1993). People with health problems thus may consume greater amounts of health-care resources than others without being unfairly privileged.

For Richard Arneson, the question of justice is what we owe to people whose well-being is compromised by ill health regardless of the excellence of their access to opportunity. Moral value is maximized by making gains in the expected well-being of such individuals, who are disadvantaged by health problems. Applications of health-care resources can sometimes reconfigure the circumstances that determine their lifetime allotment of well-being. Such social intervention promotes a fairer distribution of well-being. To be deserving, beneficiaries must be blameless for their deficits (to discourage people from being careless about their health in the expectation of receiving reparative care) and able to benefit from the receipt of extraordinary resources (Arneson, 1988).

Individualized judgments are required to determine how well each particular person with an illness or disability meets these criteria. Elizabeth Anderson criticizes Arneson for basing justice for ill and disabled people on particularized demonstrations of individual neediness rather than on improving the condition of their class. She is also concerned that only those individuals with the proper personal traits and character are considered deserving of compensatory health care. For it seems mean-spirited, to say the least, to reserve the advantage of just treatment for patients of good character and promising potential (Anderson, 1999).

Treatment allocation schemes implemented through inquiries into patients' character traits and personal values appear to ration justice itself by granting just treatment only to people whose personal traits make them eligible for justice. Nevertheless, indiscriminately blocking all consideration of patients' characters and other personal traits when determining eligibility for medical care may be too extreme. This matter of the weight properly afforded to patients' characters should be further explored, but first we should examine an alternative approach to justice, one that shifts the focus from equalizing individuals' welfare to equalizing collective opportunity.

Health Is Good for Justice: Equalizing Opportunity

This latter approach promotes the view that health care contributes to justice most directly by facilitating equal opportunity for different groups, rather than by securing equal outcomes for each individual. Securing justice for the group of people known as "the disabled" means offering this group equitable social participation. Social participation—the ability to exercise the prerogatives of citizenship with the potential for reaping benefits for oneself—is predicated on normal functioning, and nor-

mal functioning is imagined to secure a "normal" opportunity range. Normal functioning—performing not only at ordinary levels but also in commonplace modes—is empowered by good health. Illness or accident can impair normal functioning and thereby result in abnormally deficient opportunity. Reduction of mobility, sight, hearing, cardiac capacity, cognitive proficiency, hormone production, and so on can compromise normal functioning by diminishing it or by forcing functions to be performed in an anomalous way, making them disabled. Programs that restore disabled people to normal functioning thus appear to increase this group's opportunity (Daniels, 1987; see Chapter 1 of this volume)

Norman Daniels, for example, views health care that restores normal functioning as an affirmative measure for furthering fair access to the range of satisfactory opportunities or life plans reasonable people would want to have available (Daniels, chapter 1). The responsibility for maintaining equality of opportunity is collective. Therefore, the burden of restoring anomalously functioning people to normality should not rest disproportionately on those individuals themselves but should be supported by society as a whole.

To take the maintenance of normality as the goal of health care for society as a whole is to abstract from a wide variety of personal goals that patients might articulate. Daniels (1987), a proponent of this standard, explains:

I abstract from the special effects that derive from an individual's conception of the good. This level of abstraction seems appropriate given our search for a measure of the social importance, for claims of justice, of impairments of health. My conclusion is that we should use impairment of the normal . . . as a measure of the relative importance of health care needs. (p. 306)

But what qualifies as normal functioning? An initial inclination is to identify it with a set of biologically mandated performances, those so successful that their levels and modes have come to typify human activity. Thus, Daniels has imagined that "where we can take as fixed, primarily by nature, a generally uncontroversial baseline of species-typical functioning," we can show "which principles of justice are relevant to distributing health care services" (Daniels, 1987, p. 303). That is, the way the species typically functions constitutes a natural standard in respect to opportunity. Meaningful access for exercising the capabilities of citizens is predicated on citizens satisfying this standard.

However, as Ron Amundson observes, the idea of normal function has no foundation in objective biological fact because very large amounts of heritable variation occur in natural species (Amundson, 2000). Furthermore, nature does not issue an imperative to normalize individuals by altering them so that they perform in the most familiar way. In modern biology, dogmas about determinate species design have given way to appreciation of rich ranges of variation. That we think of certain modes and levels of human performances as typical, common, or average for our species does not make these the normal or natural modes and levels for humankind (Sober, 1980, 2000). Nor does turning to nature as a standard provide an apt basis for a health-care allocation scheme, for biology tends to eliminate dysfunctional individuals, not to cure or otherwise repair them.

From the perspectives of both individual and society, being a normally functioning citizen appears eminently socially desirable. In the United States, at least, being normal and thereby unobtrusive is sound strategy for social preservation. As Tom Smith, director of the General Social Survey for the National Opinion Research Center at the University of Chicago, observes: "We penalize . . . people who are extreme" (Carter, 2000, p. B9).

As Norman Daniels notes (Daniels, Chapter 1, this volume), to keep people (close to) normal functioning means that individuals maintain enjoyment of political, social, and economic participation. From the perspective of the state normally functioning people maintain the ability to be contributing citizens rather than burdensome ones. Hence, the standard of maintaining normal functioning preserves parity between the two objectives of "bedside justice" that Cassell identifies. Restoring a patient to normal functioning appears to acquire a fair share of opportunity for that individual and simultaneously to secure a productive member for the society.

Adopting this goal appears to withhold medical treatment only from those who already function within normal range and consequently do not need it. Thus, the line between deserved and undeserved treatments derives not from personalized differences (such as between considerate and nasty, industrious and lazy, or responsible and irresponsible persons) but instead depends on whether the individual's capabilities are defective when judged by the impersonal standard of normal functioning. Daniels believes that the class of deserving patients so delineated will be co-extensive with the categories of seriously diseased or disabled people. Such individuals should be returned to normal functioning or as close an approximation of it as possible. There is no similar imperative, however, to elevate the capabilities of people who function at the bottom of the normal range or who desire to improve on nature. Adopting the maintenance of normal functioning as the goal of just health care appears to offer an impersonal criterion for determining the kinds of medical treatment to be allocated, and for selecting the recipients of treatment as well.

ALLOCATING REHABILITATIVE CARE

Pursuing the Goal of Normal Functioning

If the normal functioning of all citizens is health care's goal, we can see how health care facilitates achieving a society where citizens are equally functional and equally capable of social contribution. To secure normal functioning appears to be a generally appealing and benign health-care goal. We should not, however, assume that maintaining or restoring normality is the direct or immediate goal of all medical interventions. Even if securing normal functioning seems to be a goal in some areas of medicine, we cannot assume this to be an unquestionable standard for success in allocating medical services generally, or for achieving beside justice.

Medicine can be conceived as practiced across three (overlapping) domains: preventative, acute, and rehabilitative care. While acknowledged as a value, normalcy is not the preeminent value in preventative and acute care. However, in the last of these domains—rehabilitation—the goal of achieving normal functioning, or approximating it as much as possible, is applied immediately and directly in determining whether or not resources will be allocated. Assessments of patients, made for the purpose of deciding whether to admit the patient to a rehabilitation unit or to continue his or her treatment there, typically assign importance to the patient's personal attitude toward normalcy. As Arthur Caplan (1988) observes, "Motivation is rarely used as a criterion for initiating health care" in acute cases. In contrast, the procedure for allocating rehabilitative care "is fraught with value judgments as to what constitutes sufficient levels of [the patient's] compliance, cooperation and enthusiasm [and] may even masquerade for other more subtle value judgments" (p. 9).

There are further reasons for believing that preventative and acute medicine do not have normal functioning as their direct goal, whereas rehabilitation medicine does. In preventative care, the immediate goal is to stimulate those mechanisms that promote the most robust health, even if doing so involves enhancing patients by inducing them to function superlatively rather than normally. An important strategy used in preventative care alters people so that rare but advantageous biological conditions become common. For example, immunity to smallpox was once a rare and happy competence acquired by milkmaids and some few other fortunately situated people. Subsequently, as a result of extensive vaccination programs, having effectively protective antibodies against smallpox came to be typical of many populations. Were precluding illness not the direct goal of preventative practice, and were preserving the normal state of a population its goal instead, we would hardly have embarked on programs of inoculation.

Acute care likewise differs from rehabilitative care in ways that indicate a divergence of direct goals. As Caplan points out, the criteria for deciding to cease treatment diverge in these two domains. "In acute care, cure or death may be signposts for stopping treatment . . . [but] the language used by rehabilitation professionals to describe this phase of care is 'plateauing' " (Caplan et al., 1987, p. 11). "The concept of plateauing is one that seems particularly unique to rehabilitation medicine" (Caplan et al., 1987, p. 13) To assess a patient as having plateaued "did not mean he was incapable of further progress, but that the rate of progress was deemed inadequate relative to the level of resources required to achieve it" (p. 11). This is to say that the direct and immediate justification for allocating rehabilitative treatment is to enable the patient to attain or move toward normal functioning. As the promise of progress toward that goal subsides, the justification for allocating the treatment weakens. "Patients in . . . rehabilitation settings are expected to make constant and steady progress toward attaining the goals set by the rehabilitation team. When progress slows . . . the health care team may raise questions as to whether further . . . therapy [is] worthwhile" (p. 13). Unlike acute care, failure to progress to normalcy is the signpost for withdrawing treatment in rehabilitation medicine.

Referring to Patients' Personal Traits and Values

In acute care there is "no need to ascertain the patient's values" (Caplan et al., 1987, p. 5. In contrast, "one of the most distinctive aspects of rehabilitation . . . is that practitioners choose their patients. . . . Clinical practitioners . . . review potential patients in order to select those who . . . receive treatment" (Caplan et al., 1987, p. 7). According to a *Hastings Center Report* on the ethics of rehabilitation medicine, patients and health-care professionals often are driven by different values, and "the fact that medical care in rehabilitation is unavoidably value-laden creates a variety of ethical questions of a kind that rarely arise when health care providers and patients agree about the goal of care" (Caplan et al., 1987, p. 7).

Rehabilitation through physical medicine treats patients whose impairments result from disease, accident, or congenital anomaly (Haas, 1993, p. 228). While its goal is to restore or approximate normal functioning in patients, there are various ways of characterizing this result. Among the aims mentioned prominently in the rehabilitation literature are enabling the patient to function with a high level of community participation (Kotke, 1980), improving biological function, and inducing environmental adjustment so that patients have purposeful, gratifying lives (Spencer, 1970), and maintaining a lifestyle sufficient to achieve productivity (Treischman, 1974).

However, "since patients and providers bring different values to . . . rehabilitation, disagreements may arise concerning goals" (Caplan et al., 1987, p. 6). Ten percent of the working-age U.S. population reports having a dysfunction that reduces the ability to work (Caplan et al., 1987, p. 17). "Should rehabilitation specialists stress the value of work in designing treatment plans for patients for whom employment may not be of great personal value?" ask the authors of the *Hastings Center Report* (Ca-

plan et al., 1987, p. 7) Professionals who accept the socially preeminent value of productivity may find themselves assessing patients who believe that, on balance, reentering the work force will not benefit them. Patients who express this belief tend to be described in the rehabilitation literature as "malingering" individuals whose personal character justifies withdrawing services from them. But "[i]n rehabilitation there is always the chance that more therapy will increase function, even if marginally." Moreover, what is "marginal to the provider may be of major significance for the patient or the patient's family" (Caplan et al., 1987, p. 11). So, for instance, a patient may wish to attain a mode or level of functioning that increases personal satisfaction but not social productivity. Such patients may be denied rehabilitation because they seek to retrieve capabilities valuable to them personally but insignificant from professional or social perspectives.

About a third of patients who receive rehabilitation services for physical dysfunctions have some kind of neurological anomaly, another third have skeletal or muscular anomalies, and the remainder have physical performance limitations resulting from cardiopulmonary or other chronic illnesses (Caplan et al., 1987, p. 4). Some patients can be rehabilitated so as to perform both at the level and in the mode they functioned prior to illness or injury, or would have functioned were it not for a congenital anomaly. For others, however, rehabilitation restores function by enhancing compensatory performances and imparting strategies for surmounting environmental barriers.

In treating patients in the latter category, ethical questions about the appropriateness of different functional goals arise. Patient and professional may differ about the relative merit of walking with difficulty, as compared with wheeling with ease in a world not readily accessible to wheelchair users. What "patients . . . can do is not necessarily what they will choose to do. When freed from the constraints of the treatment team, countless patients have discarded . . . prostheses . . . or convinced others to perform their daily care activities" (Hass, 1993, p. 231). However, patients may be considered to be unsuitable for care when their goals diverge from those of their care providers. To illustrate, a recent textbook for physical therapists discusses a college student, a full-leg amputee, who discards a prosthesis and chooses to mobilize by wheelchair for long distances and crutches or hopping for short ones: According to the text, this patient is stubborn, is behaving regressively, or is seeking a safer existence by "settling" for a wheelchair. Continued rehabilitation is recommended only if the patient agrees to psychological counseling. (Davis, 1994, pp. 36).

No consideration is given, however, to the likelihood that this choice of modes for mobilizing stems from the college student's rationally valuing moving efficiently more than moving in species-typical mode. Instead, the choice is described in terms of the college student's weaknesses of character and psyche. Could a preference for mobilizing in a mode that does not approximate the normal one be rational? A cluster of studies shows that disabled people's self-reported satisfaction with their lives is not associated with the individuals' degree of impairment. Instead, it is inversely associated with the extent of their exclusion from participation in the domains of occupation and social integration (Fuhrer, 2000, p. 485) Given the design of many U.S. universities (dormitories and classrooms generally are accessible, but classes may be scheduled at great distances from one another and from residences), wheelchair use may secure more effective access to the many sites with opportunities to participate in pre-professional educational and social functions than an unskilled user of a full-leg prosthetic otherwise could attain.

Adults with congenitally anomalous upper limbs, such as those occasioned by the prenatal presence of thalidomide, often believe themselves to have been injured as children by being fitted with dysfunctional artificial arms and forbidden to develop the much more functional method of manipulating objects with their feet. Adults with similar anomalies of the lower limbs have like complaints about being allocated dysfunctional artificial legs instead of useful wheelchairs because health-care professionals believed such individuals would be more socially acceptable by walking than by wheeling (Baughn et al., 2000). Of course, we must be cautious about assenting to patients' adaptations to onerous circumstances that could be mitigated by effective rehabilitation services (Fuhrer, 2000, p. 488). Nevertheless, we need to avoid pursuing medical interventions that are less effective than patients' nonmedical adaptations.

Rehabilitation is a medical intervention, and as such almost always costs the patient some pain and risk. Further, choices of rehabilitative strategies may have repercussions for the direction of a person's future. For example, choosing to rely on a certain type of durable medical equipment may increase an individual's current options by decreasing the time needed to reach certain functional goals. Yet the same choice may limit future options if the equipment only works well in the ideal conditions of a rehabilitation setting, or is difficult and expensive to maintain, or is likely to become unrepairable or unreplaceable. In view of rehabilitation's personal cost to the patient and enduring influence on the patient's future, rehabilitative strategies should reflect, rather than ignore or controvert, patients' own experiences of the value or valuelessness of possible outcomes. Some patients may place less importance on their level of functionality than on their appearing normal in whatever they can do, whereas others may give effective functioning so much priority they do not care how odd their performance of functions appears.

Just as they may differ about the value of normal-appearing functioning, patients and professionals may not value the goal of normal independence equally (Wear, 1988). Patients might fear that demonstrating independence will prompt their families to abandon them, whereas professionals may disapprove of patients who impose the burden of their care on their families. Authors of the *Hastings Center Report* note that the values of nondependence and productivity emphasize on the acquisition of self-care and employment skills. The authors then ask whether "rehabilitation advocates [should] advocate the availability of more assistance to those who are homebound rather than to teach people to live as independently as they can without the assistance of others?" (Caplan et al., 1987, p. 7)

The *Hastings Center Report* assents that an especially important ethical challenge confronting health-care providers in rehabilitation settings is to obtain agreement from those in their care as to what abilities and capacities constitute an acceptable quality of life. The authors of the report attribute to rehabilitation professionals the "most arduous" task of achieving accommodation between patients, families, and (sometimes) insurers "as to what constitutes an acceptable quality of life" and insist that "rehabilitation professionals have little difficulty in identifying central components of this concept" (Caplan et al., 1987, p. 6) Nonmedical factors such as the patient's social and personal characteristics are considered in screening for admission to rehabilitation programs (Rao et al., 1996, p. 113). Agreement between professionals and patients as to goals is imposed when rehabilitation professionals screen prospective patients and admit those whose personal characteristics will facilitate their realizing the values that inform prevailing rehabilitation protocols.

The practice of rehabilitation is framed by an acceptance of the social tendency to exclude from social opportunity those people who do not perform in species-typical fashion. In turn, people who do not value species-typical functioning sufficiently may be excluded from rehabilitative services that could help secure goals that are more important to them than seeming normal. The *Hastings Report* authors do not underestimate the importance, "at least in some facilities," of patients appearing to embrace these values in order to be admitted to or continue in rehabilitation programs (Caplan et al., 1987, p. 9). They note that "it is not clear that patients ought to be persuaded to accept such limits or to what extent persuasion lapses over into coercion" (Caplan et al., 1987, p. 9).

GIVING SOME SWAY TO PATIENTS' PERSONAL VIEWS OF THE GOOD

What is not clear is whether an allocation system can remain just when assigning so much influence to patients' paying allegiance to the values of professionals. As our discussion has shown, although rehabilitative medicine paradigmatically takes normal functioning as its standard and goal, the distribution of rehabilitative services and equipment is far from impersonal. Patients' personal values and character traits clearly influence their access to resources. Patients, especially those with disabilities of long duration, may not agree with professionals about the importance of approximating the appearance of normality. Nevertheless, they still may desire access to the therapies or durable medical equipment that rehabilitation professionals have the prerogative to dispense.

Can a system that extracts personal allegiance to a particular vision of the good life as the price of access to medical resources be a just one? Marcus Fuhrer reports that "commentators have pointed out that many of the outcome measures in current use reflect the hegemony of providers' and payers' values, and only equivocally those of patients" (Fuhrer, 2000, p. 487). Yet critics of attempts to direct the distribution of health-care services on the principle of equalizing individual welfare object to giving a central role to the exercise of patients' personal values. (Daniels, this volume, chapter 1). For example, Daniels argues that we must abstract from individual conceptions of the good in order to determine what justice decrees as the goal of systematic health-care provision. He believes that seeking normal functioning for everyone impartially protects opportunity for everyone alike with no need to invoke personal references.

As we have seen, however, even if we adopt the standard of normal functioning, as in rehabilitation medicine, we by no means rule out personal reference. In rehabilitation medicine, references to patients' personal characteristics play a powerful role in deliberations about allocating interventions, even though these interventions are aimed at the purportedly impersonal goal of restoring normal functioning.

Patients' individual conceptions of the good affect what responsibility the patient accepts for pursuing normality, and what energy the patient devotes to doing so. Consequently, patients' personal conceptions of the good can influence whether allocating rehabilitation resources to them will achieve the goal of normal functioning. The goal itself is far from universal, however. A distributive system that presumes or imposes it is not impartial. Such a system fails to protect everyone alike. Nor will patients perceive the share of resources they receive to be fair if the allocated medical services fail to advance them toward goals they personally take to be good. Medical service allocation systems thus do not achieve impartiality by ignoring different patients' individual conceptions of the good. Bedside justice cannot be achieved by blurring, distancing, or abstracting from patients' personal convictions. Fuhrer (2000), for instance, supports "taking into account the subjective judgments of rehabilitation patients . . . based on the primacy of the 'insider's viewpoint' of the individual patient" (pp. 487–88).

The idea of giving sway to a patient's personal beliefs about the good to be secured through medical interventions may seem to give patients too active a role. Daniels is not the only bioethicist to balk at

increasing the sway of patient's personal goals on the allocation of medical services. For instance, after noting that the procedures of rehabilitative medicine invite discord between patient and health-care professional, and raising the ethical issues so occasioned, the *Hastings Center Report* authors vote in favor of professional judgment. They do so by casting doubt on patients' deliberative capacities. They suggest that rehabilitation patients' affirmations of personal values be discounted because their sense of personal identity has been disrupted by the experience of disability. "The challenge facing medical professionals in rehabilitation is . . . not how to respect autonomy . . . but . . . what degree of persuasion or even coercion [is] morally permissible in the hope of restoring autonomy" (Caplan et al., 1987, p. 11).

This line of argument is a dubious strategy for giving the values of professionals pre-eminence over those of patients. Granted that the professionals' partiality for pursuing species-typical modes of functioning reflects society's preference for normality. It takes less effort to provide equitable opportunity to a homogeneously functioning population than to a diversely functioning one. But a patient's choice to pursue professionally or socially disregarded goals in therapy is no evidence of the patient's inability to make informed, voluntary decisions about the course and direction of life.

Further, authors of the *Hastings Center Report* restrict the scope of the model in which patients are imagined to be too shattered personally to direct their lives onto "patients who have no prior experience with impairment or disability" (Caplan et al., 1987, p. 12). We might be led to discount the personal values of rehabilitation patients because they have not yet had time to recalibrate the basis for their choices (Fuhrer, 2000, p. 484). But choices such as the determination to mobilize by rolling on wheels rather than by walking on prosthetic legs are made as often by those who have long functioned successfully with disability as by those new to it. It therefore is illegitimate to invoke choosing anomalous modes over species-typical modes of functioning as evidence of rehabilitation patients' devastated personalities and debilitated autonomy.

Rather, the health care system should acknowledge with impartiality the diversity of values that inform patients' goals. Rehabilitation medicine most clearly takes normal functioning to be the preeminent goal. As we have seen, however, even in rehabilitation medicine the distributive system should incorporate a commitment to multifunctionalism, meaning that appreciation of the equal value of different modes of performing human functions should be inherent in the way medical services and durable equipment are allocated.

CONCLUSION: CLEAR-SIGHTED BEDSIDE JUSTICE

Over the last decade, liberal theories of justice have affirmed the importance of giving equal status to the values of cultural majorities and minorities (Young, 1990, 1997; Taylor et al., 1992). Justice theory thus has made room for the divergent views of the good that are embraced by different cultures. In this spirit, medical professionals now are educated to be sensitive to the cultural backgrounds of their patients.

Similar arguments can be made for like acknowledgment of patients' personal values about functioning in anomalous rather than species-typical modes. Multiculturalism personalizes justice, yet simultaneously expands the scope of impartiality to embrace alternative value systems. The analogous affirmation of multifunctionalism would make room for alternative valuations of anomalous and species-typical modes of functioning.

Abandoning the belief that health-care justice requires allegiance to the abstraction of uniform functioning, and adopting instead the particularized perspectives promoted by multifunctionalism, would be important steps to ensure that bedside justice proceeds with clear vision. A theoretical commitment to multifunctionalism will save us from blurring the personal differences that individuate patients. Appreciating multifunctionalism will pave the way for providing just health care in a liberal society, where equitable medical treatment requires seeing patients in the full light of their individualized approaches to life. (See Silvers, 2000, for further discussion of the injustices associated with the rejection of multifunctionalism.)

NOTE

1. See also Fuhrer (2000) for a discussion of single and multiple perspective quality of life scales; Murray and Lopez (1996) for a discussion of disability adjusted measures; Groce et al. (1999) for an analysis of the problems with applying disability-adjusted life year measures to people with disabilities; Gill and Feinstein (1997) for a discussion of problems with quality of life measurement; and Bickenbach, this volume (chapter 30) for a detailed exploration of the injustices of disability-adjusted and quality of life measurement schemes.

REFERENCES

Amundson, R. (2000). Against normal function. *Studies in History and Philosophy of Biological and Biomedical Sciences* 31, 33–53.

Anderson, E. (1999). What is the point of equality? *Ethics* 109, 287–337.

Arneson, R.J. (1988). Equality and equal opportunity for welfare. *Philosophical Studies* 54, 79–95.

Baughn, B., Degener, T. and Wolbring, G. (2000). E-mails 1/11/2000, 1/12/2000, 1/18/2000. On file with the author.

Caplan, A., Callahan, D. and Haas, J. (1987). Ethical and policy issues in rehabilitation medicine: A Hastings Center Report. *Hastings Center Report*, Special Supplement/August.

Caplan, A. (1988). Commentary on the Case of Stan. In J. Haas, A. Caplan, and D. Callahan, (eds.), *Case Studies in Ethics and Medical Rehabilitation*. Briarcliff Manor, NY: The Hastings Center, pp. 8–12.

Carter, B. (2000). Big Brother hopes to engineer an exit, then add a face. *New York Times*, September 4, pp. B1, B9.

Cassell, E.J. (2000). The principles of the he Belmont Report Revisited: How have respect for persons, beneficence, and justice been applied to clinical medicine? *Hastings Center Report* 30 (4), 12–21.

Cole, R. (1996). After two rejections, Activist for disabled receives transplant. *Philadelphia Inquirer*, January 24.

Daniels, N. (1987). Justice and health care. In D.V. DeVeer and T. Regan (eds.), *Health Care Ethics: An Introduction*. Philadelphia: Temple University Press, pp. 290–325.

Davis, C. (1994). Influence of values on patient care: Foundation for decision making. In S. O'Sullivan and T. Schmitz (eds.), *Physical Rehabilitation: Assessment and Treatment*. Philadelphia: F.A. Davis, pp. 31–37.

Fuhrer, M. (2000). Subjectifying quality of life as a medical rehabilitation outcome. *Disability and Rehabilitation* 22 (11), 481–89.

Gill, T.M. and Feinstein, A.R. (1997). A critical appraisal of the quality of the problem of quality of life in medicine. *JAMA* 278, 619–26.

Glatzer, J. (1999). The value of a life. Adapt Z.com. Download of website posting on file with the author.

Groce, N.E., Chamie, M., Meroce, A., Chamie, M. and Me., A. (1999). Measuring the quality of life: Rethinking the World Bank's disability adjusted life-years. *International Rehabilitation Review* 99 (49) issues 1/2, 12–15.

Haas, J. (1993). Ethical considerations of goal setting for patient care in rehabilitation medicine. *American Journal of Physical Medicine and Rehabilitation* 72 (4), 228–32.

Kotke, F.J. (1980). Future focus of rehabilitation medicine. *Archives of Physical Medicine and Rehabilitation* 61, 1–6.

Moss, A. and Siegler, M. (1991). Should alcoholics compete equally for liver transplantation? *JAMA* 265 (10), 1295–97.

Murray, C. and Lopez, A. (1996). *The Global Burden of Disease*. Cambridge, MA: Harvard School of Health.

Rao, P.K., Palenski, C. and Gibson, C.J. (1996). Inpatient rehabilitation: Psychiatric and nurse practitioner admission assessment of stroke patients and their rehabilitation outcomes. *International Journal of Rehabilitation Research* 19 (2), 111–22.

Satz, A. and Silvers, A. (2000). Disability and biotechnology. In M. Mehlman and T. Murray (eds.), *The Encyclopedia of Biotechnology: Ethical, Legal, and Policy Issues*. New York: John Wiley, pp. 173–87.

Sen, A.K. (1980). Equality of what? In S. McMurrin (ed.), *Tanner Lectures on Human Values*. Cambridge: Cambridge University Press.

Sen, A.K. (1992). *Inequality Reexamined*. Cambridge, MA: Harvard University Press.

Sen, A.K. (1993). Capability and well-being. In M. Nussbaum and A.K. Sen (eds.), *Quality of Life*. Oxford: Clarendon Press.

Silvers, A. (2000). The unprotected: Constructing disability in the context of anti-discrimination law. In L. Francis and A. Silvers (eds.), *Americans with Disabilities: Implications of the Law for Individuals and Institutions*. N.Y.: Routledge, pp. 126–45.

Sober, E. (1980). Evolution, population thinking, and essentialism. *Philosophy of Science* 47, 350–83.

Sober, E. (2000). The meaning of genetic causation. In A. Buchanan, D. Brock, N. Daniels, and D. Wikler (eds.), Appendix One in *From Chance to Choice*. Cambridge: Cambridge University Press, pp. 347–70.

Spencer, W.A. (1970). A new use for the rehabilitation process—Introspection. *Archives of Physical Medicine and Rehabilitation* 51, 187–97.

Taylor, C., Gutmann, A., Rockefeller, S., Walzer, M. and Wolf, S. (1992). *Multiculturalism and "The Politics of Recognition."* Princeton, NJ: Princeton University Press.

Treischman, R.B. (1974). Coping with a disability: A sliding scale of goals. *Archives of Physical Medicine and Rehabilitation* 55, 458–62.

Wear, S. (1988). Commentary on the Case of Tony. In J. Haas, A. Caplan, and D. Callahan (eds.), *Case Studies in Ethics and Medical Rehabilitation*. Briarcliff Manor, NY: The Hastings Center, pp. 3–6

Young, I.M. (1990). *Justice and the Politics of Difference*. Princeton, NJ: Princeton University Press.

Young, I.M. (1997). "Asymmetrical Reciprocity: On Moral Respect, Wonder, and Enlarged Thought." *Constellations*. V. 3.

20

The Medical, the Mental, and the Dental: Vicissitudes of Stigma and Compassion

Michael Teitleman

In late 1999, the Surgeon General of the United States issued *Mental Health: A Report of the Surgeon General* (hereafter MHR). The report is a comprehensive survey of current scientific understanding of the major mental disorders, the therapeutic tools available to help affected individuals, and the clinical services that are needed by each age group across the life span. The report also articulates a vision of a system of mental health care with a broad range of programs to meet the needs of children, adolescents, adults, and elders through schools, nursing homes, prisons, residential programs, shelters, home-visit agencies, and community centers as well the usual hospital, clinic, and office sites.

The outlook of the Surgeon General's report is generally rosy. It touts the growth in knowledge and the clinical advances of the last three decades. The picture is less rosy when it turns to the gap between the mental health needs of the population and the delivery of mental health services. The gist of the Surgeon General's outlook is that more is known about mental disorder than ever before, more effective treatment is available than ever before, but most of those who need help do not receive it.

A major epidemiological study and a mountain of smaller studies demonstrate that clinically significant mood, anxiety, eating, attentional, substance abuse, and psychotic disorders have substantial prevalences in the population (Blazer et al., 1994). Approximately one in five individuals experiences a diagnosable mental disorder in a year. The more serious of these disorders have a deleterious impact on the quality of life comparable to cancer and cardiovascular disease (MHR, p. 4).

Clinical needs are substantial, but they are poorly met. Of the 28% of the population with a diagnosable mental disorder, only 8% made use of mental health services. Two-thirds of those with a disorder did not receive treatment (MHR, pp. 408–09).

Obviously, the explanation of this gap is complex. Failure by affected individuals to recognize the presence of a disorder and reluctance to seek help play a part. However, a recent national survey shows that the cost of treatment is actually the principal deterrent. Understandably, 83% of the uninsured said that cost was the most important reason for not getting help, but so did 55% of the insured population, suggesting that health insurance does not fully open the door to people who desire treatment.

This chapter focuses on how and why health insurance functions as a barrier to mental health treatment; it explores the current effort to remedy this through mental health parity legislation, and it examines the cultural and ideological obstacles to improving access to the mental health treatment system.

INSURANCE REIMBURSEMENT DISPARITIES FOR MEDICAL AND MENTAL HEALTH CARE

When it comes to the issue of access, mental health treatment is identical to medical treatment in one simple and important respect. The key determinant of access to care is health insurance. However, mental health treatment needs to be considered on its own, as a distinct issue, because the health insurance system differentiates between mental health treatment and medical treatment, and the system reduces access to mental health treatment in comparison to medical treatment.

Patients pay a higher proportion of the cost of their mental health care than they do for their medical care. Insurance policies set higher deductibles and/or co-payments for mental health services than for medical care. For instance, Medicare, the government insurance program for the disabled and for people over 65, reimburses patients 80% of the cost of their medical care but only 50% of their outpatient mental health treatment.

In addition to higher deductibles and co-payments, annual and lifetime limits on reimbursement for in-hospital psychiatric treatment protect insurance companies against the costs of caring for people with serious, persistent mental illnesses, such as schizophrenia and bipolar disorder, which frequently necessitate repeated and prolonged hospitalizations. Exceeding an annual limit can impose severe financial burdens on patients and their families. Reimbursement for medical–surgical care sometimes has lifetime limitations, but these are substantially more generous than limits on reimbursement for mental health care (MHR, pp. 426–27).

Policies also set annual reimbursement and visit limitations for outpatient treatment. Patients pay 100% of the cost after the limit is reached. This is especially burdensome on patients who need intensive individual, group, and psychopharmacological outpatient treatment for seriously disabling, chronic disorders, such as schizophrenia, obsessive-compulsive disorder, or bipolar disorder. Reimbursement for clinically indicated treatment ceases at a point in the year that is determined by the frequency and cost of the treatment regardless of the condition or the resources of the patient.

Annual limitations are not exceeded in brief outpatient treatments, such as crisis intervention or short-term psychotherapy, but they are readily exceeded in insight-oriented psychotherapy involving one or more sessions per week over an extended period. Patients with sufficient economic resources pay the bill themselves once the limit is met. Others must either limit or terminate treatment because they cannot afford it, or they may not seek treatment in the first place.

No comparable annual limitations exist on reimbursement for outpatient medical treatment. Reimbursement does not cease if a medical problem requires numerous visits to physicians and/or expensive diagnostic testing.

Over time, an additional advantage of annual reimbursement limitations accrues to insurance companies if the limitation is held constant or rises more slowly than the cost of services. Twenty years ago, policies with mental health coverage had annual limitations on outpatient treatment in the $750 to $1500 range, and they have largely stayed at this level. My own psychoanalysis, which began in 1975, was reimbursed annually to a limit of $1000. My current health insurance policy has a $1500 annual cap, a 50% benefit increase despite a 500% increase in prices in the intervening 25 years.

Before the era of managed care, disparities in reimbursement for medical and mental health treatment were the norm (except for policies that excluded mental health coverage altogether). In the managed care era, disparity continues to be the norm for point of service plans in which there is unrestricted choice of clinicians and for preferred provider plans when a clinician is selected who is not on the insurance company's panel.

Other disparities exist between medical and mental health insurance coverage, but for several reasons I shall focus on reimbursement limitations in this discussion of access to care. These limitations impose clear and distinct barriers to mental health care. They are not a recent innovation that arrived with managed care; they have been part of our health-care insurance arrangements for a long time.

Recently, these disparities in coverage between mental and medical care have become a focus of social criticism; they are viewed as unfair because they discriminate against those who seek help for mental disorders and psychosocial problems. Political pressure to reduce barriers to mental health care has led to legislative reform aimed at establishing parity in insurance coverage for mental health treatment.

The federal Mental Health Parity Act, passed by Congress in 1996, principally focused on protection from catastrophic costs for mental health care by prohibiting unequal annual and lifetime limits for mental and medical reimbursement (MHR, pp. 427–28). Unfortunately, the impact of the legislation is limited. It only covers firms that are exempt from state legislation. It does not apply to the largest insurance

program in the country, the government's own Medicare system. It exempts companies with fewer than 50 employees, and it does not address other mental health benefit restrictions such as higher co-payments, higher deductibles, and annual limits on visits. Moreover, even when policies are in compliance with the legislation, it does not regulate the use of managed-care cost-control mechanisms. And, of course, benefit parity does nothing for the uninsured.

Despite its practical shortcomings, the principal moral virtue of the Mental Health Parity Act is its expression of society's recognition of the inequity of making it harder for people to get mental health care than to get medical care. Politically, it breaks new ground in enhancing access to treatment and provides a model for legislative reforms; many state governments have enacted similar mental/medical parity measures. Moreover, in 2001, benefit parity was being extended to civilian employees of the federal government (Goode, 2001).

DEINSTITUTIONALIZATION AND INSURANCE REIMBURSEMENT DISPARITIES

The economic objective of reimbursement disparities is crystal clear: reducing the cost of mental health care to insurance companies by shifting costs to patients and deterring use of benefits. What is not apparent is why a health insurance system with separate and unequal reimbursement policies for medical and mental health care was not viewed as ethically problematic as it came into being after World War II. Addressing this question requires a brief survey of the state of the mental health system and of its subsequent development in those early postwar years.

At the end of the war, the mental health system consisted of large, underfunded state psychiatric hospitals. The heyday of insulin shock therapy and malarial fever therapy had passed; use of psychosurgery was in disfavor and declining. Effective clinical tools for treating severe mental illness were nugatory. Long-term hospitalization was the recourse for severely disturbed individuals who could not be maintained by themselves or their families. Commitment to an asylum was unimpeded by the niceties of civil liberties or judicial review (Grob, 1994).

Institutional care of the mentally ill had been recognized as a societal responsibility ever since the early days of the Republic. Asylums were first established by local governments; they were superseded by larger, custodial mental hospitals built and operated by state governments. It hardly needs stating that inadequate financing, appalling conditions, and eagerness to sequester deviance took the moral sheen off the recognition of this responsibility by society.

The employment-based system of private health insurance first took shape at the zenith of the century-old state hospital system. Reimbursement limitations on hospital treatment imposed a stiff price on the transfer of treatment to private hospitals and kept treatment of severely ill patients in the state hospitals where governments would foot the bill. In this institutional context, instead of blocking access to hospital treatment, annual and lifetime reimbursement limitations channeled patients into the existing publicly supported system, which was cost free to both patients and insurance companies.

Deinstitutionalization transformed the clinical landscape (Grob, 1994). Care of individuals with severe mental illness began to shift away from state hospitals to a nascent (and utterly inadequate) system of community hospitals, private and public psychiatric hospitals, community mental health centers, clinics, and office practice. Deinstitutionalization was planned and underway before the advent of antipsychotic medications, whose entry into clinical use accelerated the process by enabling clinicians to achieve some degree of control of the symptoms of previously untreatable disorders, principally schizophrenia and other psychotic afflictions.

As deinstitutionalization proceeded, both medical and psychiatric hospitals in the community replaced the state hospitals as the locus of treatment for acutely disturbed patients. Reimbursement limitations for hospital care had a quite different impact in this new clinical context. Instead of channeling patients into state hospitals, reimbursement limitations shifted costs of hospital treatment to patients and families. As a result, patients with serious lifelong psychiatric disorders requiring prolonged and/or repeated hospitalizations were sometimes threatened with impoverishment.

Outpatient treatment modalities were limited in variety, scope, and effectiveness during the early postwar period. Medications were ineffective, counterproductive, and sometimes downright dangerous. In the heyday of psychoanalytic psychology and therapy, clinical work largely consisted of psychodynamic psychotherapy or psychoanalysis, which would occur one to five times a week often for several years. In this clinical context, insurance companies used reimbursement disparities to reduce their share of the costs of treatment modalities that were both intensive in their use of clinician time and long in duration.

To some extent, outpatient reimbursement limitations channeled people to training institutions and public sector clinics with sliding fees adjusted to the patient's income. But in the main, relative to medical care, these limitations raised the cost of treatment and shut out people whose other needs in life had a stronger claim on their resources than did mental health care. The advantage to the insurance company was clear. The drawback was that some who needed and would benefit from help did not (and still do not) receive it.

STIGMA AND THE ETHICAL VALIDATION OF INSURANCE DISPARITIES

There is no mystery as to why insurance companies used mental health reimbursement disparities to reduce their costs. This is understandable corporate behavior. The question here is why these practices were ethically acceptable. Indeed, by 1965, these reimbursement practices were so completely normative that they were incorporated into the Medicare system—a system in which profit seeking is not even a factor—and concern about cost control lay far in the future.

The answer encompasses ethics and social psychology; it touches on societal perceptions of and attitudes to mental illness and also on the vicissitudes of political ideology. The U.S. Surgeon General, along with mental health professionals and advocates, maintains that the stigmatization of mental illness accounts for the unwillingness of society to finance mental health care adequately (MHR, pp. 6–8, 454ff). By implication, stigmatization would also account for society's ethical equanimity regarding discriminatory insurance practices. However, this is not simply a matter of the social acceptance of discrimination against a stigmatized population. It also serves to validate insurance discrimination against people who seek treatment when they are not severely afflicted.

The cultural stigmatization of mental illness depicts a world of the ill and the well. Mentally ill people differ from well people because there is "something really wrong with them." They are different from the rest of us because they have a real affliction: madness, or in clinical terms, psychosis. One function of stigmatization is to validate the segregation of the afflicted. Another function is protective: to assure the rest of us that the psychological and behavioral disarray of the mad is different in kind from the emotional turbulence we may experience from time to time in life.

Until deinstitutionalization relocated the treatment of the mentally ill into the community, this clinical/metaphysical categorization mapped onto a moral geography. State hospitals were institutions for the sequestration of madness. Supported by society, their doors were open regardless of ability to pay. At the outset, insurance discrimination against the mentally ill was not seen as ethically problematic because it did not create an obstacle to the principal modality in the management of severe psychiatric disorders, sequestration of the mad in state hospitals. The moral geography of managing madness was left intact.

In this cultural schema, normality and self-mastery are the counterparts to madness and sequestration. Normality is the absence of madness, of "real" illness. If the mad are fundamentally different from the rest of us, then the psychological distress the rest of us experience does not result from "real" illness or disorder.

Normality encompasses all the conditions of life that befall people who are not afflicted with "real" illness—well-being along with misery. The problems that motivate people to seek professional help are the "normal" stuff of daily life. Depression, anxiety, insecurity, phobic inhibitions are different in degree but not in kind from the unhappiness, disappointment, worry, grief, fear, and stress that everyone must contend with at some time in life. Unhappiness, stress, and anxiety have an inevitability akin to the skin wrinkles and tooth loss that come with aging. Depression, stress, and anxiety at some time or other are the human lot. Only the beatifically tranquil are spared.

Maladaptive behavior, disturbed relationships, and noncompliance with social norms are manifestations of immaturity, a difficult personality, or of moral failure. These are seen as problems of living, not manifestations of illness or disorder.

In an individualistic society that places a high value on self-reliance and independence, the burden of normality is self-mastery. The mad are sequestered because their illness has undermined their capacity for self-governance; they need others to be in charge of them. Normal people must live with, work through, and master their problems of living. On this view of life, individuals must "tough-out" their problems on their own. Independence and self-reliance are virtues; dependence on others falls short of the mark.

This synthesis of stigmatization and individualism has had a deleterious impact on attitudes toward mental health care beyond the walls of the hospital. It is a perspective that fosters shame and self-reproach in people who need the help of others. It inclines some to experience their desire for help as moral weakness and guilt-inducing dependence. For others, it fosters fear. It is not uncommon in clinical practice to encounter patients who have resisted acknowledging their suffering and have postponed seeking help because of fear of the madness they have seen in parents or siblings. They reassure themselves of their normality by avoiding treatment and suffering on their own.

This pervasive outlook provided the moral warrant for insurance reimbursement practices that discouraged treatment and legitimated the demotion of mental health care relative to medical care. Seeking medical help for symptoms of physical illness was viewed as a matter of rational prudence. But seeking a therapist because of psychological distress was a matter of choice, almost as a luxury, one way among many that a person might choose to deal with distress. Mental health treatment is seen as on a par with taking a long vacation to relieve depression or cosmetic surgery to improve self-esteem. Its inclusion in health insurance may be a boon to those who want treatment, but there is nothing ethically objectionable about diminished reimbursement.

This hostile view of seeking help was reinforced by skepticism about outpatient clinical practice. This was the heyday of psychoanalytic theory and practice that enjoyed limited acceptance beyond the cultural and social elite. Moreover, because psychoanalysis did not have intellectual roots in medicine or an institutional base in medical schools and teaching hospitals, there was little advocacy for increased access to treatment from the medical establishment.

These various threads—the legitimacy of sequestering the severely ill, the denial of mental disorder among the nonpsychotic,

the social norm of self-mastery, the devaluation of seeking help for psychological problems, and skepticism about the available therapies—served to legitimate the distinction between medical and mental health care in insurance reimbursement. Reimbursement limitations on hospital care channeled severely ill patients into institutional sequestration, which is where a stigmatizing culture thought they ought to be. Reimbursement limitations on outpatient treatment deterred people from seeking help, fostered independence, but did not, in any event, keep people from treatment that was considered effective.

CLINICAL RESEARCH AND THE DELEGITIMATION OF INSURANCE DISPARITIES

Over the last 25 years, progress in both basic and clinical research has fundamentally transformed the intellectual and clinical landscape. Basic neuroscience is assembling an understanding of neurons and brains that guides the development and use of diagnostic technology and psychotropic medications. Clinical psychiatry operates with a nosology grounded in a substantial body of epidemiological and clinical information. Highly prevalent disorders such as major depression, bipolar disorder, panic disorder, eating disorders, and obsessive-compulsive disorder have been shown to have characteristic symptomatic presentations, clinical courses, psychosocial sequelae, family histories, and treatment responses. In this respect, they do not differ from clinical syndromes in medicine.

With the development of a scientifically validated diagnostic framework, it is possible to test the safety and effectiveness of psychopharmacological interventions with a degree of scientific rigor that matches the rigor of medical research in general. Disorders that afflict substantial numbers of people can now be reliably recognized and distinguished from one another. A growing array of medications is being used with increasing sophistication. Appropriate pharmacological treatments can be offered to many people in distress, and with a reasonable prospect of success.

Progress in developing individual, family, and group psychotherapies has paralleled the growth of biological therapeutics. Psychoanalytic psychotherapy and psychoanalysis are still widely practiced, but they are now just two of many psychotherapeutic modalities. Treatment combining therapy and pharmacology is commonplace. Specialized treatment programs have been developed for mental disorders that take a substantial toll on a person's prospects in life, such as eating disorders, posttraumatic stress disorder, and borderline personality disorder.

The design of mental health services has also become more sophisticated; treatment programs are tailored to the needs of special populations. There are supervised residences and day programs for patients with chronic psychotic disorders. Community mental health centers provide treatment and services across the life span. School systems have programs for the assessment, counseling, and referral of children and adolescents. Crisis intervention programs aid people who have been acutely traumatized by catastrophic loss or violence. There are mental health programs in prisons to treat the mentally ill who migrate between the mental health system and the criminal justice system. The skeleton of the Surgeon General's vision of an ideal mental health care system has been (very partially) put in place. The skeleton, however, is shamefully underfunded and inaccessible to many.

The accretion of this research-based perspective over the last two decades has fostered societal recognition of mental disorders as real afflictions and acceptance of the need for expert help and the wisdom of seeking it. The denial of nonpsychotic mental disorder has been supplanted by a much more complex landscape. "Normal" people suffer from all kinds of maladies that qualify as clinical syndromes because of their characteristic presentations among many people over time. Mood and anxiety disorders are real; they are distinguishable from the stress, unhappiness, worry, and disappointment that life dishes out. For instance, it is now widely understood that major depression is a malady, an illness that psychiatrists and therapists can help with, and not just a particularly tough time in life that one needs to endure. Moreover, effective treatments exist for many disorders. They reduce symptomatic distress and improve psychosocial functioning; they can terminate a clinical episode or stabilize a chronic condition.

This scientific and clinical progress has provided an intellectual foundation for combating long-entrenched stigmatizing judgments about mental illness and treatment. Mental health insurance disparities have been dislodged from their normative status; they have become ethically problematic. If the maladies are real, and the treatments are effective, then it is neither rational nor benign to discriminate between medical and psychiatric disorders or to discourage or close the door to treatment.

Whatever its utility as a mechanism of cost control, reimbursement discrimination is unfair to people in two ways. First, it reduces access to care for individuals with disorders that are as real and debilitating as are medical disorders but just happen to be on a reduced insurance reimbursement list. There is no basis in scientific knowledge or clinical experience to differentiate between bipolar affective disorder or obsessive-compulsive disorder, which are on the reduced reimbursement list, and diabetes, cancer, or fungal infections of toenails, which are not. Second, those who can afford the unreimbursed costs of treatment are able to obtain partial reimbursement, whereas those whose resources and circumstances prevent them from bearing their share of the costs must forgo treatment. Insurance disparities create a pool of underinsured people who cannot utilize their benefits. Those who cannot afford the unreimbursed costs of treatment subsidize those who can.

STIGMA, COMPASSION, AND ACCESS TO MENTAL HEALTH CARE

The parallel delegitimizations of stigma and of insurance disparities have not come about through the spontaneous diffusion of scientific and clinical information. Since the end of World War II, professional mental health organizations have been advocating for public investment in psychiatric research and treatment programs. The Institute for Mental Health owes it creation to psychiatric lobbying to include mental health in the postwar acceleration of research investment by the federal government (Grob, 1994).

Even more importantly, over the last 10 or 15 years, the dispersal of information has been driven by the public discussion of mental illness by patients and their families. In both print and broadcast media, they have spoken movingly of their suffering, have fostered public understanding of mental disorder, lobbied for increased social investment in research and treatment, and fought politically for increased access to treatment. Patient advocacy groups provided a major impetus for passage of the Mental Health Parity Act. Public figures, such as Tipper Gore, Mike Wallace, and Betty Ford, have made mental health treatment a matter of everyday discourse. The acceptability of treatment has reached the point that medications for depression and social anxiety are advertised on television.

The issues of stigma and access have been intertwined in the public and professional discussions of mental illness. The campaign against stigma through the dispersal of scientific and clinical information has been based on the assumption that a better understanding of mental illness will have three salutary results: greater tolerance for the severely mentally ill; greater recognition of and willingness to seek treatment; and support for increased spending for mental health treatment. As the U.S. Surgeon General stated, "As stigma abates, a transformation of public attitudes should occur. People should become eager to seek care. They should be more willing to absorb its cost" (MHR, p. 9).

Studies of attitudinal change about mental illness suggest that the campaign against stigma has had mixed results. People now understand that mental disorder encompasses more than just psychosis and are able to recognize a range of mental afflictions. People also now believe that the severely mentally ill are prone to violence, a perception that reflects the growth of a patient population that cycles among states of incarceration, hospitalization, and homelessness.

The campaign against stigma has resulted in less irrational denial and fear of mental illness, and greater willingness to seek help and recommend it to others, but it has not led to increased support for social investment in treatment (MHR, pp. 8–9).

It is understandable that the abatement of stigma aided the mobilization of opposition to health insurance disparities for mental health. This reform was congenial to an insured population that became persuaded of the advantages of having its insurance upgraded. However, upgrading access through the elimination of reimbursement disparities does not entail expansion of mental health services to encompass the large unmet needs of the uninsured and the poor. As the Surgeon General noted, the small cost of the Mental Health Parity Act made its passage politically feasible, but its low cost also indicates how little change it accomplishes (Goode, 2001).

The Surgeon General is mistaken when he ties the eradication of stigma to support for public investment in mental health services. His rosy reformist optimism is refreshing, but the data suggest an error in inference. The Surgeon General reasonably assumes that when people relinquish irrational fears about mental illness and appreciate the effectiveness of treatment in the alleviation of suffering, they will want treatment to be available to both themselves and those they care about should illness befall them. But it is an error to suppose that they will also desire society to ensure access to treatment for anyone with a psychiatric affliction.

The inferential gap can be bridged by an assumption of compassion: Understanding that there is real and remedial suffering in mental disorder will stimulate concern that help should be available to anyone who is afflicted. Because compassion—empathizing with, and being moved by the suffering of others—is not one of the cardinal social virtues of a competitive, individualistic, nonegalitarian society, this is hardly a safe assumption.

COMPASSION AND URGENCY: THE DENTAL

Compassion is not plentiful in a cruel world, but neither the world nor American society is devoid of it. The value of compassion is woven into our moral thinking about access to health care in complex ways. Compassion pushes open the door to medical care when it is tied to urgency. For instance, it figures into the legal and ethical requirement that people in extremis may not be turned away from hospital emergency rooms because they cannot pay for care. In the first horrible decade of the AIDS epidemic, compassion and urgency also opened the door to health care for people who would otherwise have been shut out. The desperation of the afflicted and those who loved them evoked compassion in many (but not all) and built up pressure on governmental agencies to ensure access to care through health insurance programs for people with AIDS.

Compassion may be ubiquitous in a Buddhist monastery, but it is patchy and selective in our culture. It takes special circumstances for it to be evoked widely and deeply. When it is not a fundamental social value, the circumstances that evoke it must be invested with urgency and profound need. While a major social benefit of universal health care is prevention and management of chronic disease, this cold epi-

demiological fact is not what the advocates of health-care reform drew on during the Clinton administration to garner support for universal health insurance. To stir up compassion for the uninsured and evoke a political passion for change, health-care advocates broadcast the narratives of parents with sick children and of people with terrible diseases fighting to stay alive. In the absence of compassion, complacency and indifference set the tone of debate over access to care.

The issue of access to dental care bears out this idea quite nicely. A few months after issuing his mental health report, the U.S. Surgeon General (2000) weighed in with *Oral Health: A Report of the Surgeon General* (hereafter OHR). This reports offers a detailed, comprehensive review of the role of oral health in overall well being, the health problems that arise within the oral cavity, the epidemiology of dental disease, and the maldistribution and unavailability of dental care.

Not everyone suffers from cancer, heart disease, or depression. But dental disease is universal. Each of us, sooner or later, has problems with teeth or gums. Everyone, sooner or later, needs to sit in a dentist's chair. The report reviews clinical problems that all people encounter in life and the preventive, curative, and restorative clinical services that are needed to maintain oral health (OHR, p. 63)

Despite this universal need, access to dental care has been totally absent from the public discussion about health care over the last 15 years. The inaccessibility of dental care dwarfs the problem of the medically uninsured. The dentally uninsured are 2.6 times more numerous than the medically uninsured: 16% of the American population are without health insurance; more than 50% are without dental insurance. Medicare does not cover dental care for the elderly. Medicaid for the very poor includes dental coverage, but reimbursement rates are so low that clinical services are either in short supply or unavailable.

Far more than most disorders that befall

the human organism, dental disease is strongly correlated with socioeconomic status. Across all ages and ethnic groups, income is inversely correlated with the number of cavities and extent of gum disease. Untreated tooth decay and loss of periodontal attachment, both of which lead to loss of teeth, is greatest among the poor (OHR, p. 80) Fewer adults are edentulous than two decades ago, but this boon of dental progress has principally been enjoyed by the well off. At age 65, adults with low income and education are nearly nine times more like to be edentulous than those in the upper reaches of the social pyramid (OHR, p. 66)

Oral health status is strongly associated with access to dental care. Because dental problems are rarely self-corrective, people will find some kind of care for acute, emergent problems. However, emergent interventions are not sufficient to maintain oral health and preserve dentition. The Surgeon General cites a national health survey in which adults who have made a dental visit within the last twelve months are 4.4 times more likely to have complete dentition (OHR, p. 81) The evidence that clinches the connection between access to care and oral health comes from the United States military. Military personnel see dentists at very high rates (99.2% within a 2 year period; 80% in a 1 year period). They receive regular prophylaxis and treatment of detected caries. Edentulism is non-existent in this population; their overall oral health status is superior to an age-matched non-military population (OHR, p. 83). If you want to keep your teeth into old age, join the Marines.

There is nothing esoteric about dental disease. It does not take an extensive educational campaign for people to understand that teeth can become diseased and be lost. Nor does it take a leap of empathic imagination to comprehend what dental pain is like. By some point in early adulthood, everyone has either experienced such pain or directly witnessed it. There is widespread awareness of the availability of techniques to preserve and replace dentition, which those with insurance and resources utilize to preserve their teeth.

Apart from concern about children's health and development, access to dental care is simply not on society's moral horizon. There is a straightforward explanation of this at the level of moral psychology. Preventing tooth loss, which is the principal goal of dental treatment, is not a matter of urgency nor does the loss of teeth evoke compassion. Until recently, most people could expect to be edentulous if they lived long enough. Thirty years ago, nearly 50% of people 65 to 74 years old were toothless. It is "natural" outcome of aging, which good dental care can stave off. Those who can afford care are free to purchase it. But because ending up edentulous is neither life-threatening, intrinsically painful, nor seen as psychologically unbearable, inadequate and unequal access to dental care does not make it onto the agenda of health care reform.

THE MEDICAL, MENTAL, AND DENTAL

On the spectrum of compassion and urgency, the mental is probably now located somewhere between the dental and the medical. At the dental end of the spectrum, moral pressure to provide universal access to care is nonexistent because dental disease does not have outcomes that touch us deeply. At the medical end, disease carries the threat of pain, disfigurement, incapacity, fear, and extinction. We cannot be indifferent to the possibility of these eventualities for ourselves. And, sometimes, the contemplation of other enduring these tribulations without access to medical treatment calls forth caring and compassion. This was an indispensable but underutilized element in the Clinton administration's mobilization of popular support for healthcare reform.

As the stigmatization of mental illness has abated, there is a growing recognition that mental disorder brings with it real suffering, but this does not evoke a compassionate response with the power to foster social change. Psychological suffering is no longer on a par with edentulism as an ineradicable part of living that must be endured. But as a culture, we do not yet let our appreciation of suffering in the mind move us to the point of deciding that the door to treatment should be open to all who need it. This may be disturbing, but it should not be surprising. After all, if our knowledge of the afflictions of the body has not yet moved us to make treatment available to all out of compassion for their suffering, we should not expect that dispelling the fog of stigmatization would make the difference for mental health care.

The Surgeon General and the mental health professions are not wrong to combat the stigmatization of mental illness, but the problem of access is different and deeper than that. What needs to change in a so-ciety that does not care enough about all of its members is not just knowledge of disease and treatment but indifference. And that is a political matter.

REFERENCES

Blazer, D., Kessler, R. and McGonagle, J. (1994). The prevalence and distribution of major depression in a national community sample: The *National Comorbidity Survey*. *American Journal of Psychiatry* 151, 970–86.

Goode, E. (2001). 9 Million gaining upgraded benefit for mental care. *New York Times*, January 1, p. 1.

Grob, G. (1994). *The Mad Among Us: A History of the Care of America's Mentally Ill.* New York: Free Press.

Mental Health: A Report of the Surgeon General (1999). Washington, DC: Department of Health and Human Services.

Oral Health in America: A Report of the Surgeon General (2000). Washington, DC: Department of Health and Human Services.

21

Children's Right to Health Care: A Modest Proposal

Loretta M. Kopelman

There seems to be a consensus that our children deserve the best we have to offer, but what do our deeds show? A test of our commitment to this lofty ideal might be to see whether state-funded health-care programs exclude children based solely on their age. I will argue that unless a special case can be made, whatever state-funded health-care treatments, specialists, diagnostic strategies, special-duty nurses, innovative care, painkillers, dental care, experimental treatments or other health care available for adults should also be available to children on the same basis. Because different programs benefit adults and children differently, however, subtle but important age biases may exist even in programs where the same benefits are provided to them. Children, for example, rarely need treatment for dementia or prostate cancer, or require long-term nursing care. In addition, systems have age biases against children when they discount long-term future benefits (Brock, 2001; 1995).

Bias can also exist in the relative ease of access to gain benefits for adults and children. For example, programs for poor and near-poor children in the United States are confusing even to professionals as they try to understand the different criteria in different locations; bewildered parents can face a frustrating series of barriers when trying to use these programs for their youngsters (Pear, 2000; Schroeder, 2001). In contrast, access to Medicare, a program for older adults, is simple and effective. Upon reaching their 65th birthday, those eligible for Medicare receive a card in the mail easily used for that purpose. They can then obtain an array of federal- or state-supported programs and purchase heavily subsidized additional insurance as well. Rather than take benefits from older persons, we should at least extend them to children and test out systems for biases against children.

Good reasons can sometimes exist for providing government-funded health care available to adults and not to children. It might be justified to give soldiers scarce resources during war because they must defend the nation, or to provide clinicians rare inoculations during epidemics because they must provide care for everyone. Additional benefits to some people, including children, then might sometimes be justified but, of course, it would be ideal if everyone has access to good health care.

AN ARGUMENT FROM ANALOGY

In what follows, assume that adults are entitled to whatever state-supported health-care benefits they receive; and the relevant reasons for providing these benefits are to promote (a) empathy and sympathy, (b) social utility and efficiency, (c) equality of opportunity, or (d) the best interest of vulnerable people. These reasons, I argue, are at least as persuasive when considered in relation to children. Consequently, without some compelling justification, any government-funded health care available to adults should be available to children (Kopelman, 2001). This is an argument from analogy. Such arguments establish their conclusions from their premises not with certainty but with greater or lesser degree of probability based upon the degree of similarity or differences among the things compared.

The success of this or other arguments from analogy depends, in part, on agreement about what things constitute relevant similarities and differences for our comparison. Some differences between adults and children seem irrelevant from the point of fairness in allocation of health-care resources. Unlike adults, for example, children cannot vote. Whereas this difference may explain why children sometimes lack benefits available to adults, it seems irrelevant with respect to the fairness of health-care distributions. Consider policies denying reconstructive surgery to children with congenital craniofacial anomalies while offering comparable care for adults who have been in car accidents. Although the causes differ, obvious similarities exist between the needs of those in both groups to restore

their function and appearance. The social utility of well-adjusted and productive citizens should easily justify such expenditures for children as well as adults. Moreover, added years of benefit for children illustrate why the case for their access is often at least as good as it is for adults. If it is good for adults to have easily accessible federally or state-funded health and dental care, then a useful working model should provide such services and benefits in the same easily accessible way to children.

LIMITING THE FOCUS

The focus of my remarks concern inequalities in the United States. The first reason for concentrating on the United States is that it has organized its health-care systems to respond to personal choice and market forces. As other countries are hard-pressed to stretch their resources, they too may be tempted to adopt some such features. Yet this arrangement creates an unjust bias against children based upon many theories of formal justice, or so I have argued elsewhere (Kopelman, 1995; Kopelman and Palumbo, 1997). In terms of a utilitarian theory of justice, it does not produce the greatest good for the greatest number. In terms of an egalitarian theory of justice, it does not promote equality of access or equality of opportunity. In terms of a libertarian theory of justice, it constitutes an unjust seizure of property to provide state-funded benefits to competent and sometimes even wealthy adults while neglecting incompetent persons.

A second reason for focusing on the United States is that intergenerational inequities exist despite the government spending more per capita on health care than any other country, with disparities greatest for children (Starfield, 2000). Health outcomes in the United States were compared to 13 other industrialized countries that spend far less. It ranks the worst for low birth-weight infants, for neonatal and infant mortality, and in years of potential life lost. Moreover, it ranks near the bottom for postneonatal mortality, as well as for almost all categories of life expectancy. Paul Newachecket and colleagues (2000) found that unmet health needs affect children's long- and short-term health status and function. They analyzed four years of the National Health Interview Survey data from 1993 to 1996 (sponsored by the National Center for Health Statistics) and surveyed 97,206 children under the age of 18. They found that 7.3% (4.7 million) of children in the United States had at least one unmet health-care need, with the most prevalent being dental care. Not surprisingly, poor and uninsured children were both three times more likely to have unmet needs. Poor children in the United States are two to three times as likely as children in higher-income homes to be of low birth weight, to get asthma and bacterial meningitis, to have delayed immunizations, and to suffer from lead poisoning (Starfield, 1991).

Eleven million, or one in four, of those without health insurance in the United States are children (Pear, 2000). In contrast, many adults, including all those over 65, some of whom are extremely wealthy, receive high quality health care at government expense. Moreover, optional programs for these adults are often heavily subsidized. For example, Part B of the U.S. Medicare program offers those adults over 65 who can afford it supplemental health-care insurance at low cost. They are not really "paying their own way" in buying into these state-supported insurance programs, but paying disproportionately little for a great deal more in the way of potential services (Kopelman and Palumbo, 1997).

Four reasons for providing many older persons with access to good health care also justify giving this to children when society can afford it. They also show that we should be motivated to provide good care for children and that without good and sufficient reason, it is shameful to provide health care benefits to adults and not to children.

EMPATHY AND SYMPATHY

Many older citizens have access to state-supported, health-care programs unavailable to others, based, in part, on empathy, sympathy or concern for their well being. Similar reasoning also offers a good case for not excluding children based upon their age. Consider first the case for relating empathy or sympathy to just distributions generally.

Empathy and Sympathy as a Grounding for Justice

The eighteenth-century philosopher David Hume ([1752], 1958, [1739], 1998) argued that sympathy served as the basis for justice and social solidarity generally. Hume maintained that the origin of morality and just systems is grounded in our common psychological and social natures. Although personal relationships are inherently partial, they are preconditions of morality and just systems. Hume argued that moral reasoning originates in our common human nature, which is inherently social, and in our capacity for limited but educable benevolence. Aggregate data and abstract notions of public interest, he posited, do not affect us in a forceful way, especially when they seem contrary to our own interests. Yet our awareness of the plight of particular individuals can be deeply moving.

Hume argued that self-interest and concern for others are linked, because our private interests include not only some narrowly understood partiality for oneself, but also a natural partiality for family, friends, and members of our community. We learn, moreover, that it is in our long-term interest and happiness to deny some of our desires and to support morality and just systems so as to live in a peaceful and orderly society. In the end, morality and systems of justice are so advantageous that we support them even when they occasionally thwart us or cost us more in taxes. Hume argued that our natural sympathy for others was the basis for our systems of justice where adults obtained liberty rights and the right to be provided with certain goods, services, and benefits. Promoting sympathy for children has been the key to establishing rights for them.

Empathy and Sympathy as a Basis for Children's Rights

As the twentieth century progressed, so did the awareness that many children were neglected or abused by parents. This realization became a basis for social change, limiting parents' rights to control the lives of their children. Access to good parenting, education, food, housing, and sanitation remains the most immediate means to enhance children's well being and opportunities. The consensus that children should also have basic health care and social services as a matter of justice developed during the last century as concern for them grew. Initially, advocates for better health and social care for the many impoverished, neglected, abused, and exploited children included those in the women's rights movement, doctors in the newly recognized specialty of pediatrics, and nurses who were a part of the visiting home-health programs. In addition, lawyers and social scientists joined the reform movement. They attacked the long-dominant view that children were the property of their parents or guardians, and that the state had no authority to intervene even if the children were abused or neglected (Kopelman, 1995). Children gained rights to certain kinds of medical care and to be protected from abuse, neglect, and exploitation; adolescents gained certain liberties such as the right to consent for certain kinds of treatments or services without parental approval or notification (Holder, 1985, 1989). Scientists further helped transform children's programs through study of children's growth, development, needs, experiences, illnesses, and perspectives, showing the importance of candor and respect for children's views. A distinctive feature of advocacy for improved health and social care for children remains: Others make most decisions for minors, both in terms of their

personal care and in allocation of funds for their programs.

A Need for More Empathy and Sympathy

Historically, empathy and sympathy for children helped generate social change, but there seems too little awareness of their current unmet health needs. Although the United States spends an unprecedented 14% of its gross national product (GNP) on health care, many American children do not receive basic health services. By the middle of the 1990s, 15% of the United States population lacked health insurance (40 million), with 25% of them children (10 million); many of the uninsured are less than three years of age (Berman, 1995; Kogan et al., 1995). The proportion of children in this country who are uninsured has steadily grown over the last decade (McDonough et al., 1997) as the United States health delivery systems turned to market forces to solve problems of cost containment and limiting access (Kilner, 1995; Budetti, 1997). Families of the working poor suffered most from these cost-cutting efforts, as more employers sought savings by providing health-care insurance for employees but not their family members, and fewer of these families could afford to buy insurance on their own; this trend may continue (Bodenheimer, 1999).

A recently adopted program was intended to help the millions of uninsured children who were ineligible for Medicaid. The Children's Health Insurance Plan (CHIP) passed by the U.S. Congress in 1997 gave states an opportunity to provide insurance for many more youngsters of the working poor (U.S., Title XXI, 1997). The CHIP program provides $48 billion over 10 years and $4 billion in annual grants for states to provide coverage for uninsured children either through Medicaid expansions or other state plans. These changes in the law make it possible for states to receive five-year block grants of 3:1 matching funds to cover the uninsured.

Many states do a poor job implementing or even informing families of these programs. In 1996, 23% of the children who were eligible for Medicaid (3.4 million) were uninsured (USGAO, 1998). To build more support for change, the public needs to realize the difficulties faced by children with unmet health needs. Programs available to underinsured children as well as the 11 million children currently uninsured are so complex that federal funds for them often go unspent (Pear, 2000). Parents may not be to blame for not taking advantage of these programs simply because they are so complex and difficult to access. Working-poor parents must traverse a maze of hard-to-navigate plans with different standards in different regions. These plans leave many children uninsured and, because of serious gaps in coverage, they also leave children with serious unmet health-care needs. The complexity of these programs, when contrasted to the ease of access to Medicare for people over 65, raises issues of fairness.

A key to building social support for good health and dental care for underinsured and uninsured children may be to make their needs more visible. This will motivate people to act in their best interest. Not only will providing good health care help children flourish and enhance their opportunities, but it is also efficient and socially useful. Improving public health, and preventing later costly illnesses, fosters a healthy, stable, and productive work force now and in the future. In addition, we need to build in more concern for parents of these children. Some parents cannot leave work, others cannot leave their homes, and still others lack resources for transportation or must rely on baby-sitters. The plight of many of these families and children is too frequently hidden from the general social view to make an impact on social policy. Creating good social polices to help children, however, requires empathy for them, as well as data showing which polices would be socially useful, would honor social commitments to fair equality of opportunity, and would fulfill duties to act in their best interests.

EQUALITY OF OPPORTUNITY

Equality of opportunity has been an important reason to justify people's health-care rights (Daniels, 1985). The kind of health care available to children may have a profound impact on their lives, so a society committed to equality of opportunity for children should provide adequate health care for them. Norman Daniels (1985), building on Rawls's work (1971, 1993), argues that while we should provide basic care to all, we should redistribute health-care benefits more favorably to children. The moral justification for giving children access to basic health care, argues Daniels, rests on social commitments to what he and Rawls call "fair equality of opportunity" (or affirmative action). Health-care needs are basic insofar as they promote fair equality of opportunity. Health care for children is especially important in relation to other social goods, because diseases and disabilities inhibit children's capacities to use and develop their talents, thereby curtailing their opportunities.

Daniels holds that we have to use objective ways of characterizing medical and societal needs. The ranking of needs helps determine what is basic and who profits most from certain services. Using the "difference principle," free and additional health services might be provided to the poorest children so they could compete more effectively with those from more affluent homes. Clearly, sick children cannot compete as equals in school or athletics, and illness endangers their chances to develop their capabilities or talents.

Studies show a relationship between heath outcomes and income, both in terms of wealth itself and how the wealth is shared (Daniels et al., 1999). This has an observable impact on children's health. The data show that children living in low-income homes in the United States have fewer opportunities because they get sick more often and stay sick longer when they become ill (Starfield, 1991; Berman, 1995).

Children from families of the poor and working poor bear the worst of such inequalities, adding harms of lost opportunities from poor health care to their social disadvantages (Starfield, 1991, Berman, 1995). Children's main health problems often arise from lack of basic and inexpensive care, including dental pathology, vision impairment, meningitis, allergies, asthma, hearing loss, and other chronic illnesses. Consequently, many children in the United States suffer not only loss of well-being from poor health care, but also lost opportunities.

Some state-supported programs that exclude children, such as health care benefits to veterans or members of Congress, seem to honor people's special contributions to society. Yet these benefits may be regarded as state-supported prizes for which everyone should be able to compete fairly. However, sick children cannot compete as equals with healthy children. During children's crucial and most vulnerable early years, health care may determine their later opportunities. Children living in low-income homes are more likely than richer children to suffer ill health, become seriously ill and get multiple illnesses when they do get sick (Starfield, 1991). Children cannot compete fairly if they are sick, in pain, or cannot hear or see their teacher. Children are rarely responsible for their illnesses, affluence, or social class, yet health varies directly with affluence and social class (Daniels et al., 1999). So if some state-supported health care should be regarded as prizes for people's special contributions, and if all should be able to compete for these awards fairly, then fair competition may require good health care for children.

SOCIAL UTILITY AND EFFICIENCY

Another persuasive reason for providing adults access to basic health care is that it has great social utility since a healthy population maximizes productivity. This reasoning applies to children as well.

Common Problems That Are Inexpensive to Treat

Relatively inexpensive interventions can alleviate many problems common in children, including impaired vision, hearing loss, dental pathology, allergies, asthma, and a variety of chronic disorders that can cause considerable functional impairment (Starfield, 1991; Newachecket et al., 2000). Some of the least expensive and most beneficial interventions, moreover, are education about the benefits of exercise, a good diet, prevention of teenage pregnancy, and avoidance of alcohol, tobacco, and harmful drugs (USDHHS, 1992). Providing good health care to children would not only greatly increase their overall well being and opportunities, but also would be socially useful and cost-effective. It improves public health, prevents later costly illnesses, and benefits the current generation of adults who, when aged, will need support from a healthy, stable, and productive work force.

In many cases, early intervention may prevent morbidity that plagues people for life. For example, prevention of childhood caries and common dental problems is cost-effective for society as well as extremely important to the individual. Dental pathologies represent some of the worst and most common childhood infections, and those most apt to suffer are poor and minority children. Yet our own health-care system and insurance plans tend to discount the importance of good dental health. While Medicaid technically covers dental care, poor reimbursement policies are discouraging.

Efficiency

In some countries, children receive dental care unavailable to adults because the treatments have lifelong benefits and avoid later costly problems. Providing children with routine care, mass screening, prevention, and other programs routinely available to older adults also offers society great benefits. Interventions that can benefit both children and adults generally provide longer benefits to children. Schemes that favor efficiency by means of cost-benefit (where costs and benefits are reduced to monetary considerations) or cost-effectiveness analyses (which consider in addition to monetary costs, the person's quality of life and number of healthy years) generally favor interventions and policies that target children (Mackie et al., 1996). Advocates for using such analyses assess costs and benefits to set priorities in terms of quality-adjusted life years (QALYs) and that measure the "number of years someone will likely live after the intervention multiplied by a percentage reflecting the quality of life to be experienced during those years" (Kilner, 1995, p. 1073). Those who favor setting priorities in this way, argue that the QALY method is fair and would allocate resources more equitably to children (Mackie et al., 1996).

Maximizing the good would disallow many current policies which provide care for adults but not for children. Thus maximizing the good might not always justify an age bias toward children, but it would certainly disallow the age bias against children that we have in the United States (Kopelman, 1995; Kopelman and Palumbo, 1997). Furthermore, arbitrarily discounting long-term effects creates an unjust age bias against children in these calculations (Brock, 2001).

DUTIES TO PROTECT THE BEST INTEREST OF INCOMPETENT PEOPLE

Societies recognize the duty to act in the best interest of incompetent people and children, our most vulnerable citizens. They cannot handle their own affairs in a competent manner and, therefore, need to be protected. In the United States, market forces and parental choices about how to use their money often shape children's access to health care. But even if children's health care is largely the responsibility of their guardians, society recognizes responsibilities to ensure that guardians are adequately providing for their children's best interests, including health care. Special government protections for children include a "safety net" of health care and social services for all children—albeit inadequate protection (Pear, 2000).

The use of the "best-interest" standard in medical and other decision making for incompetent persons illustrates that society recognizes special duties to them. This is a widely used ethical, legal, and social basis for policy and decision making involving children and other incompetent persons. Although this standard is used in a number of ways, two are particularly relevant to our discussion. First, the best-interest standard is used as a threshold for intervention and judgment. Second, it serves as an ideal to establish policies or duties (Kopelman, 1997).

A Threshold for Intervention and Reasonable Judgment

First, in some cases, the best-interest standard is used as a threshold for intervention and judgment, as in child abuse and neglect rulings. Suppose that clinicians believe a child's parent makes choices falling below some acceptable cut-off point with regard to the child's good; they should seek state intervention to protect the child's interests. Parents endangering their children, even for religious reasons, may find the courts willing to take custody temporarily or permanently to serve the best interest of the child. To override parental authority the state must prove, often by clear and convincing evidence, that the child has suffered or is in danger of suffering serious harm (Krause, 1986). Once the threshold has been met, the courts apply a second test that can be couched in terms of the child's best interests to determine what to do with the child (Kopelman, 1997). For example, a parent who denies a life-saving transfusion to his child would meet the two-step test: First, a judge would decide that the child is in danger within his parent's care, and, second, that having transfusions is in his best interest. The use of the best-interest standard as a threshold for intervention and reasonable judgment shows that society recognizes duties to protect children from abuse or neglect. The basis for this policy is that children are vulnerable and dependent on adults. Consequently, we should attend to the health-care needs of children based on what is in their best interest and include them in programs available to many less vulnerable or less needy adults.

Best-Interest Standard as an Ideal

Second, the best-interest standard can serve as an ideal or goal to help foster children's best interests. Even if ideals can never be perfectly fulfilled, establishing goals can help direct actions, set priorities, and establish policies. Such norms are related to assumptions about what constitutes acceptable parenting, duties of the state, professional responsibilities, unacceptable danger to children, good health care, and so on. Ideals help us shape our decisions and priorities, even if they cannot be entirely fulfilled. Balancing ideals helps forge our actual duties. Clearly, one important ideal would be to provide everyone with good health care, or at least not exclude children from programs based on their age.

BETTER, BEST, OR BIAS? "THE LEAD ABATEMENT AND REPAIR & MAINTENANCE STUDY"

I have argued that unless a special case can be made, whatever state-funded health-care programs are available for adults should also be available to children on the same basis. One such special circumstance is that policies to enroll children as research subjects are different from those for adults and this has far-reaching consequences in their therapy. An example may show the complexity of this issue.

Even though children and adults often have the same diseases and are treated with the same interventions, few modalities have been well tested on pediatric populations, and a majority of marketed drugs are unlabeled for children's use. Given this lack of information about safety and efficacy, clinicians face difficult choices. If they use untested interventions, they may endanger their patients. Yet if clinicians only use tested interventions, they are severely limited in their treatment options. This gap between research for adults and children needs to be addressed. Yet consider how bias against children may spring from research policies intended to protect them.

A recent decision from the Maryland Court of Appeals on children's participation in nontherapeutic studies concludes: "We hold that in Maryland a parent, appropriate relative, or other applicant surrogate, cannot consent to the participation of a child or other person under legal disability in nontherapeutic research of studies in which there is any risk of injury or damage to the health of the subject" (*Grimes*, 2001, p. 89). The motion for reconsideration was accompanied by an impressive array of critical commentaries (Brief of Amici Curiae, AAMC, AAU, JHU, et al, in Support of the Appellees Motion for Reconsideration, 2001). They worry that, if adopted, this holding could paralyze many important and safe research projects, thus harming children as a group in its attempt to protect the rights and welfare of research subjects. In the motion for reconsideration (2001), however, the *Grimes* court clarified that its holding did not mean "no risk" of any kind, as critics had charged. Rather it prohibited "any articulable risk beyond the minimal kind of risk that is inherent in any endeavor." Nonetheless this holding is still more restrictive than the federal regulations, so critics are unlikely to be entirely satisfied.

The Maryland Court of Appeals (its highest court) was asked to consider whether investigators or research entities, such as the Kennedy-Krieger Institute (KKI), have a special relationship with subjects, thereby creating a duty of care that could, if breached, give rise to an action in negligence. The controversy involves a $30 million study of lead poisoning conducted at the KKI, a Johns Hopkins University affiliate. This study, conducted between 1995 and 1996, was done in four sites and involved 780 children. Those children, identified as having moderate lead poisoning, were given either a placebo or the drug succimer to determine whether this medication prevented brain damage (it did not). Some parents sued the investigators and the KKI for allegedly inducing them to keep the children in houses having lead hazards while promising that their homes would be cleaned, repaired, and made safe; the parents alleged this was not done and that their children were harmed. The Court of Appeals ruled that investigators and KKI owed a duty to the plaintiffs, and the parents could sue. It not only remanded the cases to the trial court, reversing a lower court ruling that there was no such duty, but also condemned the study as unethical.

The Court of Appeals refers to the Code of Federal Regulations at 45 CFR 46. The standard in 45 CFR 46 sometimes permits local Institutional Review Boards (IRBs) to approve studies that do not hold out direct benefit to the children if they have no more than a minor increase over minimal risk. The *Grimes* court indicated this limit had been exceeded and that the risk to the children was unacceptably high, and also that the parents were not fully informed when they gave consent: "Children should not have been used for the purpose of measuring how much lead they would accumulate in their blood while living in partially abated houses to which they were recruited initially or encouraged to remain because of the study" (*Grimes*, p. 72).

The consent form fails to clarify the study's goals, including that the purpose was to measure the success of the abatement programs by measuring the degree to which the children got lead poisoning. Nor is it clear from the consent form that the repeated sampling of children's blood is essential to the study, not just a free service. Investigators, according to the Maryland Court of Appeals, may have even had some

role in placing young children in these older homes, thus increasing their danger of lead exposure and brain damage: "The project required that small children be present in the houses. To facilitate that purpose, the landlords agreeing to permit their properties to be included in the studies were encouraged, if not required, to rent the properties to tenants who had young children. In return for permitting the properties to be used and in return for limiting their tenants to families with young children, KKI assisted the landlords in applying for grants or loans to perform the levels of abatement required by KKI for each class of home (*Grimes*, pp. 19–20). The investigators and KKI contend that the subjects benefited from the study and that only a few subjects had an increase in lead blood levels. They maintain that they were not responsible for protecting the children who were in the study from unreasonable harm or the delays in complete and prompt reporting of potential hazards.

Although there are controversies about the lead-abatement study, the holding in *Grimes* is even more controversial. It contains a standard with implications for many medical and public health studies of children. Nontherapeutic research cannot be guaranteed to be safe. Grave consequences, for example, might result from unforeseen violations of confidentiality, unanticipated complications, or accidental exposure to pathogens in a clinic setting.

The initial justification for excluding individuals who lack the capacity to give informed consent from certain research was to honor their rights and to protect their welfare. Forbidding safe and important studies on people who lack the capacity to give consent does not promote their rights or welfare. Rather, it seems unfair to disallow such studies as it fails to give full consideration to their needs. The standard set forth in the *Grimes's* conclusion would, if adopted, make it more difficult to conduct non-therapeutic or "no-benefit" pediatric studies (studies designed to gain knowledge but not to benefit the subjects directly) since it restricts these to minimal-risk investigations (Kopelman, 2002). Investigators have argued that this would create a further age bias against children by making it very difficult to conduct many important studies. Critics charge that the *Grimes* holding, which sought to protect children, could have the unfortunate result of stopping most medical and public health research, inhibiting medical progress, and restricting children's opportunities for health and well-being. Defenders say it is needed to protect children.

A narrow path runs between too much and too little protections in making progress for children while protecting individual subjects. The *Grimes* holding should promote public discussion about how best to promote the well-being, opportunities and best interest of children through good research, and yet not open the door to unwarranted risks of harm to children in studies. Without good research their health care suffers, but as the *Grimes* Court indicates, nonnegotiable standards exist about how to treat children.

This case illustrates the complexities involved in good faith attempts to bring the sort of health care available to adults to children. The elimination of age-based bias against children is an important commitment. Yet implementation involves only the resources at hand and an array of other important ideals. Consequently, reasonable and informed people of good will may reach different conclusions.

CONCLUSION

Competition for limited health-care resources is likely to intensify as populations age and as the demand for expensive medical technology soars. Because children cannot advocate for themselves in struggles for funds and programs, adults will have to advocate for them if children are to get their fair share of these resources. But what is children's fair share of health-care resources and how can we motivate adults to act in children's best interest? It is certainly

not fair that children are routinely and without compelling justification excluded from state-supported health-care programs available to many adults. It may even be fair to give children additional benefits. The burden of proof for any lesser allocation should be on those arguing in favor of state-funded health care for adults that excludes children.

This conclusion is based upon an argument from analogy that assumes that adults should have this health care to foster the following values: (a) empathy and sympathy, (b) the social utility and efficiency of such arrangements, (c) social commitments to equality of opportunity, or (d) special duties to act in vulnerable people's best interest. These four arguments justify social duties to provide good health care for people to the extent that a society can afford it. But they also show that children deserve these benefits at least as much as adults in the usual case. Without good and sufficient reason, it is shameful to provide health care benefits to adults and to make them unavailable to children. If these are good arguments for giving benefits to adults, they offer at least as much reason for giving them to children.

REFERENCES

Berman, S. (1995). Uninsured children: An unintended consequence of health care system reform efforts. *JAMA* 274, 1472–73.

Brief of Amici Curiae, AAMC, AAU, JHU, et al. in support of the Appellees Motion for Reconsideration of *Grimes v. Kennedy-Krieger*, September 17, 2001.

Brock, D.W. April (2001). Children's right to health care. *Journal of Medicine and Philosophy* 26(2), 163–70.

Brock, D.W. (1995). Some unresolved ethical issues in priority setting of mental health services. In P.J. Boyle and D. Callahan (eds.), *What Price Mental Health?: The Ethics and Priority of Priority Setting.* Washington, DC: Georgetown University Press, pp. 216–32.

Bodenheimer, T. (1999). The American health care system: Physicians and the changing medical marketplace. *New England Journal of Medicine* 340, 584–88.

Budetti, P.P. (1997). Health reform for the 20th century? It may have to wait until the 21st century. *JAMA* 277(3), 193–98.

Daniels, N. (1985). *Just Health Care*. Cambridge: Cambridge University Press,

Daniels, N., Kennedy, B.P. and Kawachi, I. (1999). Why justice is good for your health. *Daedalus* 128(4), 215–51.

Grimes v. Kennedy Krieger Institute, Inc., In the Court of Appeals of Maryland, September term, 2000, no. 128, *Erica Grimes v. Kennedy Krieger Institute, Inc.*, et al., On Motiom for Reconsideration, Per Curiam, Raker, J. Dissents, Filed October 11, 2001.

Grimes v. Kennedy Kriegar Institute, Inc., Case no 24-C-99-00925 and 24-C-95066067, (August 16, 2001), unpublished.

Holder, A. (1985). *Legal Issues in Pediatrics and Adolescent Medicine*, 2nd ed. New Haven, CT: Yale University Press,

Holder, A. (1989). Children and adolescents: Their right to decide their own health care. In L.M. Kopelman and J.C. Moskop (eds.), *Children and Health Care: Moral and Social Issues*. Dordecht, The Netherlands: Kluwer, pp. 161–72.

Hume, D. (1739/1958). *Treatise Concerning Human Nature*. Edited by L.A. Selby-Bigge. Oxford: Clarendon Press.

Hume, D. (1752/1998). *An Enquiry Concerning the Principles of Morals*. Edited with introductory material by Tom L. Beauchamp. Oxford: Oxford University Press

Kilner, J.F. (1995). A health care resources, Allocation of I, Macroallocation and Allocation of II, Microallocation. In *Encyclopedia of Bioethics*, rev. ed. New York: Simon & Schuster, pp. 1067–84.

Kogan, M.D., Alexander, G.R., Teilelbaum, M.A., Jack, B.W., Kotelchuckl, M. and Pappas, G. (1995). The effect of gaps in health insurance on contiguity of a regular source of care among preschool children in the United States. *JAMA* 274, 1429–35.

Kopelman, L.M. (1995). Children/III. Health care and research. In *Encyclopedia of Bioethics*, rev. ed. New York: Simon & Schuster, pp. 357–68.

Kopelman, L.M. (1997). The best-interests standard as threshold, ideal, and standard of reasonableness. *Journal of Medicine and Philosophy* 22(3), 271–89.

Kopelman, L.M. (2001). On duties to provide basic health and dental care to children. *Journal of Medicine and Philosophy* 26(2), 193–209.

Kopelman, L.M. (2002). Pediatric research regulations under legal scrutiny: *Grimes* narrows the interpretation. *Journal of Law Medicine & Ethics* 30, 38–49.

Kopelman, L.M., and Palumbo, M.G., (1997). The U.S. health delivery system: Inefficient and unfair to children. *American Journal of Law and Medicine* 23 (2–3), 319–37.

Krause, H.D. (1986). *Family Law in a Nutshell*, 2nd ed. St. Paul, MN: West Publishing.

Mackie, J., Kuhse, H., Richardson, J. and Singer, P. (1996). Allocating healthcare by QALY: The relevance of age. *Cambridge Quarterly of Healthcare Ethics* 5, 534–45.

Maynard A. and Bloor, K. (1996). Introducing a market to the United Kingdom's National Health Service *New England Journal of Medicine* 334, 604–608.

McDonough, J.E., Hager, C.L. and Rosman, B. (1997). Health care reform stages a comeback in Massachusetts. *New England Journal of Medicine* 336(2), 148–51.

Newachecket, P., McManus, M., Fox, H.B., Hung, Y.Y., Halfon, N. (2000). Access to Health Care for Children with Special Health Care Needs. *Pediatrics* 105(4), 989–97.

Pear, R. (2000). 40 States forfeit health care funds for poor children. *New York Times*, September 24, p. 1.

Rawls, J. (1971). *A Theory of Justice*. Cambridge, MA: Harvard University Press.

Rawls, J. (1993). *Political Liberalism*. New York: Columbia University Press.

Schroeder, S.A. (2001). Prospects for expanding health insurance coverage. *New England Journal of Medicine* 344(11), 847–51.

Starfield, B. (1989). Child health and public policy. In L.M. Kopelman and J.C. Moskop (eds.), *Children and Health Care: Moral and Social Issues*. Dordrecht, The Netherlands: Kluwer, pp. 7–22.

Starfield, B. (1991). Childhood morbidity: Comparisons, clusters, and trends. *Pediatrics* 88(3), 519–26.

Starfield, B. (2000). Is U.S. health really the best in the world? *JAMA* 284(4), 483–85.

U.S. Title XXI Children's Health Insurance Program, from the Balanced Budget Act of 1997 (P.L. 105–33). August 5, 1997.

U.S. Department of Health and Human Services (DHHS) (1992). *Healthy People, National Health Promotion and Disease Prevention Objectives*. Full report with commentary. Publication No. (PHS) 91–50212.

U.S. General Accounting Office (USGAO) (1998). *Report to the Honorable John McCain, U.S. Senate. Medicaid: Demographics of Nonenrolled Children Suggest State Outreach Strategies*. March 1998. GAO/HEHS 98–93.

22

Age Rationing Under Conditions of Injustice

Leslie Pickering Francis

How can an egalitarian justifiably reject age rationing in health care, if rationing is necessary at all? The elderly have had more of the good of life, a "fair innings" in British parlance, so it would seem to follow that they should be of lower priority when it comes to fulfilling health care needs. Or so Daniel Callahan contends (1998). And so Norman Daniels (1985) also contends, but for different reasons. Daniels's view is Rawlsian: If we do not know our circumstances with respect to health, we would choose health care for ourselves that attempts to further the normal opportunity range over a life span, rather than care extending life beyond that range. Perhaps Daniels is right, and we would so choose.

In the real world, however, we do not have the luxury of choosing a health-care system for a complete life, at least for those who are already in the middle of life or nearing life's end. Instead, we must think about how to apply whatever system turns out to be in place to a wide variety of individuals, some of whom will have enjoyed relative wealth and good health care over a life span but others of whom will not have been so fortunate. The suggestion on which this discussion is based is that Callahan and Daniels consider the problem of age rationing as a problem of "ideal theory." Daniels, for example, argues that age rationing is justified as a choice made within individual lives, not among lives. Choosers behind the veil of ignorance can expect that earlier benefits will follow them across a lifetime.

Suppose, instead, that we consider the problem of age rationing as part of the problem of how to distribute health care in a world both of prior injustice in health care and of social injustice more generally. In other words, suppose we ask whether the problem of age rationing raises different concerns if we view it as a problem of what has been called, by John Rawls and others, "partial compliance theory," rather than as a problem of ideal theory.[1] Surely any proposal to ration health care by age in the United States today must confront not only the question of age rationing in ideal theory, but also the question of age rationing in a society that is less than ideal with respect to ideal justice.

For purposes of this discussion, I will leave open many questions about the relative severity of injustice as well as the forms of injustice in contemporary America. Several rough, basic observations might be in order, however. I am assuming at least some injustice in the basic institutions that affect the opportunities people have to lead their lives: employment, property arrangements, and housing, for instance. I am also assuming that injustice in these institutions affects health, and that there may be injustice in the distribution of health care. Finally, I am assuming injustice that is sufficiently pervasive and systematic to require institutional correction from the point of view of justice—not simply injustice that is episodic or localized, such as problems of injustice with particular people that can be corrected individually (as an unjust conviction might be corrected to the extent possible with a pardon and compensation).

At the present time in the United States, those who are elderly have done relatively well—well enough to survive, that is. If anything, the elderly are better off than many other Americans with respect to health care. At least for those who qualify, there is the social safety net of the Medicare program, although with significant gaps such as the lack of coverage for prescription drugs or for long-term care, and the elderly now pay a proportionately higher share of their medical care than at the time when Medicare was originally introduced. Those who do not qualify for Medicare are those who have not paid into the Social Security system for the requisite number of quarter-years (40), most likely those in underground industries such as domestic or agricultural work, or those who immigrated to the United States too late in life to accumulate 40 quarter-years. Indeed, it is likely that background injustices of race, gender, and class are at least, if not more, severe

than injustices of age. There are significant differences in life expectancy by race particularly in the United States. At the same time, age may compound these other injustices. To a woman who has been a caregiver for most of her life—first for children, then for elderly parents, and perhaps then for an ill husband—the thought of age rationing might seem at best a cruel loss of the only turn she might ever have. In short, partial compliance theory in the United States must deal with overlapping patterns of injustice. Some elderly are poor, others are not. Some live with the ability to pay for almost all of their own health care. Of others, the best that can be said is what William Faulkner said of the fictional African-American, Dilsey, "They endured."[2]

PARTIAL COMPLIANCE THEORY

Let me begin with some general observations about *partial compliance theory*, starting with the extent to which claims of partial compliance theory can be defended independently of commitments to particular theories of justice. These remarks will be skeletal, for the goal of this contribution is to employ rather than defend some contentions of partial compliance theory, but I hope they are sufficiently developed to be helpful. Although I do think that some points of partial compliance theory hold across theories of justice, ranging from libertarianism to fair equality of opportunity to egalitarianism, I will not make such bold claims here. Establishing this larger point would require examining what each of these kinds of theories of justice would say about partial compliance problems. A typical example would be the problem of understanding what libertarians might conclude about entrenched property rights with historical antecedents of force or fraud, such as claims now being challenged in Eastern Europe over 50 years after the end of World War II. It may indeed be that this examination would reveal that different theories of justice would agree about points of partial compliance theory, but the work to establish this far exceeds the scope of this brief discussion.

The observations about partial compliance theory that I will offer are made within the different theories of justice that assume a commitment to a minimally decent package of opportunities for everyone. This commitment is that each person should be afforded a minimal set of basic opportunity goods, goods that are critical to living a wide range of lives in the society in which he or she dwells. Examples of such basic opportunity goods in the United States include education and a minimally decent health-care package. There are, of course, many different opportunity-based theories, differing in the opportunity goods they identify, in the level at which they set the basic minimum, and in whether they insist on further levels of equality beyond the basic minimum. The observations about partial compliance theory made here are based on theories of justice that are committed to a basic package of opportunities for everyone.

The structure of the relation between partial compliance theory and a preferred ideal theory is another important threshold issue. There are many plausible ways the two might be related. One possibility is that the relation is linear: that the only question we should ask in circumstances of injustice is how to move society along a trajectory toward ideal justice. Another possibility is a derivative relationship: that the principles of partial compliance theory are inferred from ideal theory, in conjunction with relevant facts about the circumstances of injustice. Still another possibility is that the principles of ideal theory set side-constraints on the principles that may be adopted in contexts of partial compliance. For example, if ideal theory is committed to certain basic rights, perhaps the principles of partial compliance theory are constrained by the requirement that these rights be given particular importance.

A final possibility is that the two theories are entirely independent—that the principles of justice that apply under circumstances of injustice simply differ from the principles that apply under circumstances of ideal justice. This possibility may seem surprising, but it is perhaps not so odd if we reflect that a number of theorists have suggested that their views about ideal justice simply do not apply when circumstances of justice proposed by David Hume are not met.[3] The views that follow rest on questioning the model of linear progression toward absolute justice; partial compliance theory is more complicated than simple linear progression toward ideal justice. The views do not, however, make further assumptions about the structure of the relationship between the two.

Some Claims of Partial Compliance Theory and How They Confound the Issue of Age Rationing

Now let me lay out some more particular claims that opportunity-based theories of justice should find relevant in circumstances of partial compliance, together with what they might reveal about the age-rationing problem. I contend only that these are principles of partial compliance that would be appealing to someone who thinks in terms of an opportunity view of justice. More generally, they yield some useful suggestions about age rationing and health policy toward the elderly; and they indicate a cautious case for expanding Medicare under the current circumstances, rather than a case for age rationing.

First, in situations of partial compliance, consider whether acting in a certain way aimed toward ideal justice nevertheless risks making the situation appreciably worse from the point of view of ideal justice, and why it might do so. This suggestion seems to hold across theories of ideal justice; for opportunity-based theories, it would direct us to consider whether actions today would make it more difficult to achieve basic opportunities in the future. One concern might be that a policy would diminish opportunities, leaving us with further to go along the trajectory toward ideal justice. Another concern might be that a policy would set up moral roadblocks that would ultimately need to be undone if progress toward ideal justice is to occur.

An example would be the creation of obligations that stand in the way of eventual progress, such as commitments to provide health care that literally break the bank. Arguably, the commitment to add end-stage renal disease to the Medicare program, while defended as a step toward a more just health care system, in the end proved so costly that it has made it more difficult to secure extended funding for other programs. There may be a lesson here for other proposals to expand Medicare. For example, if pharmaceutical coverage is offered under Medicare, and proves even more expensive than current projections indicate, it might derail other efforts to expand publicly provided health care. The situation would be even worse if the expansion contributes to further entrenching problematic features of the current situation, such as questionable practices in the advertising of prescription drugs. These risks do not, to be sure, argue for age rationing per se, but they do suggest caution in the assumption that every expansion of care that is apparently a linear move toward justice is thereby fully warranted.

Yet another concern about effects on progress toward justice is the creation of attitudes that make justice harder to achieve—what might be called "backlash attitudes." Policies might foster attitudes of resentment that slow progress or feed political opposition to movement toward justice. Backlash attitudes, although not morally worthy in themselves, surely at least risk detouring progress toward justice; they are, as it were, additional blocks in the moral road.[4] Backlash attitudes toward affirmative action, such as the tendency to regard with suspicion the qualifications of all minorities in prominent positions, are a notorious example.[5] It seems unlikely that resentment toward the elderly per se might

be created by a failure to age-ration. At the same time, it seems at least possible that attitudes of resentment fostered by the half-hearted expenditure of resources on long-term care might underlie at least some of the elder abuse that is now reportedly widespread. What this suggests is the need for expending resources in a way that provides adequate support rather than problematic dependency.[6]

Second, in circumstances of injustice, more fundamental commitments of ideal moral theory should be protected instead of less basic ones, unless there is strong reason to the contrary. This suggestion can apply only when an ideal theory ranks commitments, as does a hierarchical theory of rights. The argument for this suggestion is that a reason that counts for ranking priorities in the ideal context should at least be brought into play in the nonideal context. The suggestion that ideal rankings should be brought into play in nonideal contexts does not mean that they are conclusive: just that some countervailing reason from the nonideal context is required to displace the ideal priorities.

In some circumstances, giving priority toward ideal rankings might raise questions about policies that otherwise would appear to be justified as linear movements toward ideal justice. For example, consider the concerns that have been raised about physician aid-in-dying and vulnerable populations. Suppose we think that from the point of view of justice, it is not wise to introduce aid-in-dying in the United States until we have achieved relatively universal health care. The concern here is that people might be coerced by unjust allocations of health care to choose aid-in-dying, when they would not have opted for this alternative under allocations that were just. Advocates for the elderly such as the American Bar Association on the Legal Problems of the Elderly have voiced the concern in this way.[7]

Conversely, suppose we also believe that a failure to permit aid-in-dying with proper safeguards is a serious violation of autonomy. In an ideal world, in which the injustice of manipulating deaths too soon by the curtailment of resources did not occur, we would not face this choice. In a nonideal world, we probably do. What this suggestion about partial compliance theory would recommend is that we consider which of autonomy or distributive justice is the more important moral commitment in ideal theory and then give that commitment priority in the partial compliance context, unless there is strong reason to the contrary. And there might well be. Suppose that autonomy is indeed the more fundamental moral commitment, yet we suppose that the risks of injustice are very significant indeed; then we would have reason to reorder the commitments in a partial compliance context. In contrast, if the risks of slippage in justice are relatively slight, we might countenance these slippages to preserve the more important ideal value of autonomy. Situations of injustice, if sufficiently severe, may demand temporary realignment of the priority of ideal values.

A third claim of partial compliance theory is that in situations of injustice, we should develop strategies that spread the burdens of moving toward justice. The argument for considering burden-sharing strategies begins with the observation that it is morally unfortunate for progress toward justice to impose burdens on anyone; all things being equal, it would be preferable (and simpler) to achieve justice in a costless manner. If burdens are unavoidable, however, it is preferable for them to be shared than to be borne by one or a small group of individuals, unless there is some moral reason, such as individual fault, for localizing them. Without a reason to localize, and so without a reason for picking out a particular individual to bear the burdens of achieving justice, sharing the burdens is fairer; no one is disproportionately disadvantaged without good reason. Moreover, the impact of a widely shared burden on any given individual's opportunities in life is likely to be less than the impact of a concentrated burden.

In the health-care context, burdens are not shared when they fall on individuals, such as sick patients or the families who care for them. They are shared when they are paid for through tax dollars or community-rated insurance. This suggests that we should continue to pursue progress toward justice through the expansion of public programs such as Medicare, rather than through private funding or support. We might, however, note that the current tax structure that funds Medicare, namely FICA, does not represent an optimal sharing strategy, as it does not apply to unearned income.[8] Burden-sharing also suggests favoring community rating in insurance, avoiding the concentrated burdens when health insurance costs rise precipitously for individuals or small employers based on experience rating. Pie-expanding strategies (that is, strategies aimed at expanding the availability of a scarce resource) are another important way of spreading the burdens of achieving progress toward justice. Of course, pie-expanding strategies are the antithesis of rationing. This last observation may count directly against age rationing. The elderly are relatively powerful politically and enjoy the benefits of Medicare. It may be that the only way that it is politically feasible to move toward a more just health-care system for younger Americans is to expand Medicare as well. An illustration of how factors may be delicately balanced in partial compliance theory, however, is the risk of backlash when expansions are not carefully considered.

Fourth, in partial compliance contexts, honor legitimate expectations, to the extent possible, when lives are disrupted, and regard compensation as a particularly weighty consideration when such expectations cannot be honored. (This principle might be limited by the recommendation that the commitments of ideal theory come first; but if the case for expectations is sufficiently strong, it might override the commitments of ideal theory.) Expectations are beliefs about the future that people count on when planning their lives; honoring expectations is thus part of what is involved in treating people as autonomous beings who order their own lives.

Expectations generate reliance, but naturally not all such reliance is "legitimate."[9] By "legitimate expectations," I mean expectations that carry independent moral weight—that is, there is at least some moral reason to satisfy expectations in their own right. Expectations are legitimate when they are reasonable, when they have been deliberately encouraged or fostered by long-term social arrangements, and when they are not the product of injustice or other moral wrongs on the part of those who hold them. The moral case for honoring expectations is strongest when they concern individuals' basic needs or central aspects of their lives, and when inadequate time is available for readjustment if they are disappointed.

On all these counts, health benefits often are an excellent example of legitimate expectations. Consider, for example, the expectations created by many early retirement packages which promised health benefits until the age of eligibility for Medicare, and perhaps Medigap insurance thereafter. At the time these agreements were entered, the expectations founded upon them seemed reasonable. They were deliberately fostered by employer promises and inducements, promises that were at the time seen to be in the employer's interests. Such expectations are not the product of injustice on the part of their holders—if anything, they might be the product of predatory behavior by employers. They surely concern basic needs: health care. And there is little or no time, after retirement, for readjustment by reentry into the work force. The expectation of receiving Medicare benefits is an even more persuasive example. Here the expectation has been fostered by government policy since the 1960s. Although there are periodic expressions of concern about the long-term viability of Medicare, political rhetoric promises efforts to shore it up rather than

to dismantle it. And there is even less time for readjustment after retirement than before.

Of course, concern for protecting legitimate expectations is a two-edged sword. After all, if there are no legitimate expectations, there is no case for protecting them (although there might be a case for creating them). Commitment to protecting expectations might, therefore, also suggest caution about creating them. There is a lesson here for Medicare as well: Show restraint about promising more than can be delivered.

Finally, in partial compliance situations we should be especially wary of strategies that impose disproportionate burdens on vulnerable individuals or groups. By vulnerable groups I do not necessarily mean the economically worst off, but those who are most susceptible to losing whatever position they have. Legal immigrants, for example, are not necessarily the poorest of residents in the United States, yet their vulnerability was clear in the 1997 welfare reforms, which stripped them of eligibility for Medicaid benefits.[10] My defense of this suggestion is pragmatic: It is no doubt easier to try to achieve justice by making trade-offs among groups who cannot really protect themselves, so the pressures here might be particularly intense. It is also moral: It is especially unjust to prey on the vulnerable, even in the name of justice. When we are having difficulty achieving justice, we should pay particular attention to what kind of community we are, and to values such as solidarity.

The frail aged may be among the most vulnerable in American society. So in partial compliance circumstances, we should be particularly careful of the burdens of moving toward justice by imposing burdens on them. This vulnerability is deepened for the elderly who are poor, or disabled. It may have been complicated by earlier experiences of discrimination. Moreover, vulnerability may be still worse if earlier features of discrimination in health care are factored in. Just as critics of the Oregon health plan argued that it increased benefits for the near-poor by rationing care on the back of the poor, so critics of rationing within Medicare might raise the concern that it keeps Medicare afloat by rationing on the backs of the vulnerable elderly.

But there are other vulnerable groups who also might be considered: children, people with disabilities, people of color—all the other subjects of injustice considered in this volume. In health care, another example of the vulnerable might be those who are too old or sick to work, but who are not yet eligible for Medicare: the cohort aged in their late fifties or early sixties. Health status might be particularly precarious for this age cohort. Medicare should not be saved by means of strategies that deny benefits to these other vulnerable groups. Indeed, one strategy might be a gradual expansion of Medicare to provide coverage for groups such as those nearing retirement who are not able to work.

Some elderly, however, are not vulnerable at all. These predominate among the elderly who are quite well off. However, as it is currently structured, Medicare does not have a means test. One suggested modification of Medicare that might help spread the costs of expansion, without unduly burdening expectations or risking vulnerable populations, would be the introduction of a moderate means test into Medicare premiums, co-payments, and deductibles.

CONCLUSION

If we consider age rationing as a problem of partial compliance theory, its desirability does not seem so obvious as it might if we consider it as a matter of ideal theory. It is quite different to bring age rationing into play in a world of people who have already suffered from injustice, than to consider it for people who will live their full lives in a just society. Perhaps we will be at that point someday; perhaps we are even trying to phase it in with better health care for children. One can only hope.

In the meantime, however, several arguably important features of partial compliance theory count against age rationing. It is especially unjust to make progress toward justice by disadvantaging the vulnerable, and at least some of the elderly are among the most vulnerable. Legitimate expectations should be protected to at least some extent from the disruptions of progress toward justice, and expectations of Medicare and other retiree health benefits are among such expectations. Burdens of moving toward justice should be shared, and Medicare is a good example of such burden-sharing through tax dollars, although one that might be arranged in an even better way.

At the same time, there are reasons for caution. Other vulnerable populations are also at risk and might reasonably be added to Medicare; the near-elderly who are unable to work are a good example. Yet too rapid expansion of Medicare might risk the creation of roadblocks that make it more difficult to move toward a more just health-care system. At least some of the elderly are quite well off, and it might be appropriate to finance at least some expansion of Medicare through at least some means testing. In short, the view from partial compliance theory favors more caution in expanding Medicare benefits than in expanding the reach of the Medicare program. But then, partial compliance theory is always messy.

NOTES

1. See Rawls, *A Theory of Justice*, pp. 245–46. I hold the view that some of the most important contemporary issues of justice are problems of partial compliance theory, and that those of us who are deeply interested in these issues would do well to explore partial compliance theory in a serious way. Indeed, problems of applied ethics quite typically are problems of partial compliance; we must act under real world constraints when we face real world problems. To the best of my knowledge, there have been very few discussions of partial compliance theory; a noteworthy exception is Holtman, "Kant, Ideal Theory, and the Justice of Exclusionary Zoning."

2. William Faulkner. *The Sound and the Fury.* New York: Random House, 1956..

3. See, e.g., Rawls, *Theory of Justice,* pp. 126–27.

4. The extent to which the roadblocks outlined here should be taken into account morally is a difficult question. If these roadblocks involve complicity in injustice, or are fostered in injustice, that is a moral reason for not giving them any moral weight. Backlash attitudes towards affirmative action that are rooted in discrimination are examples of attitudes that are not morally worthy but are politically very troublesome. Some roadblocks may arise without complicity on the part of their beneficiary. Bona fide seniority rights are a likely example.

5. For a description of the demoralizing effects of such backlash attitudes in affirmative action, see Steele, *The Content of Our Character.*

6. For a discussion of dependency, see Kittay, *Love's Labor,*

7. See Francis, "Assisted Suicide." 1998.

8. "FICA" refers to the Federal Insurance Contributions Act, originally Title II of the 1935 Social Security Act. There are two FICA taxes. The Social Security tax, 6.2% of earned income, matched by an additional 6.2% of earned income paid by employers, had a 2000 to 2001 ceiling of $72, 600. (That is, no income over $72,600 was subject to the tax for Social Security.) The Medicare tax, an additional 1.45% of earned income, also matched by employers, has no ceiling but is only levied on earned income.

9. For a more critical account of the legitimacy of expectations, see Munzer, "A Theory of Retroactive Legislation."

10. This provision of the Personal Responsibility and Work Opportunity Act of 1997 (PROWRA) was later amended to grandfather immigrants in the country legally as of August 1997. The amendment followed the recognition that PROWRA would strip many elderly nursing home residents of Medicaid coverage; the image of many incompetent or ill elderly persons literally turned out on the streets was a powerful factor in lobbying for the amendment. See Francis, "Elderly Immigrants."

REFERENCES

Callahan, D. (1998). *False Hopes.* New York: Simon & Schuster.

Daniels, N. (1985). *Just Health Care.* New York: Cambridge University Press.

Francis, L. (1997). Elderly immigrants: What should they expect of the social safety net? *The Elderlaw Journal* 5, 229–50.

Francis, L. (1998). Assisted suicide: Are the elderly a special case? In P. Battin, R. Rhodes, and A. Silvers (eds.), *Physician-Assisted Suicide.* New York: Routledge.

Holtman, S.W. (1999). Kant, ideal theory, and the justice of exclusionary zoning. *Ethics* 110, 32–58.

Kittay, E. F. (1999). *Love's Labor: Essays on Women, Equality and Dependency.* New York: Routledge.

Munzer, S.R. (1982). A theory of retroactive legislation. *Texas Law Review* 61, 425–80.

Rawls, J. (1971). *A Theory of Justice.* Cambridge, MA: Harvard University Press.

Steele, S. (1990). *The Content of Our Character.* New York: St. Martin's Press.

23

Just Expectations: Family Caregivers, Practical Identities, and Social Justice in the Provision of Health Care

James Lindemann Nelson

For some decades now, dampening the explosive growth of health-care costs has been a matter of pressing concern in the United States.[1] While the recent lengthy cycle of economic expansion in this country significantly tempered the rate at which health-care expenditures had been eating up the gross domestic product (GDP), costs in this area remain dynamic, fueled by the wide dissemination of new technologies (Levit et al., 2000; Freudenham, 2000).

Not that the health-care industry has put its faith solely in the hope of a permanent economic boom. The dizzying upward spiral of medical costs that characterized the 1980s and early 1990s has been flattened out in important part by a sort of semivoluntary conscription of unpaid health-care workers, who generally lack any professional training for their tasks. This new "draft" has largely escaped attention because of just who is being pressed into service. Responsibilities have been shifted from professional caregivers working in hospitals and other such sites, to *caregiving relatives* whose work largely takes place at home. This trend has been coupled with a reduction of home-care benefits available through insurers or public programs (Levine, 1999a).

There is every reason to believe that increasing reliance on family caregivers will continue to be an attractive tactic. Increasingly complex forms of medical technologies are being more or less adapted to home use, and spouses, parents, and children remain inexpensive compared to registered nurses or respiratory technicians. Employment of advanced technologies can now be directed and monitored remotely, via "telemedicine," speeding the process of turning homes into *faux* hospitals, and their inhabitants into health-care professionals *manqué* (Arras, 1995; Bauer, 2001).

It will be interesting to see what kind of impact on the quality of patient care emerges from this progressive deprofessionalization of health-care provision. Diverting responsibilities for patient well-being from highly trained and experienced professionals (who have tolerably clear role-related limits to the extent of the services they are supposed to provide), to an amateur population, often otherwise employed, and with no clear and socially recognized limits to their responsibilities, looks very much like a type of rationing. Though it does not require that any particular health-care service be denied, or any special population be excluded (except, perhaps, those who lack families)—thus avoiding the most visible and controversial forms of rationing—deprofessionalizing the health-care work force achieves cost savings at the risk of a more generally distributed dilution of the quality of care available to patients.

Nor are the consequences for family members, pressed into intense and prolonged caregiving roles, likely to be benign. In a recent discussion of the increased role of informal caregivers in the new health economy, Carol Levine summed the matter up with bleak pith: "Individuals and families will be under increased pressure to pay more direct costs; families will be expected to provide more hands on, often technologically complex care; undertake greater burdens for longer times; and forgo more educational, career and social opportunities" (Levine, 1999a, p. 342).

Both questions of possibly decreased quality of care for patients (particularly if construed as a form of rationing) and questions concerning the "increased pressures" on caregiving individuals and families raise issues of distributive justice that have been largely overlooked by bioethicists. I will focus on the impact of these changes on care providers, in part because of their particular philosophical interest. Surely, it is only the fact that informal caregivers are typically family members that explains why they are so employed with only the faintest whimpers of protest; even in a culture with a notoriously spotty record of respect for women and people identified with ethnic or racial minorities, the notion that any other group could be expected to take on such tasks *gratis* is not credible. At the same

time, at least some family caregivers who shoulder extreme burdens apparently find great value in the provision of hands-on care to those they love, and they are reluctant to turn to whatever alternative sources of care might still be available. Despite some recent attention to the ethical character of intimate associations, we still lack fully mature accounts of what societies may justly expect of families, and of what family members may justly expect of each other. In what follows, I aim to contribute to the development of such an account, and to trace out some implications bearing on whether the "impressment" of families into more, and more intensive, health-care responsibilities is defensible.

ARE FAMILIES BEING UNJUSTLY DONE BY?

Is it consistent with a defensible account of distributive justice to constrain health-care costs by established policies that transfer prolonged or intensive health care responsibilities from professionals to family members? This is a complicated question, in part because the trend has not resulted from some central planning agency that might reasonably be held accountable for the systematic effects of its decisions—in this respect, the "conscription" metaphor employed earlier is misleading. Rather, the migration of increasingly burdensome health-care responsibilities from professionals to family members is a function of many decisions made by federal and state governments, by different private insurers, and, perhaps, even by those insurance consumers who may have some measure of realistic choice about the kind of coverage to elect. This ambiguity about agency makes it tougher to determine who bears what responsibility for any resulting harms. It hardly seems plausible that *any* reliance on family for *any* kind of care constitutes an injustice, and so decisions tending to contribute to this trend incrementally may seem more or less innocent.

Acknowledging that it is appropriate to

expect families to sacrifice to at least some extent for their needy members introduces what I believe the most vexing complication. Assessing the justice of this kind of deprofessionalization of health-care provision is caught up with the question of what family members are entitled to expect of one another, and of what kinds of contributions to social goals such expectations license.

Suppose, for example, one turns to some of the currently leading understandings of distributive justice. Philosophical reflection about distributive justice is often depicted as a matter of discovering and motivating ways of allocating the benefits and burdens involved in social arrangements that do not run afoul of some special moral character that human beings are thought to have. The special character is often indicated with notions like "inviolability" or "separateness." John Rawls, is fond of both notions; inadequate respect for the "distinction between persons" (Rawls, 1971, p. 27) is at the heart of his objection to utilitarian allocation schemes, and, in one of his memorable ringing phrases, he observes: "Each person has an inviolability founded on justice that even the welfare of society as a whole cannot override" (p. 3). Justice, then, is thought to involve considering people as individuals with certain moral prerogatives that must be respected, even if doing so should make everyone worse off than they otherwise would be.

Consider people as members of a large, "impersonal" social arrangement, in which the exploitation of variously marginalized groups and individuals endures, and the intuitive appeal of notions such as separateness and inviolability may seem compelling. Consider people as members of families—in which exploitation, while surely present, often coexists with affirmation, caring, and love—and the appeal flags. This shift in our intuitions may reflect the conviction that the relationships between members of tolerably intimate families are significantly different in morally important ways from those between people

qua citizens of a state, or *qua* economic agents in a marketplace.

In reasonably well-functioning families, people will generally find something more than opportunities to amuse or aggrandize themselves though interchanges with similarly motivated others. Such families are places where selves are, in important senses, formed, maintained, and shared. Individual interests abound in families, but so do shared interests, and even what might be called the interests of the family as a whole (Minuchin, 1974; H. Nelson and J. Nelson, 1995). Acknowledging that such shared and interdefined interests are often importantly characteristic of families does not require allegiance to any strong form of communitarianism, or any overly roseate view of families as homogenous and ideal havens; the presence of joint interests does not exclude the possibility of distinct and oftentimes conflicting interests.[2] But the significance of such shared interests as there may be calls into question the suitability of conceptions of distributive justice that are predicated on the primary significance of individuality and distinctness to clarify who is indebted to whom for what.

The theoretical emphasis on the "distinctness of persons" is not the only problem in sorting out what family members do and do not owe to each other. Just as one does not have to be a communitarian to acknowledge morally relevant differences between personal relations *qua* citizen and personal relations *qua* family member, neither does one have to be a moral particularist to allow that families are rife with morally relevant particulars. Families tend to endure over significant periods of time, involve people in strong emotions, and play important and varied roles in how people understand themselves and others. The patterns of feeling and action, of duties and of disappointment, and of what goes beyond both duty and disappointment pertinent to sorting out claims can differ from relationship to relationship within a family, from time to time within one family,[3] and certainly from family to family. To know, for example, whether some assignment of burdens and benefits in a family is morally defensible, one is going to have to know a good deal about the particular family under consideration.

Despite these difficulties, I want to argue that the shift of health-care responsibilities to families does raise questions of justice that are both deeply serious and potentially tractable. There are features of families that make treating them as a standing reserve of labor for the health-care system morally problematic, and which, in addition, render them particularly vulnerable to exploitation.

My argument has two stages. First, I want to call attention to some specific and serious kinds of vulnerability that families generally have to the shifts of health-care responsibilities. Second, I will argue that these vulnerabilities are salient from the point of view of distributive justice; there is reason, that is, to see the community as having a duty to deploy its resources to avoid, or at least ameliorate, the harms associated with intensive or prolonged family provision of health care.

THREE THREATS TO FAMILIES

I will employ three considerations to help illuminate what is at stake for families in current trends in health-care delivery. The first is their *propensity for exploitation*. It follows fairly directly from the ways in which family members in many instances do not regard their own interests as altogether distinct from each other's. Families, although not outside the "circumstances of justice," are institutions in which other kinds of value, and hence other reasons for action, are extremely powerful. A nation, for example, might come to the reasonable conclusion that supplying the resources needed to satisfy certain citizens' needs was an unreasonable or even flatly unjust drain on the common pool. Having decided that it need not or even ought not meet such needs, a nation might, in fact, simply let them go unmet; charity (or shame), although playing some role in public policy, is not an overwhelmingly strong motivator. Families might confront similar situations and engage in analogous reasoning leading to the same conclusion. Some of its members may have needs that are simply too great for others to be expected to fulfill. But there are also considerations apart from justice—considerations of love, to take a prominent example—that may lead families to provide care over and above what could be expected of them as a matter of justice. This inclination to supererogation makes families prime targets for exploitation.

The second consideration highlights an important feature of the kind of risk that families face. In supplying care that is prolonged and intensive, family members can put in harm's way what I will call (following Christine Korsgaard) their *practical identities*. A practical identity is "a description under which you find your life to be worth living and your actions to be worth undertaking" (Korsgaard, 1996, p. 101). Korsgaard (1996) speaks of people having a "jumble" of such identities ("a human being, a woman or a man, an adherent of a certain religion, a member of an ethnic group, a member of a certain profession, someone's lover or friend"), and regards those identities as providing reasons and obligations: "Your reasons express your identity, your nature; your obligations spring from what that identity forbids" (p. 101).

Some practical identities seem to make more central contributions to our overall sense of self than others; some are more inextricably caught up with our convictions about the worthwhileness of our lives and actions. Further, our grasp on any of our practical identities is surely contingent; misadventure and mortality can take them all away. However, when human agency is involved in wrenching away cherished practical identities from us, the agents are at least presumptively culpable, as they would be for intentionally or negligently causing any serious harm.

Reflecting on the importance of practical identities is on point because the kind of intensive caregiving increasingly demanded of families is not merely a matter of shifting resources from one area of an organization's endeavors to another. Rather, it is very likely to involve a restructuring of people's most basic projects—those activities that are deeply implicated in some of the most fundamental and personally significant ways that people identify themselves. One's ability to take on and maintain an identity as, say, a breadwinner, a professional, a student, or even a spouse, may be impaired or blocked. Sufficiently burdensome caregiving requirements also threaten to harm the character of both the family itself and its ability to discharge competently a central function: nurturing those capacities required for people to take on and pursue their practical identities.

This is clearly the case for children being brought up in families: A family unable to foster the ability of its young to form practical identities, because all its energies are channeled into providing intensive health care or for any other reason, is truly a dysfunctional family. It is not, however, just the young who are vulnerable; a family's adults, too, depend on each other to maintain their practical identities. Families typically provide some of the crucial material and expressive resources that enable people to form, consider, endorse, revise, and live out their conceptions of themselves. The significance of practical identities reflects the extent to which people, even in close, interdependent, and intimate families, have distinct identities and basic projects. Indeed, reflection on practical identities calls attention to the way in which families actually contribute in important ways to the distinctiveness of their members.

The third consideration I want to examine is the tendency of families to *embody patterns of injustice*, and for that tendency to be exacerbated by increased caregiving demands. Families are hardly immune from objectionable uses of gender and age as the basis for assigning duties and benefits to their members. The shift of health-care responsibilities from professional to intimate realms threatens to worsen these biases. Women continue to be disproportionately assigned primary caregiving tasks, rendering them especially prone to further exploitation in circumstances that involve prolonged or intensive caregiving for family members (Brody, 1990). As women are typically the "least well off" in families when it comes to having discretionary time and energy after responsibilities at home and in the workplace, social practices that make them still worse off in these respects are particularly suspicious.

While all these considerations will figure in the development of my position, I will concentrate on harm to practical identities, in part because it provides ways of thinking about "distinctness" and the forms of value characteristic of intimate associations, and in part because gender and generational justice issues in families can be vividly appreciated by deploying the notion of practical identities; oppression can be understood in terms of the links between the practical identities out of which goals and values emerge, and the social practices that constrict a person's ability to form, pursue, and modify those identities.[4]

THE SOCIAL CONSTRUCTION OF FAMILY CAREGIVING, AND THE CONSTRICTION OF PRACTICAL IDENTITIES

In a pair of remarkable recent articles, Carol Levine has vividly illustrated ways in which these considerations can play themselves out in families confronting serious health-care problems. In her *New England Journal of Medicine* "Sounding Board" essay, "The Loneliness of the Long-Term Care Giver," Levine (1999b) writes of nearly a decade's experience of being a family caregiver to her husband, gravely injured in a car accident early in 1990. She tells us of her nightmares of disconnections and strained connections with the health care system, nightmares that have haunted her awake, as well as asleep. Despite the fact that she is herself a distinguished bioethicist and health policy analyst, it took Levine years to appreciate that her nightmares stemmed not from any inadequacy of her own, but from a "system" that is decidedly unsystematic, and badly out of order to boot.

A chilling sentence occurs early in the essay: "During my nine year odyssey, I stopped being a wife and became a family care giver" (Levine, 1999b, p. 1587). What is perhaps most striking about this radical shift in one of Levine's central practical identities is that she does *not* link it to the pervasive changes in her profoundly disabled husband, but rather to how *she herself* has been reconfigured by the set of social practices and understandings with which the health-care system (and the broader society in which it is nestled) responds to the chronically ill and those whose lives are most closely caught up with the ill.

During the weeks of her husband's stay in the hospital's intensive care unit, Ms. Levine reports that she remained a wife, treated with "kindness and concern." Then came something of a liminal period, when her husband's life was no longer in immediate danger, and she effectively disappeared from the attention of his professional caregivers. When the extent and permanence of her husband's disabilities became clear, she reemerged into view, but under a decidedly different aspect. She was now only the manager and the hands-on provider of his care. During her husband's stay in a rehabilitation facility ("boot camp for care givers," Levine labels it) she was initiated into her new role—the performer of "an unrelieved series of nasty chores," expected to impoverish herself to procure Medicaid funding for the home care needed by her husband. One anecdote is particularly telling:

A nurse stuck my husband's soiled sweat pants under my nose and said, "Take these away. Laundry is your job." A woman whose husband had been at the same facility later told me the same story—different nurse. (Levine, 1999b, p. 1588)

Mr. Levine was sent home from "rehab" a poorly treated, poorly diagnosed man, profoundly physically handicapped, cognitively challenged, emotionally labile—"not the same person in any sense." And, in at least some important senses, neither was Ms. Levine.

I have lingered on this difficult story because it powerfully shows how deeply the experience of chronic illness and disability can penetrate the lives not solely of patients, but also the lives of those most closely bonded to them. It is not hyperbolic to claim that the Levines' story indicates how current social arrangement for providing care to those with serious and chronic illnesses and disabilities can be life threatening for family caregivers, in a biographic, if not a biological sense. It shows how relatives and other bonded intimates pressed into extensive caregiving responsibilities risk the persistence of their central practical identities. It is worth underscoring that this damage is caused not by the flow of funding (although that is surely crucial), but by the way in which family caregivers are portrayed by the health-care system with which they interact. In a companion article recently published in *Ms.* magazine, Levine gives another, more gender specific, illustration of disparaging attitudes:

When my husband's prognosis became clear, and the long future stretched ahead of us, I looked for help. None was forthcoming. Even more appalling, the most judgmental responses came from women—nurses and social workers. Some nurses, admittedly overworked, were so resentful of my continuing to work [in her "outside" job] and failing to relieve them of their duties that I had to hire a "companion" to be with my husband in the rehab center until I arrived each day at 4 P.M. to feed him. When he screamed for help (regularly) or was uncooperative (even more frequently), I was blamed. (Levine, 2000, p 44)

Levine goes on to note that the spouse of another patient, who visited with fanfare and flowers every few evenings, was effusively greeted by the nurses. This patient was a woman; her "wonderful" spouse, a man. When Levine noted the discrepancy, she was told by a nurse: "You don't realize how rare it is for men to stay involved" (Levine, 2000, p. 44).

Carol Levine's articles distinctively highlight two interrelated dimensions of the damage that family caregivers face. One of these dimensions is material—family caregivers do not generally command the financial resources to enable them to both care for their relative and maintain and develop the range of practical identities they previously enjoyed. The other is expressive: Family caregivers—particular women—are caught up in socially enacted narratives that tend to silence the diversity of caregiver identities and emplot them as caregivers plain and simple.[5]

There is nothing fundamentally idiosyncratic about Carol Levine's experience. For example, in the United Hospital Fund of New York's recent Special Report, *Rough Crossings: Family Caregivers' Odysseys through the Health Care System*, the derangement of practical identities caused by family-provided health care is plain in case after case.[6]

Consider the story of Theresa and Robert Smith and their 18-year-old daughter, Jill, for instance. Jill was struck by a delivery van and suffered severe neurological trauma. She remained in a coma for two weeks, and when she emerged, she was unable to speak or control her limbs, bladder, or bowels. Jill needed to be strapped into her bed so that she would not injure herself.

When inpatient insurance ran out after the second month, Theresa and Robert decided to care for Jill at home, finding themselves immediately caught up in a grueling caregiving practice that seemed to have no end. They campaigned tirelessly for a range of service for their daughter, including physical, occupational, and speech therapy, nursing care and equipment. They also tried to secure good home-health aides to help care for Jill.

Taking on these responsibilities required significant and systematic changes in the Smiths' lives. Theresa cut her out-of-the-home job to part time, devoting the rest of her day to Jill's needs, including overseeing the stream of home attendants who passed into, and then quickly out of, their lives. In the discussion of this case, we read:

Robert received little attention from his wife. During evening meals, which were usually takeout, she would engage him in decisions about Jill's care, and conflict often erupted. After a long day at the office he didn't want to think about or second guess his wife's preferences. Tension grew between them until they seldom spoke. They stopped going out alone together. Their intimate life ended. (Levine, 1998, p. 24)

In the story of the Smiths, the threat to practical identities posed by inadequate material support is plain. And, although no one in particular is identified as propagandizing for a narrative of (female) caregiver self-abnegation, it is clear that the Smiths have imbibed a toxic dose of the culture's general stories about who draws the lot for caregiving. It is Theresa who cuts back on her job; it is Robert who seems to think that he is effectively released from sharing his wife's responsibilities. Even the way the story is told seems influenced by these stereotypes. We are informed that "Robert received little attention from his wife," when the opposite might seem more accurate— Theresa did try to interact with Robert, but not in the way he preferred, so that he withdrew *his* attention. The Smiths' spousal identities, as well as Theresa's work-related identity, eroded.

More general results point in the same direction. Social scientists studying "the caregiving career" have noted that caregiving not only exerts significant pressure on the array of identities that family members maintain, but does so in a dynamic and steadily expanding fashion. In their study, *Profiles in Caregiving: The Unexpected Ca-*

reer, Aneshensel and colleagues (1995) note that "[typically] the caregiver role keeps expanding in its demands so that even with adjustments in other areas, it keeps a steady pressure on the boundaries of other roles in the constellation" (p. 37). Thus, even creative accommodation to new demands is not sufficient to ensure that the integrity of a family caregiver's other practical identities is preserved. At the same time, the stories of the Smiths and the Levines also suggest that families regard the immense burden of intense, prolonged, and exacting care as worth bearing. This willingness can also be understood as a testimony to the importance that people place on the maintenance of practical identities. For if home-based care can erode and transmute family relationships, causing, for example, distinctively spousal identities to fail, alternative institutional care carries dangers of its own. It seems fair—indeed, important—to ask whether the Smiths would have been likely to hang onto any remnant of their identities as parents if their daughter had been institutionalized.

IS THERE A RIGHT TO "FAMILY CARE"?

I have aimed to illuminate various dimensions of harm that intensive and prolonged health-care provision can pose to families, while acknowledging that such care can have value to families as well. Yet, the kinds of goods that many families find in providing care to ill or disabled relatives, along with at least some of the social savings to be had from their involvement, do not require that lives and identities be as deeply harmed as in the stories retold here.[7] More generous and generously available benefits allowing family-care providers respite from their tasks would help; greater acknowledgment on the part of the health-care professions and of society of the important and expanding role of family in health care would also help. The imperative to spend resources down to the poverty

level to qualify for Medicaid's long-term care benefits seems a Draconian measure in an affluent society; need, rather than penury, could be the chief eligibility criterion. Family leave provisions, such as those guaranteed by the Family and Medical Leave Act, could be extended and strengthened; those who must relinquish or cut down on paid employment for caretaking purposes could be extended taxation and retirement fund support to ease the fiscal costs of substituting one sort of socially significant work for another.

In addition, home-based care providers need information and a sense of connection and appreciation; the Internet might help with these things (assuming caregivers have sufficient time and energy to take advantage of it), and access might be subsidized for those family care providers not now on line. If telemedicine can add to the momentum behind refiguring the health-care roles of family members, telecommuting might allow more family members to express their practical identities as workers, and enjoy the stress-reducing benefits that out-of-the-home work apparently can afford.[8]

Most of these proposals most directly target "material" conditions of the sort that imperiled some of the Smiths' practical identities; others speak to the "expressive" conditions that damaged Carol Levine, the withdrawal of the community "up-take" that diluted her social standing as a wife. Changing the social perception of family caregivers is likely to require also changing their material conditions; if greater economic support for family caregivers made it easier for them to continue to lead rich and varied lives, it would be harder to view them as simply and solely the performers of those "unrelieved nasty chores." The inverse may tend to be true as well: Although caring relatives ought to be cherished by health-care professionals as the key allies they have become, such a reworking of attitudes is not likely to take place without a change in the material substrate.

Yet life is full of misfortunes, and not all

misfortunes implicate questions of justice and injustice. Many of the proposals canvassed above could reduce the savings drawn from increased reliance on family caregiving, and tempering health-care spending is a significant matter, particularly as the health care inflation engine seems to be shifting back into high gear (Rosenbaum, 2000). What is it about those misfortunes faced by family members in providing health care to their relatives that distinguishes them from, say, finding one's self locked into a tedious job owing to an inability to get health insurance elsewhere? Practical identities can be constrained or withheld if your salary is too small to satisfy your deep interest in contemporary art, or if your vertical leap is too short to play in the National Basketball Association or dance with the American Ballet Theater.

One conditional line of argument that family caregiving should be subvened by social resources is suggested by what seems a ready analogy between caregiving and illness. It is relatively commonplace among bioethicists—and apparently among most of the people of the developed world outside the United States—to think that health-care needs are in some morally significant way among the most important human requirements, more akin to the need for education than to a penchant for collecting 18th century violins or taking ski vacations. Maintaining my health, curing my illnesses, repairing my dysfunctions, easing my pain, staving off my mortality—all these tasks are caught up with a class of possible misfortunes that it is seemingly appropriate to provide for out of a community's joint resources; health, or at least access to the health system, is a kind of good that a just society will make available to all its members.

Among the misfortunes people face, why is health care reasonably thought to enjoy this special status? One popular argument is that health care aims at securing a *primary* good—a good that aids us in the pursuit of every more specific vision of the good. I may, for example, pin my hopes on

acquiring a gracious home, a prestigious job, and a charming and compliant spouse; you may regard all this as so much fluff, as a frivolous or even as an immoral set of goals for a human life, preferring to build communities of resistance to entrenched powers and practices, to undermine patriarchal and capitalist systems. But we will both do better in achieving our aims if we are healthy, and we both have a better chance of being healthy if we have reliable access to health-care resources. A society professedly neutral among its members' conceptions of the good might justify ensuring access to health care by trading on the "plasticity" of the benefit of health.

A related, although distinguishable idea—the notion that health care is key to the maintenance of a "normal opportunity range"—has been prominently advocated by Norman Daniels (1985). Noting that some people (a rare few, presumably) may hold conceptions of the good that are not abetted by health, he argues that the ability to change one's plan of life within a range normal for one's species and to which we are otherwise suited is also rationally regarded as a significant good. If anyone were indifferent to it, that would presumably be because she either had no interest in how she lived at all, or because she was absolutely convinced that her present plan of life was in no need of assessment or improvement. Holding appropriate allocation of social resources hostage to nihilism seems too strong a requirement, and it is unlikely that assumptions of infallibility are consistent with practical rationality. If the ability to revise one's plan of life is an especially significant good, then interventions designed to maintain or restore normal species function (i.e., health care) may well be required for one to have that kind of opportunity. Neither notional nor practical revision may be possible if one is seriously ill.

The analogous argument for socially supporting family health care provision hinges on the view that the ability to form and to maintain a practical identity is as likely to be a primary good as is health. Close ties exist between the idea of practical identity and the notion of a normal opportunity range. Illnesses and traumas are not the only impairments in our normal species function that can block our revising (or living out) a conception of the good. Forming practical identities is part of what is normal to our species, and the ability to do so is intimately caught up with our opportunity range.

Indeed, one might think of the collection of practical identities open to a person as a way of specifying the range of opportunity normal to our species and to which the individual is otherwise suited. While some practical identities will be less significant to a person than others, the same could be said about the impairments caused by different illnesses. Accordingly, what undermines a person's ability to form or maintain central practical identities is therefore, in general terms, as morally significant as what threatens her health. If the appeal to primary goods or normal opportunity ranges makes the provision of health care a matter of justice, then, by parity of argument, it would motivate a similar conclusion with respect to provision of support for family-based care providers, at least in a society whose health-care system relies on exacting forms of family-provided care.

It might be argued that, whereas a person cannot simply walk away from her ill body, one can refuse family caregiving responsibilities and their potential risks to practical identities. Such a position, however, both understates our freedom with respect to ourselves, and overstates our freedom with respect to our families. Failure to provide care needed by a family member may be, for many people, little more consistent with the maintenance of central practical identities than would be suicide.

I conclude that if arguments based on such notions as "primary goods" or "normal opportunity ranges" are successful in showing that access to a reasonable level of health care is guaranteed by an appropriate understanding of distributive justice, then access to a reasonable level of support for families providing burdensome health care is equally strongly supported. In the United States, of course, such arguments have not been effective politically, regardless of their philosophical merits.

But the conditional argument sketched here is also more ambitious than strictly required to show that "drafting" families to replace health-care professionals is unjust. Considerations of ambiguous agency notwithstanding, the increasing threat of constriction of opportunities to form, revise, and live out practical identities is not the result of natural causes. Rather, it results from a collection of decisions to shift costs from government or private insurers to families, an inexpensive and readily available labor source. That some family members may see themselves as having a moral obligation to take on these jobs does not imply that the social arrangements that put them in such positions are acceptable.

There are, as I have tried to show, serious considerations justifying socially funded effort to ameliorate the burdens of family caregivers quite apart from schemes that rely on their propensity for exploitation. However, the fact that the particular situation facing American families now is a result of the efforts of morally responsible agents—insurers, employers, employees—trying to make their own lot easier needs a positive moral justification that has not been forthcoming. Ignorance about the impact of these decisions is an increasingly implausible plea.

At least when prolonged and intense family-care provision is at issue, then, reasonably affluent societies have as stringent a duty to provide families with the kind of support that will make such caregiving compatible with a reasonable chance for caregivers maintaining central practical identities, as they do to provide basic health care. Further, if people in the United States benefit by the kind of care increasingly loaded onto family members—and even in the absence of a nationally insured system of universally accessible health care, it seems that we do—then we have a justice based reason to keep the provision of that care from being gravely harmful to features of human life that are very widely and very deeply valued.

Sadly, appeals to justice sometimes lack pragmatic clout. Yet where justice flags, prudence sometimes prevails. Many of us will find ourselves called upon to provide prolonged, difficult health care to those we love. We all have reason to assure that our identities will remain rich and varied, that our lives as caregivers will not need to be lives of heroic sacrifice.[9]

NOTES

1. And not solely in the United States, although conditions in America will serve as the context of this chapter.

2. Some theorists of the family are quite convinced, however, that there are no good moral reasons for families not to become more formal, their interchanges governed by contract rather than implicit patters of understanding and practice. See, for instance, Okin, 1989.

3. What constitutes "one family" is itself also open to debate. Late-appearing "long-lost relatives" who assert authority over health-care decisions, and homosexual or otherwise queer partners, are just two fairly prominent instances where who is "really family" is sometimes disputed.

4. More direct discussions of gender justice in families can be found in Okin, 1989, and H. Nelson and J. Nelson, 1995, among other sources; a good recent discussion is Kittay, 1999. For an extended discussion of the relationships among identity, agency, and justice, see Nelson, 2001.

5. This analysis is much influenced by H. Nelson, 2001.

6. The literature on family caregiving and dementia is also full of similar stories. For representative examples, showing families seeking ways to both care for and to preserve other significant features of their lives, see J. Nelson and H. Nelson, 1996.

7. A fuller story of the impact on families and on practical identities of intensive tending for ill relatives would require the input of those who have studied family caretaking for disabled children, and of those family members themselves. Some have maintained that families involved in this type of caregiving do not fare notably worse than families otherwise engaged. See, for instance, Philip Ferguson, Alan Gartner, Dorothy Lipsky, "The Experience of Disability in Families: A Synthesis of Research and Parent Narratives."

8. See Levine, 2000, p. 45.

9. I am most grateful for the thoughtful comments and editorial observations provided by Hilde Lindemann Nelson, and Margaret Pabst Battin, and most particularly for a rich set of ideas owing to Joel Frader; I only wish I could have pursued more of them.

REFERENCES

Aneshensel, C., Zarit, S., and Whitlach, C. (1995). *Profiles in Caregiving: The Unexpected Career*. San Diego: Academic Press.

Arras, J. (1995). *Bringing the Hospital Home: Ethical and Social Implications of High-Tech Home Care*. Baltimore: Johns Hopkins University Press.

Bauer, K. (2001). Home-based telemedicine: A survey of ethical issues. *Cambridge Quarterly of Health Care Ethics* 10, 137–46.

Brody, E. (1990). *Women in the Middle: Their Parent-Care Years*. New York: Springer.

Daniels, N. (1985). *Just Health Care*. Cambridge: Cambridge University Press.

Ferguson, P., Gartner, A. and Lipsky, D. (2000). The experience of disability in families: A synthesis of research and parent narratives. In E. Parens and A. Asch (eds), *Prenatal Genetic Testing and the Disability Rights Critique*. Washington, DC: Georgetown University Press.

Freudenham, M. (2000). HMO costs spur employers to shift plans. *New York Times*, September 6, Section A p. 1.

Kittay, E. (1999). *Love's Labor*. New York: Routledge.

Korsgaard, C. (1996). *The Sources of Normativity*. Cambridge: Cambridge University Press.

Levit, K., Cowan, C., Lazenby, H., Sensenig, A., McDonnell, P., Stiller, J. and Martin, A. (2000). Health spending in 1998: Signals of change. *Health Affairs* 19, 124–32.

Levine, C. (1998). *Rough Crossings:Family Caregivers' Odysseys Through the Health Care System*. New York: United Hospital Fund.

Levine, C. (1999a). Home sweet hospital: The nature and limits of private responsibilities for home health care. *Journal of Aging and Health Care* 11, 341–59.

Levine, C. (1999b). The loneliness of the long-term care giver. *New England Journal of Medicine* 340, 1587–90.

Levine, C. (2000). Night shift. *Ms.* magazine, Vol. 10, p. 44.

Minuchin, S. (1974) *Families and Family Therapy*. Cambridge, MA: Harvard University Press.

Nelson, H. (2001). *Damaged Identities, Narrative Repair*. Ithaca, NY: Cornell University Press.

Nelson, H. and Nelson, J. (1995). *The Patient in the Family*. New York: Routledge.

Nelson, J. and Nelson, H. (1996). *Alzheimer's: Answers to Hard Questions for Families*. New York: Doubleday.

Okin, S. (1989). *Justice, Gender and the Family*. New York: Basic Books.

Parens, E. and Asch, A. (eds.) (2000). *Prenatal Genetic Testing and the Disability Rights Critique* Washington, DC: Georgetown University Press.

Rawls, J. (1971). *A Theory of Justice*. Cambridge, MA: Harvard University Press.

Rosenbaum, D. (2000). What if there is no cure for health care's ills? *New York Times*, September 10, Section 4, p. 1.

24

Caring for the Vulnerable by Caring for the Caregiver: The Case of Mental Retardation[1]

Eva Feder Kittay

> The ward for the profoundly retarded had been built in a pentagon shape with a nurse's station in the center surrounded by five locked, barred rooms. The nurse's station was empty—the hospital has just six ward aides for the 58 retarded patients, and the aides spend all day either feeding them or cleaning them.
>
> (Description of a "psychiatric hospital" in Guadalajara, Mexico. From "The Global Willowbrook," Michael Winerip, *New York Times Magazine*, January 16, 2000, p. 61)

> The corpse measured 66 inches from blue toes to jutting ears. . . . The body in plaid pajamas was that of a 57-year-old retarded ward of the District of Columbia . . . Frederick Emory Brandenburg . . . He blanketed old telephone directories with that name, covered the TV Guides . . . glutted the fly leaves of his large-print Living Bible. . . . In this way Brandenburg, . . . impressed the fact of his existence on his world. In January 1997, that existence was obliterated by his caretakers. Today, in the name of the privacy and dignity of the retarded, top city officials say they can't publicly acknowledge that a man named Fred Brandenburg was ever in their care.
>
> ("Invisible Deaths: The Fatal Neglect of D.C.'s Retarded," Katherine Boo, *The Washington Post*, December 5, 1999, p. A1)

The stories from which these paragraphs are taken have served as the inspiration for this chapter. What I set out to do here is to consider how it is that vulnerable people come to suffer, rather than thrive, in the hands of those to whom their well-being is entrusted. Frequently those who attempt to answer this question delve into the darker recesses of people's hearts. What evil demons dwell there, they ask? While I do not doubt that sadistic impulses reside in us, and in some of us far more than in others, this is not the sort of answer I am interested in here. I want to ask about the social conditions that allow for the persistent and widespread neglect and abuse of some of the most vulnerable among us. What social conditions and social understandings exist that make certain persons "moral others," that is, persons not included within the community of moral beings? Are some of these understandings lodged in the very conceptions meant to bind people to certain duties—that is, to a conception of justice? Are some of these conditions embedded in the circumstances in which people provide care?

I answer the latter two questions in the affirmative. I take certain presuppositions in our understanding of justice to exclude some from the realm of justice—to make of certain vulnerable people, moral others. And I believe that the circumstances in which we are expected to provide care bear heavily on the sort of care we can give and receive. Furthermore, the two questions are related. For I take it that certain dominant conceptions of justice abet the social neglect of the conditions under which individuals give and receive care—primarily, but not exclusively, those in marginalized and stigmatized groups.

I not only want to ask about the social circumstances and understandings that facilitate the sort of neglect and abuse the passages above indicate, I want to begin to consider what sorts of understandings regarding justice and conditions of care will help to rid our world of such moral indignities. Toward this end, I envision a public ethic of care in which care is just and justice is caring. If we can elaborate these notions for those who are moral others—for those who have stood outside the dominant articulations of morality and justice, then the task for those who are already deemed moral agents is made much easier. For this abstract reason, and for a very personal reason, I begin the task I have set for myself by considering people with severe cognitive impairments, the mentally retarded.

People with severe and profound intellectual disabilities are people in need of care. The need is "inevitable" when the individual cannot fend for herself, not because her particular social setting is inhospitable to her form of impairment, but because she lacks the ability to do some of the most basic tasks of self-care needed to sustain life. While all needs, no matter how fundamental, are shaped by historical and cultural circumstances, those that come from "inevitable dependency" will not disappear with different social arrangements. These are dependencies that arise from infancy and childhood, frail old age, acute illness, chronic infirmity, or severe impairments.[2] When we are inevitably dependent, we are dependent on a caregiver and on the adequacy of the caregiver's care.

Care is multifaceted: a labor, an attitude, a virtue. As a labor, caregiving requires[3] heeding the needs of another, putting aside one's own needs for someone more vulnerable, and becoming intimate with the body and the bodily functions of the cared-for. Without the attitude of care, the open responsiveness to another—so essential to understanding what another person requires—care is never *good* care. Care as a virtue is a disposition manifested in caring behavior (the labor and attitude). One characteristic of care is the "shift [that] takes place from the interest in our life situation to the situation of the other, the one in need of care" (Gastmans, 2000).

The skills and virtues of caregiving are many, and the degree to which the caregiver must become enmeshed in another's needs in order to adequately meet those needs vary with both the urgency and extent of the other's dependency and with the degree to which one has cultivated the virtue of care. Because care involves a shift from one's own interests to those of the person in need of care, it often requires the caregiver to defer the fulfillment of his or her own needs. Where the deferral lasts long enough, as it does with someone who is extremely (and inevitably) dependent, the deferral changes into loss unless a third party comes to the aid of the caregiver. In this way, the caregiver herself becomes dependent on someone who will look after her interests and meet her own needs.

However, the person charged with another's care may do her job poorly. She may give preference to those of her own interests and desires that are detrimental to her charge. She can meet the other's needs inadequately, or not at all, becoming neglectful and even abusive. She may see in the vulnerability of the other, not a vested trust, but an opportunity to exert her dominance over another, causing physical or psychological injury. Sara Ruddick has spoken of the temptations of care, among which are the temptation to dominate a vulnerable other. To think about caregiving is to consider what sort of power the caregiver can exercise over another. But we also need to consider the sorts of powers to which the caregiver can become subjected. To think about caregiving is to contemplate what is morally demanded of the caregiver, but it is also about what is morally required of those upon whose support the caregiver (and her charge) must depend. Finally, to think about caregiving is to consider the reason resources are to be devoted to the care of the charge and the support of the caregiver. The case of giving care to the severely mentally retarded person, one who is totally dependent and who does not emerge from his or her dependency, shows us the moral dimensions of caregiving in its most stark form.

ADVOCACY—A VOICE FOR CARE

Mentally retarded people come to the public's attention in sensational stories that expose appalling forms of lack of care, of abusive or neglectful treatment by those charged with their care. The mentally retarded have, at times, been objects of pity, compassion, indifference, fear or abuse. They have rarely been seen as subjects, as citizens, as individuals entitled to the same fulfillment as any other person.

Mental retardation is the disablement that other disabled persons do not want attributed to them. It is the disability for which prospective parents are most likely to use selective abortion.[4] It is the disability that prompted the great Oliver Wendell Holmes to declare that "three generations of idiots were enough,"[5] and so justify the forced sterilization of a mentally retarded woman. And mental retardation, especially in its more severe forms, is the disability least amenable to the inclusion fought for, and the advances made by, the disability community (Ferguson, 1994).

Those with physical disabilities have had some success in getting heard, but many with severe mental retardation cannot speak, or they communicate in a language different from and demeaned by those who speak in the language of the public sphere.

Theirs is a most disabling disablement, for whatever voice they have remains without authority.

To be heard, to be recognized, to have one's needs and wants reckoned along with those of others, the mentally retarded individual requires an advocate—a role that has voice at its center. This has been my role for my daughter, Sesha. I have considered how to interject my daughter into a public discourse. She cannot speak, so I must speak for her. How do I speak about her and for her? Notice that I have already begun by speaking of her—in the negative—by saying that she cannot speak. This deficit is part of a larger picture of all that she is unable to do: feed herself, dress herself, toilet herself, walk, talk, read, write, draw, say Mama or Papa. I would have preferred to start by speaking of her positively, conveying another picture: the picture of a lovely and intense 30-year-old woman, one with boundless affection, an exuberant enjoyment of the sensuous feel of water, and an abiding and profound appreciation of music and musical performances. Yet for me to adequately communicate to another person about my daughter, indeed, to adequately speak *for* her, the reader needs to know what she cannot be because of her profound cognitive limitations, her cerebral palsy, and her seizure disorders. My reader needs to know that although I speak of a 30-year-old woman, her chronological age fails to reflect her level of functioning and her total dependence.

The positive ascriptions are truer to who she is. Her limitations are manifest in the face she shows to those who do not know her, but they also convey the ways she cannot make her own way in the world. Describing her capabilities gives a glimpse into the richness of her life and the remarkable quality of her very being. Nonetheless, the limitations shape her life and ours, so we must address them if we are to make it possible for her beauty to flourish. Conversely, only by considering her in the fullness of her joys and capacities can we view her impairments in light of *her* life, *her* interests, *her* happiness—and not as projections of her "able" parents or of an able-biased society. Caring for her properly means attending to her own personhood and agency. An exclusive focus on her limitations sets her outside most current definitions of personhood and citizenship, for these are fixated on intellect, independence, and productivity. These values throw into question her entitlement to the resources she needs for her full development and her flourishing.

Among her many needs is the need for care. If she is to flourish, she needs *good caring* care—and lots of it. Because her survival and flourishing depends on caregivers who are genuinely devoted to her well-being, to advocate for my daughter without also advocating for those who are entrusted with her well-being fails to accomplish its original aim. It is also unjust and uncaring toward the caregiver. That, at least, is a thesis I wish to maintain—all the while recognizing that the interests of my daughter and those of her caregivers (my own or others) are not *always* aligned, and that the interests of her paid caregivers are not infrequently at odds with those of her familial caregivers. Nonetheless, to give voice to one who cannot speak, whose very agency appears so attenuated, means to pay utmost heed to what I have called elsewhere "the dependency relation": that is, the relation between one who gives care and one who is dependent.

INTELLIGENCE AND MORAL STATUS

A certain level and kind of intellectual and physical capacity is critical to negotiating any environment in which we live. When that capacity is impaired, we become dependent on another to provide for us what we cannot manage ourselves. So much is obvious. Less obvious are the ways in which impaired capacities render us dependent *by virtue of* the particular environments in which we find ourselves—environments that are shaped by human

activity and social values. Less obvious still are the ways in which these humanly constructed environments create dependencies *whether or not* our faculties are impaired. The last are hidden dependencies. When we look at the environments we inhabit with an eye to hidden dependencies, it is clear that we are all dependent to some degree on the physical and intellectual capacities of others. The dependencies have different valuations—they are stigmatized to the extent to which they are visible. But even among those that are visible, there is a hierarchy. To depend on another person to carry a heavy package is hardly viewed as a problem—it is even a sign of status not to have to do certain physically demanding tasks. But to depend on another person to perform mental labor is another matter altogether.

Intellectual capacities, and so mental incapacity, have special significance in defining an individual's value: that is, the value of the person's contribution to society and the person's standing in the moral community. In the philosophical tradition that dominates the Western world, humans acquire a unique moral status by virtue of their intelligence and capacity for rational deliberation. By virtue of a base line of intelligence and capacity for rational deliberation, people are viewed as being able to participate in a just assignment of burdens and benefits of a social life. Such a view is not limited to philosophers from Aristotle to Rawls. It seeps through to the culture at large: to the doctors responsible for providing health services, to the legislators who appropriate funds for services, to the citizens who watch over the ways in which their taxes are spent.

In this moral universe—and in a social/political world so represented—there is little room for those whose rational, reasonable, and reasoning capacities are impaired. It is not even clear that justice applies to them. Given their tenuous relation to the moral community, it becomes important to ask on what basis those with significant intellectual impairments can make claims for care and on what basis their families and caregivers can make claims on the larger community for caring for those with such disabilities. Are there any claims from justice to care for those with significant cognitive impairments and to extend public provision for families to lighten the extra demands of raising a child with cognitive deficits so severe that no education or habilitation will turn their child into a future taxpayer? Or are there any claims *from justice* that we, as a society, should be providing the means necessary for caregivers in group settings to be well-supervised, well-trained and well-paid?

Those with significant mental disabilities still fall within the purview of the legal protections provided by the Americans with Disabilities Act, yet health providers, legislators, and taxpayers alike see little need to be open-handed in assigning funds for the care, health, and well-being of this populations. For those with intellectual deficits who are poor or members of minority groups devalued by the dominant group, the case is aggravated—so much so that the consequence of inadequate care is easily measured in gross disparities in life expectancy.[6] Where the value of those cared for is diminished, their care is seen as unearned and something to which they have no title and for which there is little reward.

In a society that places little value on the mentally retarded, care will be minimal, and callous caretakers will be an inevitability. A society that values only things precluded by mental retardation not only will fail to see any goodness in the lives of the mentally disabled, it will not value those charged with their care. Such an attitude is reflected in the minimal pay and low status of those who care for the intellectually disabled. They, like their charges, are treated as expendable; such caregivers come to partake in the marginalization of those for whom they care.[7]

Caregivers do, however, have a modicum of power. Given the responsibility to care for those who cannot care for themselves, caregivers frequently have the power of life and death over their vulnerable charges. When those who are vulnerable are also valued, there is oversight and accountability, which holds such power in check. But when caregivers can exercise their power and others are indifferent to their charge, the oversight is spotty, and the responsibility with which dependency workers are entrusted is rarely matched with means to do the work well. Their power resides more in their ability to deny care than to provide it. Where caregivers share society's negative views of retarded people, and they have the opportunity and latitude to violate the trust given to them, we have a potent recipe for neglect, and even abuse. Sheer coercion and policing could perhaps serve as a guarantee against maltreatment, but the vigilance required makes such a means mostly ineffective. The caring caregiver must battle against expediency and avoid the temptations of domination. It is she who goes against the tide, not the callous one.

When we moved large numbers of institutional residents into group homes, we thought we left behind the appalling conditions of the Willowbrooks[8] of the world. But the mistreatment, which had largely been attributed to the systemic inadequacies of what Goffman had called "total institutions," resurfaces today in group homes (Goffman, 1961), as the *Washington Post* story cited at the outset indicates. The group homes in Washington, DC, which testify to the persistent nature of the problem of good care for the mentally retarded, is only one case among many. [9] A change from institution to group home is helpful, but the form of the residence cannot compensate for the lack of regard suffered by those who live within its walls if those who are charged with their care are as abject as their inhabitants.

THE MORAL IMPORTANCE OF DEPENDENCY RELATIONSHIPS

In a previous work, *Love's Labor* (Kittay, 1999), I argued that not only are dependents effectively left out of the social contract, but the "dependency workers" who care for them are implicitly excluded as well. Even as they advocate for their kin, their own interests—whether these arise because of, or irrespective of, caregiving responsibilities—become eclipsed.

Under fortunate circumstances, the person responsible for the well-being of the mentally retarded person is a parent, or close family member, although it need not be. When an individual is placed in residential care, there tends to be an alienation between child and family.[10] It requires the active attention of the residential facility to sustain the tie between family and resident. The logic of Goffman's "total institution" is, instead, to strip individuals of their individuality and to sever ties between the individual and the outside world. In the case of group homes within the community there is a better likelihood that the protective connections will be retained, but not for individuals whose families have already lost touch.

While familial caregivers are as capable of neglect and abuse as are strangers paid to give care, affective bonds that normally form between family members offer important defenses against the harmful behavior, especially when supports are available to ease hardships. The affective bonds are themselves subject to stress when supports are not in place. Expenditures that aided mothers, fathers, grandmothers, other close family members, or "fictive kin" would be especially well spent.

Today, government funding for families who want to keep their mentally disabled family member at home is very limited and tends to be means-tested, providing (some, but inadequate) relief only for families who are below a certain income.[11] We could instead provide families with income to care for the disabled relative (or to pay another to do so), respite time to ease physical and emotional depletion, job training for when the care work ceases (ensuring that the caregiver does not become dependent on the dependency of the disabled relative or the income she brings into the family).

What if a family did not have to worry about spending money for medical, including psychiatric, services, or for a clothes washer for an incontinent family member, a specially equipped van, a stair elevator, counseling, or a support group? What if there was a strong information network available to caregivers about medical, habilitative, and therapeutic services? Families that have been fortunate enough to procure such supports for themselves have found them as life-sustaining as we have in our relationship with Sesha. Families that are supported and encouraged to be involved with the facility where a family member resides are far more likely to be vigilant in overseeing the care of the residents. Government oversight would not become irrelevant, but it could become a second, rather than a first, line of defense. Furthermore, families would be there to hold governments accountable when they fail in their duties.

If unpaid familial caregivers need assistance in maintaining their relationship to their mentally disabled family member and keeping ties alive for the long haul, caregivers who work for pay need support in forming the bonds in the first place. Earlier I argued that abusive behavior by caregivers is facilitated not only by the social devaluation of persons with mental disabilities, but also by the devaluation of the caregivers themselves. If we want to remove the prejudice and lack of understanding that blights the lives of people with mental retardation, we can begin by treating those to whom we entrust these vulnerable individuals as if their work mattered—because it does—and as if they mattered—because they do. To do this we need to provide caregivers with appropriate training, the opportunity to grow in their work, a voice in the care of their charges, compensation that matches the intensity of the labor, and encouragement in their sympathetic and empathic responses to their charges (see Bogdan and Taylor, 1992).

In *Love's Labor* (Kittay, 1999), I argue

that we need a conception of reciprocity in which the obligation falls to a third party. I have called this form of reciprocity *doulia*, after the Greek term *doula*,[12] which refers to the contemporary postpartum caregiver who cares for the mother so that the mother can care for her new infant. In a public conception of doulia, the larger society supports those who care for the inevitably dependent. I conceive of this as a principle of justice, one that incorporates those whom the standard contractual model of reciprocity excludes. *Doulia* provides a principle of justice that is caring by insisting that caring be justly compensated and supported.

JUSTICE AND INEVITABLE DEPENDENCY

Thomas Pogge has argued that there are two dominant strains of thought among egalitarian liberals. On one view, "an ideal social state" is one in which "no person is worse-off than others except as a consequence of (free and informed) choices this person has made" (Pogge, 2000, p. 30). This he calls a *full consequentialist view*. On the second view, "a social order is . . . unjust insofar as it treats some of its participants worse than others. . . . Personal . . . differences among persons—however unchosen—are not seen as a collective responsibility and are not required . . . to be corrected or compensated at public expense" (Pogge, 2000, p. 30). The latter he calls a "semi-consequentialist" position.[13]

The interpretation of the Americans with Disabilities Act (ADA) for which Anita Silvers (Silvers et al., 1998) has argued may be said to be semi-consequentialist. Silvers holds that justice does not demand that we devote resources that will *equalize* the condition of those with disabilities (regardless of whether we understand the benchmark of equality to be resources, capabilities or welfare).[14] Rather, as Silvers insists, the ADA is antidiscrimination legislation that requires only that past injustices in constructing the social environment be recti-

fied, because the dependency of the disabled is socially constructed.

A semi-consequentialist position such as Silvers necessarily leaves the severely mentally retarded worse off than others unless they have a family or loved ones who will take care of them throughout their lives. Even the mildly mentally retarded could not compete for well-paying, prestigious jobs, for example. To leave the entire burden of the well-being of the severely mentally retarded in the hands of those who privately assume the job will leave many uncared for, or cared for poorly, or take its toll on those families or individuals who assume the care. They are left out of the semi-consequentialists' conception of a just state of affairs.

Robert Veatch (1986), who advocates a full consequentialist position, is one of the few investigators who have specifically addressed the question of just demands for the mentally retarded. He argues that the differences between even the weakest and most powerful among us are negligible compared to the greatness and power of God. Although Veatch justifies his claims on theological grounds, he could be understood as arguing for an equality of capabilities similar to that of Amartya Sen and Martha Nussbaum.[15] Veatch insists that if we are to be a just society, we have to bite the bullet of equality and commit ourselves to devoting as many resources as are required to equalize the life prospects of the mentally retarded. Thus, for example, we may need to spend more on educating the cognitively disabled child than the able one, and may even have to limit some of the latter's educational enhancements to provide for the retarded youngster.

Silvers asks why those who are in no way responsible for another's disability should be compelled to use their own resources to equalize the disabled person's life prospects, beyond the call for fairness that antidiscrimination demands. This concern is not fully answered by invoking a theological conception, it is merely stipulated.[16]

Second, Silvers identifies another difficulty in the fully consequentialist position. Silvers worries, rightly I think, that the demand to equalize is a black hole into which infinite resources could be poured. What, for example, would constitute an "equal education" for a severely retarded person and one without any intellectual impairments? How many resources ought we devote to bringing a person with mental retardation to a level of functioning that is equal to an nonimpaired individual before we determine his or her limits?

Contractarianism, such as that proposed by Scanlon, (1998), may perhaps be useful when addressing these concerns. Such a contractualist could justify her position by appealing to reasonableness. A retarded child is first of all *someone's child*. If we agree that the means to provide nurturing care is a demand any parent can reasonably make of others, the ensuing obligation would then be on par with other similar obligations such as the obligation to provide support and education to the child of poor parents who would similarly justify their demand.

This justification runs into serious difficulty. An objection to this line of reasoning by those who have had no experience with retardation may well focus on the dissimilarity between the wishes of the parent of the able and the disabled child. It is reasonable, they may object, to want support and education for your own child if that will equalize the child's opportunity to compete for resources in adulthood and to contribute to the community in ways that others do. A child with significant retardation (and perhaps even mild retardation) cannot contribute, and, therefore, devoting resources to such a child's education cannot be justified in the same way.

A Scanlon-type contractarian justification may not uphold an obligation to retarded individuals because, like other forms of contractualisms, it does not reach into the difficult question of how to include those who lack a full measure of rationality into a moral community when the qualification for membership is rationality. The contractarian position provides grounds for what is owed to the rational moral agent, the parent, not for what is owed to the retarded person. What we are owed *qua* parent, however, is importantly tied to the idea that the relation of parent to child is between full members of the moral community or one full member and one who is a member *in potentia*. But if nothing is owed to the retarded person, the grounds on which the parent or caregiver can argue become tenuous at best.

The principle of *doulia* that I invoke indicates the need to move beyond semi-consequentialism and contractarianism, for caregiver and cared-for alike. While my fellow citizens may in no way be responsible for the disability of my daughter, we invoke a principle of *doulia* that situates us in nested relations that begin with the relation between a dependent person and her caregiver. We have each been dependent, and so we have each been cared for in such a relation. The nested relations are arranged to come to our aid as we become needy on our own account or because we care for others. Without some such expectation the human species could not sustain itself. The requirement to move beyond semi-consequentialism and contractarianism arises from such a condition, a circumstance of justice, if you will—one that is universally applicable.

But I too worry that equality requires some benchmark. Veatch's theological conception provides none. I noted earlier that a contractualism such as Scanlon's would put the obligation for quality care and education of the retarded child on par with other similar obligations, say the obligation to provide a good education for a poor child. But these can be viewed as competing obligations, where a fixed pool of resources is made to serve different obligations without setting forth criteria by which to adjudicate competing claims.

In contrast, in a relatively affluent society such as ours, we could demand that resources be made available for quality care and quality education for both retarded persons and for poor children. This is to say that a just society will provide care and resources necessary for its dependents and those who care for them so as to promote a level of well-being commensurate with that of those who (at this time of their lives) neither require care nor are expected to provide care. The prospects for a rich and satisfying life ought to be independent of inevitable dependencies and responsibilities to care for those who are inevitably dependent. Let us dub this understanding "dependency consequentialism." In the case of the severely retarded person, for example, the dependency is so deep that the effort would not be to achieve independence, but to assure the care needed to flourish, *and* to provide for the caregiver so that the caregiver's personal prospects will not be blighted by unmanageable caregiving burdens.

Dependency concerns ought not to be seen as competing with other circumstances that merit attention, for dependency is frequently a condition that modulates and inflects situations requiring social resources. Dependency interacts with racism, poverty, education, and the various sorts of devastation that need urgent social attention. Whereas people of all races and economic classes experience inevitable dependencies, the consequences of unmet dependency needs is intensified by racial exclusion and economic deprivation, as studies revealing the different life expectancy of people with mental retardation so dramatically indicate (see note 6 above). When dependency needs go unmet, income is reduced, poverty deepens, and natural catastrophes become exponentially more catastrophic. Furthermore, the consequences of allowing inevitable dependencies to remain unaddressed by the wider society can lead to some of the worst sorts of abuse and neglect—the sort a decent society ought not to tolerate.

Dependency concerns also require a central place in considerations of justice because most social relations are so constructed as to include and incorporate all sorts of dependencies. Inevitable depend-

encies, however, have been largely confined to private relations, so that we have come to discount them and the integral part of social life they in fact constitute. Doing so permits us to avoid our collective responsibility to maintain dependents and dependency workers. We forget the extent to which we need social organization to assure that should we become dependent, we will have the assistance we need; and to assure that should we have to care for dependents, we ourselves will not come to bear the full burden and become unable to meet our own needs.

CONCLUSION

A way to understand the point I have been pressing is to say that when caregiving for the most highly dependent, among whom are the mentally retarded, is deemed a matter of mere charity, not justice, it is seen to have a very low priority on social resources. Inadequately supported caregivers caring for people who are on the margins of the moral community too easily become neglectful and even abusive. By keeping the level of compensation for caregiving minimal—itself a direct consequence of depending on charity and benevolence rather than on the claims of justice—we promote conditions that make a mockery of the benevolence on which we make retarded people depend. The consequence is the blighted fate of those in the global Willowbrooks and the Washington DC group homes. These are intolerable in a just and decent society.

Not all of us will remain in a state of dependency as profound as that of my daughter. But any of us could become so— an illness or an accident could make us so. From the vantage point of our socially constructed independence, we might think, "Oh, but should that happen, I would rather be dead." From the vantage point of my daughter, that is wasteful of what life has to offer, a failure to appreciate the gifts of being.

Hiding dependency, stigmatizing it, ignoring its frequency, valorizing only a particular segment of human possibility leads to the avoidance of our collective responsibility to take care of one another and to see that we are well cared for by someone for whom our well-being matters deeply. Seeing dependence as constructed and failing to see independence as still more constructed will only reinstate prejudices against disability. This time the prejudice falls most heavily on the shoulders of the severely and profoundly mentally retarded, those who are the most vulnerable, and for whom no environmental modifications can nullify their dependency. We exclude concerns of dependency from matters of justice at a cost. That cost is the denial of the dependent animals we are. It is a condition no amount of rationality can alter. Justice that begins with acknowledging our dependency and that seeks to organize society so that our well-being is not inversely related to our need for care makes caring itself a mode of just action.

NOTES

1. This chapter is a revised and shortened version of "When Caring Is Just and Justice is Caring: Justice and Mental Retardation," *Public Culture*, vol. 13, no. 3, September 2001, 557–73. A version was read at the Feminist Bio-Ethics Association, Imperial College, London, September 19, 2000. The term "mental retardation" is sometimes in disrepute. I frequently use "mental disabilities" but this includes those who have mental illnesses. The term "cognitive disability" includes disabilities such as autism, among whom are highly intelligent persons who can, with some supports, function well in the able-minded world. "Developmental disability" again can include disabilities that are not primarily cognitive. I vary the terms I use with a sensitivity to the over- or under-inclusiveness for the condition I am trying to address.

2. See Kittay, 1999; also Fineman, 1995.

3. See also Macintyre, 1999; Gastmans, 2000.

4. See Wertz, 2000, esp. Tables 4 and 5.

5. *Buck v. Bell*, 274 U.S. 208 (1927).

6. According to a study conducted at the Centers for Disease Control and Prevention, white individuals with Down syndrome live twice as long as blacks and four times as long

as that of Asians, Hispanics, and Native Americans. In the 1960s the life expectancy of an individual with Down syndrome was not much more than two years of age. Today, whites with Down syndrome live till to be 50, but the life expectancy for blacks is 25 years and "others" is 11. There was no improvement for blacks or other racial groups until the 1990s, whereas improvement for whites began in the 1970s. When you compare the life expectancy of whites and blacks in the same socioeconomic class the disparities are not nearly so great, indicating that class and social standing, not the genetic features of racial difference, are at play. ("All Things Considered," June 18, 2001; also "Down syndrome longevity seen linked to race," M.A.J. McKenna, *The Atlanta Journal and Constitution*, June 8, 2001.

7. See Lundgren and Browner, 1990.

8. In 1972, Geraldo Rivera brought television cameras into the Willowbrook State School and Letchworth Village, thereby broadcasting on national television the unimaginably dreadful conditions of state schools for retarded people. The exposes lead to the movement to close state institutions and replace them with more community based services and residences, such as group homes. "Willowbrook" became synonymous with the wretched conditions of large institutions for the mentally retarded.

9. See the account of group homes in Ohio (Ohlemacher, 2000) and in Queens, New York City (Tully, 1999), for other instances.

10. This has been reported to me in a discussion with the director Patrick Dollard of the Sullivan County Treatment and Diagnostic Center in upstate New York, an organization that works hard to prevent this alienation.

11. Wealthy as well as poor families find themselves overwhelmed with medical and caretaking responsibilities. For an account of such a family, the Kelsos, see Jacobs, 1999. The Kelso case in the context of the many families raising children with serious medical, physical, and mental difficulties can be found in Manning, 2000.

12. *Doula* originally meant *slave* or *servant* in Greek. I find it intriguing to redirect the concept of servant or slave, to reappropriate, if you will, the very significance of serving. The service in *doulia* reestablishes our interdependence and the indispensability of us being of service to one another.

13. Both positions have prioritarian versions. These permit strict equality of well-being or strict equality of treatment to be compromised if the outcome will benefit the least well off more. I ignore the prioritarian versions for now.

14. Silvers joins her argument with efforts on the part of many in the disability community to

resist the characterization of the disabled as more needy than others.

15. While they briefly refer to disability, they do not expand their arguments or focus specifically on cognitive disabilities. A capability approach such as Nussbaum's (1999, 41–42) is promising but some of the capabilities in her list, for example "practical reason," are of questionable or limited applicability to the profoundly retarded. It may be possible to amend the list. I worry that any list will favor some and exclude others. There are so many ways in which people may be incapable of functioning, so many capabilities will not be realized, even in a society geared to treat disabled people with the full measure of justice.

16. While Veatch recognizes the difficulty of basing the secular conception on the theological one, he claims that the secular conceptions are not more grounded in reason than the theological. Both involve a "faith move."

REFERENCES

Bogdan, R. and Taylor, Steven J. (1992). The social construction of humanness. In D.L.F. Philip M. Ferguson, and Steven J. Taylor, *Interpreting Disability*, eds. New York: Teacher's College, Columbia University, pp. 275–94.

Boo, K. (1999). Invisible lives: Troubled system for the retarded. *Washington Post*, December 5, (p. 3, Section A1).

Ferguson, P.M. (1994). Abandoned to Their Fate: Social Policy and Practices toward Severely Retarded People in America. Philadelphia: Temple University Press.

Fineman, M.A. (1995). The Neutered Mother: The Sexual Family, and Other Twentieth Century Tragedies. New York: Routledge.

Gastmans, C. (2000). The (altruistic) virtue of care. Presented at the Feminist Approaches to Bioethics Conference. London, September 19.

Goffman, I. (1961). *Asylums; Essays on the Social Situation of Mental Patients and Other Inmates*. New York: Anchor Books.

Jacobs, A. (1999). Pennsylvania couple accused of abandoning disabled son. *New York Times*, December 29, National Page.

Kittay, E.F. (1999). *Love's Labor: Women, Equality, and Dependency*. New York: Routledge.

Kittay, E.F. (2000). At home with my daughter.,

ed. In L.P. Francis and A. Silvers, *Americans with Disabilities*. New York: Routledge, pp. 64–80.

Kittay, E.F. (2000a). Relationality, impairment and Peter Singer on the fate of severely impaired infants. *The APA Newsletter on Philosophy and Medicine* 99 (2) (Spring), 253–56.

Kittay, E.F. (2001). A feminist public ethic of care meets the New Communitarian family policy. *Ethics*, April, pp. 523–547.

Levine, C. (1990). AIDS and changing concepts of the family. *The Milbank Quarterly* 68 (Suppl 1), 33–57.

Lundgren, R.I and Browner, C.H. (1990). Caring for the institutionalized mentally retarded: Work culture and work-based social support. In E. Abel and M.K. Nelson (eds.) *Circles of Care: Work and Identity in Women's Lives*, Albany: State University of New York Press, pp. 150–72.

Macintyre, A. (1999).*Dependent Rational Animals*. Peru, IL: Carus Publishing.

Manning, A. (2000). Quietly overwhelmed. *USA Today*, January 17, p. 1.

Nussbaum, M. (1999). *Sex and Social Justice*. Oxford: Oxford University Press.

Ohlemacher, S. (2000). Retarded patients lack protection, study finds. *The Plain Dealer* (Cleveland) January 8, p. 1A.

Pogge, T. (2000). Justice for people with disabilities: The semiconsequentialist approach. In L.P. Francis and A. Silvers, (eds.), *Americans with Disabilities*. New York: Routledge, pp. 34–53.

Scanlon, T.M. (1998). *What We Owe to Each Other*. Cambridge, MA: Belknap Press, Harvard University.

Silvers, A., Wasserman, D. and Mahowald, M.B. (1998). *Disability, Difference, Discrimination*. Baltimore: Rowman and Littlefield.

Trent, J.W.J (1994). *The Invention of the Feeble Mind*. Berkeley: University of California Press.

Tully, T. (1999). Retarded are found living in squalor. *New York Daily News*, July 12, p. 7.

Veatch, R.M. (1986). *The Foundations of Justice*. New York: Oxford University Press.

Wertz, D.C. (2000). Drawing lines: Notes for policy makers. In *Parental Testing and the Disability Rights Critique*, ed. E. Parens and A. Asch. Washington, D.C: Georgetown University Press, pp. 261–87.

25

Justice, Health, and the Price of Poverty

Patricia Smith

Poverty, health, and health care, or rather poverty, *ill* health, and *lack* of health care are intimately connected. In this chapter I review some of the ways this is true and some major arguments about why or whether we should care. I first consider the issue of health itself, and whether a society is responsible for the conditions under which its members must live. Next, I examine the issue of health care, and whether a society has any obligation to provide it.

HEALTH IN POVERTY

There is no question that poverty is a health hazard. For some time now it has been statistically verified beyond any doubt that the poor get sick more often, stay sick longer, and die younger than those who are financially better off. They are also at higher risk of accidents, and are exposed to worse environmental conditions than those with greater wealth.[1]

These facts, while well established, are also widely disregarded. For example, if one were to follow the extensive media coverage one might well assume that hypertension and heart disease are primarily afflictions of high-level executives in high-pressure positions. Statistics indicate otherwise: namely that the incidence of high blood pressure and heart attack increases as the levels of wealth and power decrease. Similar patterns have been shown for many (although not all) other problems of health and physical well-being. Some researchers have concluded that social class or inequality itself is a powerful health factor.[2] Without question the farther you descend the economic ladder, the more likely you are to suffer from ill health.

There is a troubling chicken-and-egg problem here: Poverty increases the risk of bad health, and bad health increases the risk of poverty. Each aggravates the other condition, so it is impossible to say (except in particular cases) which way the causal direction runs. Ill health was named as the leading cause of bankruptcy in the past three years.[3] Among the homeless, two thirds suffer from chronic illness or infectious disease and fully 57% from mental illness.[4] Obviously those in ill health are less able to work, less able to work full time if they do manage to work part time, and less able to compete with healthy workers if they do manage to work full time. Naturally, they have more trouble paying their rent and other debts.

One major flaw (or limitation) of the recent "welfare to work" reform movement has been the failure to acknowledge that a certain percentage of long-term welfare recipients have suffered from long-term poor health; consequently, they make unattractive, indeed implausible, job candidates.[5] Badgering a 50-year-old, overweight grandmother with high blood pressure and arthritis to compete in the job market at minimum wage is not realistic, cost-effective, or humane, for it fails to take into account why she is where she is. Most people lack jobs for a reason, and the reason is often ill health.[6]

Thus, poor health often leads to poverty, especially among those (40 million or so working men and women) who were only marginally above the poverty level in the first place.[7] That is to say, bad health is a leading cause of poverty.

Looking from the other direction, poverty is a leading cause of bad health. The reasons are many, some more obvious than others. The poor tend to live in substandard housing where walls may be damp, mold content high, sanitation poor, ventilation worse, and heating sporadic. They are exposed more often to smog, bad water, toxic environmental or hazardous work environments.[8] It is poor children who suffer from exposure to lead paint, asbestos, and poor nutrition. The babies of poor mothers (teenage or otherwise) are more susceptible to low birth weight, leading in turn to further health and developmental problems.[9] The incidence of asthma in poor children is five times that of their wealthier counterparts.[10] While all this is deplorable, it is well established.

What more recent studies have shown is the health toll taken by the mental drag of poverty (or class) itself. The rate of depression and stress-related illness in poverty-stricken adults is much higher than it is in wealthier people, and the connection between stress or depression and other illness (ranging from heart disease and hypertension to susceptibility to virus and bacterial infection) previously thought unrelated is being increasingly demonstrated.[11] The poor lack the resources to avoid or correct hazardous conditions or to treat illness and injury. All they can do is worry about illness or repress it, either of which is health impairing. As recent studies show, poor living conditions, dearth of resources, constant worry and frustration at the lack of control over one's life produce stress and depression that are strongly associated with health problems.[12] Poverty makes people sick.

I raise these points merely to show that health and health care issues are embedded in the larger issue of distributive justice. Not only is health care unevenly distributed in this country, but health itself is unevenly distributed. Those who are most deprived of other basic goods—wealth, position, opportunity, security—are also most likely to be deprived of health as well. Conversely, those suffering ill health are also more likely to be deprived of other basic goods. This is not just a vicious circle; it is a vicious downward spiral.

Of course, the very idea of distributive justice can be and has been challenged, thus, as a strategic matter connecting the specific issue of health care to larger issues of distributive justice could be considered a tactical error. It is likely that more people favor universal health care than the redistribution of wealth in general. In fact, most people in the United States do favor universal health care.[13] (They just cannot agree on how to accomplish it.)

Still, the strong links between poverty and health have implications for reasonable judgments about eliminating poverty. If the causal connection runs from poverty to ill health, doesn't that provide a strong reason for combatting poverty? If we know that poverty is actually a health hazard, isn't requiring some people to live in poverty rather like requiring them to live in a toxic environment?

It might be; yet some respond that in a free country, no one is banned from rising out of poverty; therefore no one is required to live in it. But if we are talking about populations rather than individuals, then we do require a percentage of our fellow citizens to live in poverty just as long as a percentage of our jobs do not pay enough to allow the entire population to cross over the poverty line, and our government programs (such as food stamps, rent subsidies, or health care) are not adequate to make up for the shortfall. Thus, the very structure of our society itself condemns some of us to live in poverty and sickness.

Conversely, if the causal direction runs the other way—from ill health to poverty, how can we possibly square the existence of preventable poverty with the requirements of fairness? What excuse can we give ourselves for not eliminating it? In my view, we cannot reasonably say that the poor deserve to be poor if the reason they are so is that they are sick. This is true even if the sick are less productive (which they usually are). Almost no one believes that sick people are less worthy or deserving of a decent life because they are less productive.

Consequently, whichever way the causal connection runs the recognition of the connection itself between poverty and poor health provides a powerful reason for greater efforts to reduce poverty. Indeed, I want to suggest that taking steps to reduce poverty would be both more efficient and more fair than the current status quo.

That it would be more efficient is obvious. Preventing conditions that make people sick in the first place is more efficient than providing them with health care after subjecting them to unhealthy conditions. This point merely takes the well-known arguments for the efficiency of preventive medicine just one logical step further. Of course, it could be argued that we have no obligation to provide health care to the sick at all, and if so the efficiency claim fails. But the fact is that we do not just let poor people die, intentionally, nor could we stomach a public policy that openly advocated doing so. Consequently, sooner or later the impoverished sick wind up in emergency rooms across the country, and we all then pay dearly for health care delivered in the least efficient, least effective, and perhaps least humane manner we could possibly devise. Thus, preventive measures would clearly benefit all of us.

The fairness claim raises more objections, but it does seem to me that knowingly subjecting some percentage of the population to high risk of bad health is unfair, at least if it can be avoided. It can be avoided if and only if all people have other options, that is to say, options that would enable all of them to avoid the most unhealthy conditions.[14]

Some years ago when I was a struggling assistant professor with two children to support, my son got work in a tobacco warehouse because it paid better than anything else available to him. His job scared me to death because although he wore a mask, he went to work every day with the mask white and came home every day with it black. We were lucky. He only worked there for a summer, but what do you suppose a job like that does to someone who stays on for five or ten years or a lifetime? And who do you suppose would stay? Someone with no other options. Most of the people working in that warehouse were not kids on summer vacation, and they were not on their way to something better. If they are still alive, they still work in the warehouse. This is as good as it gets for them, so they trade their lungs for money. It is not even very good money by middle-class standards, but it is good enough to be their best option.

We call America a free country, and so it is on many measures. But if some people have no viable options, how free is that? If we still call it free, we cannot call it just;

not in a nation that has so much to offer others.

Workers across this country are not receiving just compensation for their contribution to the national product. More than 34 million people live in poverty today, and most of them work for a living.[15] They are not receiving their fair share for what they do. If they did we would go a long way toward eliminating poverty and many of the health problems it fosters.

Of course, there are long and ongoing debates over how a fair share should be determined. Currently favored is the market theory of value, according to which a commodity or service is worth no more and no less than the price it brings in an open market.

There is much to be said for a market economy—it encourages and rewards creativity, initiative, energy, drive, freedom, and enterprise. It has a proven record of productive results. But not all its tendencies and effects are good. Even under an ideal interpretation it tends to disadvantage the poor, the weak, the vulnerable, and the sick. It feeds on vice, while penalizing altruism. And it makes selfishness the ultimate virtue.

As the foundation for a theory of justice or morality, then, it leaves much to be desired. Consequently, it should be recognized that the market theory of value is not a theory of *moral* value. When economists substitute wealth maximization for utility (because the former is easier to calculate) they transform a moral theory into a nonmoral (economic) theory.[16] A market theory of value (along with supply-side economics) has produced America's current economic situation which on some measures (such as GNP) is almost as good as it has ever been, but is also more polarized than it has ever been.

A recent study[17] (using figures corrected for inflation)showed that the lowest one-fifth of the nation now earns $900 (or 6%) less than it did in 1978. The second-lowest one-fifth dropped by 1%, while the middle fifth gained only 5% over 20 years. By con-trast, the average income of the top quintile increased by 33%, and the richest 5% of the population increased its income by 55%. For three-fifths of the population, wages have been stagnant or worse for 25 years, and although the average wage increased to $7.78 an hour over the past two years (because of low unemployment) that wage is still considerably less than the average of $8.50 an hour in 1973.[18] During this same time government benefit programs have been cut to their lowest levels since the 1970s.[19] In fact, average Americans are not doing better than they did two years ago, the poverty rate has recently increased, the poorest Americans are worse off than they were in the 1970s, and half of us are not doing as well as our parents did 25 years ago, when an ordinary family could still live on one salary.

Statistics again: Does any of this show that our economic system is unjust? Only if you believe there is such a thing as distributive justice. If you agree that this concept is meaningful, then you must agree that every member of society is entitled to some reasonable share of the economic pie. We may debate forever what that share should be, but current data are enough to give one pause. For at least the past 15 years, 20% of the population controled 80% of the wealth, while 80% of the population shared the other 20%. In 1997, 5% of our households controled 21.7% of our income, whereas the bottom 20%—one-fifth of our population—eked out a miserable 3.6%.[20] And we now also know that those at the bottom suffer proportionally worse health than do those who are better off. By allowing inequality to increase we allow ill health to grow. Whatever our concept of distributive justice might be, it surely cannot be that.

HEALTH CARE AND JUSTICE

Assuming that we will not adjust our wage and tax structure to correct these grave imbalances any time soon, should at least health care be a universal benefit? In many societies it is assumed that access to basic medical care should not depend on the ability to pay. In fact, all industrialized nations (except the United States) have instituted universal health-care systems of one sort or another to guarantee basic care to all. But the commitment to equal access without regard to wealth can be disputed.

"Why is this principle appropriate for health care when it has been rejected for vacation homes and fast cars?" legal scholar Richard Epstein asked provocatively in his recent book.[21] According to Epstein, health care is a commodity to be distributed like any other commodity in an open market; and he offers a systematic set of arguments against universal access by government provision. Relying on the common-law tradition that limits collective responsibility for individual well-being, he argues, first, that there is not and cannot be a universal positive right to health care, and second, that in the long run an unregulated free market in health care will provide greater access to quality care for more people. Thus, the two issues he isolates are justice and efficiency.

Given limitations of space and the focus of this text, I will consider only the issue of justice. Rather than becoming entangled in the possibility of positive rights I will look directly at the question of collective responsibility.[22] Epstein admits that his position denying a collective responsibility for health care is a minority view. Most people think that there is a collective (or governmental) responsibility—that a society should provide its members with equal access to basic health services.[23] Yet the question is one of justification. Epstein effectively demonstrates that the common law provides no basis for a collective (legal) responsibility to aid strangers, but, then, it would be surprising if anyone thought it did. The ground for collective responsibility is legislative. However, the bounds of legislative legitimacy can always be questioned. So the issue remains: What justifies recognizing a collective responsibility to provide health care for all?

Numerous arguments have been offered, but most philosophers and advocates have focused on health care (or health) as a basic need or primary good. Like food or freedom, the loss of health seems to impair all other values. So it would seem that basic health care is necessary to the enjoyment of our other rights: life, liberty and the pursuit of happiness, for example.[24]

Epstein, while acknowledging that health care is indeed a very basic need, argues that mere need in itself has never been sufficient to generate a responsibility on the part of one individual to provide for another—certainly not in American common law.[25]

It should be recognized, however, that the claim at issue here is not that need generates a (legal) responsibility for any particular individual to aid any other particular individual. Rather, it is that basic need may generate a collective responsibility for all (who are able) to contribute to a common fund that ensures (at least some) basic necessities for all. That is not the same kind of claim. The latter may entail only that legislative action creating common obligations for the common good is legitimate. To deny that claim in general is to deny the foundations of democratic government. So the denial would have to be more specific, such as: Funding for health care (or schools, or roads, or whatever) is not a common obligation or a legitimate legislative objective for reason X, Y, or Z.[26]

Indeed, no one supposes that there is a social responsibility to provide everything that anyone needs. Thus, again, the question remains: What makes health care in particular a common responsibility? Consider the nature of some other basic needs: National security, clean air, and perhaps clean water are known as public goods.[27] No one can have them unless everyone has them. If they are necessities, they must be provided for all. Health care then is obviously not a public good, except for the prevention of highly contagious diseases (such as smallpox or diphtheria). Prevention of epidemics is arguably a public good, but other than that, health care can easily be provided for some and not for others. There is nothing indivisible about it, so it is not in general a public good.

Consider another sort of basic need: food, clothing, shelter, some means of income. These are certainly basic needs that are just as important as health care. People die or are seriously impaired without them. We might call them "constant needs." All people need them all the time in order to function in ordinary life. It is currently thought that the best way to provide for these needs is to develop a society that enables all to participate in the economic system in such a way that each can provide for him- or herself by ordinary exchange of goods and services.[28]

By contrast, medical care is not something that most people need all the time. It is usually an abnormal need, rather like fire or police protection, an uncommon need, but one that is of vital importance when it arises. We might call this a "need for special risk insurance." Also like fire and police protection, health care may be extremely expensive, so that sharing the cost and pooling the risk seem to make sense. Finally, it requires special expertise and equipment to handle medical problems. Like fire and police protection, it is a service not just anyone can provide.

Of course, the analogy is far from perfect. Some people have chronic disorders with daily costs; most people have sporadic ailments with occasional costs; and all people need preventive health maintenance that generates some regular costs.[29] Even so, it is the emergency aspect and potential catastrophic cost of medical need that sets it apart from constant normal needs like food and shelter.

Is that enough to make it a basic need that should be provided for all? Is it enough to generate a collective responsibility? I believe it is. It certainly is enough to make it a focus of common concern. As is widely recognized, any one of us could be struck without warning by a sudden, severe, urgent medical need that is costly enough to bankrupt even the wealthy, and is far beyond the reach of most. The obvious way to handle a problem of this sort is by pooling resources. That would be practical and efficient.

Furthermore, the only way to prepare for medical needs in the long run is by means of very expensive research and training that would be completely out of reach for any single individual. Public funding has always been crucial to the development of these resources. Consequently, it is reasonable to view them as common assets to be shared by all in need.

Yet Richard Epstein denies any collective responsibility for individual health care. He would presumably distinguish police and fire protection from medical care by claiming that the former are inefficient to provide privately and in that sense are somewhat akin to public goods (like clean air or national defense). Medical care, Epstein would argue, is more like food or housing: best supplied by private enterprise. Thus, he might conclude, the comparison to quasi-public goods is inappropriate because medical care (and medical insurance) can be and have been supplied by individual participants in a competitive market. As it is possible and efficient to supply these goods in an open market, any other mode of distribution unnecessarily restricts the freedom and rights of individuals to run their own lives and make their own choices.

The objection to this line of argument on the basis of justice is that the market would not distribute health care efficiently to *all* members of society, but at best only to those who can pay. A competitive market, by its nature, tends to exclude the poor. There is no reason to think it would function differently in this case.[30]

In fact, the analogy to food and shelter provides some interesting points worth noting. American society (and all other societies that can afford it) do, actually, recognize a collective responsibility to provide food and shelter for those who are so unfortunate as to lack even these basic necessities. We have publicly funded homeless shelters, housing subsidies, food stamps, welfare programs, social security, and other programs. Thus, despite the usual distribution of food and shelter by market forces, the fact that we recognize them as basic necessities is reflected in supplementary programs to provide for them where the market fails. Consequently, to treat health care as analogous to food or shelter we would need to supplement market distribution wherever it failed.

In fact, the general presupposition underlying this conclusion leads to more or less the system we currently have: a private system supplemented by governmental programs and incentives designed or intended to extend coverage to those who would otherwise be excluded. It also explains complaints about the inadequacy of this system. If there were no presumption that everyone should be covered, then there would be no complaint about the failure to do it. All this suggests a general recognition of a social responsibility to provide the most basic necessities to all people.

Epstein objects vigorously to this idea. Instead, he argues that those who cannot pay are best served by charity. (Presumably he would argue the same with regard to food and shelter.) Is anything wrong with the capitalism plus charity model? Charity in itself is a very good thing, but as a model for supplying basic necessities it has several drawbacks, especially as applied to medical needs. I cannot pursue this matter comprehensively here, but I will discuss three major considerations.

The most fundamental issue raised is what the proper attitude should be about basic necessities: Is there a social responsibility to see to it that all members of society are able to receive the most basic necessities of life, or is this a matter of good fortune and grace—the benevolence of one's family or neighbors, the good luck of fortunate birth? If there is no social responsibility, it means that justice requires no particular

minimum on the distribution of social burdens and benefits, and charity for the downtrodden is the view that seems to follow.

My own view is that society is a collective enterprise; all inhabitants are members and participants, each person significant in her own right. Some may contribute more than others and some may benefit more than others. That is inevitable. But the point of living in a society rather than existing in isolation is that human beings do better by cooperating than any person can do alone. Everyone benefits and everyone owes a return on that benefit.

Consequently, I believe that distributive justice does apply to such groups, and therefore that each member is responsible to contribute to a common fund that ensures basic necessities to every member. If that is a better view of society, then charity is not enough as applied to necessities.[31]

A further issue, one specific to medical care, is that it is potentially so expensive that many people (especially those who need it most) will not be able to afford it, and there is no way to tell with certainty which person will need it. As a result, unlike food or shelter, which can generally be planned for, predicted, and pretty easily provided for by most people at a basic level, any one of us might confront catastrophic medical costs that almost none of us could meet without an insurance plan. Theoretically, one could go off into the wilderness and build a home and grow food, but you cannot provide your own medicine (except at a very primitive level). Similarly, within a society, acceptable low-cost versions of food and shelter are generally available for most people. Those who are able to spend more receive more luxurious versions. But the cost of medicine has almost nothing to do with luxury. There is no low-cost version if you need heart surgery or cancer treatment. And from the point of view of health, the most expensive treatment may be as much a necessity as the least expensive. Cost does not track luxury in medicine. It is this realization that creates the need for insurance.

Consequently, provision of medical care is essentially social; almost no one can have it without being in the pool. To exclude some people from the pool is like denying them police or fire protection. It is to require some people to bear their own risks alone when others have the benefit of sharing assets.

Finally, good health is a social benefit, and ill health is a social drain. Those who are sick are not productive. In this sense (universal) health care is like (universal) education. The better off each individual is, the better off society as a whole is, because each individual can contribute more to society if healthy and well educated rather than the reverse.

Are these views of society unusual or ideosyncratic? I believe that they are very widely accepted, although perhaps grudgingly, and with qualifications in some quarters. The fact that they are widely accepted is reflected in the supplementary programs I mentioned earlier. Very few Americans think any of their fellow citizens should have to beg for food or sleep on the streets; much less should anyone have to beg for medical treatment. But that is what charity means. It is to rely on the good grace of someone to give you that to which you are not entitled.

Perhaps, then, the issue of positive rights is not avoidable. Let me just say this for the present. There are two questions relevant to addressing the issue of rights in this context. (1) Is there a right to health care? (2) Is there a right not to be taxed for the purpose of providing universal health care?

I have been arguing indirectly for a "yes" to question (1) by arguing that there is a social responsibility to provide basic necessities for all, and that health care is a basic necessity. If there is such a responsibility, then there is also a right correlative to it. But this is a very controversial set of claims. Not everyone will agree with the position laid out here. What can be said to those who remain unpursuaded?

Given general attitudes about health care there is a sense in which it is not necessary to argue for (1) because under the circumstances denying (2) may be sufficient, and denying (2) involves a much weaker claim. Question (2) shifts the burden of pursuasion. It asks whether, in the face of majority agreement, there is some reason why taxation to pay for health care in particular should be excluded from the democratic process as a matter of justice. Is it like free speech or the exercise of religion that should be protected for each individual from majority rule? Hardly. From all appearances, it is a mainstream legislative issue regarding the allocation of resources, exactly the kind of thing that a legislature is supposed to handle for the benefit of the people at large.

So, shifting the burden of pursuasion back to Richard Epstein, what reason can there be for restricting this issue in particular from the democratic process? Presumably, there is none. The only possible argument against a (legislatively, or self-imposed) collective responsibility for universal health care (or a correlative right to it) on the basis of a claim of justice is the general position that the redistribution of wealth is unjust in itself.[32] Of course, that takes us back to the general redistribution issue, well known, long debated, and discussed here as well as in the previous section. I cannot pursue it further at this point, but the general obligation to support the common good has been assumed or defended by great philosophers, from Aristotle to Rawls. If their efforts have not been conclusive, neither have the arguments of those who seek to deny collective responsibility.

Unless it can be shown that redistribution of wealth is unjust in any form whatsoever, there is no reason to find it so in the case of health care in particular. Why not?

To summarize my previous arguments, first, health care is a basic necessity, and no one in a reasonably successful and minimally just society should be deprived of basic necessities.

Second, even if the first point is not accepted as applicable to all basic necessities, health care is potentially so costly to random individuals that pooling resources is the only secure way to provide it, and there is no justifiable reason to exclude some people from the pool. Such exclusion is unjustified because doing so requires some, specifically those who can least afford it, to face alone a risk that has been effectively socialized otherwise. This is like basing police or fire protection on the ability to pay.

Third, even if some individuals do not agree with the previous two points, given that a majority of people in this country accept them, it is more cost-effective and more fair to provide universal access to health care without regard to ability to pay. It is more cost-effective, first, because preventive medicine is more cost-effective than emergency treatment or intensive care, and second, because a healthy population (like an educated one) is much more productive than the opposite. Hence, general good health is a common benefit. It is more fair because if we rely on private charity alone to provide this common benefit, only some will contribute, allowing others to have a free ride on the charitable impulses of their fellow citizens.

While Richard Epstein has shown that there is no common law basis for a responsibility to provide health care to all, he certainly has not shown (nor could anyone show without undermining the foundations of democracy) that there is any legal basis whatever to deny that a democratically elected legislature is lawfully empowered to create such a collective responsibility on behalf of the people for the common interest. Furthermore, if the arguments just given are correct, a responsible legislature should do so.

It follows that health care should not be denied on the basis of poverty (or in other words, allocated on the basis of ability to pay) assuming that it is not in the common interest to do so. Is that a reasonable assumption? This is, admittedly, a question of efficiency, something I cannot address

here, but let me conclude this chapter with a few suggestive words.

SOME CONCLUSIONS ABOUT JUSTICE AND EFFICIENCY

The United States remains the only major industrialized nation not to offer universal health care to its citizens even though it spends more on health care than any other country in the world. Despite its expenditures, America is ranked 54th out of 191 countries by the World Health Organization. Our infant mortality rate and rate of low birth weight are no better than that of some third-world countries.[33] One cannot help but notice that this is not exactly Pareto Optimal.

Fully 42.6 million people or 15.5% of the U.S. population was uninsured in 1999, and the rate of coverage was directly related to wealth. More that one-fifth of our poor children and almost one-half of all poor people were uninsured. Nearly half of our working poor were without insurance in 1999. This also correlated with race, in that one third of Hispanics and one-fifth of blacks and Asians were without coverage, while only 11% of (non-Hispanic) whites were without insurance.[34]

A recent report by Consumers Union found that the uninsured receive second-class care, if any, depending on where they live (better to live in Minnesota than Texas, for example), what health problems they have (better to have a contagious disease than a degenerative one), and how much money they can pay up front. For example, there may be money to diagnose a disease, but no money to treat it: money for mamograms but none for breast cancer, money for a free clinic visit but not for prescription medicine.[35] The efficiency of laying out money to diagnose diseases that will not be treated is highly questionable. Diagnosis without treatment is not prevention; it is just wasted (and stress-producing) information.

Not only is it inefficient, but inhumane and unjust, and given the current system can only be expected to get worse. Private insurance and health maintenance organizations (HMOs) have financial incentives to insure the healthy and avoid the sick, and/or to cut benefits in order to cut costs. The sick and the poor (especially racial minorities), namely those with the fewest resources, are the least likely to be insured, and those who are poor and uninsured are the least likely to receive care and the most likely to need it.

Epstein suggests that this situation is best handled by charity, but nothing prevented it from being handled by charity today, or last week, or last year or 10 years ago, or in 1999 when Epstein published his book. There is no law against charity, nor any tax disincentive, nor moral disapproval. We have no reason to believe that if medicine were more rather than less privatized, charity would increase.[36] But we might well wonder whether a capitalistic economy that relies on pervasive mass marketing to promote material consumption, competition, envy, and greed is really an environment that is most likely to foster an attitude of charity.[37]

Not everything is best viewed as *simply* a commodity like any other. Health care is not like a vacation home or a luxury car. The world is not simply a market, nor are human beings nothing but consumers. We love and hate; we suffer and die; we care and struggle; and none of that is best represented as buying and selling. The attempt to capture human life in a single metaphor is inevitably deficient and sometimes dangerous, but always an intellectual lure.

In the eighteenth century the universe was a clock. Newtonian physics was all the rage, and the world and humanity were expected soon to be deciphered with clocklike precision. There were both benefits and costs to this picture of reality, and the same is true of our twentieth century vision of the "world as a market." One of the greatest costs may well be its comprehensive application to medicine.

Is the ideology of the market compatible with the Hippocratic oath, or the ancient tradition of unselfish concern for human health? This is not to say that doctors should be saints or that medical technology is evil if profitable, but the sole pursuit of profit cannot be the foundation of medicine. Perhaps it is worth noting that our two top pharmaceutical companies earned an average net profit of 229% over the past five years, while raising prices so high as to cause even the wealthy to blink.[38] This is captialism par excellence, but where is there any commitment to health left in this scenario or others like it? The trouble is that medicine is not and cannot ever be a truly open market. Sick people are so vulnerable that to follow the capitalist maxim to charge the highest price the market will bear is inevitably extortion. Consequently, the natural limits of the market will never be fully operative in the medical context, and we end with a system both inefficient and unjust.

To base health care on the ability to pay and to deny that sick people are equally entitled to care is to deny a piece of our common humanity and to erode one of the few traditions we got right for several thousand years. Medicine should be dedicated to health without qualification. That includes the qualification of poverty.

NOTES

1. See, e.g., Wilkerson, *Unhealthy Societies*; *New York Times*, "In Health It Helps to Be Rich and Important," June 1, 1999, p. F9.

2. Ibid. Hadley and Osei, "Does Income Affect Mortality?" p. 901.

3. See, e.g., Reinhardt, "Employer-Based Health Insurance: A Balance Sheet"; Bernstein, "Deep Poverty and Illness Found Among Homeless," citing HUD surveys 1995–1996.

4. See NY Times 12-8-99.

5. See DeParle, "Project to Rescue Needy Hits Persistence of Poverty," reporting on Milwaukee Project New Hope; DeParle, "What Welfare to Work Really Means," p. 50ff. See also Solow, *Work and Welfare*.

6. Of course, I am not suggesting that ill health is the only reason for unemployment, yet it is a major contributing factor that remains underestimated.

7. *Center on Budget and Policy Priorities:*

Analysis of Census Bureau Income and Poverty Report, October 10, 1999; http://www.cbpp.org/9-30-99pov.htm.

8. The hazards of slum living and the deficiencies of substandard housing are well known. See Carson, *Rachel and Her Children*; and Wilson, *The Truly Disadvantaged*.

9. See, e.g., *New Jersey Star-Ledger* August 16, 2000; Wilkerson, note 1 *supra*; Sewell, Price, and Karp, "The Ecology of Poverty, Undernutrition and Learning Failure"; and Smeeding and Torrey, "Poor Children in Rich Countries," pp. 873–77.

10. See, e.g., *New York Times*, March 23, 2000, p. B1; or Leivick, "Helping Children—and Their Families—Breathe Easier."

11. See references in note 1 *supra*.

12. See, e.g., Wilkerson, note 1 *supra*; or *New York Times*, January 14, 1997, p. C1; Vockovic, "Self-Care Among the Uninsured," pp. 197–201.

13. Providing universal health care has been a major issue in the United States at least since the 1992 presidential election, when Bill Clinton made it his campaign centerpiece. Since his election, numerous polls have shown that at least a majority of Americans favor universal health care, but reaching agreement on how to provide it is another matter.

14. Of course, some people still would not function well enough to stay out of poverty. I am not suggesting that utopia is possible, but only that reasonable social structures would not condemn over a tenth of our population, millions of people, to live in or near poverty.

15. One-half of the working poor are uninsured, along with their dependents. See, e.g., *New York Times*, September 29, 2000, p. A16.

16. This move is accepted common practice among many economists. See, e.g., Posner, *Economic Analysis of Law*, or Epstein, *Mortal Peril: Our Inalienable Right to Health Care?*

17. *New Jersey Star-Ledger*, May 16, 1999, sec.3, pp. 1,3, citing Census Bureau figures; *New York Times*, January 19, 2000, p. B5, on stagnant wages.

18. See Callahan, *False Hopes*, p. 177, also Kolahan and Kim, "Why Does the Number of Uninsured Americans Continue to Grow?" pp. 188–96; also Phillips, *The Politics of Rich and Poor*, p. 88.

19. See, e.g., *New York Times*, February 21, 1999, p. A1; June 3, 1999, p. A22; April 21, 2000, p. A1; or Kolahan and Kim, note 17 *supra*.

20. *New Jersey Star-Ledger*, May 16, 1999, sec.3, p. 3.

21. Epstein, note 16 *supra*, p. 112.

22. On the possibility of positive rights, see Smith, *Liberalism and Affirmative Obligation*; Shue, *Basic Rights*; Wellman, *Welfare Rights*, among others.

23. In this context, the notion of collective responsibility means governmental responsibility, although this is not always the case. See, e.g., May, *The Morality of Groups*; and French, *Collective and Corporate Responsibility*, on group responsibility.

24. See Rawls, *A Theory of Justice*, on primary goods.

25. See Epstein, note 16 *supra*, p. 243.

26. Libertarians, like Epstein, respond that the only legitimate legislative goals are the protection of negative rights, which must be universalized to be effective and which create no extravagant costs by being universal. While in the abstract this argument is conceptually defensible, in practice it will not do. In practice, negative rights must be enforced and protected, which generates huge social costs and requires extensive social institutions at least as complex as any needed to supply positive rights. The United States currently spends much more on national defense and the federal court system (to protect negative rights) than anyone proposes to spend on positive rights of any sort, including health care. See Shue, note 22 *supra*.

27. Water is controversial as a public good because it can be bottled and shipped in for the wealthy. Still, protecting pure water sources is arguably a public good. In any case, it is not necessary to refine the notion of a public good, for I will not argue that health care falls in that category.

28. This is not the only possibility, of course. A society, especially a small one, could be much more communally organized, among other things.

29. This could still be made analogous to people who live in higher-and lower-risk areas, or who engage in higher-risk activities, and thus need more fire or police protection. Banks and forests, for example, could be characterized as existing in states of chronic risk, thus preserving the analogy. It is not a particularly helpful analogy, however.

30. See Buchanan, "Privatization and Just Health Care," pp. 220–39, or Rowman and Allenheld, *Ethics, Efficiency and the Market*.

31. I argue this view at length in *Liberalism and Affirmative Obligation*, note 22 *supra*; see especially chaps. 8 and 9.

32. This is exactly the position Epstein in fact takes; namely that there are no positive rights, and so no positive right to health care.

33. See *New Jersey Star-Ledger*, "Report Disparages Health Care for Poor," August 11, 2000, p. 44.

34. *New York Times*, "Number of Insured

Americans Up for First Time Since '87," September 29, 2000, p. A16.

35. See note 33, *supra*; see also Spillman, "Adults Without Health Insurance: Do State Policies Matter?"

36. The one thing that does seem to increase the charitable impulse is a clear and dramatic emergency, such as a fire, a hurricane, the attack on the World Trade Center. But chronic conditions, even deadly ones, do not trigger this impulse. Apparently, people get used to problems (like poverty) that are ongoing. It is interesting to note that the outpouring of charity to the World Trade Center victims was accompanied by a dramatic drop in charitable gifts to virtually all other relief funds.

37. Interestingly, Epstein notes (his informal impression) that charitable provision of health care has declined since the 1940s and 1950s. He attributes that decline to the rise of governmental programs, but why suppose that? The impulse for profit is encouraged much more by capitalism than by social programs. And if professional charity were so effective in the 1950s why were social programs thought necessary? The real danger is the attitude encouraged by viewing medicine as a business rather than a profession or even a calling.

38. See *Value Line Investment Survey*, Edition 8, April 28, 2000, pp. 1264, 1271; see also www.valueline.com.

REFERENCES

Bernstein, J. (1999) Deep poverty and illness found among homeless, *New York Times*, December 8, 1999.

Buchanan, A. (1995). Privatization and just health care, *Bioethics* 9, pp. 86–103.

Buchanan, A. (1985). *Ethics, Efficiency and the Market*, Totowa, NJ: Rowman and Allenheld.

Callahan, D. (1998). *False Hopes*, New Brunswick, NJ: Rutgers University Press.

Carson, R. (1988). *Rachel and Her Children*, New York: Routledge.

Center on Budget and Policy Priorities: Analysis of Census Bureau Income and Poverty Report (1999).; http://www.cbpp.org/9-30-99 pov.htm.

DeParle, J. (1999). Project to rescue needy hits persistence of poverty, *New York Times*, May 12, 1999.

DeParle, J. (1998). What welfare to work really means, *New York Times Magazine*, December 20, 1998.

Epstein, R. (1999). *Mortal Peril: Our Inalienable Right to Health Care?* Cambridge, MA: Perseus Publishers.

French, P. (1984). *Collective and Corporate Responsibility*, New York: Columbia University Press.

Hadley, C. (1982). Does income affect mortality? *Medicare Care* 20, pp. 152–159.

Holahan, J. and J. Kim, "Why does the number of uninsured Americans continue to grow? *Health Affairs*, 19 (4), pp. 188–197.

Leivick, L. (2000). Helping children and their families breathe easier, *Folio*, New York, NY: CUNY Graduate Center.

May, L. (1986). *The Mortality of Groups*, Notre Dame, IA: Notre Dame University Press.

Phillips, K. (1990). *The Politics of Rich and Poor*, New York: Random House.

Posner, R. (1992). *Economic Analysis of Law*, Chicago: West Pub.

Rawls, J. (1971). *A Theory of Justice*, Cambridge, MA: Harvard University Press.

Reinhardt, U. (1999). Employer-based health insurance: a balance sheet, *Health Affairs*, 18 (6), pp. 124–132.

Sewell, J., L. Price, and S. Karp (1993). The ecology of poverty, undernutrition and learning failure, In S. Karp, ed., *Malnourished Children*, New York: Springer Press.

Shue, H. (1996). *Basic Rights*, Princeton, NJ: Princeton University Press.

Smeeding, K. and L. Torrey (1988). Poor children in rich countries, *Science* 242, pp. 240–244.

Smith, P. (1998). *Liberalism and Affirmative Obligation*, New York: Oxford University Press.

Solow, L. *Work and Welfare*, Princeton, NJ: Princeton, University Press.

Spillman, B. (2000). Adults without health insurance: Do state policies matter? *Health Affairs* 19 (4), pp. 178–188.

Value Line Investment Survey, (2000). Edition 8, April 28, 2000, pp. 1264, 1271; see also www.valueline.com.

Vockovic, N. Self-care among the uninsured: You do what you can do," *Health Affairs*, pp. 197–201.

Wellman, C. (1996). *Welfare Rights*, New York: Oxford University Press.

Wilkerson, J. *Unhealthy Societies*, New York: Routledge.

Wilson, W. (1987). *The Truly Disadvantaged*, Chicago: Chicago University Press.

IV

DILEMMAS FOR MEDICINE AND HEALTH-CARE SYSTEMS: ASSESSMENT AND PRIORITIES

Although different theories of justice offer general views on how to allocate goods within a society, none reaches so far as to give specific advice on the details of allocating specific treatments and services among competing individuals with rival claims for health care. And while the health-care systems that have developed around the world can be seen as attempts to justly allocate their society's medical resources, the problems they create and the needs they fail to address show that they all have to go further toward creating equitable systems. The discussions of the distinctive needs of various social groups illuminate their special medically related concerns and how social arrangements contribute to the complexity of designing and implementing a socially just health-care system. Yet, the insight from appreciating problems of particular social groups tells us little about how to order their distinctive priorities when limited resources make it impossible to satisfy everyone's desire for medical treatment and health services.

In Part II Tony Hope, John Reynolds, and Siân Griffiths explained the details of how decisions are made for allocation of services within their local British health council, the Oxfordshire Priorities Forum. The chapters in Part IV move on from the discussion of the practical decision-making process to address a range of dilemmas that arise when health systems have to set priorities in allocation. The authors writing for this section draw on a range of theoretical tools and challenge some of their implications in speaking directly to the kinds of issues that must be confronted when health-care systems make policy decisions about which treatments or individuals should be given priority. These chapters address dilemmas about which differences between patients deserve special consideration and which should be ignored, which treatment outcomes should be weighed in allocation decisions, and which needs or desires should be satisfied by using medical resources. These are sub-tle but significant issues with great relevance in determining the justice of health-care systems.

In Part IV, the opening chapter by E. Haavi Morreim discusses justice in funding for alternative medicine while the chapter by Rosamond Rhodes examines justice in transplant organ allocation. Both authors identify the kinds of extraneous ideas and agendas that can and do infiltrate systems that are supposed to allocate medical care justly. The chapters by Dan Brock, F.M. Kamm, and Jerome Bickenbach raise important questions of how a just system should treat background differences in health status. The importance of these issues may not be apparent until we actually try to assess a system that allocates medical resources or try to apply theoretical positions in allocating medical care. Even then the problems are hard to identify and the solutions even harder to find. Lance K. Stell's chapter raises the question of how health systems should respond to differences in health status that could be seen as an individual's own responsibility. And the concluding chapters by Mary Anne Warren, Ian R. Holzman, and Leonard Fleck encourage thoughtful attention to the place of desire, as opposed to need, in setting priorities for the allocation of a society's medical resources.

In "Alternative Health Care: Limits of Science and Boundaries of Access," E. Haavi Morreim identifies the sometimes unfounded bias that paints all alternative medicine as quackery and the sometimes unwarranted exaltation that paints all conventional medicine as science. Morreim argues that the gulf between the two is sometimes far less than claimed by those who discredit alternative medicine. Thus, the reasons for allocating resources to conventional medicine, but not offering patients the choice of alternative medicine, are not as strong as we might have thought. Morreim shows that in many respects conventional medicine does not meet its own scientific ideals: Much cannot be studied, research to translate the discoveries of basic science into clinical practice has been very limited, the complexity and uniqueness of patients narrows the applicability of study findings, and the clinical practice of doctors varies widely with much documented overuse, underuse, and misuse of recognized therapies. Morreim argues that to respond appropriately to the health-related needs of patients, health-care financing plans must avoid a double standard by using the same criteria for evaluating conventional and alternative modalities. An equitable (just) system should promote good care within prudent limits by avoiding waste and harm and by requiring empirical substantiation of the value of all interventions, the conventional as well as the alternative ones.

Systems for allocating organs for transplantation vividly exemplify another facet of the problem of justice. In transplantation of vital solid organs, the scarcity of what is to be distributed is glaringly obvious, while the political forces that affect allocation policy are hard to see and the injustices that result even harder to discern. In "Justice in Transplant Organ Allocation," Rosamond Rhodes explains the complex national system for allocating transplant organs in the United States. She argues that a just system should attend to the most important concerns of those whose interests are relevant. In transplantation the relevant parties are those who need a transplant organ, and their priorities consist of getting an organ, having a successful transplant, and receiving fair treatment from the system. Yet, the dramatic disparity in waiting times for transplantation and the disparate treatment for groups of people who need a transplant organ indicate the injustice of the current United Network for Organ Sharing system despite its rhetorical commitment to justice, equity, and efficacy. The author explains how policymakers and other interested parties subvert justice by supporting policies that promote their private and irrelevant agendas at the expense of those who are entitled to justice. These agendas of other parties have

to be identified, discounted, and not allowed to intrude on the design and implementation of organ allocation policy. In view of how crucial medical resources are to the well-being of the individuals who depend upon the system for distributive justice, those who assess systems need to be alert, vigilant, and wary of how statements of goals, surveys, and data can disguise injustice and make it look like justice.

Some people are better off than others. With respect to health, some are worse off in that they have some disability or some congenital or acquired chronic disease that is thought to make their quality of life worse than other people. In allocating medical care and in assessing the justice of health-care systems, we have to decide how such differences in background health should be weighed. Does being worse off merit higher priority in the allocation of medical resources as a means of compensation? Or, instead, should those who are worse off have lower priority because a year of their lives seems less valuable than an equally long life for people without disabilities or chronic illness? Or should the deciding factor be the significance of the difference that treatment could make in the patient's life, rather than how healthy the person will be compared to others?

Dan Brock responds to three questions about this issue in his chapter titled "Priority to the Worse Off in Health-Care Resource Prioritization." Brock considers various moral justifications for giving priority to the worse off, and he points out the differences in the goals of improving the condition of the worse off, improving outcomes for the worse off, responding to different reasons for the disadvantages of the worse off, enhancing equality of opportunity for the worse off, and other ways of understanding these issues. He also raises the question of who the worse off are—those who are sicker? those with overall worse health? those with life-threatening conditions? those with chronically poor health? Brock then considers how priorities should be set among them and how great the priority given to the worse off should be—a mild preference? a sizable advantage? a trump card over all other claims? Although Brock does not defend any particular solution to the questions he raises, he does make a strong case that justice requires paying special attention to these issues in the development of health-care allocation systems. In the end, we are left with the sense that Brock is convinced by the work of philosophers Rawls, Daniels, Parfit, Scanlon, and Nagel that the worse off, but perhaps not the worst off, have some claim to priority in the allocation of medical resources.

F.M. Kamm raises the question of priority in her discussion of how a health-care system should make choices between individuals in its allocation of scarce and expensive resources. In "Whether to Discontinue *Non*futile Use of a Scarce Resource," Kamm specifically discusses the use of the drug clozopine in the treatment of schizophrenia, but her arguments can be extrapolated to decisions about the allocation of any scarce and expensive resource, such as the limited number of beds in an intensive care unit, and to broader issues of system design and assessment. Appealing to both intuition and reason in considering a range of relevant cases, Kamm holds that the extent of needs of patients who are worse off than others, the outcomes of treating them, and the urgency of doing so should all be considered. Nevertheless, Kamm ultimately concludes that we should take into account only the likelihood for significantly better outcomes, but not for small improvements, when it comes to making decisions between individuals who have a similarly urgent need for medical resources.

Jerome Bickenbach argues against those who oppose "prioritarianism" and who, instead, adopt the utilitarian economic position that discounts years of suboptimal life. In his chapter on "Disability, Justice, and Health Systems Performance Assessment," Bickenbach discusses the justice of the framework that supports the *World*

Health Report issued by the World Health Organization (WHO) in 2000. After carefully explaining how the report integrates the assessment of (1) the health of a population, (2) responsiveness in terms of treating people promptly with respect for their dignity and their wishes, and (3) fair financing in its evaluation of the health systems of 191 countries, Bickenbach questions whether the framework disadvantages people with disabilities, with chronic illness, and the elderly. He argues that by focusing on economic costs, the *World Health Report* undervalues fairness and other important human values. Reading what Bickenbach has to say in light of Brock's discussion of those who are worse off than most others, and Kamm's point about the importance of distinguishing significant from insignificant differences and only taking significant ones into account in the allocation of health care, suggests that disability-adjusted life expectancy (DALE), which is the performance matrix adopted in the WHO *Report*, makes unjust distinctions by discounting the value of every suboptimal life.

Lance K. Stell focuses on a different issue in his chapter on "Responsibility for Health Status." Some people are good stewards of their health; others abuse their bodies, take large risks, and fail to adhere to recommended medical protocols. Stell questions whether society or health-care systems have the same responsibility to the responsible as they do to the irresponsible. He points out many philosophical difficulties in drawing a sharp line between action for which individuals are accountable and behavior that has an involuntary component and, therefore, makes the individual seem less culpable. While the cost of holding people strictly accountable for their health status would be the denial of treatment in a huge number of cases, Stell points out that there also are serious costs in not holding people responsible. Lack of accountability tends to make people less risk averse, therefore increasing the burdens on the system and forcing more rationing on other grounds. From a moral point of view, because expecting accountability and respecting autonomy go hand in hand, forgoing accountability involves the sacrifice of respect. Stell's discussion shows how the tension in moral philosophy between respect and benevolence recurs for decisions about the just allocation of medical resources.

Mary Anne Warren argues that the importance most people place on procreation supports the claim that a just distribution of medical resources should provide resources for assisted reproduction. In her chapter, "Does Distributive Justice Require Universal Access to Assisted Reproduction?," she comes to the conclusion that because of the high cost and low rate of in vitro fertilization (IVF) success, distributive justice does not require universal access to all forms and unlimited tries at assisted reproduction. Nevertheless, because most people see great value in having children, at least a modest subsidy should be universally provided. Furthermore, Warren argues that any limitations on access to assisted reproduction must not be discriminatory. Denials should only be grounded on differences in efficacy or on the inability of individuals to provide responsible parenting.

Ian R. Holzman discusses the medical treatment that is provided and withheld from seriously compromised newborns. As Holzman explains in "Premature and Compromised Neonates," the decision about whether or not to provide or continue aggressive care for such infants often turns on the parents' desire to either pursue treatment because they value the small chance of success or to withhold or withdraw treatment because they see the burdens of treatment as not being worth the small possibility of limited success. Although neonatal intensive care is expensive, decisions about treatment provision or limitation frequently reflect the family's desires as well as the more typical standards of need, urgency, and cost containment. Holzman notes, however, that any policy to limit treatment for neonates in the United States will have to address racial, cultural, and religious concerns as well as desire, need, urgency, and costs. Because there is a higher incidence of prematurity among the urban poor, particularly among the urban African-American poor, any limitation on treatment for seriously compromised neonates would fall disproportionately on that population.

Part IV concludes with Leonard M. Fleck addressing issues that will arise with the dawn of genetic medicine. In his chapter, "Just Caring: Do Future Possible Children Have a Just Claim to a Sufficiently Healthy Genome?," Fleck focuses on preimplantation genetic diagnosis (PGD), a genetic technology that is already available. Couples who know that they are at risk of having a child with a serious genetic disorder can use IVF technology to create embryos that can be tested for the specific genetic defect. Only embryos without the defect would be candidates for implantation. Fleck argues that support for PGD is warranted by justice because having a child without a serious genetic disorder reflects equal access to effective procreative liberty and the social commitment to preventing deep human suffering. At the same time, Fleck argues that commitments to liberal pluralism require that resources should be made available to support the choices of both couples who choose to employ the technology and couples who choose to take their chances without it. An equitable health-care system is committed to tolerance and respect and, therefore, accommodates diverse reasonable conceptions of a good life.

26

Alternative Health Care: Limits of Science and Boundaries of Access

E. Haavi Morreim

The past decade has witnessed a rapid growth of interest in complementary and alternative medicine—approaches to health, illness, and healing that often differ markedly from conventional Western medicine. The range is broad, from spiritual and mind–body approaches, to manual healing approaches, to dietary and nutritional emphases and beyond.[1] Eisenberg and colleagues found that in 1990 Americans spent nearly $14 billion on such alternatives, three-quarters of that sum out of pocket. There were more visits to unconventional providers than to all primary care physicians combined, and the people most commonly using alternatives were relatively affluent and well educated.[2] By the time Eisenberg and co-workers revisited the question in 1997, there had been a 47% increase in the number of visits to alternative practitioners, and a 45% increase in spending. The great majority of people declined to tell their regular physicians about their use of alternatives.[3]

Commentators point to a variety of factors behind this rising interest. Medical science achieves dazzling rescues for life-threatening illnesses, but it offers rather less for debilitating chronic illnesses. Moreover, some of the alternatives at which Western medicine once scoffed are now seen to have merit, including acupuncture, chiropractic, guided imagery, support groups, nutrition, herbs, even leeches.[4] Additionally, with managed-care organizations imposing "productivity" expectations, physicians have less time for the personal touch many patients deeply desire. Partly through these limits, and partly through headlines trumpeting medical errors and malpractice litigation, the physician's halo seems a bit tarnished.

Across the spectrum of these changes, society faces some interesting issues. On the one hand, many people believe they should have better access to alternatives, and some health plans and even legislatures have expanded financial coverage for patients to visit nonmedical providers.[5] On the other hand, with annual costs of health care over

319

a trillion dollars, and with around 40 million Americans still uninsured, many critics caution against wasting money on alternatives that may be quackery.[6]

As we assess such criticisms and consider whether society should accept or even fund alternatives, we need to look at a few issues more deeply. In particular, it will be important to examine the view, articulated by some critics, that alternatives should be accepted—or more commonly, rejected—on the basis of their scientific validity. As this chapter will argue, such critics tend to overestimate the extent to which traditional medical practice is science-based, while potentially underestimating the value of at least some alternative modalities. Instead, a temperate approach should guide our decisions about whether and when society should accept or fund access to alternative health care.

I do not purport to resolve these difficult issues here. Nor should this chapter be read as an assault against conventional Western medicine. Rather, the goal is to dislodge a few preconceptions and thereby to enable a fresher, more carefully reasoned assessment as we weigh profoundly different healing approaches against one another.

RADICALLY DIFFERENT PERSPECTIVES

Perhaps the most common complaint about alternatives is that these approaches typically embrace metaphysical entities and forces that cannot possibly be evaluated scientifically. For instance, "[i]n many traditional medical systems, the primary explanation for biological phenomena is based on the existence of a 'vital force,' an elusive entity designated *Qi* in China, *Ki* in Korea and Japan, *prana* in India, and *vital force* in Western traditions (e.g., homeopathy)."[7] In Chinese medicine, *qi* is said to move "through the body along invisible meridians. Good health depends on the proper flow of this energy; disease and pain are the result of qi out of kilter."[8]

Such invisibles, postulated to be the foundation of both wellness and disease, intrinsically elude the scientific study that is the hallmark of Western medicine, thus inviting some commentators to conclude they must surely be fictional.[9] Moreover, critics argue, such fantasies can usually be explained much more straightforwardly. Where that is the case, then "we have wasted a lot of time and effort. The time has been wasted on all the people who have spent years learning falsehoods about acupuncture points and the principles of homeopathy. And the patients have wasted their time, money, and efforts receiving treatments that were not what they were represented to be or were harmful."[10]

Such criticisms seem to presuppose that medicine itself is free of metaphysics—that the science on which it relies is the direct, unencumbered product of observation available to all who care to look, leading to conclusions that are available to anyone who cares to be rational. No unseen Mysterious Forces.

On closer inspection, however, medical science has a metaphysic of its own. It presupposes a certain picture of the way the world is and functions. That picture has its distinctive epistemology (i.e., its own approach to how we identify and gather knowledge), and on the whole is just as unprovable as any spiritual entity or lifeforce. Several elements in this implicit picture can be identified.

First, the world is seen to be finite and sensible. Its constituent entities are observable to the senses, and can be measured and counted. If something cannot be observed, measured, and counted, then it is "off the radar screen," at least from the perspective of medical science.

Second, it is assumed that all people with the requisite sensory capacities have basically the same sensory experiences of the world, so that observations about the world's phenomena are intersubjectively confirmable. Thus, what I personally experience in association with the words "blue" or "acrid" is essentially the same as your experiences. A phenomenon or experience that only one person can perceive is relegated to the domain of anecdote or even illusion, not a fit object of scientific knowledge.

Third, the world is orderly, and this order persists through time via immutable laws of nature. Tested generalizations will be just as true tomorrow as they are today—otherwise there would be no point in doing science at all, because we could not build our knowledge over time by relying on yesterday's observations as we add today's. In this way, the truths of science are found in reliable patterns, not lone events.

Finally, science holds that understanding the laws of nature gives us predictability and control. We can use the forces of nature as tools to make things happen the way we want them to, at least up to the limits of our knowledge and power.

Although these precepts are regarded as obvious and immutable truths, however, such empiricism and materialism[11] are no more "provable" than *qi, prana*, or any other metaphysic. Philosophers have long pointed out, for example, that no argument or evidence can possibly justify our presumption that the world is orderly or that this order must persist over time. Illustrating this "problem of induction,"[12] as it is called, they note that we cannot conclude the sun will rise in the east tomorrow by pointing to the fact that it always has done so in the past. After all, the reliability of the past as a predictor of the future is the very issue in question. Neither can we prove that everything in the world is (at least in principle) available to human empirical observation and measurement, because we cannot see what is beyond human vision or hear what is beyond our auditory apparatus in order to document that "there's nothing more out there."

The upshot is that, for any healing approach, whether religious or scientific, certain fundamental beliefs must simply be taken as "givens" without any possibility

of conclusive proof, lest we land in an infinite regress of proofs-for-the-proof. Accordingly, on the metaphysical and epistemic plane at least, we are left with a collection of irreducible contrasts. Just as science assumes everything is controlled by natural laws, a religious approach will hold that its healing God is not obligated to follow laws of nature, because God made those laws and can change or override them at will. For medicine, even thousands of years of accumulated experience within a given tradition, such as Aryuvedic medicine, will not count as evidence in the absence of properly controlled trials to distinguish between a law-governed pattern and pure happenstance. In contrast, many alternatives are willing to find knowledge in received traditions, in lone events, or in subjective experiences like personal revelations from a deity.

Each perspective then interprets its successes or failures from within the rules and framework of that perspective. The faith healer will confront a failure with "he just needed a little more faith" or "God works in mysterious ways." He will not conclude, if his patient dies, that "there is no God, after all." By the same token, the physician whose patient dies will not conclude that "science is bogus." He will say "we just need a little more data" or a better theory. By the same token, where an alternative approach ostensibly cures a patient whom medicine had declared to be incurable—the "miracle" cancer cure—the medical scientist will not conclude the alternative approach is correct after all. Rather, he will question the original diagnosis or call the healing unexplained, with the proviso that one day it will be scientifically accounted for.

In this way, conventional medicine stands philosophically more on a par with alternatives than its proponents may recognize. If medicine can criticize Chinese medicine or faith healing because it "violates fundamental scientific laws,"[13] an alternative can criticize medicine for its own failure, e.g., to honor the supreme principles of balance and harmony in the universe. Each criticism is made from within a framework that is itself presupposed as true.

MEASURING UP TO SCIENCE

Proponents of conventional medicine have sometimes proposed that alternatives might be acceptable, but only if they measure up to the rigorous standards of science. There are two problems with such a requirement. First, many alternatives are not conceptually oriented toward the tidy world of measurability, quantifiability, orderliness, predictability, and control embodied in a scientific approach. To require them to do so would be to distort their essential character. Second, medicine itself often cannot measure up to its own scientific standards, for reasons of both principle and practicality. Hence, this section will suggest that a rigid demand for thoroughgoing science cannot be met even by medicine, and should not necessarily be required of alternatives.

Science and Alternatives

From the perspective of some alternatives, gathering empirical data is a fundamentally wrongheaded way to search for truth. Spiritual healing, for instance, may emanate from historic teachings or divine revelations that come through opening one's heart rather than opening one's eyes, ears, or toolbox.

Other kinds of alternative medicine are more amenable to tracking empirical connections between healing inputs and patients' outcomes, but they do not necessarily lend themselves well to classic science, in which study subjects are narrowly selected to exclude confounding factors, and in which all study subjects receive the same inputs to facilitate the cleanest statistical analysis. Homeopathy, for instance, emphasizes highly individualized diagnoses and treatments—not really compatible

with the standard randomized, controlled trial (RCT) in which everyone in a given group receives exactly the same dose of the same treatment.[14] Similarly, acupuncture cannot easily accommodate classical placebo controls without introducing conceptual distortions into its theory and practice.[15]

Accordingly, to require alternatives to meet medicine's criteria of scientific validity may do them an injustice. A science-style "controlled evaluation of alternative medicine therapies may require its practitioners to undertake a fundamental conceptual shift from a view of patients as requiring individualized treatment that may vary at each session to one in which trial participants are regarded as members of an equivalence class, defined by the diagnosis, who all will be given a standard prescribed treatment."[16] Again, this does not entail that alternatives are excluded from science altogether. More will be said on this below. But it may mean that the science by which they are evaluated will look more like paleontology or geology than like highly controlled laboratory experiments.[17]

Science and Medicine

If various alternatives do not quite fit with classical bench science, conventional medicine actually shares that difficulty. There are many respects in which medical practice does not, and in important respects can never, meet its own scientific ideal. The reasons are both philosophical and practical.

Philosophical obstacles to science in medicine
Science's focus on that which can be defined, observed, measured, enumerated, and statistically analyzed tends to leave out whatever is not amenable to such precision. If something cannot be counted, it does not count. And yet even devoted scientists recognize that this rigorous standard leaves out many factors that can be important in medicine and other human endeavors.[18] For instance, one obviously important as-

pect of health and health care is quality of life. Although various measures are available, none are entirely satisfactory.[19] As a result, many studies of medical interventions look only at the intervention's effects on major morbidity and mortality, while those that do assess quality of life (QL) are subject to criticism because the QL measures are so flawed.

An even more potent example is the *placebo effect*. Although placebos usually take the form of a pill, injection, or infusion with no medically active ingredient, the more important factor is the placebo effect, i.e., the power of belief, expectation, hope, trust that comes with the patient's anticipation of healing. With placebo alone, patients can experience marked improvement in their condition, or can even suffer significant side effects.[20] That much is well documented. This effect it so powerful it can confound any research if not appropriately controlled for. Hence, gold-standard science requires double-blinding: Where neither the investigator nor the subject knows which treatment the subject is receiving, it is more difficult for the hopes and expectations—the states of mind of both sides—to precipitate biological changes that could distort any findings regarding the drug, device, or other intervention under study.[21]

Interestingly, however, once controlled research has deemed an intervention effective, the placebo tends to be regarded essentially as "nothing," so that conclusions from the research typically imply that the intervention is better (or not) than no treatment at all. Sullivan (1993) explains the implications:

The healing power of the placebo arises from the therapeutic encounter and alters the physiology of the body according to the nature of that encounter. It is unlikely that this power has any single biochemical identity within the body throughout its varied applications. It is thus essentially different from the specific/pharmacological healing proffered by orthodox medicine. ... Within placebo-mediated healing, knowing

and healing are directly linked. A shift in beliefs is therapeutic. . . . [Thus] placebo-induced therapeutic changes are specifically those successes which are illegitimate for orthodox scientific medicine.[22]

The result is almost paradoxical. On the one hand, medical science recognizes the extraordinary power of placebo, and must design research around its potentially confounding effects. On the other hand, in the aftermath of those studies, medicine relegates this avowedly powerful mode of influencing body processes to the "art" of medicine. It is not an art that many physicians study or cultivate, and when alternative healers harness it effectively, it is usually dubbed "mere" placebo.[23] Reciprocally, if a patient is made considerably better by placebo, a common inference is that the problem must not have been "real" to begin with. So, one wonders, which is it: a force so powerful it can thwart the best research and overshadow powerful medicinals, or a meager result that alternatives produce because they cannot cause "real" healing.

Aside from discounting whatever cannot be precisely measured and enumerated, medical science faces other philosophical limits. Ethical constraints, for instance, restrict research topics and methods. Theoretically, the best way to learn how a new drug treats an illness would be to give people the disease—exactly the same strain of the bacterium or virus to each person—and then administer the drug. But such a research design is ordinarily unethical, and so we must find people who already have the illness in question. And then we can only request, not require, them to participate. In the same vein, randomization is sometimes precluded by patients' preferences. In studies comparing lumpectomy with mastectomy for breast cancer, women's refusal to leave such an important choice to chance required modification of the usual randomization procedures.[24] Ethical concerns also have restricted testing potentially harmful drugs on children and pregnant women, and have limited the use of placebo ("sham") arms in surgery trials. Requirements are now emerging to improve the rigor of surgical research and to test products more thoroughly on women and children before offering them for widespread use, because where they are untested, then in essence the intervention is experimental for everyone.[25] Still, such research can only place limited risk on study subjects.[26] In all these instances, the rigor of research designs must be attenuated to accommodate other values.

In sum, science cannot, even in principle, tell us about everything that is significant in illness and healing. Important factors will always be left out, namely those that are not amenable to satisfactory quantification and those that cannot be studied for other reasons, such as ethical constraints.

Practical obstacles to science in medicine
Science in medicine also faces practical constraints. For instance, it is impossible to do double-blinded trials in surgery, for obviously the surgeon must see what he is doing. Likewise, differences in skills among practitioners, and evolution of each practitioner's skills over time, are difficult to control for. The same is true for psychotherapy, which is additionally complicated by variations in the interpersonal chemistry between individual therapists and patients.

Research is also very costly, particularly because studies must usually be large in order to attain statistical significance. We cannot afford to study everything that needs scientific evaluation, nor to replicate important results, nor to undertake new studies every time a technology or its use is revised. Further, funding for the great majority of medical research comes either from manufacturers of drugs, devices, and other products, or from government. Thus, a research proposal must usually be either commercially or politically attractive if it is to be funded.[27] Garas and others have observed this close connection between science and funding in conjunction with clon-

idine, a very effective and inexpensive drug for congestive heart failure:

[D]espite multiple efforts, there has been no interest so far from anyone to fund large controlled studies to demonstrate the long-term impact of these alterations on patient outcome. The clinically observed benefits of clonidine in heart failure are known to a small circle of academic cardiologists, but the primary care physicians who treat 90% of patients with chronic heart failure are totally unaware of them.[28]

As a result of these myriad impediments, many important topics in medicine have never been studied, or are not studied soon enough.[29] For instance, as of 1988, a national conference on antithrombotic therapy (anticlotting treatments used to prevent stroke, pulmonary embolism, and the like) evaluated the scientific foundation for various recommendations on which physicians based treatment. The American College of Chest Physicians found that only 24% of those recommendations were based on appropriately scientific studies, whereas 55% were based on uncontrolled clinical observations. Ten years later, 44% of the recommendations were science-based, though this was largely because of Food and Drug Administration (FDA) requirements for the testing of new drugs.[30] Similarly, although coronary artery bypass surgery was first performed in 1964, its efficacy was not scientifically evaluated until 1977. Likewise, angioplasty to open up clogged arteries in the heart was "performed in hundreds of thousands of patients prior to the first randomized clinical trial demonstrating efficacy in 1992."[31] "When The U.S. Preventive Services Task Force reviewed more than 6,000 studies on 200 clinical preventive practices, it concluded that very few are supported by sound scientific evidence."[32] The now-defunct Office of Technology Assessment "estimated that fewer than 30% of procedures currently used in conventional medicine have been rigorously tested," and some other assessments conclude the figure is even smaller.[33]

Aside from these significant limits on the content and scope of scientific research, the translation of research into the clinical care of individual patients deviates even further from science. On the whole, the more pristine the science, the less it is applicable to actual clinical care. This is because, to test strictly for the effects of a specific drug or procedure, study design must be limited to patients fitting a narrow set of eligibility criteria—typically, patients with a minimum of other diseases and medications that could confound the findings.[34] Once the study is complete, however, its results are applied to all those complex patients who would never have been eligible for the study.[35] Thus, the more perfectly scientific and highly controlled a study is, the less its enrolled subjects resemble the ordinary souls, with their multiple problems, for whom ordinary physicians care.

One result of this misfit between the research populations and the broader clinical population is that sometimes even well-researched new drugs and procedures must be quickly withdrawn from the market because of unanticipated problems. Between September 1997 and September 1998, five FDA-approved drugs were removed from the market because of unexpected side effects or interactions with other medications. For instance, by the time mibefradil (Posicor) was removed, it was known to interact with 26 different drugs.[36]

Implications

Between the dearth of studies and the finite applicability of existing studies to the care of individual patients, physicians would be hard-pressed to claim that their care is exclusively or even always primarily a direct application of science to clinical practice. This is not to deny that clinical medicine is science-based in many respects. Physicians are increasingly practicing "evidence-based" medicine, in which the routine care of routine situations is based on the most up-to-date, scientifically validated approaches to a given problem. Additionally, many illnesses and injuries exist for which

a broad consensus guides care. In puzzling situations physicians can also, of course, refer to their basic knowledge of human physiology, anatomy, and the like, to hypothesize what should, in theory at least, be the right approach for the patient.

Though important and useful, these strategies cannot entirely compensate for the lack of studies or for the inapplicability of existing studies to individual patients. In actual practice, "doctors usually rely on a combination of habit and casual intuition, using tests and treatments they are familiar with, have heard good things about, or seem to work in test tubes or laboratory animals."[37]

Moreover, treating patients on the basis of hypotheses, absent real research, can be disastrous. Recently, two theoretically attractive interventions have shown those hazards. Pulmonary artery catheterization, widely in use for three decades, is only now coming under scientific scrutiny as recent reports suggest it may actually do more harm than good.[38] Similarly, autologous bone marrow transplant was used to treat breast cancer for more than a decade. There was never any real evidence the treatment would work,[39] only a bit of theory and physicians' desire to do something—anything—to help patients for whom they had little to offer. Not until 1999, when studies were finally completed, did it become evident that the treatment is no better than conventional chemotherapy.[40] Numerous treatments in the history of medicine have been widely adopted and then later found to be ineffective.[41]

The upshot is a mixed review. Medicine can justly pride itself on a wide array of stunning successes, attributable in large part to scientific research. At the same time, science cannot possibly be the sole basis on which physicians care for patients. There is too much that has never been studied and too much that, for many reasons, can never be adequately studied. Much research leaves out or vastly underrates avowedly important aspects of illness and healing, and even the best studies cannot be applied in any straightforward way to individual patients. Physicians' practices vary widely, in ways that cannot be explained by differences among patients.[42] As a further practical reality, physicians' actual practices often do not implement what science is available. Overuse, underuse, and misuse of recognized treatments is now recognized as a major problem throughout medicine.[43] Although best-evidence approaches are steadily improving clinical care, large portions of medicine are not, and never will be, scientific.

Interestingly, many practicing physicians have articulated a similar conclusion when protesting managed-care efforts to reduce the variation in clinical practices or to control costs.[44] Partly they note that many of the guidelines on which health plans rely are not based on good science.[45] But even with scientifically credible guidelines, medicine cannot be practiced by "cookbook," they argue, because no guidelines can be sufficiently accurate, complete, up-to-date, and detailed to dictate the care of specific patients; care must be individualized.

This becomes, perhaps, the most important conclusion from all of the foregoing discussion: Medical research and clinical care, while related, are very different enterprises. While the former can strive for great precision in the strongest traditions of science, the latter will forever be a far more intuitive, use-your-best-judgment, rely-on-experience kind of enterprise—the "art" of medicine. It is the very sort of cumulative experience-based healing on which many alternatives also heavily rely.

ADDRESSING THE TENSIONS: HOW SHOULD HEALTH PLANS RESPOND

At this juncture, important questions arise concerning how society, and its health plans in particular, should respond to the public's increasing interest in alternatives. Simplistic answers will not suffice because, as observed above, medicine cannot conform fully to its own scientific ideal, and in any case science cannot likely claim a mo-

nopoly on effective healing. A temperate approach thus seems appropriate, acknowledging that there may be more than one way to understand what illness is, and that healing might come through a diversity of avenues.

As an initial move, it is important to avoid double standards that would hold alternatives to a standard of proof that medicine itself cannot meet.[46] When alternative providers emphasize individualizing care they should not be called "unscientific" if, at the same time, clinical physicians who likewise individualize their interventions are approvingly regarded as practicing the "art" of medicine.[47] The successes of alternatives cannot be dismissed as mere "anecdotes" and "testimonials," if we accept as authoritative statements by physicians that "my patients have done well/poorly with this treatment," or "in my clinical experience X has worked well." When alternative providers invoke the power of belief and expectation it should not be dubbed "mere placebo," if at the same time we permit doctors to invoke the "power of the white coat" or to foster "a certain mystique" in the physician–patient relationship. An alternative is not "peddling false hope" if, in a comparable situation, physicians might paint overly optimistic pictures on the ground that "we can't take away the patient's hope."[48]

At the same time, even an open-minded approach to alternatives does not resolve the challenges that health plans and society now face. If some alternatives offer bona fide help for some patients and some conditions, there is also undoubtedly a significant measure of quackery and sheer hucksterism in the current turbulent health-care market. Society thus faces an array of questions, such as whether to regulate alternatives, requiring them to demonstrate that they are at least safe if not also effective; whether to license alternative practitioners such as homeopaths or acupuncturists and, if so, how to set the applicable standards; whether to add any alternative healing modalities to government-sponsored health plans such as Medicare, or to require such coverage in federal employees' health plans.

Such societal issues are beyond the scope of this chapter, but it would be useful to explore a related question, namely how health plans should respond to increasing pressures to cover alternatives. The issues will not be resolved in this brief forum, but a few basic considerations can be suggested. We will first consider benefits and harms, then economic concerns.

Benefits and Harms

Perhaps the most powerful reason Western medicine has such preeminence is the simple fact that, for many diseases and injuries, its treatments often work so well.[49] Infectious diseases are a classic example: A pathogen is identified and drugs are developed that literally, dramatically, save a life. Organ transplants with antirejection treatment, joint replacements, and limb reattachments are but a small sampling from the rest of the list.

Still, it is widely agreed that there are many problems, particularly those involving chronic illness, that medicine does not address so well. Moreover, treatments sometimes carry a terrible price. A recent meta-analysis found that more than 100,000 people die annually from adverse drug reactions in U.S. hospitals, placing these events between the fourth and sixth leading cause of death.[50] Many of those drug reactions are not the product of error, but rather are side effects of known incidence whose possibility has been accepted as part of a risk-benefit assessment. In a related area, a recent study by the Institute of Medicine estimates that as many as 98,000 individuals per year may be dying from medical errors—ranking medical error as the eighth leading cause of death, killing more Americans than motor vehicle accidents, breast cancer, or AIDS.[51] To be sure, one cannot blame conventional medicine per se for these errors, and yet health care delivery has become so complex that quite likely some significant level of error

will always be a problem, even if that level can be reduced from present levels.

On the other side of the coin, relatively few data have been gathered regarding the risks of various alternatives, though surely there are some hazards. Herbal preparations, for instance, can react with other drugs, although exact profiles have yet to be established. Manufacturing problems can adversely affect quality, and there may be toxicities that have not yet been precisely identified.[52] In the same vein, chiropractic, improperly applied, can sometimes cause serious injury. Nevertheless, many alternative approaches, such as acupuncture, homeopathy, biofeedback, or guided imagery,[53] use such noninvasive, benign modalities that they pose few obvious risks as long as they do not prompt patients to forgo treatments of proven value.

At the same time, many patients have found great benefit in alternatives—enough value that in 1997 they were willing to invest over $20 billion in alternatives, including more than $12 billion out of their own pockets—more than the out-of-pocket expenditures for all U.S. hospitalizations.[54] Willingness to pay does not equate with successful outcomes, of course, yet it is reasonable to suppose that some significant measure of value was perceived, else these figures would not have risen so markedly since 1990.[55]

If this risk–benefit picture is anywhere near accurate, it is difficult to argue that alternatives should be simply forbidden, or even that people should always be required to try Western medicine first. Autonomous adults are entitled to make their own choices for their own reasons, even if sometimes foolishly.[56] In fact, use of alternatives seems to be quite judicious thus far. Most people still seek out Western medicine where it offers clear, major benefits, and they turn to alternative treatments where medical science has the least to offer—chronic illnesses, disabling conditions, medically incurable diseases, and the like.[57] The major exceptions are people with univocal dedication to a faith tradition such as

Christian Science. Accordingly, as long as an alternative is not demonstrably harmful or fraudulent it ought, prima facie at least, to be permitted.

If various alternatives should still be freely available in the marketplace, the more pressing question is whether and under what conditions health plans should cover them.[58]

Costs and Coverage

As we consider whether health plans should cover alternatives, and if so which ones, several potential criteria come to mind. As a first attempt, if one wants to be sure that the common funds that health plans use for all their enrollees are not wasted, one might propose that plans should only cover interventions that are shown to be of value by the best-quality science. Such a stiff criterion must quickly be discarded, however. As noted above, many areas of medicine, from surgery to psychiatry to epidemiology, do not always lend themselves to classic "gold-standard" RCTs. And much of clinical medicine can make only limited use of RCT science, since ordinary patients are more complex than the narrowly chosen subjects of research trials. This first criterion would surely save money, but only by denying patients a wide array of helpful care—hardly the purpose of a good health plan.

An alternative, looser criterion might require that there be at least some science to substantiate the value of an intervention, or a healing approach, before it will be covered. There is much to recommend such an approach. One reason an empirical, science-based approach is attractive is its intersubjectivity. We need not simply trust one person's report that something works or doesn't; we can use a fairly clear set of rules for gathering evidence via shared observation, and for discerning which conclusions are warranted by that evidence. We can be reasonably confident that treatments passing such a test will work for many people, even if there is no guarantee. When common funds are involved, that in-

tersubjective agreement is appealing because we want shared resources to be used well.

In that spirit, recent studies suggest that, under such a criterion, health plans might be obligated to cover a number of alternatives. Recent research suggests that:

- transcendental meditation appears to be just as effective as drugs in the treatment of mild hypertension[59]
- spinal manipulative therapy may be the most effective, cost-effective treatment in many cases of acute low back pain[60]
- auricular acupuncture appears to be of significantly greater value in treating cocaine dependence than relaxation treatment or "sham" needle insertion[61]
- individualized Chinese herbal preparations are of significant value in treatment of irritable bowel syndrome[62]
- a yoga-based regimen is more effective than wrist splinting or no treatment in relieving symptoms and signs of carpal tunnel syndrome[63]
- saw palmetto extract produces similar improvement with fewer side effects in the treatment of benign prostatic hypertrophy, compared with the drug finasteride[64]
- asthma patients who wrote about their stressful experiences in a journal experienced significant, clinically relevant changes in their health status[65]
- horse chestnut seed extract is significantly effective in treating chronic venous insufficiency[66]
- willow bark extract may be safe and effective for exacerbations of low back pain[67]
- a specific nutrition regimen cannot only stop but reverse some coronary artery disease[68]
- aroma therapy has shown success in treatment of alopecia areata[69]
- remote intercessory prayer appears effective in improving the overall condition of critically ill patients and may be an effective adjunct to care[70]
- weekly support groups and self-hypnosis

were associated with doubling the survival of women with advanced breast cancer.[71]

This looser criterion would admit a much wider array of care, both conventional and alternative, than the first one. Yet even here, some very helpful modalities might still be excluded. After all, conventional Western medicine unavoidably goes well beyond the limited number of studies for which scarce research funding is available, and a mandate to provide specific scientific backing for each intervention—even shy of gold-standard RCTs—would obligate us to throw out a substantial portion of day-to-day medicine. Up to a point, such pruning would be desirable. The quest for evidence-based medicine is grounded on a growing recognition that medical care could and should be more effective, and that ineffective care can cause harm as well as waste resources.

Still, a requirement that every intervention have at least some specific scientific support would arguably be hasty. From the bare fact that "there is no evidence" it is simply fallacious to conclude "there is no value." There is simply not enough money to study everything that merits research, whether conventional or alternative. And so it is assured that some useful interventions will never have their value adequately documented. However, once we embrace unsubstantiated conventional medicine, it is not clear on what grounds we can exclude equally unsubstantiated alternatives. As pointed out earlier, some alternatives such as spiritual healing do not lend themselves to standardization and quantification, yet this does not entail that they are worthless. We remain in a quandary, then, if our objective is to draw some sort of fairly "bright line" between that which health plans should fund and that which they should not.

A third criterion might focus on avoiding waste and harm. There is wide agreement that conventional medicine has enormous benefits for most people, and thus is un-

likely to waste much money. In contrast, as long as alternatives have only minimal scientific documentation, the argument might go, they should find their own funding. If and when a particular alternative approach gains scientific ascendancy by proving its worth, then health plans can accept it for coverage.

This approach may sound initially attractive, because it resembles quite closely what most health plans already do. However, its problems quickly become evident. A closer look at conventional medicine suggests that the vast amounts of money it sometimes wastes can make the costs of alternatives pale by comparison. During the decade in which 30,000 women received bone marrow transplant for breast cancer, over $3.4 billion was spent on this nonbeneficial, often harmful, treatment.[72] In the process, additional enormous sums were spent on hundreds of lawsuits that often required health plans to pay for the treatment and in some cases levied millions of dollars in punitive damages against plans.[73] Many families incurred overwhelming personal debts, sometimes losing their homes and retirement funds,[74] to pay for the treatment because doctors said it represented the patient's best or only hope.

Other once-popular, later-disproven treatments tell similar tales of wasted money, from glomectomies for asthma, to photodynamic therapy and organic solvents for herpes simplex infection, to gastric freezing for ulcers.[75] To these we can add ongoing instances of overuse,[76] such as prescriptions for antibiotics that are either clearly unnecessary or more powerful/costly than the patient's illness requires. As also noted above, physicians' clinical practices vary widely, in ways not justified by differences in patients' conditions.[77] While we cannot be certain "which rate is right"[78] for various surgeries, diagnostic interventions, and drug prescriptions, it is safe to suppose that at least some of this variation represents unnecessary care and thereby additional wasted money. Decades of generous fee-for-service funding, combined with defensive medicine and other inflationary pressures, have almost certainly raised medical customs to a level above that which is truly useful.

If high-technology Western medicine is thus capable of such unwise expenditures, it would be awkward to conclude that alternatives should be automatically excluded from coverage simply because they might waste money. At the same time, a reciprocal point should also be emphasized. The bare fact that an alternative may be cheaper does not mean it should be endorsed. As health plans, and the governments and employers who purchase most of them, face relentless pressures to contain the costs of care, and as more information comes to light about the limited evidentiary basis on which conventional medicine must often practice, the possibility exists that plans will not only cover alternatives, but might even mandate or at least encourage their use in cases where there is no evidence to show a superiority of costlier conventional modalities. However, just as "no evidence" does not mean "no value," neither can we conclude that, where two interventions are equally unsupported by evidence, the two must be equally good.

Accordingly, perhaps the proper task should not be understood as a need to identify some criteria by which health plans will "correctly" include or exclude this or that healing modality. Rather, the proper task should be for health plans to find ways to shepherd their resources prudently, whether for conventional or for alternative remedies, while maximizing the good those funds do.

Promoting Good Care Within Prudent Limits

A balanced approach would seem to require several elements. First, plans should leave room for patients themselves to define what constitutes the "good" that health care will provide for them. As long as the evidence is equivocal regarding the benefits and harms of so many modalities, and as long as some of the alternatives that people find very helpful are not amenable

to scientific quantification, across-the-board exclusions of alternatives seem inappropriate. Perhaps a reasonable approach might use the test of time. Long-standing traditions with widespread support, such as acupuncture or chiropractic, might be more readily embraced, while giving "overnight sensations" less credence if they cannot provide more substantial evidence of value. Such an approach would essentially be equivalent to the "physician acceptance" standard on which many plans currently rely for determining whether a new intervention is "medically necessary" or is instead "experimental."

Second, health plans need not all have identical coverage. For a variety of reasons,[79] plans should be permitted openly to provide varying levels of coverage, ranging from basic care to more generous packages. In this setting, the most basic plans might limit coverage—whether of medical or of alternative interventions—to care that has been reasonably well demonstrated to be safe and effective. Broader packages might include various alternatives, alongside broadening access to less well-proven medical procedures.

Third, plans can institute some of the same kinds of cost containment for alternatives, ranging from incentive systems to utilization management and fee scales, that they now exert upon conventional medicine. Admittedly, there is hot debate concerning how appropriate these economic measures are, and yet with the rising cost of care, and millions still uninsured, some kind of cost control is as appropriate as it is inevitable.

Arguably, patients should play a role in the cost containment that governs their own care.[80] In a system where patients share in the costs of their own choices, they have reason to be prudent about the value and the cost of their requests. These financial incentives should not pose barriers to needed care, but they should provide rewards for prudence and an opportunity to consider carefully which care is worthwhile. Various alternatives have been described, from graduated co-payments for prescription medications, to medical savings accounts,[81] to other options. Via whatever plan, the more patients take responsibility for their own utilization management, the less health plans will need to dictate, detail by detail, what they will receive, and the less plans may feel impelled to give physicians incentives to work against their own patients.

Where patients have access to alternatives, combined with incentives to be prudent, health plans can conduct a further kind of research, assessing which alternatives their enrollees actually prefer, whether those modalities produce favorable outcomes, and how the cost for patients who use alternatives compares with those who use only conventional providers. It might be found that a fairly broad access to alternatives can actually save money—for instance, if people suffering from vaguely defined conditions like fibromyalgia find better and cheaper relief from massage than from costly drugs.

With a combination of prudence and open-mindedness, coverage for a reasonable range of alternatives might enhance patients' outcomes and satisfaction without necessarily increasing health-care costs.

CONCLUSION

This is a time of extraordinarily turbulent transition throughout health care. From within and from outside conventional medicine, traditions hitherto unquestioned are being challenged. Although deeply unsettling for many people, wonderful opportunities are also emerging that can improve medicine through its encounters with the strangers from outside and, perhaps even more so, by examining its own most cherished assumptions.

Acknowledgment

The author acknowledges with gratitude the very helpful comments provided on earlier drafts of this chapter by Lawrence J. Schneiderman, M.D., Rosamond Rhodes, Ph.D., and Anita Silvers, Ph.D.

NOTES

1. A lengthy but still incomplete list would include chiropractic, massage, exercise therapy such as Tai Chi or yoga, acupuncture, coining, cupping, homeopathy, naturopathy, herbal medicine, self-help groups, folk remedies, energy healing, relaxation techniques, guided imagery, therapeutic touch, spiritual or faith healing, nutrition and special diets such as macrobiotics or megavitimin therapy, self-help groups, biofeedback, hypnosis, root medicine, aromatherapy, reflexology, prayer, and purification ceremonies.

2. Eisenberg DM, Kessler RC, Foster C, et al. Unconventional medicine in the United States. *New England Journal of Medicine* 1993; 328:246–52 (hereafter *NEJM*).

3. Eisenberg DM, Davis RB, Ettner SL, et al. Trends in alternative medicine use in the United States, 1990–1997. *JAMA* 1998; 280: 1569–75.

4. See below, pp. 328–29.

5. The state of Washington, for instance, has mandated that health plans cover some forms of alternative health care—a statute that courts have upheld. See Wash. Rev. Code § 48.43.045. For cases concerning this statute see *Hoffman v Regence Blue Shield*, 991 P.2d 77 (Wash. 2000); *Washington Physicians Services Ass'n v. Gregoire*, 967 F.Supp. 424 (W.D. Wash. 1997). See also Grandinetti DA. 'Integrated medicine' could boost your income. *Medical Economics* 1997;74(8):73–99, at 74; YaDeau R. Cost-effectiveness and complementary medicine. *Am J Managed Care* 1996; 2: 460; Grandinetti DA. Your newest competitors: Alternative-medicine networks. *Medical Economics* 1999;76(10):44–51.

6. "Roughly a third of unconventional practices entail theories that are patently unscientific and in direct competition with conventional medicine." Campion EW. Why unconventional medicine? *NEJM* 1993;328:282–83, at 282.

"It is time for the scientific community to stop giving alternative medicine a free ride. There cannot be two kinds of medicine—conventional and alternative. There is only medicine that has been adequately tested and medicine that has not, medicine that works and medicine that may or may not work." Angell M, Kassirer JP. Alternative medicine—the risks of untested and unregulated remedies. *NEJM* 1998; 339:839–41, at 841.

7. Eskinazi DP. Factors that shape alternative medicine. *JAMA* 1998; 280: 1621–23, at

1621; see also Kaptchuk TJ, Eisenberg DM. The persuasive appeal of alternative medicine. Ann Intern Med 1998;129:1061–65.

8. Kanigel R. Taking acupuncture seriously. *Hippocrates* 1998;12(5):23–24, at 24.

9. "Most alternative systems of treatment are based on irrational or fanciful thinking and false or unproven factual claims. Their theories often violate basic scientific principles and are at odds not only with each other, but with current knowledge of the structure and function of the human body as now taught in our medical schools." Relman AS. Is integrative medicine the medicine of the future? *Arch Intern Med* 1999; 159:2122–26, at 2123. Relman continues: "Alternative medicine stands apart from modern science, challenging many of its assumptions and methods and depending for its verification largely on personal belief and subjective experience . . . alternative medicine teaches that faith in a method will make it effective and that the strongest kind of evidence is the patient's belief that a treatment is working."

10. Schneiderman LJ. Alternative medicine or alternatives to medicine? A physician's perspective. *Cambridge Quarterly of Healthcare Ethics* 2000;9:83–97, at 91.

11. Eskinazi summarizes the metaphysics of medical science:

Biomedicine is founded in part on materialism (in contrast to the vital force explanation). Materialism in this context refers to the theory that "physical matter is the only or fundamental reality, and that all beings and processes and phemonema are manifestations or results of matter." While biomedicine does not necessarily reject religion or spirituality, it does not routinely incorporate these aspects into diagnosis and treatment. . . . Consistent with this philosophical theory, biomedicine considers biological entities more or less as equal to the sum of their anatomic parts . . . and endeavors to elucidate molecular, physiological, and pathological mechanisms believed to form the basis of biological processes. Allopathic medical treatment often logically consists of interventions chosen to interfere with identified pathological molecular processes.

Eskinazi DP. Factors that shape alternative medicine. *JAMA* 1998;280:1621–23, at 1621–22.

12. Black M. Induction. In: Edwards P, editor-in-chief. *The Encyclopedia of Philosophy*. New York: Macmillan, 1967, vol. 4, pp. 169–81.

13. Angell M, Kassirer JP. Alternative medicine—the risks of untested and unregulated remedies. *NEJM* 1998;339:839–41, at 839. See also Boozang KM. Western medicine opens the door to alternative medicine. *Am J Law & Medicine* 1998; 24: 185–212, at 204, defining quackery as any treatment that:

a. is implausible on *a priori* grounds (because its implied mechanisms or putative effects contradict well-established laws, principles, or empirical findings in physics, chemistry or biology),
b. lacks a scientifically acceptable rationale of its own,
c. has insufficient supporting evidence from adequately controlled outcome research (i.e. double-blined, randomized, placebo-controlled trials), or
d. has failed in well-controlled studies done by impartial evaluators and has been unable to rule out competing explanations for why it might *seem* to work in uncontrolled settings.

14. "[H]omeopathic treatments are highly individualized and homeopaths do not comply with orthodox diagnostic criteria. This can create problems when conducting a standard randomized clinical trial." Ernst E, Kaptchuk T. Homeopathy revisited. *Arch Intern Med* 1996; 156:2162–64, at 2164. "Homeopaths often claim that modern trial methods are not applicable to homeopathy" and that " 'controlled, randomized, double-blind studies have little significance with respect to homeopathic medical therapy.' " Id., at 2164.

"[T]he efficacy of its therapies is intrinsically unmeasurable because therapy for every individual patient is, by definition, unique, an assumption that makes it difficult if not impossible to assemble meaningful study cohorts." Davidoff F. Weighing the alternatives: Lessons from the paradoxes of alternative medicine. *Ann Intern Med* 1998;129:1068–70, at 1069.

15. Margolin A, Avants SK, Kleber HD. Investigating alternative medicine therapies in randomized controlled trials. *JAMA* 1998;280: 1626–28. Traditional Chinese medicine does not have the concept of "placebo," and it is difficult for practical as well as philosophical reasons even to construct a viable concept of "sham" insertion points for the needles. Moreover, within this approach there is no biochemical "marker" for active treatment, "nor is there one that would differentiate an active from a control treatment." Id., at 1627.

16. Margolin A, Avants SK, Kleber HD. Investigating alternative medicine therapies in randomized controlled trials. *JAMA* 1998;280: 1626–28, at 1627–28.

17. Kaptchuk TJ, Eisenberg DM. The persuasive appeal of alternative medicine. *Ann Intern Med* 1998; 129: 1061–65.

18. For instance, we have little understanding about the nature of consciousness, of how it is that brain, or any other sort of matter, can have awareness. As suggested by one observer, "[n]obody has the slightest idea how anything material could be conscious." Dossey L. Prayer and medical science: A commentary on the prayer study by Harris et al and a response to

critics. *Arch Intern Med* 2000;160:1735–38, citing philosopher Jerry A. Fodor, at p. 1736.

Science remains similarly puzzled over other mental/physical issues, such as evidence indicating that psychokinesis—the apparent ability of a human mind to affect physical events at a distance—may be a bona fide phenomenon.

"For example, in *Foundations of Physics*, one of physics' most prestigious journals, Radin and Nelson reported a meta-analysis of 832 studies from 68 investigators that involved the distant influence of human consciousness on microelectronic systems. They found the results to be "robust and repeatable." In their opinion, . . . "there is no escaping the conclusion that [these] effects are indeed possible." While these hundreds of studies do not involve actual prayer, they nonetheless deal with whether human intention can, in principle, affect the physical world at a distance. In recent years, researchers have also studied the effects of mental efforts to change biological systems. Scores of controlled studies have examined the effects of intentions, often expressed through prayer, on biochemical reactions in vitro, on the recovery rate of animals from anesthesia, on the growth rates of tumors and the rate of wound healing in animals, on the rate of hemolysis of red blood cells in vitro, and on the replication rates of microorganisms in test tubes. Testing prayer in lower organisms makes sense for the same reason we test drugs in nonhumans. We share physiological similarities with animals and bacteria; if prayer affects them, it may affect us as well." Id., at 1735.

19. For discussion of the difficulties in measuring quality of life, see, e.g.: Morreim, EH. The impossibility and the necessity of quality of life research. *Bioethics* 1992; 6(3): 218–32; Leplege, A, and Hunt, S. The problem of quality of life in medicine. *Journal of the American Medical Association* 278, 47–50; Morreim, EH. Quality of life in health care allocation. In: *Encyclopedia of Bioethics*, 2nd edition, edited by Warren Thomas Reich; New York: Simon & Schuster MacMillan, 1995; Volume 3, 1358–61; Morreim, EH. Computing the quality of life. In: *The price of health: Cost benefit analysis in medicine*. Agich G, Begley C. Dordrecht: D. Reidel Pub. Co, 1986, pp. 45–69; Testa, MA, Simonson, DC. Assessment of quality-of-life outcomes. *New England Journal of Medicine* 1996; 334: 835–40; Coates, A, Gebski, V, Bishop, JF, et al. for the Australian-New Zealand Breast Cancer Trials Group, Clinical Oncological Society of Australia. Improving the quality of life during chemotherapy for advanced breast cancer. A comparison of intermittent and continuous treatment strategies. *New England Journal of Medicine* 1987; 317:

1490–5; Gill, TM, and Feinstein, AR. A critical appraisal of the quality of quality-of-life measurements. *Journal of the American Medical Association* 1994; 272: 619–26; Lehman AF. Measuring quality of life in a reformed health system. *Health Affairs* 1995; 14(3): 90–101; Smith A. Qualms and QALY's. *Lancet* 1987; May 16: 1134–6; Guyatt, GH, Feeny, DH, and Patrick, DL. *Measuring health related quality of life. Annals of Internal Medicine* 1993; 118: 622–9; LaPuma J, and Lawlor EF. Quality adjusted life-years: Ethical implications for physicians and policymakers," *Journal of the American Medical Association* 263 (1990): 2917–21.

20. "The record of medical treatments is largely the chronicle of placebos. When subjected to scrutiny, the overwhelming majority of treatments, old and new, turn out to have no inherent therapeutic activity. And it is worth remembering that treatments now known to be of questionable value, from bloodletting to routine tonsillectomy, rested on compelling theories. Each theory may have been invalid, even wacky, but it made sense at the time. . . . But placebo treatment is not the same as no therapy. Studies have shown that although up to 70 percent of depressed patients improve after taking a placebo, depressed patients rarely improve while awaiting treatment. And in a placebo-controlled study assessing propranolol's effect on mortality in myocardial infarction survivors, patients who took a placebo regularly (more than 75 percent of the prescribed dose) had half the mortality rate of those who took it less steadily. Finally, a recent study showed that people with schizophrenia who took placebos were less likly to relapse than those who didn't receive any treatment." Brown WA. The power of the placebo. *Hippocrates* 1998;12(6):47–52, at 48–49. See also Jaret P. The mind has the power to heal. *Hippocrates* 1997; 11(5): 71–77. See also Horwitz RI, Horwitz SM. Adherence to treatment and health outcomes. *Arch Intern Med* 1993; 153:1863–68; Brody H. Placebos and the Philosophy of Medicine. Chicago: University of Chicago Press, 1980.

21. A further purpose of blinding is also to minimize the chance that the perceptions and the reports of scientists and of research subjects will be shaded by the goals they hold for participating in the research.

22. Sullivan MD. Placebo controls and epistemic control in orthodox medicine. *J Med & Phil* 1993;18:213–31, at 223–25.

23. Schneiderman LJ. Alternative medicine or alternatives to medicine? A physician's perspective. *Cambridge Quarterly of Healthcare Ethics* 2000;9:83–97, at 94.

24. Angell M. Patients' preferences in ran-

domized clinical trials. *NEJM* 1984;310:1385–87.

25. Merkatz RB, Temple R, Sobel S, et al. Women in clinical trials of new drugs. *NEJM* 1993; 329: 292–96; Bennett JC. Inclusion of women in clinical trials—policies for population subgroups. *NEJM* 1993; 329:288–92; Freeman TB, Vawter DE, Leaverton PE, et al. Use of placebo surgery in controlled trials of a cellular-based therapy for Parkinson's disease. *NEJM* 1999;341:988–92; Macklin R. The ethical problems with sham surgery in clinical research. *NEJM* 1999; 341:992–96.

26. Freeman TB, Vawter DE, Leaverton PE, et al. Use of placebo surgery in controlled trials of a cellular-based therapy for Parkinson's disease. *NEJM* 1999; 341: 988–92; Macklin R. The ethical problems with sham surgery in clinical research. *NEJM* 1999;341:992–96.

27. The manufacturer of a costly new drug for arthritis is hardly likely, for instance, to do a scientific comparison between its products and copper bracelets. Even a remote possibility of finding such an inexpensive remedy to be effective is enough to discourage such a study from being undertaken. And because copper is so inexpensive, the bracelet manufacturers cannot make enough profit to justify the expense of the research—particularly because they are not required to do any science as long as they make no health claims. Indeed, science is not merely unlikely in such scenarios. History has shown that sometimes even when high-quality scientific trials have been done, their results may not see the light of day if they are unfavorable to the study's sponsor. See Rennie D. Thyroid storm. *JAMA* 1997;277:1238–43.

28. Garas I, Manolis AJ. The economics of therapeutic advances: The paradigm of sympathetic suppression in chronic heart failure. *Arch Intern Med* 1999;2634–36, at 2635. Others have likewise observed that inexpensive, effective therapies tend to be ignored. See Goodwin JS, Goodwin JM. The tomato effect: Rejection of highly efficacious therapies. *JAMA* 1984;251:2387–90; Goodwin JS Goodwin JM. Failure to recognize efficacious therapy: The history of aspirin treament for rheumatoid arthritis. *Perspect Biol Med* 1981;25:78–92; Lederle FA, Applegate WA, Grimm RH, Jr. Reserpine and the medical marketplace. *Arch Inter Med* 1993; 153:705–6.

29. As noted by Feinstein, clinical research, as opposed to basic science and laboratory research, has long been looked down upon as being somehow inferior "applied" work. As a result, until recently funding has focused mainly on the latter and not on the former. Feinstein AR. Clinical judgment revisited: The distraction of quantitative methods. *Ann Intern Med* 1994;

1230:799–805. And as noted by other commentators, those who use guidelines "cannot help but notice that guideline developers must often reckon with research that is modest in rigor, discordant, or nonexistent. Although most guidelines are an amalgam of evidence and expert opinion, methods of integrating knowledge and experience into guidelines, particularly when data are sparse, are neither as mature nor as transparent as methods of incorporating research results." Cook D, Giacomini M. The trials and tribulations of clinical practice guidelines. *JAMA* 1999;281:1950–51, at 1950.

30. Dalen JE. "Conventional" and "unconventional" medicine. *Arch Intern Med* 1998;158:2179–81, at 2179.

31. Id., at 2180.

32. Berwick DM. We can cut costs and improve care at the same time. *Medical Economics* 1996;73(15):180–87, at 186.

33. Relman AS, Weil A. Is integrative medicine the medicine of the future? *Arch Intern Med* 1999;159:2122–26, at 2125. Another estimate puts the figure even lower. "Richard Smith, editor of the *British Medical Journal*, [states that] 'only about 15% of medical interventions are supported by solid scientific evidence. . . . This is partly because only 1% of the articles in medical journals are scientifically sound and partly because many treatments have not been assessed at all.' " Dossey L. Prayer and medical science: A commentary on the prayer study by Harris et al and a response to critics. *Arch Intern Med* 2000;160:1735–38, at 1736.

34. In scientific research, evaluation of diseases and treatments "generally requires a priori hypotheses, randomization (to eliminate selection bias and confounding), homogeneous patients at high risk for the outcome, experienced investigators who follow a protocol, a comparative measure such as a placebo (if ethical), and intensive follow-up to ensure compliance. Under these circumstances, if a treatment proves to be better than a placebo (or a comparative measure), one can be reassured that the treatment can work. However, questions may remain about the ability of the treatment to work adequately in a broader range of patients and in usual practice settings in which both patients and providers face natural barriers to care." Epstein RS, Sherwood LM. From outcomes research to disease management: A guide for the perplexed. *Ann Intern Med* 1996;124:832–37, at 833. See also Feinstein AR, Horwitz RI. Problems in the "evidence" of "evidence-based medicine." *Am J Med* 1997;103:529–35; Wells KB, Sturm R. Care for depression in a changing environment. *Health Affairs* 1995;14(3):78–89, at 80.

"Clinical trials are not real life. To assess efficacy in as unconfounded a manner as possible, trials sometimes exclude certain patients (e.g., the elderly, the very young, those too sick, or those taking certain other medications). Any special vulnerability to adverse events in those groups will be missed." Friedman MA, Woodcock J, Lumpkin MM, Shuren JE, Hass AE, Thompson LJ. The safety of newly approved medicines: Do recent market removals mean there is a problem? *JAMA* 1999;281:1728–34, at 1733.

35. Epstein RS, Sherwood LM. From outcomes research to disease management: A guide for the perplexed. *Ann Intern Med* 1996;124:832–37.

"The failure to account for the effects of comorbid and associated conditions on the clinical outcome of chronic diseases is reflected in the common disjunction that occurs between the efficacy of an intervention, such as a drug used in a clinical trial, and the lack of effectiveness of the same drug used in clinical practice. For example, as many as 60% to 80% of patients with heart failure have been excluded from clinical trials of angiotensin-converting enzyme inhibitor therapy owing to comorbid and associated conditions that tend to obscure the efficacy of the drug in improving functional capacity or prognosis. This standard practice in research has a rational basis. However, the clinician must treat 100% of the patients with heart failure, not just the 20% to 40% who are free of comorbidities and associated conditions. Moreover, the clinical effectiveness of drug therapy is often limited by the very comorbid and associated conditions for which patients were excluded from drug trials." DeBusk RF, West JA, Miller NH, Taylor CB. Chronic disease management. *Arch Intern Med* 1999;159:2739–42, at 2740.

Regarding coronary bypass surgery, Gellins et al observed that "only 4 to 13 percent of the patients who now undergo this operation would meet the eligibility criteria for the randomized controlled trials that established its efficacy." Gellins AC, Rosenberg N, Moskowitz AJ. Capturing the unexpected benefits of medical research. *NEJM* 1998;339:693–97, at 694. See also Feinstein AR. Clinical judgment revisited: The distraction of quantitative methods. *Ann Intern Med* 1994;1230:799–805.

36. Friedman MA, Woodcock J, Lumpkin MM, Shuren JE, Hass AE, Thompson LJ. The safety of newly approved medicines: Do recent market removals mean there is a problem? *JAMA* 1999;281:1728–34, at 1729.

37. Zugar A. New way of doctoring: going by the evidence. *Physician's Management* 1998; 38(2):41–44, at 42.

As Eisenberg notes, "There is sufficient evidence to suggest that most clinicians' practices do not reflect the principles of evidence-based medicine but rather are based upon tradition, their most recent experience, what they learned years ago in medical school, or what they have heard from their friends." Eisenberg, JM. What does evidence mean? Can the law and medicine be reconciled? *Journal of Health Policy, Politics & Law* 2001;26:369–81.

See also Mold, JW, and Stein, HF. The cascade effect in the clinical care of patients. *New England Journal of Medicine* 1986;314:512–14; Fisher, ES, and Welch, HG. Avoiding the unintended consequences of growth in medical care. How might more be worse? *Journal of the American Medical Association* 1999;281:446–53; Franks, P, Clancy, CM, and Nutting, PA. Gatekeeping revisited—protecting patients from overtreatment. *The New England Journal of Medicine* 1992;327:424–9; Burnum JF. Medical practice a la mode. *New England Journal of Medicine* 1987;317:1220–1222; Hardison JE. To be complete. *New England Journal of Medicine* 1979;300:193–4.

38. Hall JB. Use of the pulmonary artery catheter in critically ill patients: Was invention the mother of necessity? *JAMA* 2000;283:2577–78; Rapoport J, Teres D, Steingrub J, Higgins T, McGee W, Lemeshow S. Patient characteristics and ICU organizational factors that influence frequency of pulmonary artery catheterization. *JAMA* 2000;283:2559–67; Bernard GR, Sopko G, Cerra F, Demling R, et al. Pulmonary artery catheterization and clinical outcomes: NHLBI and FDA workshop report. *JAMA* 2000;283:2568–72.

39. ECRI. High-dose chemotherapy with autologous bone marrow transplantation and/or blood cell transplantation for the treatment of metastatic breast cancer. Healthy Technology Assessment Information Service: Executive Briefings, February 1995.

40. Stadtmauer EA, O'Neill A, Goldstein LJ, et al. Conventional-dose chemotherapy compared with high-dose chemotherapy plus autologous hematopoietic stem-cell transplantation for metastatic breast cancer. *NEJM* 2000;342:1069–76; Lippman ME. High-dose chemotherapy plus autologous bone marrow transplantation for metastatic breast cancer. *NEJM* 2000;342:1119–20.

41. For example, Roberts et al "carefully examined the data obtained from open studies at a time when they were considered highly effective by the patients as well as their physicians. They analyzed the use of glomectomies as a treatment for asthma, levamisole as an immunomodulator, photodynamic therapy and organic solvents for herpes simplex infection, and gastric freezing for ulcers. Seventy percent of the almost 7000 patients who participated in these open studies in the 1960s and early 1970s were

found to have obtained good to excellent results from these modalities. This report shows that belief and expectancy of patients, and especially of their health care providers, played a critical role in determining the effectiveness of treatments later found to be nonspecific by scientific measures." Tausk FA. Alternative medicine: Is it all in your mind? *Arch Dermatol* 1998;134: 1422–25, at 1423 (citing Roberts AH, Kewman DB, Mercier L, Hovell M. The power of non-specific effects in healing: implications for psy-chogocial and biological treatments. *Clinical Psychology Review* 1993;13:375–91).

42. Though physician practices vary rela-tively little in situations where strong consensus guides practice, as in the treatment of hip frac-tures, in areas where there is little consensus, practices vary widely, in ways not correlated with differences in patients' condition. "The re-cent Dartmouth Atlas details less than a 2-fold variation in the treatment of hip fractures—30% higher than the national average to 25% below the average—most likely because there is strong evidence about the most effective inter-ventions, and the medical community agrees on this evidence. . . . On the other hand, Wennberg also found an almost 6-fold variation in the rates of carotid duplex diagnostic procedures, from 20 to more than 115 per 1000 Medicare enrollees, due largely to 'no consensus among physicians about which patients would be screened with carotid duplex.' In another ex-ample, there was a 5.5-fold variation in the use of coronary angiography, from 9.6 to 53.1 per 1000 Medicare enrollees, because 'physicians disagree about how severe patients' symptoms must be to warrant' its use." Eisenberg, JM. Ten lessons for evidence-based technology assess-ment. *Journal of the American Medical Associ-ation* 1999;282:1865–9, at 1866.

See Wennberg, JE. Which rate is right? *New England Journal of Medicine* 1986;314:310–311; Chassin, MR, Brook, RH, and Park, RE, et al. Variations in the use of medical and sur-gical services by the medicare population. *New England Journal of Medicine* 1986;314:285–290; Wennberg, JE, Freeman, JL, and Culp, WJ. Are hospital services rationed in New Haven or overutilized in Boston? *Lancet* 1987;1:1185–8; Welch, HG, Miller, ME, and Welch, WP. An analysis of inpatient practice patterns in Florida and Oregon. *New England Journal of Medicine* 1994;330:607–612; Wennberg, JE. The para-dox of appropriate care. *Journal of the Ameri-can Medical Association* 1987;258:2568–9; Chassin. MR, et al. Does inappropriate use ex-plain geographic variations in the use of health care services? *Journal of the American Medical* 1987;258:2533–7; Wennberg, JE. Outcomes re-search, cost containment, and the fear of ration-

ing. *New England Journal of Medicine* 1990; 323:1202–4; Leape, LL, Park, RE, Solomon, DH, et al. Does inappropriate use explain small-area variations in the use of health care services? *Journal of the American Medical Association* 1990;263:669–72; Leape, LL, Park, RE, Solo-mon, DH, et al. Relation between surgeons' practice volumes and geographic variation in the rate of carotid endarterectomy. *New En-gland Journal of Medicine* 1989;321:653–7; Wennberg, JE. Unwanted variations in the rule of practice. *Journal of the American Medical Association* 1991;265:1306–7; Cleary, PD, Greenfield, S, Mulley, AG, et al. Variations in length of stay and outcomes for six medical and surgical conditions in Massachusetts and Cali-fornia. *Journal of the American Medical Asso-ciation* 1991;266:73–9; Fisher, ES, Welch, HG, Wennberg, JE. Prioritizing Oregon's hospital re-sources: An example based on variations in dis-cretionary medical utilization. *Journal of the American Medical Association* 1992;267:1925–31; Greenfield, S, Nelson, EC, Subkoff, M, et al. Variations in resource utilization among medical specialties and systems of care: Results from the medical outcomes study. *Journal of the American Medical Association* 1992;267:1624–30; Welch, WP, Miller, ME, Welch, HG, et al. Geographic variation in expenditures for phy-sicians' services in the United States. *New En-gland Journal of Medicine* 1993;328:621–27; Miller, MG, Miller, LS, Fireman, B, and Black, SB. Variation in practice for discretionary ad-missions. *Journal of the American Medical As-sociation* 1994;271:1493–8; Detsky, AS. Re-gional variation in medical care. *New England Journal of Medicine* 1995;333:589–90; Guad-agnoli, E, Hauptman, PJ, Avanian, JZ, et al. Variation in the use of cardiac procedures after acute myocardial infarction. *New England Journal of Medicine* 1995;333:573–8; Pilote, L, Califf, RM, Sapp, S, et al. for the GUSTO-1 In-vestigators. Regional variation across the United States in the management of acute myo-cardial infarction. *New England Journal of Medicine* 1995;333:565–72; Ashton, CM, Pe-tersen, NJ, Souchek, J, et al. Geographic varia-tions in utilization rates in Veterans Affairs hos-pitals and clinics. *New England Journal of Medicine* 1999;340:32–9; O'Connor, GT, Quin-ton, HB, Traven, ND, et al. Geographic varia-tion in the treatment of acute myocardial in-fraction: the cooperative cardiovascular project. *Journal of the American Medical Association* 1999;281:627–33; Wennberg JE. Understand-ing geographic variations in health care delivery. *New England Journal of Medicine* 1999;340: 52–3.

43. For an extensive discussion of the ways in which actual clinical practices can constitute

overuse, underuse, and misuse of available diagnostic and therapeutic interventions, see Morreim EH. Playing doctor: Corporate medical practice and medical malpractice. *Michigan Journal of Law Reform* 1999;32(4):939–1040, at 989–98. See also Chassin MR, Galvin RW, National Roundtable on Health Care Quality. The urgent need to improve health care quality. *JAMA* 1998;280:1000–1005; Bodenheimer T. The American health care system: The movement for improved quality in health care. *NEJM* 1999;340:488–92; Chassin MR. Is health care ready for six sigma quality? *Milbank Quarterly* 1998;76(4):565–91.

44. In some cases clinicians point out, quite correctly, that the guidelines imposed by health plans sometimes have a very poor scientific basis. And yet other times the protests, based on an insistence that "every patient is individual" and "my patients are different," amount to a claim that clinical medicine cannot be scientific in any thoroughgoing way. At this point the clinical physician begins to resemble alternative providers.

45. For further discussion on the limits of guidelines' scientific basis, see Morreim EH. Playing doctor: corporate medical practice and medical malpractice. *Michigan Journal of Law Reform* 1999;32(4):939–1040, at 981–89.

46. "[M]ainstream medicine can be criticized for overselling its own scientific legitimacy. It's reasonable to say that much of existing medicine has not met the standards that alternative medicine is being asked to meet." Brown C. Alternative medicine comes to the OR. *Medical Economics* 1995;72(17):207–19, at 218–19.

47. As one commentator observed, one view holds that everything that makes an individual an individual is outside of science. This is the art of medicine. However, as an alternate view has noted: "Art kills. It was the art that gave us purging, puking, leeches, the gastric freeze, all that sort of stuff. There's a science to the art of medicine." Zugar A. New way of doctoring: Going by the evidence. *Physician's Management* 1998;38(2):41–44, at 44.

48. Accordingly, the scorn that sometimes marks medicine's appraisals of alternatives should be avoided. In a variety of instances, derision has been used as a weapon where better-quality arguments are unavailable. Through the 1950s, 1960s, and 1970s, for instance, standard medical textbooks like Harrison's and Cecil's treated vitamin therapy with a scornful, dismissive tone, using terms like "massive," "carelessness," "useless," "indiscriminate," "false," "indefensible," "wasteful," "insidious," "unnecessary," "deplored." Goodwin JS, Tangum MR. Battling quackery: Attitudes about micro-nutrient supplements in American academic medicine. *Arch Intern Med* 1998;158:2187–91.

Similarly, in the mid-1980s, one article in the New England Journal of Medicine scoffed at the notion of "antioxidants" (Gillick MR. Common-sense models of health and disease. NEJM 1985;313:700–1703), while another in the same journal pronounced dead the idea that human emotions have a causal role in illness. "[I]t is time to acknowledge that our belief in disease as a direct reflection of mental state is largely folklore." Angell M. Disease as a reflection of the psyche. *NEJM* 1985;312:1570–72, at 1572. Subsequent research findings have challenged such dismissals with considerable force.

"[O]ne should remain humble about physicians' own mixture of art and science. Not so long ago, leeches and frozen stomachs were in their domain, and many of their beliefs today must remain tentative." Delbanco TL. Bitter herbs: Mainstream, magic, and menace. *Ann Intern Med* 1994;121:803–4, at 804.

49. As noted by Paul Starr, medicine's dominance of the health care market is also a political phenomenon. Starr P. *The Social Transformation of American Medicine.* New York: Basic Books, 1982.

50. Lazarou J, Pomeranz BH, Corey PN. Incidence of adverse drug reactions in hospitalized patients. *JAMA* 1998;279:1200–12205.

51. Institute of Medicine. *To Err Is Human: Building a Safer Health System.* Washington, DC: National Academy Press, 1999.

52. Coppes JM, Anderson RA, Egeler RM, Wolff JEA. Aternative therapies for treatment of childhood cancer (letter). *NEJM* 1998;339:846; Ko RJ. Adulterants in Asian patent medicines (letter). *NEJM* 1998;339:847; LoVecchio F, Curry SC, Bagnasco T. Butyrolactone-induced central nervous system depression after ingestion of RenewTrient, a "dietary supplement" (letter). *NEJM* 1998;339:847–48; Angell M, Kassirer JP. Alternative medicine—the risks of untested and unregulated remedies. *NEJM* 1998;339:839–41; Winslow LC, Kroll DJ. Herbs as medicines. *Arch Intern Med* 1998;158:2192–99.

53. See note 1 *supra*.

54. Eisenberg DM, Davis RB, Ettner SL, et al. Trends in alternative medicine use in the United States, 1990–1997. *JAMA* 1998;280:1569–75.

55. In 1990, the estimated total expenditure for alternatives was $13.7 billion, of which $10.3 billion was out of pocket. Eisenberg DM, Kessler RC, Foster C, et al. Unconventional medicine in the United States. *NEJM* 1993;328:246–52.

56. In the very different case of children,

mandates for medicine can indeed be appropriate in cases where the illness or injury is life-threatening, and the ability of medical treatment to help is clear and substantial. Issues regarding children and alternatives would take this chapter too far afield, however, and will thus at this point be left for another forum.

57. In recent studies, alternatives were mainly used for chronic conditions such as back problems, headache, anxiety, and depression. Eisenberg DM, Davis RB, Ettner SL, et al. Trends in alternative medicine use in the United States, 1990–1997. *JAMA* 1998;280:1569–75; Campion EW. Why unconventional medicine? *NEJM* 1993;328:282–83; Eisenberg DM, Kessler RC, Foster C, et al. Unconventional medicine in the United States. *NEJM* 1993;328:246–52.

58. Exceptions can be made if some particular alternative were shown to be clearly, seriously harmful and without redeeming benefit—just as some drugs are removed from the market when their risks are determined to exceed their potential benefits.

59. Herron RE, Schneider RH, Mandarino JV, et al. Cost-effective hypertension management: comparison of drug therapies with an alternative program. *Am J Managed Care* 1996; 2:427–37.

60. Micozzi MS. Complementary care: When is it appropriate? Who will provide it? *Ann Intern Med* 1998;129:65–66.

61. Avants SK, Margolin A, Holford TR, Kosten TR. A randomized controlled trial of auricular acupuncture for cocaine dependence. *Arch Intern Med.* 2000;160:2305–12.

62. Bensoussan A, Talley NJ, Hing M, et al. Treatment of irritable bowel syndrome with Chinese herbal medicine. *JAMA* 1998;280: 1585–89.

63. Garfinkel MS, Singhal A, Katz WA. Yoga-based intervention for carpal tunnel syndrome. *JAMA* 1998;280:1601–3.

64. Wilt TJ, Ishani A, Stark G, et al. Saw palmetto extracts for treatment of benign prostatic hyperplasia. *JAMA* 1998;280:1604–9.

65. Smyth JM, Stone AA, Hureswitz A, Kaell A. Effects of writing about stressful experiences on symptom reduction in patients with asthma or rheumatoid arthritis. *JAMA* 1999;281:1304–9.

66. Pittler MH, Ernst E. Horse-chestnut seed extract for chronic venous insufficiency. *Arch Dermatol* 1998;134:1356–60.

67. Chrubasik S, Eisenberg E, Balan E, et al. Treatment of low back pain exacerbations with willow bark extract: A randomized double-blind study. *Am J Med* 2000:109:9–14.

68. Gould KL, Ornish D, Scherwitz L, et al. Changes in myocardial perfusion abnormalities by positron emission tomography after long-term, intense risk factor modification. *JAMA* 1995;274:894–901; Ornish D, Scherwitz LW, Billings JH, et al. Intensive lifestyle changes for reversal of coronary heart disease. *JAMA* 1998; 280:2001–7.

69. Hay IC, Jamieson M, Omerod AD. Ramdomized trial of aromatherapy: Successful treatment for alopecia areata. *Arch Dermatol* 1998; 134:1349–52.

70. Byrd R. Positive therapeutic effects of intercessary prayer in a coronary care unit population. *South Med J* 1988;81:826–29; Harris WS, Gowda M, Kolb JW, et al. A randomized, controlled trial of the effects of remote, intercessory prayer on outcomes in patients admitted to the coronary care unit. *Arch Intern Med* 1999;159:2273–78.

71. Spiegel D, Kraemer HC, Bloom JR, Gottheil E. Effect of psychosocial treatment of survival of patients with metastatic breast cancer. *Lancet* 1989; 334: 888–91. See also the effects of psychiatric interventions in prolonging the lives of patients with other malignancies: Fawzy FI, Fawzy NW, Hyun CS, et al. Malignant melanoma: Effects of an early structured psychiatric intervention, coping, and affective state on recurrence and survival 6 years later. *Arch Gen Psychiatry* 1993;50:681–89. But see Spiegel D. Mind matters–group therapy and survival in breast cancer. *NEJM* 2001; 345: 1767–68.

72. Mello MM, Brannan TA. The controversy over high-dose chemotherapy with autologous bone marrow transplant for breast cancer. *Health Affairs* 2001;20(5):101–118, at 110.

73. Peters WP, Rogers MC. Variation in approval by insurance companies of coverage for autologous bone marrow transplantation for breast cancer. *NEJM* 1994;330:473–77. See also Ferguson JH, Dubinsky M, Kirsch PJ. Court-ordered reimbursement for unproven medical technology: Circumventing technology assessment. *JAMA* 1993;269:2116–21.

74. Hoffman S. A proposal for federal legislation to address health insurance coverage for experimental and investigational treatments. *Oregon Law Review* 1999;78(1):203–74.

75. Tausk FA. Alternative medicine: Is it all in your mind? *Arch Dermatol* 1998;134:1422–25, at 1423, citing Roberts AH, Kewman DB, Mercier L, Hovell M. The power of nonspecific effects in healing: Implications for psychogocial and biological treatments. *Clinical Psychology Review* 1993;13:375–91.

76. Chassin MR, Galvin RW, National Roundtable on Health Care Quality. The urgent need to improve health care quality. *JAMA* 1998;280:1000–1005; Bodenheimer T. The American health care system: The movement for

improved quality in health care. *NEJM* 1999; 340:488–92.

77. See note 42, *supra*.

78. Wennberg JE., Which rate is right? *NEJM* (1986); 314:310–11.

79. Morreim EH. Playing doctor: Corporate medical practice and medical malpractice. *Michigan Journal of Law Reform* 1999;32(4):939–1040; Morreim EH. Medicine meets resource limits: Restructuring the legal standard of care. *University of Pittsburgh Law Review* 1997; 59(1):1–95, at 47–52; Morreim EH. Moral justice and legal justice in managed care: The ascent of contributive justice. *Journal of Law, Medicine, and Ethics* 1995;23(3):247–65; Morreim EH. Diverse and perverse incentives in managed care; bringing the patient into alignment. *Widener Law Symposium Journal* 1995; 1(1):89–139; Morreim EH. Saving lives, spending money: Shepherding the role of technology. In: *Ethical Issues in Health Care on the Frontiers of the Twenty-First Century*. Wear S, Bono JJ, Logue G, McEvoy A, editors; Philosophy and Medicine Series. Dordrecht, The Netherlands: Kluwer Academic Publishers, 2000, pp. 63–110; Havighurst CC. *Health Care Choices: Private Contracts as Instruments of Health Reform*. Washington, DC: AEI Press, 1995; Kalb PE. Controlling health care costs by controlling technology: A private contractual approach. *Yale Law Journal* 1990;99:1109–26; Hall MA, Anderson GF. Health insurers' assessment of medical necessity. *University of Pennsylvania Law Review* 1992;140:1637–1712, at 1689–93.

80. Morreim EH. Redefining quality by reassigning responsibility. *American Journal of Law and Medicine* 1994;20(1–2):79–104; Morreim EH. Diverse and perverse incentives in managed care; bringing the patient into alignment. *Widener Law Symposium Journal* 1995;1(1):89–139; Morreim EH. Saving lives, spending money: Shepherding the role of technology. In: *Ethical Issues in Health Care on the Frontiers of the Twenty-First Century*. Wear S, Bono JJ, Logue G, McEvoy A, editors; Philosophy and Medicine Series. Dordrecht, The Netherland: Kluwer Academic Publishers, 2000; pp. 63–110.

81. Morreim EH. Diverse and perverse incentives in managed care; bringing the patient into alignment. *Widener Law Symposium Journal* 1995;1(1):89–139.

REFERENCES

Angell, M. (1984). Patients' preferences in randomized clinical trials. *New England Journal of Medicine* 310, 1385–7.

Angell, M. (1985). Disease as a reflection of the psyche. *New England Journal of Medicine* 312, 1570–72.

Angell, M., and Kassirer, J. P. (1998). Alternative medicine—the risks of untested and unregulated remedies. *New England Journal of Medicine* 339, 839–41.

Ashton, C. M., Petersen, N. J., Souchek, J., et al. (1999). Geographic variations in utilization rates in Veterans Affairs hospitals and clinics. *New England Journal of Medicine* 340, 32–9.

Avants, S. K., Margolin, A., Holford, T. R., and Kosten, T. R. (2000). A randomized controlled trial of auricular acupuncture for cocaine dependence. *Archives of Internal Medicine* 160, 2305–12.

Bennett, J. C. (1993). Inclusion of women in clinical trials—policies for population subgroups. *New England Journal of Medicine* 329, 288–92.

Bensoussan, A., Talley, N. J., Hing, M., et al. (1998). Treatment of irritable bowel syndrome with Chinese herbal medicine. *Journal of the American Medical Association* 280, 1585–9.

Bernard, G. R., Sopko, G., Cerra, F., et al. (2000). Pulmonary artery catheterization and clinical outcomes, NHLBI and FDA workshop report. *Journal of the American Medical Association* 283, 2568–72.

Berwick, D. M. (1996). We can cut costs and improve care at the same time. *Medical Economics* 73(15), 180–7.

Black, M. (1967). Induction. In: Edwards P, ed. *The Encyclopedia of Philosophy*. New York: Macmillan Publishing Co., vol. 4, pp. 169–81.

Bodenheimer, T. (1999). The American health care system, the movement for improved quality in health care. *New England Journal of Medicine* 340, 488–92.

Boozang, K. M. (1998). Western medicine opens the door to alternative medicine. *American Journal of Law & Medicine* 24, 185–212.

Brody, H. (1980). *Placebos and the Philosophy of Medicine*. Chicago: University of Chicago Press.

Brown, C. (1995). Alternative medicine comes to the OR. *Medical Economics* 72(17), 207–19.

Brown, W. A. (1998). The power of the placebo. *Hippocrates* 12(6), 47–52.

Burnum, J. F. (1987). Medical practice a la mode. *New England Journal of Medicine* 317, 1220–2.

Byrd, R. (1988). Positive therapeutic effects of intercessary prayer in a coronary care unit population. *Southern Medical Journal* 81, 826–9.

Campion, E. W. (1993). Why unconventional medicine? *New England Journal of Medicine* 328, 282–3.

Chassin, M. R., Brook, R. H., Park, R. E., et al. (1986). Variations in the use of medical and surgical services by the medicare population. *New England Journal of Medicine* 314, 285–90.

Chassin, M. R., et al. (1987). Does inappropriate use explain geographic variations in the use of health care services? *Journal of the American Medical Association* 258, 2533–7.

Chassin, M. R. (1998). Is health care ready for six sigma quality? *The Milbank Quarterly* 76(4), 565–91.

Chassin, M. R., and Galvin, R. W. [National Roundtable on Health Care Quality] (1998). The urgent need to improve health care quality. *Journal of the American Medical Association* 280, 1000–5.

Chrubasik, S., Eisenberg, E., Balan, E., et al. (2000). Treatment of low back pain exacerbations with willow bark extract, a randomized double-blind study. *American Journal of Medicine* 109, 9–14.

Cleary, P. D., Greenfield, S., Mulley, A. G., et al. (1991). Variations in length of stay and outcomes for six medical and surgical conditions in Massachusetts and California. *Journal of the American Medical Association* 266, 73–9.

Coates, A., Gebski, V., Bishop, J. F., et al. [for the Australian-New Zealand Breast Cancer Trials Group, Clinical Oncological Society of Australia] (1987). Improving the quality of life during chemotherapy for advanced breast cancer. A comparison of intermittent and continuous treatment strategies. *New England Journal of Medicine* 317, 1490–5.

Cook, D., and Giacomini, M. (1999). The trials and tribulations of clinical practice guidelines. *Journal of the American Medical Association* 281, 1950–1.

Coppes, J. M., Anderson, R. A., et al. (1998). Aternative therapies for treatment of childhood cancer (letter). *New England Journal of Medicine* 339, 846.

Dalen, J. E. (1998). 'Conventional' and 'unconventional' medicine. *Archives of Internal Medicine* 158, 2179–81.

Davidoff, F. (1998). Weighing the alternatives, lessons from the paradoxes of alternative medicine. *Annals of Internal Medicine* 129, 1068–70.

DeBusk, R. F., West, J. A., Miller, N. H., and Taylor, C. B. (1999). Chronic disease management. *Archives of Internal Medicine* 159, 2739–42.

Delbanco, T. L. (1994). Bitter herbs, mainstream, magic, and menace. *Annals of Internal Medicine* 121, 803–4.

Detsky, A. S. (1995). Regional variation in medical care. *New England Journal of Medicine* 333, 589–90.

Dossey, L. (2000). Prayer and medical science, a commentary on the prayer study by Harris et al and a response to critics. *Archives of Internal Medicine* 160, 1735–8.

ECRI. (1995). High-dose chemotherapy with autologous bone marrow transplantation and/or blood cell transplantation for the treatment of metastatic breast cancer. Healthy Technology Assessment Information Service, Executive Briefings, February 1995.

Eisenberg, D. M., Kessler, R. C., Foster, C., et al. (1993). Unconventional medicine in the United States. *New England Journal of Medicine* 328, 246–52.

Eisenberg, D. M., Davis, R. B., Ettner, S. L., et al. (1998). Trends in alternative medicine use in the United States, 1990–1997. *Journal of the American Medical Association* 280, 1569–75.

Eisenberg, J. M. (1999). Ten lessons for evidence-based technology assessment. *Journal of the American Medical Association* 282, 1865–69.

Eisenberg, J. M. (2001). What does evidence mean? Can the law and medicine be reconciled? *Journal of Health Policy, Politics & Law* 26, 369–81.

Epstein, R. S., and Sherwood, L. M. (1996). From outcomes research to disease management, a guide for the perplexed. *Annals of Internal Medicine* 124, 832–37.

Ernst, E., and Kaptchuk, T. (1996). Homeopathy revisited. *Archives of Internal Medicine* 156, 2162–64.

Eskinazi, D. P. (1998). Factors that shape alternative medicine. *Journal of the American Medical Association* 280, 1621–23.

Fawzy, F. I., Fawzy, N. W., Hyun, C. S., et al. (1993). Malignant melanoma, effects of an early structured psychiatric intervention, coping, and affective state on recurrence and survival 6 years later. *Archives in General Psychiatry* 50, 681–9.

Feinstein, A. R. (1994). Clinical judgment revisited, the distraction of quantitative methods. *Annals of Internal Medicine* 1230, 799–805.

Feinstein, A. R., and Horwitz, R. I. (1997). Problems in the 'evidence' of 'evidence-based medicine'. *American Journal of Medicine* 103, 529–35.

Ferguson, J. H., Dubinsky, M., and Kirsch, P. J. (1993). Court-ordered reimbursement for unproven medical technology, circumventing technology assessment. *Journal of the American Medical Association* 269, 2116–21.

Fisher, E. S., Welch, H. G., and Wennberg, J. E. (1992). Prioritizing Oregon's hospital resources: an example based on variations in discretionary medical utilization. *Journal of the American Medical Association* 267, 1925–31.

Fisher, E. S., and Welch, G. (1999). Avoiding the unintended consequences of growth in medical care. How might more be worse? *Journal of the American Medical Association* 281, 446–53.

Franks, P., Clancy, C. M., and Nutting, P. A. (1992). Gatekeeping revisited—protecting patients from overtreatment. *New England Journal of Medicine* 327, 424–9.

Freeman, T. B., Vawter, D. E., Leaverton, P. E., et al. (1999). Use of placebo surgery in controlled trials of a cellular-based therapy for Parkinson's disease. *New England Journal of Medicine* 341, 988–92.

Friedman, M. A., Woodcock, J., Lumpkin, M. M., et al. (1999). The safety of newly approved medicines, do recent market removals mean there is a problem? *Journal of the American Medical Association* 281, 1728–34.

Garas, I., and Manolis, A. J. (1999). The economics of therapeutic advances, the paradigm of sympathetic suppression in chronic heart failure. *Archives of Internal Medicine.* 2634–6.

Garfinkel, M. S., Singhal, A., and Katz, W. A. (1998). Yoga-based intervention for carpal tunnel syndrome. *Journal of the American Medical Association* 280, 1601–3.

Gellins, A. C., Rosenberg, N., and Moskowitz, A. J. (1998). Capturing the unexpected benefits of medical research. *New England Journal of Medicine* 339, 693–7.

Gill, T. M., and Feinstein, A. R. (1994). A critical appraisal of the quality of quality-of-life measurements. *Journal of the American Medical Association* 272, 619–26.

Gillick, M. R. (1985). Common-sense models of health and disease. *New England Journal of Medicine* 313, 700–3.

Goodwin, J. S., and Goodwin, J. M. (1981). Failure to recognize efficacious therapy, the history of aspirin treatment for rheumatoid arthritis. *Perspectives in Biology and Medicine* 25, 78–92.

Goodwin, J. S., and Goodwin, J. M. (1984). The tomato effect, rejection of highly efficacious therapies. *Journal of the American Medical Association* 251, 2387–90.

Goodwin, J. S., and Tangum, M. R. (1998). Battling quackery, attitudes about micronutrient supplements in American academic medicine. *Archives of Internal Medicine* 158, 2187–91.

Gould, K. L., Ornish, D., Scherwitz, L., et al. (1995). Changes in myocardial perfusion abnormalities by positron emission tomography after long-term, intense risk factor modification. *Journal of the American Medical Association* 274, 894–901.

Grandinetti, D. A. (1997). 'Integrated medicine' could boost your income. *Medical Economics* 74(8), 73–99.

Grandinetti, D. A. (1999). Your newest competitors, alternative-medicine networks. *Medical Economics* 76(10), 44–51.

Greenfield, S., Nelson, E. C., Subkoff, M., et al. (1992). Variations in resource utilization among medical specialties and systems of care, Results from the medical outcomes study. *Journal of the American Medical Association* 267, 1624–30.

Guadagnoli, E., Hauptman, P. J., Avanian, J. Z., et al. (1995). Variation in the use of cardiac procedures after acute myocardial infarction. *New England Journal of Medicine* 333, 573–8.

Guyatt, G. H., Feeny, D. H., and Patrick, D. L. (1993). Measuring health-related quality of life. *Annals of Internal Medicine* 118, 622–9.

Hall, M. A., and Anderson, G. F. (1992). Health insurers' assessment of medical necessity. *University of Pennsylvania Law Review* 140, 1637–712.

Hall, J. B. (2000). Use of the pulmonary artery catheter in critically ill patients, was invention the mother of necessity? *Journal of the American Medical Association* 283, 2577–8.

Hardison, J. E. (1979). To be complete. *New England Journal of Medicine* 300, 193–4.

Harris, W. S., Gowda, M., Kolb, J. W. et al. (1999). A randomized, controlled trial of the effects of remote, intercessory prayer on outcomes in patients admitted to the coronary care unit. *Archives of Internal Medicine* 159, 2273–8.

Havighurst, C. C. (1995). *Health Care Choices: Private Contracts as Instruments of Health Reform.* Washington, D.C., The AEI Press.

Hay, I. C., Jamieson, M., and Omerod, A. D. (1998). Ramdomized trial of aromatherapy, successful treatment for alopecia areata. *Archives in Dermatology* 134, 1349–52.

Herron, R. E., Schneider, R. H., Mandarino, J. V., et al. (1996). Cost-effective hypertension management, comparison of drug therapies with an alternative program. *American Journal of Managed Care* 2, 427–37.

Hoffman v Regence Blue Shield, 991 P.2d 77 (Wash. 2000).

Hoffman, S. (1999). A proposal for federal legislation to address health insurance coverage for experimental and investigational treatments. *Oregon Law Review* 78(1), 203–74.

Horwitz, R. I., and Horwitz, S. M. (1993). Adherence to treatment and health outcomes. *Archives of Internal Medicine* 153, 1863–1868.

Institute of Medicine (1999). *To Err is Human, Building a Safer Health System.* Washington D.C., National Academy Press.

Jaret, P. (1997). The mind has the power to heal. *Hippocrates* 11(5), 71–7.

Kalb, P. E. (1990). Controlling health care costs by controlling technology, a private contractual approach. *Yale Law Journal* 99, 1109–26.

Kanigel, R. (1998). Taking acupuncture seriously. *Hippocrates* 12(5), 23–4.

Kaptchuk, T. J., and Eisenberg, D. M. (1998). The persuasive appeal of alternative medicine. *Annals of Internal Medicine* 129, 1061–5.

Ko, R. J. (1998). Adulterants in Asian patent medicines (letter). *New England Journal of Medicine* 339, 847.

LaPuma, J., and Lawlor, E. F. (1990). Quality-adjusted life-years, Ethical implications for physicians and policymakers. *Journal of the American Medical Association,* 2917–21.

Lazarou, J., Pomeranz, B. H., and Corey, P. N. (1998). Incidence of adverse drug reactions in hospitalized patients. *Journal of the American Medical Association* 279, 1200–5.

Leape, L. L., Park, R. E., Solomon, D. H., et al. (1989). Relation between surgeons' practice volumes and geographic variation in the rate of carotid endarterectomy. *New England Journal of Medicine* 321, 653–7.

Leape, L. L., Park, R. E., Solomon, D. H., et al. (1990). Does inappropriate use explain small area variations in the use of health care services? *Journal of the American Medical Association* 263, 669–72.

Lederle, F. A., Applegate, W. A., and Grimm, R. H., Jr. (1993). Reserpine and the medical marketplace. *Archives of Internal Medicine* 153, 705–6.

Lehman, A. F. (1995). Measuring quality of life in a reformed health system. *Health Affairs* 14(3), 90–101.

Leplege, A., and Hunt, S. (1997). The problem of quality of life in medicine. *Journal of the American Medical Association* 278, 47–50.

Lippman, M. E. (2000). High-dose chemotherapy plus autologous bone marrow transplantation for metastatic breast cancer. *New England Journal of Medicine* 342, 1119–20.

LoVecchio, F., Curry, S. C., and Bagnasco, T. (1998). Butyrolactone-induced central nervous system depression after ingestion of RenewTrient, a 'dietary supplement' (letter). *New England Journal of Medicine* 339, 847–8.

Macklin, R. (1999). The ethical problems with sham surgery in clinical research. *New England Journal of Medicine* 341, 992–6.

Margolin, A., Avants, S. K., and Kleber, H. D. (1998). Investigating alternative medicine therapies in randomized controlled trials. *Journal of the American Medical Association* 280, 1626–8.

Mello, M. M., and Brennan, T. A. (2001). The controversy over high-dose chemotherapy with autologous bone marrow transplant for breast cancer. *Health Affairs* 20(5), 101–18.

Merkatz, R. B., Temple, R., Sobel, S., et al. (1993). Women in clinical trials of new drugs. *New England Journal of Medicine* 329, 292–6.

Micozzi, M. S. (1998). Complementary care: When is it appropriate? Who will provide it? *Annals of Internal Medicine* 129, 65–6.

Miller, M. G., Miller, L. S., Fireman, B., and Black, S. B. (1994). Variation in practice for discretionary admissions. *Journal of the American Medical Association* 271, 1493–8.

Mold, J. W., and Stein, H. F. (1986). The cascade effect in the clinical care of patients. *New England Journal of Medicine* 314, 512–4.

Morreim, E. H. (1986). Computing the quality of life. In: *The Price of Health: Cost-Benefit Analysis in Medicine.* Agich G, Begley C. Dordrecht, D.: Reidel Pub. Co., pp. 45–69.

Morreim, E. H. (1992). The impossibility and the necessity of quality of life research. *Bioethics* 6(3), 218–32.

Morreim, E. H. (1994). Redefining quality by reassigning responsibility. *American Journal of Law and Medicine* 20(1–2), 79–104.

Morreim, E. H. (1995). Quality of life in health care allocation. In: *Encyclopedia of Bioethics, 2nd edition,* edited by Warren Thomas Reich New York, Simon & Schuster MacMillan, Volume 3, pp. 1358–61.

Morreim, E. H. (1995). Moral justice and legal justice in managed care, the ascent of contributive justice. *Journal of Law, Medicine, and Ethics* 23(3), 247–65.

Morreim, E. H. (1995). Diverse and perverse incentives in managed care bringing the patient into alignment. *Widener Law Symposium Journal* 1(1), 89–139.

Morreim, E. H. (1997). Medicine meets resource limits, Restructuring the legal standard of care. *University of Pittsburgh Law Journal* 59(1), 1–95.

Morreim, E. H. (1999). Playing doctor, corporate medical practice and medical malpractice. *Michigan Journal of Law Reform* 32(4), 939–1040.

Morreim, E. H. (2000). Saving lives, spending money, shepherding the role of technology. In: *Ethical Issues in Health Care on the Frontiers of the Twenty-First Century*. Wear S, Bono JJ, Logue G, McEvoy A, editors Philosophy and Medicine Series Dordrecht, Kluwer Academic Publishers, pp. 63–110.

O'Connor, G. T., Quinton, H. B., Traven, N. D., et al. (1999). Geographic variation in the treatment of acute myocardial infraction, the cooperative cardiovascular project. *Journal of the American Medical Association* 281, 627–33.

Ornish, D., Scherwitz, L. W., Billings, J. H., et al. (1998). Intensive lifestyle changes for reversal of coronary heart disease. *Journal of the American Medical Association* 280, 2001–7.

Peters, W. P., and Rogers, M. C. (1994). Variation in approval by insurance companies of coverage for autologous bone marrow transplantation for breast cancer. *New England Journal of Medicine* 330, 473–7.

Pilote, L., Califf, R. M., Sapp, S., et al. [for the GUSTO-1 Investigators] (1995). Regional variation across the United States in the management of acute myocardial infarction. *New England Journal of Medicine* 333, 565–72.

Pittler, M. H., and Ernst, E. (1998). Horse-chestnut seed extract for chronic venous insufficiency. *Archives in Dermatology* 134, 1356–60.

Rapoport, J., Teres, D., Steingrub, J., et al. (2000). Patient characteristics and ICU organizational factors that influence frequency of pulmonary artery catheterization. *Journal of the American Medical Association* 283, 2559–67.

Relman, A. S. (1999). Is integrative medicine the medicine of the future? *Archives of Internal Medicine* 159, 2122–6.

Relman, A. S., and Weil, A. (1999). Is integrative medicine the medicine of the future? *Archives of Internal Medicine* 159, 2122–6.

Rennie, D. (1997). Thyroid storm. *Journal of the American Medical Association* 277, 1238–43.

Schneiderman, L. J. (2000). Alternative medicine or alternatives to medicine? A physician's perspective. *Cambridge Quarterly of Healthcare Ethics* 9, 83–97.

Smith, A. (1987). Qualms and QALY's. *Lancet*, 1134–6.

Smyth, J. M., Stone, A. A., Hureswitz, A., and Kaell, A. (1999). Effects of writing about stressful experiences on symptom reduction in patients with asthma or rheumatoid arthritis. *Journal of the American Medical Association* 281, 1304–9.

Spiegel, D., Kraemer, H. C., Bloom, J. R., and Gottheil, E. (1989). Effect of psychosocial treatment of survival of patients with metastatic breast cancer. Lancet 334, 888–91.

Spiegel, D. (2001). Mind matters—group therapy and survival in breast cancer. *New England Journal of Medicine* 345, 1767–8.

Stadtmauer, E. A., O'Neill, A., Goldstein, L. J., et al. (2000). Conventional-dose chemotherapy compared with high-dose chemotherapy plus autologous hematopoietic stem-cell transplantation for metastatic breast cancer. *New England Journal of Medicine* 342, 1069–76.

Starr, P. (1982). *The Social Transformation of American Medicine*. New York, Basic Books.

Sullivan, M. D. (1993). Placebo controls and epistemic control in orthodox medicine. *Journal of Medicine and Philosophy* 18, 213–31.

Tausk, F. A. (1998). Alternative medicine, is it all in your mind? *Archives in Dermatolology* 134, 1422–5.

Testa, M. A., and Simonson, D. C. (1996). Assessment of quality-of-life outcomes. *New England Journal of Medicine* 334, 835–40.

Wash. Rev. Code § 48.43.045.

Washington Physicians Services Association v. Gregoire, 967 F.Supp. 424 (W.D. Wash. 1997).

Welch, W. P., Miller, M. E., Welch, H. G., et al. (1993). Geographic variation in expenditures for physicians' services in the United States. *New England Journal of Medicine* 328, 621–7.

Welch, H. G., Miller, M. E., and Welch, W. P. (1994). An analysis of inpatient practice patterns in Florida and Oregon. *New England Journal of Medicine* 330, 607–12.

Wells, K. B., and Sturm, R. (1995). Care for depression in a changing environment. *Health Affairs* 14(3), 78–89.

Wennberg, J. E. (1986). Which rate is right? *New England Journal of Medicine* 314, 310–11.

Wennberg, J. E., Freeman, J. L., Culp, W. J. (1987). Are hospital services rationed in New Haven or overutilized in Boston? *Lancet* 1, 1185–8.

Wennberg, J. E. (1987). The paradox of appropriate care. *Journal of the American Medical Association* 258, 2568–69.

Wennberg, J. E. (1990). Outcomes research, cost containment, and the fear of rationing. *New England Journal of Medicine* 323, 1202–4.

Wennberg, J. E. (1991). Unwanted variations in

the rule of practice. *Journal of the American Medical Association* 265, 1306–7.

Wennberg, J. E. (1999). Understanding geographic variations in health care delivery. *New England Journal of Medicine* 340, 52–53.

Wilt, T. J., Ishani, A., Stark, G., et al. (1998). Saw palmetto extracts for treatment of benign prostatic hyperplasia. *Journal of the American Medical Association* 280, 1604–9.

Winslow, L. C., and Kroll, D. J. (1998). Herbs as medicines. *Archives of Internal Medicine* 158, 2192–9.

YaDeau, R. (1996). Cost-effectiveness and complementary medicine. *American Journal of Managed Care* 2, 460.

Zugar, A. (1998). New way of doctoring, going by the evidence. *Physician's Management* 38(2), 41–4.

27

Justice in Transplant Organ Allocation

Rosamond Rhodes

Steadily improving transplantation survival rates and transplantation becoming an accepted treatment for more lethal medical conditions mean that the demand for transplant organs is increasing. While the number of organs donated for transplantation has increased slightly year by year, the percentage of cadaveric organs that are donated for transplantation has remained about the same, and the numerical increase is not large enough to meet the growing demand despite national and local efforts to boost organ donation. About 4,000 Americans die each year for lack of a transplant organ (UNOS, 1999). This severe shortage of human organs for transplantation has created competition for the cadaveric organs that are donated, it and has made allocation policies highly controversial.

Currently, organ allocation in the United States is administered by the Organ Procurement and Transplant Network (OPTN) in accordance with the 1984 National Organ Transplant Act and with oversight for equitable allocation by the Department of Health and Human Services (DHHS). The mechanisms for organ procurement and distribution have gradually evolved and now include 11 United Network for Organ Sharing (UNOS) regions that encompass 51 Organ Procurement Organizations (OPOs) for organ retrieval and distribution. Together they serve 868 organ-specific transplant programs at 261 transplant centers and performed 22,854 organ transplants in 2000 (UNOS, 2001a). Presently, local patients are given priority for organs procured within the local OPO. When a local recipient is not found, the organs are then shared across the region, and when no recipient is found in the region, organs are made available nationally within the time constraints of effective organ survival without blood supply (i.e., cold ischemia time). When no acutely urgent recipient is identified in the local area, the organ is offered to acutely urgent patients across the region before offering the organ to chronically ill or less severely ill local patients[1] (Table 27–1). This system of local priority has created differences in the length of time that patients wait for a transplant organ and has spurred a national debate about changes that should be made in the current system.

In her June 1, 1998, letter to Congress, Donna Shalala, then Secretary of Health and Human Services, discussed a significant problem in the way organs are allocated for transplantation in the United States. Describing the effects of the UNOS policy, she explained that,

the median waiting times for the two major liver transplant centers in Kentucky were vastly different—38 days at one center, 226 at the other. Similarly, in Louisiana, the median waiting time at one center was reported to be 18 days, while at another, it was 262 days. In Michigan, the numbers were 161 days and 401 days. Although these numbers do not tell the whole story, they certainly reflect that unacceptable disparities in waiting times exist, even within States. (Shalala, 1998)

Although many disparities in what people have and get are unavoidable, other disparities can be averted, and while many disparities are ethically unproblematic, others signal serious problems of injustice. Social policies are just when they provide for equal treatment of all who are similarly situated and attend to relevant and important common human concerns. Policies are unjust when they give priority to extraneous concerns and irrelevant differences and thereby give people in relevantly similar situations inequitable treatment. For people who need an organ transplant to live or to live without significant disability, their primary concern is receiving a successful transplant. For people making an equitable allocation of transplant organs, the most appropriate considerations for distinguishing between potential recipients should be the urgency of patient need and the likelihood for success—beyond those medical standards, patients should be treated equally (Rhodes et al., 1992). However, a careful examination of UNOS allocation policies reveals that additional agendas inform their positions and practices.

Though UNOS policies are supposed to provide for the equitable (just) allocation of cadaveric transplant organs, and while they take significant steps in that direction, the disparities in waiting time suggest that UNOS policies still have some way to go in achieving justice. It is, therefore, important to appreciate precisely what the focus of a just allocation scheme should be, why and how UNOS policy falls short of the mark, and what would be required for creating a just scheme for the future. In this chapter I examine existing UNOS policies in light of their effects, that is, their creation of the disparity in waiting times for transplantation and their disparate treatment of groups of people who need a transplant organ. I also review considerations that are and should be taken into account in a just policy for allocation, spotlight factors that should not be given heed, and argue for principles to guide future organ allocation policy. With this agenda in mind, I discuss in turn society's trust as an essential requirement for the practice of organ

Table 27–1. UNOS Policy 3.6: Allocation of Livers (as of June 16, 2000)

Adult Donor Liver Allocation Algorithm

Local
  1. Status 1 patients in descending point order
Regional
  2. Status 1 patients in descending point order
Local
  3. Status 2A patients in descending point order
  4. Status 2B patients in descending point order
  5. Status 3 patients in descending point order

Regional
  6. Status 2A patients in descending point order
  7. Status 2B patients in descending point order
  8. Status 3 patients in descending point order

National
  9. Status 1 patients in descending point order
  10. Status 2A patients in descending point order
  11. Status 2B patients in descending point order
  12. Status 3 patients in descending point order

Note: Available online at <http://www.unos.org/frame_Default.asp?Category=About>

transplantation, the crucial transplantation goal of acting for the patients' good, the principle of equity, considerations of efficacy, irrelevant agendas, and the importance of trust among transplant programs.

TRUST AND TRANSPLANTATION

From the point of view of American society, the training of transplant surgeons, the establishment of centers for organ transplantation, and the national system for organ procurement and allocation are all institutions of medicine or parts of the institution of medicine. As such, they must function in ways that preserve and promote society's trust, and the institutions themselves must strive to be trustworthy.[2]

The importance of trust in medicine becomes obvious when you consider that doctors and medicine are committed to acting for the good of patients.[3] To be permitted to take histories, to perform examination, to prescribe medication, or to perform surgeries for their patients' good, doctors must be *trusted*. In other words, all reasonably farsighted physicians must recognize that, to practice medicine, they must *seek trust and deserve it*. Because this rule follows from a reasonable consideration of the basic requirements for medical practice, it is the fundamental moral imperative for doctors. Every physician who considers the context of medical practice cannot fail to acknowledge it. No patient who vividly imagines what is being undertaken would want it any other way. All prospective patients—everyone, that is—want doctors to be trustworthy.[4] And, so, all doctors must accept *seek trust and deserve it* as their moral law, as their creed. In deciding what to do and how to do it, physicians must pay attention to promoting trust and not eroding it. In molding themselves as physicians they must focus on making themselves trustworthy practitioners.

Trust dictates the necessary model for medical practice, and it plays a crucial role in explaining the ethics of transplantation. The concept of trust can tell us a great deal about the characteristics that a transplant program must embody. It can also tell us a great deal about the design of transplant policies and the ethical limits of transplantation.

Professional Competence

Because successful organ transplantation involves the collaboration of many individuals working together, a trustworthy transplant program must involve a well-staffed cooperative team of trustworthy individuals. For a transplant program to be trustworthy, members of the transplant team must, of course, be *knowledgeable and skilled*. They must be well versed in the etiology and progress of organ failure, proficient in diagnosis, fully informed of the most recent clinical studies of pre- and postoperative management of their patients, skilled in the assessment of their patients' likelihood of having a good outcome, discerning in their evaluation of a patient's anatomy, masters of technical dexterity, practiced in operative cooperation, and accomplished in recognizing and managing bouts of rejection. Without professional competence, the team is not deserving of trust. Competence, therefore, is more than a matter of competitive pride, personal curiosity, ambition, or prudence. Being knowledgeable and skilled are essential to trustworthiness and, hence, a *moral* obligation.

Caring

Because patients are more inclined to trust transplant team members who they believe genuinely *care* about their good, team members must also be compassionate. For everyone, ethical conduct involves an emotional component. Beyond the psychological appeal of a caring doctor, physicians, in particular, need to feel caring concern for their patients' well-being in order to *be* trustworthy. Caring is a prophylactic against the ethical danger of making clinical judgments that reflect self-interest rather than patient interest, and it also protects against the moral hazard of finding good excuses rather than doing what one should. Furthermore, for patients to trust their transplant surgeons and accept their recommendations, patients need to believe that their surgeons are acting from caring rather than selfishness (Rhodes, 1995).

Respect for Autonomy

To be trusted, members of the transplant team will also have to pay serious attention to the patient's view of what is good. People like to have their own way, and when decisions are intimately concerned with a patient's own body and life, differences between alternatives can be tremendously important to that patient. Sometimes a doctor's view of what is best can be at odds with a patient's view. In some circumstances a patient and doctor will give priority to various factors differently and actually consider the other's choice to be no good at all. Because doctors need their patients' trust and because patients need to feel confident that their doctors will not impose their personal values and thereby, in the patient's eyes, cause harm, the patient's ranking of goods, or *respect for patient autonomy*, has to be incorporated into the professional commitments of the physician.

In sum, for transplant teams and programs to be trusted to a degree that allows them to act for their patients' good, they are committed to making themselves professionally competent, caring, and respectful of patient values. The importance of these physician characteristics and the actions they dictate are relatively noncontroversial. To appreciate the centrality of trust and trustworthiness in transplantation policy, and in the goals and design of transplant organizations and institutions, requires some creative application of the concepts and attentive understanding.

APPROPRIATE GOALS FOR TRANSPLANTATION

Families that donate the organs of deceased loved ones do so out of appreciation of the great good that transplanted organs provide and out of trust that their gifts will be allocated justly. They expect that all those in need of organs will be treated equitably and that cadaveric organs will be allocated according to principles that reasonable people could endorse. Transplant surgery, transplant centers, and institutions responsible for organ retrieval and allocation all exist because our society acknowledges the great benefit that transplantation provides for those with end-stage organ failure and because society intends the equitable allocation of its scarce transplant organs. In general, society expects that the focus on the good of patients is the central moral goal of medicine; and in transplantation, society expects that the commitment to the good of individual patients and the good of the pool of potential transplant recipients is the guiding agenda in the establishment of organ transplant programs and the design of equitable organ allocation policies.

Individuals each have their own unique conceptions of what is good. Nevertheless, the needs that human beings share lead to a significant overlap in their appreciation of what counts as good. It is reasonable to presume that everyone who is a candidate for an organ transplant sees life, the ability to function, the enjoyment of liberty and pleasure, and the avoidance of disability as good (Gert et al., 1998). Because policies are just when they attend to people equally with respect to their most important human concerns, policies that govern allocation of vital organs for transplantation must address what is most important to potential recipients. To the extent that receiving a transplant is necessary for their enjoyment of all of the most important goods, the primary good that a just policy must provide is a transplant organ, and in the face of the current shortage of such organs, the good that policies should promote is the increased likelihood of receiving an organ and having a successful transplant.

This is not to say that other things are not important to transplant candidates as well. Candidates will want transplant policies and programs to provide respectful treatment, caring attention, honest and clear communication, clean and attractive surroundings, convenience. These various considerations will have different priorities for different individuals; some factors will be significant to some patients and trivial to others. Yet it is hard to imagine that receiving an organ and having a successful transplant is not the first priority of organ transplant candidates with respect to transplant programs and policies. Indeed, when patients understand the differences among transplant centers and have the option, we see them flocking to those programs with a proven track record of success or traveling to be listed in regions where they are more likely to receive an organ (UPMC, 1997). In life, when different options offer opportunities for satisfying different preferences, people make choices and they triage their values so they can achieve what is most important to them. Various considerations have different weight in different contexts, and what is less important is sacrificed for the sake of achieving what is most crucial.

Thus, while having a transplant center close to home may be important to some patients, it is easy to appreciate that they might be willing to travel farther for the sake of achieving other more important goals. Because of the priority that most accord to receiving an organ and having a successful transplant, reasonable transplant candidates would likely endorse policies that tend to increase organ availability and to improve the likelihood of transplant success over policies that provide greater convenience, particularly if that convenience should cost needed organs.

OTHER GOALS

In contrast, others involved in transplant programs and others who are affected by organ allocation policies may very well have different goals and different priorities. In this age of managed care and competition among medical centers for market share, there are public relations advantages to announcing that you offer technology at the cutting edge. Hospital administrators may be eager to promote their institution's "high-tech" transplant centers because the image is likely to make them generally more attractive to consumers. And when transplantation is also profitable, administrators will also be scrambling for a greater revenue share.

In addition to hospital interests, politicians stand to benefit from the luster of transplant programs in their district and also from appreciation for their support from local beneficiary medical centers. Furthermore, both the convenience and the comaraderie of coordinating organ procurement and allocation within a limited circle of people who have experience working together promote the preference of OPO staffers for sharing organs within local OPO boundaries. And certainly surgeons stand to gain glory, fame, credentialing, stature, and money by performing transplants.[5] As bioethicist Arthur Caplan has noted, transplant organ "[s]carcity means that access to the lucrative and prestigious field of transplantation is available only to a relatively small number of surgeons and an even smaller number of hospitals" (Caplan, 1992).

In any discussion of justice in the design of organ allocation policy, these conflicting interests of hospitals, OPOs, politicians, and surgeons have to be appreciated to assess their claims clearly. The appropriate goals of maximizing organ availability and improving the success of transplantation have to be maintained as the primary agenda. Allocation policies should not make sacrifices to antithetical interests, and policymakers have to be alert to the rhetoric of competing interests, particularly when it masquerades as the voice of patient interests.

Equity

Transplantation policies do not and should not treat all people equally: Everyone is not given equal access to organs for transplantation (e.g., one per person). Transplant organs, which are especially scarce and precious resources, are reserved only for those who need them. Principles for their just distribution aim at achieving equity (rather than equality) by treating relevant differences among those who need a transplant similarly. For all the differences among candidates, the crucial policy problem is specification of the relevant differences and assignment of a relative priority to each of those relevant differences. When a policy gives irrelevant differences significant weight and when that assignment results in unequal treatment of similarly situated transplant candidates, the policy is, on its face, unjust.

So far, transplant programs have treated nonmedical judgments about patients as irrelevant differences and have, for the most part, resisted the impulse to make blatant personal or relative judgments about recipient worthiness.[6] This attitude reflects medicine's general commitments to a nonjudgmental regard of every patient and a caring attitude toward each. These are professional commitments because they have an essential role in promoting the community's trust. We all want our doctors not to judge us harshly and to take good care of us regardless of who we are and what we have done. For example, in wartime, doctors have a professional responsibility to treat all medically needy combatants alike, those from their own side as well as the enemy. Medicine's implicit attachment to these principles of nonjudgmental regard and caring for all enables patients to bring themselves to physicians so that they can receive the benefits that medicine has to offer. These professional positions on the appropriate physician attitude toward patients have translated into the transplant community's reluctance to judge recipient worthiness, recipient behavioral contribution to their present need, recipient age, or even the share of good life that the patient has already enjoyed.[7]

By quantifying severity of disease, UNOS can be seen as attempting to identify and to give priority to only medically relevant differences in need so that transplant candidates can be treated equitably. The system's stated aim is to establish instruments for making uniform measurement for urgency of need (i.e., "how *soon* someone will die without the transplant" and "how *badly off* someone will be without it") so that patients who are listed for transplantation at different centers can be fairly assessed and compared (Kamm, 1993, p. 234). Although arguments persist about how much weight should be assigned to each consideration, the criteria are intended to reflect differences in urgency of need, and they can be validated with clinical data and adjusted to reflect refined understanding. Whereas the specific criteria and standards vary somewhat from organ to organ, because of immunological sensitivities and features specific to the survival of particular organs, these assessment instruments are supposed to quantify medical differences and, beyond these relatively objective criteria, leave priority to fairness as approximated by a rule of first-come first-served.

For example, the Child-Turcotte-Pugh score for listing liver transplant candidates assigns points for symptoms and biological markers of disease (Table 27–2). It is used to approximate an objective standard for assessing the seriousness of need and the urgency of liver transplantation. Patients with liver disease must have 7 points to be listed for transplantation. Then, depending on the number of points their condition merits and factors about their disease, they are assigned to a category (e.g., 1, 2A, 2B, 3) of urgency. Theoretically, those with the most urgent need are given priority for receiving an organ.[8] Organs are also matched to recipients based on biological and size compatibility so as to minimize harm and to maximize benefit.

Efficacy

Aside from urgency of need, listing criteria have focused on the medical judgment of likelihood of efficacy. Policies for or-

Table 27–2. Child-Turcotte-Pugh (CTP) Scoring System to Assess Severity of Liver Disease

Points	1	2	3
Encephalopathy	None	1–2	3–4
Ascites	Absent	Slight (or controlled by diuretics)	At least moderate despite diuretic treatment
Bilirubin (mg/dl)	<2	2–3	>3
Albumin (g/dl)	>3.5	2.8–3.5	<2.8
International Normalized Ratio (INR)	<1.7	1.7–2.3	>2.3

Note: United Network for Organ Sharing, available online September 4, 2001, at <*http://www.unos.org/frame_Default.asp? Category=aboutpolicies*>.

gan distribution take the limitations of cold ischemic time into account so as to maximize organ viability. Programs also evaluate patients for the likelihood of their long-term survival and the likelihood of post-transplant organ survival. When a potential recipient becomes so ill that the likelihood of survival is significantly diminished, the patient is not listed for transplantation or is made inactive on the UNOS organ recipient list (e.g., currently status 7 for liver transplantation).

Patients are also evaluated with respect to the likelihood of their adhering to rigorous post-transplant protocols so that the transplanted organ will not be lost to rejection. Typically, when a patient's history raises questions about the likelihood of adherence with a schedule of anti-rejection medications and post-transplantation medical monitoring, the patient is further examined and assessed by a psychiatrist or a social worker. Adherence and efficacy are reasonable and relevant medical considerations for the evaluation of individual patients because cadaveric organs are scarce and they should be allocated so as to provide significant benefit.

Incentives Opposed to Efficacy

Although UNOS proudly proclaims its commitment to efficacy as an essential feature of a just allocation system, the current system compromises the efficacy of organ allocation by giving urgently ill patients priority. Presently, there are no incentives to encourage programs to triage out the patients who are least likely to derive a significant benefit from a transplant. So long as policy validates allocation to those who are most ill, transplant teams are not likely to limit the access of their patients to organs, even when those patients have a low likelihood of long-term survival.

Policy should proscribe the behavior that the public wants avoided or provide incentives to promote the behavior that the public values. Allocation policy that focuses on urgency without also attending to efficacy is likely to provide less long-term benefit overall by promoting allocation of organs to patients with low likelihood for long-term survival. While we want transplant programs to try hard to provide benefits to all patients who have a similarly good chance for deriving significant benefit from transplantation and not to restrict the procedure only to those who will be easiest to manage or who have the greatest likelihood for survival (e.g., everyone with at least an 85% chance for long-term survival and not just those with a 95% chance of survival), we also want programs to avoid allocations to those who have a significantly diminished chance for long-term survival (e.g., those with less than a 60% chance for long-term survival). Without including some mechanism to promote efficacy, current and proposed policies pay lip-service to their commitment to efficacy in organ allocation while actually promoting the opposite behavior.

Unsupported Distinctions

Transplant policy distinctions that rest on claims about the efficacy of transplantation for groups of patients must be supported by compelling evidence. Differentiation in listing, prioritization, or allocation of organs without an adequate basis of evidence should be eyed with suspicion. Drawing distinctions based on unsupported assumptions about efficacy is likely to create injustice.

Although UNOS policy and the UNOS Liver Status categories illustrate standard considerations for recipient prioritization, they also illustrate some significant problems in liver allocation that derive from making distinctions without sufficient evidence. For example, regardless of the urgency of their need or the likelihood of their future adherence to posttransplantation regimens, UNOS policy requires at least six months of abstinence before patients with a history of drug or alcohol use can be listed for transplantation. This UNOS policy accepts the presumption that patients who are labeled "substance abusers," alcohol and narcotics users in particular, are at greater risk of nonadherence and losing transplanted organs than are other patients. Without evidence of low efficacy for transplantation of alcoholics and addicts, the listing of these patients is restricted by a waiting period and requirements for participation in abstinence support programs that are not applied to patients who are viewed without that belief.

In addition, evidence suggests that substance-abusing patients who are judged likely to comply with posttransplant regimens (including those who return to substance use posttransplant) adhere to their required posttransplant treatment and maintain their transplanted organs quite well (Osorio et al., 1994; Gerhardt et al., 1996; Tang et al., 1998; Burra et al., 2000; Pereira et al., 2000; Mackie et al., 2001). Presumptions that persist, even in the face of counter-evidence, smack of unfounded discrimination. Without evidence of a difference in outcomes, holding substance-abusing patients to a different standard from others is not medically justified. Distinguishing between patients in the face of refuted presumptions is ethically untenable.

Similarly, the 1996 rule change (starting in 1998) that gave priority to status 1 liver transplant patients (people who suddenly develop liver failure and are likely to die within a week) over status 2A patients (people with chronic liver failure who have deteriorated to the point where they are likely to die within a week) raises questions of evidence and justice. The argument for the rule change was that patients with chronic illness (status 2A patients) had a lower chance of surviving than did patients with acute liver failure (status 1 patients) who had otherwise been healthy. The implicit justification was that the change in policy would allow more people to benefit from transplantation (Showstack et al., 1999). However, opponents of the change have argued that the data do not support the distinction. If that claim is true, the change in policy unjustly disadvantages those with chronic illness. In either case, distinctions in patient treatment are only justified by a significant difference in efficacy. Until a significant disparity in outcomes can be shown, allocation policy should not distinguish between potential recipients. Hunches are not enough of a ground for medical judgment, and assumptions cannot support policy distinctions for allocation of life-preserving scarce resources. And, as Kamm has argued, very small differences may not be significant enough to justify a distinction that will leave some to die while others live or suffer a major disability (Kamm, 2002).

Another set of questionable efficacy claims are invoked to support the UNOS grant of local priority in organ distribution. Here advocates of local priority point to efficacy advantages of local distribution. They claim that by keeping organs within a local or regional geographic area they can be transplanted when they are more viable and, thereby, improve outcomes. They also claim that by transplanting organs to patients who are less seriously ill, patient survival is improved. Again, the current evidence does not support these conclusions. Today's methods of organ preservation allow for periods of cold ischemia time for kidneys and livers that are longer than they had been before the technological advances and without a diminution in organ viability (Stratta et al., 1990; Bretan et al., 1994; Porte et al., 1998; Pirenne et al., 2001). Furthermore, geographic boundaries do not always translate into shorter transport times, because the other side of the boundary could actually be closer or take less time to reach than the other side of the local area. And, as to the question of an improvement in the number of patients who survive, the 1999 Institute of Medicine (IOM) report, *Organ Procurement and Transplantation: Assessing Current Policies and the Potential Impact of the DHHS Final Rule*, suggests the opposite. According to their study,

as OPO size increases to 9 million people, . . . the number of status 2B and 3 patients receiving transplant could be reduced to allow more status 1 and 2A patients to receive transplants, without an increase in pretransplant mortality for the status 2B and 3 patients. (IOM, p. 70)

Advocates of local priority also maintain that keeping organs close to their source will increase donation, in other words, that people are more likely to donate organs when they will be used by a needy patient within the local OPO. Again, findings in the IOM study dispute these assumptions (IOM, pp. 47, 71). Without strong evidence for a significant enough difference in outcomes, drawing geographic distinctions between potential organ recipients is unjust because geographic differences are irrelevant. Donna Shalala's declaration that the disparities in waiting time are "unacceptable" amounts to a charge of injustice. And Robert M. Veatch, a former member of the UNOS Ethics Committee and author of *Transplantation Ethics*, echoes that assessment. According to Veatch,

[t]he bottom line is that local priority makes the transplant program inequitable. People who are equally sick, who have equal entitlement to a transplant, and who are equally good candidates will have significantly different probabilities for getting an organ. Because many people die while on the waiting list, a delay in getting an organ equals an increased risk of death. The moral principle of justice requires that people who are equally situated are entitled [to] be treated equally. (Veatch, 2000, p. 375)

The IOM report acknowledges the problem of injustice but defines it in terms of disparities in life risk rather than variations in waiting time. According to the IOM analyses of available data, there is a 5% variation in the transplant rates for status 1 patients in different OPOs, but a 13% variation for status 2B patients, and a 35% variation for status 3 patients. After discounting other factors that might contribute to the disparity, authors of the IOM report cautiously conclude that "smaller OPOs, by generally transplanting more statuses 2B and 3 patients than larger OPOs, may contribute to a situation in which more severely ill patients are required to wait longer for organs at increased risk of death" (IOM, p. 73)

SMALL CENTERS AND LARGER CENTERS

In light of organ scarcity and concerns about just allocation, the UNOS protective policy stance toward small transplant centers is particularly peculiar. The IOM report addresses the possibility of changes in allocation policy negatively effecting the viability of small centers and advocates monitoring the situation. It also points out that evidence from changes in New York State suggest that the viability of small centers will not be affected and, further, that there is no reason to believe that closing small centers will adversely effect minority transplant candidates (IOM, pp. 39–41). Yet concern for the viability of small centers seems to be motivating the debate over national versus local priority allocation schemes, and that attention raises the question of whether small centers should be protected.

If the goal of increasing the likelihood of patients receiving an organ and having a successful transplant and the goal of just allocation of cadaveric organs are the appropriate central agenda for national transplantation policy, concern for the viability of small transplant centers should be reconsidered. If transplantation at small centers actually diminishes the likelihood for successful transplantation, if it undermines efficient use of the current organ supply, and if it impedes future advances in transplantation, then instead of worrying about the viability of such centers, policymakers should curtail the activity of small transplant centers.

Expertise

For a transplant center to be trustworthy, it must have at least two teams of knowledgeable and skilled transplant surgeons, because transplant organs can become available at any time and there must always be a team of surgeons available to perform the transplant. A trustworthy program must also have a well-staffed cooperative team of knowledgeable and trustworthy health professionals to provide the support that assures good transplant outcomes. Beyond the surgeons, a program needs physicians who are expert in the pretransplant management of acutely and chronically ill patients, expert anesthesiologists, experts in the critical care of posttransplant patients, experts in the management of infectious disease in immunosuppressed patients, experts in the pharmacology of immunosuppressive drugs and the medications for the co-morbidity of persisting chronic diseases (e.g., diabetes), experts in the management of other organ systems for patients pre- and posttransplantation (e.g., cardiologists, nephrologists, hepatologists), and experts in the psychiatric assessment of transplant candidates and their posttransplant support.

In addition, a trustworthy program needs the assistance of nurse/transplant coordinators, trained surgical nurses, social workers, and ethicists. Without this requisite framework, a program cannot provide optimal transplantation services. It is hard to imagine that small programs have such resources and that available resources are practiced enough to provide skilled services and to manage the routine and unusual emergencies that are part of transplantation. It is, therefore, hard to imagine that small centers can match the success of larger programs, and, in fact, the transplantation literature documents the unsurprising fact that high-volume transplant centers have better results than do small programs. (Laffel et al., 1992; Hosenpud et al., 1994; Belle et al., 1995; Lin et al., 1997; Edwards et al., 1999).

Research

Transplantation owes its success to the research that has accompanied its practice. Research findings have enabled the transplant community to develop protocols for improved immunosuppressive therapy, improved pre- and posttransplant management of patients, and improved surgical techniques. Research has enabled more patients to survive transplantation, and future research promises to improve transplant outcomes even more.

Biomedical research draws conclusions from studies of significantly large numbers of subjects. In other words, medical science requires information from many patients in order to draw its general inferences. Because small centers do not have sufficient numbers of relevantly similar patients, there are many kinds of studies they cannot perform. When patients at small centers are not recruited for studies, precious opportunities for learning are lost. To the extent that transplantation research improves the success of transplantation and promotes more effective use of transplant organs, every patient who receives a transplant outside of a research center represents a loss of knowledge that could benefit those who will need transplantation or retransplantation later on.

Fairness

Current organ allocation policies that allow local priority in organ distribution make it more likely that patients at small centers will receive an organ when they are not urgently ill. Small centers prefer this arrangement because it allows them to transplant healthier patients who are likely to have an uncomplicated course. Conversely, as the IOM report makes clear, the resulting disparity in treatment of similarly situated needy patients is unfair (IOM, 1999, p. 73).

However, laws recently passed in several states (e.g., Lousiana, Oklahoma, South Carolina, Wisconsin) prohibit organs from leaving the state if patients in the state could use them. These positions are supported by the rhetoric of local politicians and transplant officials. For example, Oklahoma Governor Frank Keating (1998) complained that the federal government tries to "suck organs" from his state, and Nancy A. Kay (1998), executive director of the South Carolina Organ Procurement Agency, declared that "Our work is based on the giving of South Carolinians. . . . We like to take care of our neighbors here."[9]

While we recognize that preference for those who are near and dear is sometimes appropriate, the usual rule for when it is morally acceptable to acknowledge such priority is that other reasonable people could not object to the preferential treatment (e.g., the priority we accept for family and friends) (Scanlon, 1998, pp. 158–171). Clearly the controversy over local priority and suspicion about the motives of its advocates suggest that people have good reason for opposing local priority in organ distribution. Furthermore, laws and language that promote geographic localism are divisive and dangerous to a pluralist democratic society. They undermine our national spirit of cooperative mutual support for fellow Americans in time of need,

encourage prejudice and discrimination that is anathema to justice in allocation, and thwart the good will of those good Samaritans who donate out of love for their neighbors even when they don't live in South Carolina.

TRUST AMONG TRANSPLANT CENTERS

Given the controversy and self-serving stands that embroil transplant policy, it is easy to appreciate that transplant centers and institutions are suspicious of one another. Given the variety of competing interests and the complex incentives for self-serving rule bending, it is reasonable for each transplant center to doubt that other centers are observing the rules.

Many states allow institutions to make their own decisions about opening transplant centers, and centers everywhere are left to decide when to list patients for transplantation and the status of each listed patient. These freedoms from regulation and oversight provide opportunities for numerous questionable judgments. Institutions that are ill equipped for the task can declare themselves to be transplant centers, and centers can list patients for transplant who are not yet sick enough to meet listing criteria or exaggerate patients' need for transplant to move them to a preferential status. Such distortions can advantage a center's patients by securing them transplant organs or securing them sooner than they would be allocated otherwise. These manipulations of the system can also advantage physicians and staff as well as institutions. Each center can see the array of advantages from violating the rules when it is possible to do so without penalty. And there are no current systems for inspecting institutions for compliance with guidelines and no current national authority for penalizing institutions that flaunt or bend the rules. The absence of oversight nourishes distrust among centers and cultivates pressure to violate the rules. It is easy to imagine that other centers could be cheating because the honest center and its patients would be disadvantaged in the competition for status and scarce transplant organs when others were breaking the rules.

Still, many centers understand that their patients would be better off if they followed the rules as long as they could trust that other centers were doing the same. This is a standard "prisoner's dilemma" problem where the best outcome cannot be achieved as long as the parties lack the trust to underwrite cooperation. The solution to "prisoner's dilemma" problems always lies in creating an environment where trust is possible. The transformation from natural competition, where the prudent strategy is distrust and rule-breaking, to trusting and rule-abiding cooperation requires empowering an authority to oversee and enforce compliance.

It will be difficult for the transplant community to accomplish all of the necessary transformations because the existing organizations and their administrators already have vested interests. The structure of UNOS governance gives just one vote to each transplant center, regardless of the number of transplant programs within the center or the number of transplants performed at the center. This arrangement leaves the interests of the large numbers of patients treated at large centers seriously under-represented.

The status quo is in place because it has support from the status quo, and it perpetuates itself because its activities are designed to do just that. For example, questions on public opinion surveys employed to support policy decisions are designed to elicit responses favoring local priority and to protect small transplant centers. These survey findings are then used to make a case for those positions. Surveys are designed to be self-serving because the designers are selected by those in power and because their future service depends upon pleasing those who have engaged their services.

Nevertheless, through open public discussion that provides an opportunity for sharing reasons and exposing irrelevant private agendas, it may be possible to see through smoke screens and to achieve a consensus on the goals that are most important to transplant candidates and potential candidates—that is, receiving an organ and having a successful transplant. It is theoretically possible to authorize an agency with ample power for oversight and rule enforcement. Those who are empowered to decide will have to start with a shared commitment to the core goals of increasing the likelihood of receiving an organ and having a successful transplant. Centers will also have to be willing to yield some of their autonomy and accept oversight and rule enforcement from an agency authorized to act on equitable policies. They will also have to tolerate some disagreement as to the justice of particular rules (e.g., how many listing points to allocate for a particular symptom) and recognize that there can be a range of reasonable views. In the pursuit of justice in organ allocation policies, small differences between positions can be less important to patients and institutions than consensus and trust.

When center administrators believe that rule breaking will be discovered and that rule breakers will be seriously punished, they can trust other centers to abide by the rules because doing otherwise would be imprudent. That change would allow administrators to comfortably abide by the rules without fear of disadvantage. With oversight and enforcement in the context of consensus on reasonable goals for organ allocation, national policy can actually further justice in organ allocation.

ADVANCES IN THE JUSTICE OF LIVER ALLOCATION

The MELD/PELD Scoring Systems

The OPTN/UNOS Board of Directors has proposed a new system for liver allocation which is supposed to take affect at the end of February 2002 and replace the current categories. The Model for End Stage Liver Disease (MELD) Scoring System and the Pediatric End Stage Liver Disease (PELD) Scoring System assign points to each patient based on prognostic indicators of serious liver of disease (serum creatinine, serum bilirubin, INR). The number, a "mortality risk score," is supposed to indicate each potential recipient's urgency of need in terms of the probability of pre-transplant death. While organs will still be allocated by local and regional priority and with priority for acute illness, the MELD system is being promoted because it is supposed to make the assessment of urgency more objective than the current system and allow those in most urgent need to have priority in the allocation of cadaveric livers. Because, to some extent, time on a transplant list indicates access to medical care rather than medical need, waiting time, which had previously played a significant role in allocation, is to be discounted and only used to break a tie in MELD/PELD scores.

Although the MELD and PELD Scoring Systems do not address the problems of local and regional priority and unsupported distinctions with respect to priority for the acutely ill and discrimination against drug and alcohol users, in several respects, they express significant advances toward a just distribution system. The MELD/PELD Scoring Systems represent principles that are the outcome of a process of thoughtful discussion among a committee of professionals who are committed to making the allocation of livers more just. The Scoring Systems they have adopted are based on studies of individual indicators of the seriousness of disease and combinations of these several factors into a single rating system that has been shown to correlate with the probability of pre-transplant death. The relevant standard of avoiding deaths is the one that is most significant to potential recipients and the commitment to objective and uniform criteria makes the system fair. Yet,

the committee designing the system appreciates that end-stage liver disease is very complicated and the assessment of urgency is very difficult. Individual markers of serious disease might be more or less significant in the light of additional indicators. The policy modifications, therefore, provide a mechanism for assigning a patient Status 1 or a higher MELD score if the change in status can be justified to the Regional Review Board in terms of "a rationale for incorporating the exceptional case" into the UNOS criteria or MELD calculation. A process for addressing conflicts at the local level by appeals to the UNOS Board is built into the system. And changes in policy have to be assessed for appropriateness six months after implementation. In effect, the new policy and the rules for further modification appeal to reasons that no reasonable transplant surgeon/program should reject and the rules apply equally to all.

Furthermore, some of the MELD/PELD innovations reflect genuine concern for making allocations efficacious. Blood type compatibility is related to long-term organ survival, but that consideration has been given no weight in the allocation of organs to the acutely ill Status 1 patients. Under the new system, patients with blood types that are identical to the liver donor are given priority (i.e., an extra 10 points), those with compatible but not identical blood types are give less priority (i.e., an extra 5 points), while candidates with incompatible blood types do not receive any priority (i.e., 0 extra points). This policy modification will give priority to the acutely ill patients who are most likely to derive a long-term benefit from a particular liver. Similarly, the sickest of the chronically ill Status 2A patients have been given priority without any regard to the likelihood of their long-term survival. Under the new MELD system, scores will be limited to a maximum of 40 points. In affect, that change limits the priority for the sickest and accepts the triage of those with the least likelihood of surviving because without giving them priority, they are likely to die waiting for an organ.

As of this writing, oversight and enforcement also appear to be features in the latest version of the policy modifications. Patient data based on clinical information must be reported to UNOS according to a status re-certification schedule. Cases for which exceptions to policy have been granted must be retrospectively reviewed. Incentives are built into the system to compel timely responsiveness from Regional Review Boards and transplant programs. On-site review of particular cases and on-site audits of institutions are built into the proposal with the implicit (but unstated) threat of expulsion from the UNOS system. If these measures are implemented and enforced, they will assure compliance with UNOS policy and help to make the organ allocation system more trustworthy.

Although these are significant advantages, the MELD/PELD systems also introduce new problems. These scoring systems will be using small numerical distinctions as the basis for allocating life saving organs to one recipient rather than another. Again, without a study there is no evidence that these small numerical differences are at all significant, and, even if they are, they may not be significant enough to justify preferring one recipient over another. For example, it may be more equitable to give a liver to a patient with a MELD score of 29 who has been waiting for nine months than to a patient with a MELD score of 30 who has only been waiting for one week, particularly if a study would show that the difference in expected survival without transplantation would amount to no more than a day. In light of the important ethical distinction between any difference and a significant difference, perhaps it would be more appropriate to group patients with scores that are close but not identical (e.g., by units of five or according to cleavage planes that are predictive of some significant difference in mortality risk) and then

factor in waiting time at the group level to make the distinctions more meaningful.

Another troubling consideration is that the MELD/PELD systems require frequent recalculation of each patient's scores and even daily recalculation of scores for the sickest patients. This requirement translates into increased patient burdens in the form of more frequent unpleasant, invasive tests and increased burdens for transplant programs in terms of the time, energy, and money that will be required to update scores and to give their patients the best chance for getting an organ. Both sets of burdens raise questions about whether they are worth their anticipated advantages.

CONCLUSION

Both patients and the public are well served when they can feel secure that allocation of transplant organs is governed by a just policy and that the policy enjoys scrupulous adherence by each transplant center and every OPO. The rhetoric endorsed by UNOS espouses principles and objectives similar to those advocated in this chapter. Unfortunately, their additional inserted agendas make a significant difference in the resulting allocation policies (UNOS Principles, 2001b) To achieve justice in transplant organ allocation, the patient's good must be clearly avowed as the guiding agenda in the establishment of organ transplant programs and the design of organ allocation policies. Institutions that are responsible for organ retrieval and allocation must, therefore, commit themselves to focus on treating patients with equity and providing patients with a successful transplant. They must be discriminating in their assessment of demands and refuse to be sidetracked by other irrelevant private agendas. They must also command and wield the authority to enforce just policies in order to allow the public to be confident that transplantation is a trustworthy part of medicine.

Acknowledgment

I am grateful to Drs. Lewis Burrows, Charles Miller, Myron Schwartz, and the entire faculty of the Recanati/Miller Transplantation Institute of Mount Sinai School of Medicine for allowing me the opportunity to work with them and to learn from our numerous challenging discussions.

NOTES

1. In kidney transplantation, because of the importance of organ/recipient immunological compatibility for graft survival, exceptions to local priority rules are allowed for patients with extraordinarily sensitive immune systems and for organs that are highly compatible with a particular recipient (i.e., a six antigen match). In liver transplantation, as of 1999, an exception to local priority is made for patients in the *acutely urgent category*—that is, patients who have suddenly become ill and are likely to die within a week without receiving a liver transplant.

2. This section draws on my presentation, "Trusting Transplantation When Taking Organs from Good Samaritans and Emotionally Related Living Donors." Issues in Medical Ethics: 1999, Mount Sinai School of Medicine, December 10, 1999, New York.

3. What counts as the "patient's good," the scope of the "goals of medicine," and the purview of medicine are all interrelated subjects that significantly affect a theory of bioethics. For the purposes of this limited discussion, all of those important issues will have to be bracketed and set aside for a later, fuller elabor-ation.

4. Unfortunately, medical treatment is sometimes delivered without a climate of trust. Patients have learned to be distrustful because of unfortunate experiences with untrustworthy physicians and our untrustworthy system of health-care delivery. Distrustful patients do accept treatment when there is no better option. Examples of distrust do not refute the claim that patients would prefer to be able to trust their doctors and that most doctors would prefer to be trusted by their patients.

5. See Robert M. Veatch, 2000, pp. 368–70, who makes a similar point.

6. The transplantation stand is in opposition to the earlier stand of committees that rationed access to dialysis machines in the early 1960s according to "social worth criteria" (Jonsen, 1998, pp. 211–217). Criticism of those criteria have led to the adoption of medical criteria that focused instead on urgency of need, efficacy, and equity.

7. Kamm and others argue for the opposite view, that such considerations are relevant and should be taken into account by organ allocation policy (Kamm, 1993).

8. The 1996 rule change that gave priority to status 1 patients over status 2A patients raises questions of evidence and justice. The argument for the change was that patients with chronic illness had a lower chance of surviving and that patients with acute liver failure, who had otherwise been healthy, had a better chance of surviving. The implicit justification was that the change in policy would allow more people to benefit from transplantation (Showstack et al., 1999). Opponents of the change have argued that the data do not support the distinction and that the change in policy, therefore, unjustly disadvantages those with chronic illness.

9. Following Veatch, 2000, p. 366.

REFERENCES

Belle, S.H., Detre, K. M. and Beringer, K. C. (1995). The relationship between outcome of liver transplantation and experience in new centers. *Liver Transplantation and Surgery* 1(6), 347–53.

Bretan P.N., (1994). Characterization of improved renal transplant preservation mechanisms using PB-2 flush solution by HPLC assay. *Transplant International* 7 (Suppl 1), S465–68.

Burra, P., Mioni, D., Cillo, U., Fagiuoli, S., Senzolo, M., Naccarato, R., and Martines, D. (2000). Long-term medical and psychosocial evaluation of patients undergoing orthotopic liver transplantation for alcoholic liver disease. *Transplant International* 13 (Suppl 1), S174–78.

Caplan, A. (1992). Living dangerously: The morality of using living persons as donors of lobes of liver for transplantation. *Cambridge Quarterly of Healthcare Ethics* 1(4), 311–17.

Edwards, E.B., Roberts, J.P., McBride, M.A., Schulak, J.A., and Hunsiker, L. G. (1999). The effect of the volume of procedures at transplantation centers on mortality after liver transplantation. *New England Journal of Medicine* 341(27), 2049–53.

Gerhardt, T.C., Goldstein, R. M., Urschel, H. C., Tripp, L. E., Levy, M. F., Husberg, B. S., Jennings, L. W., Gonwa, T. A. and Klintmalm, G. B. (1996). Alcohol use following liver transplantation for alcoholic cirrhosis. *Transplantation* 62(8),1060–63.

Gert, B., Danner Clouser, K. and Culver, C. (1998). *Bioethics: A Return to Fundamentals*. New York: Oxford University Press.

Hosenpud, J. D., Breen, T. J., Edwards, E. B., Daily, O. P., and Hunsicker, L. G. (1994). The effect of transplant center volume on cardiac transplant outcome. A report of the United Network for Organ Sharing Scientific Registry. *JAMA* 271(23), 1844–49.

Institute of Medicine (IOM) report (1999). *Organ Procurement and Transplantation: Assessing Current Policies and the Potential Impact of the DHHS Final Rule*. Washington, DC: National Academy Press.

Jonsen, A. R., (1998). *The Birth of Bioethics*. New York: Oxford University Press.

Kamm, F. M. (1993). *Morality, Mortality: Vol. I*. New York: Oxford University Press.

Kamm, F. M. (2002). Whether to Discontinue *Non*futile Use of a Scarce Resource In Rhodes, R. Battin, M. P. and A. Silvers. (eds.), *Health Care and Social Justice*. New York: Oxford University Press.

Laffel, G. L. Barnett, A. I., Finkelstein, S. and Kaye, M. P. (1992). The relation between experience and outcome in heart transplantation. *New England Journal of Medicine* 327(17), 1220–25.

Lin, H.-M. Kauffman, H. M., McBride, M. A., Davies, D. B., Rosendale, J. D., Smith, C. M., Edwards, E. B., Daily, P., Kirkin, J., Shield, C. F. and Hunsicker, L. G. (1997). *Center-Specific Graft and Patient Survival Rates: United Network for Organ Sharing (UNOS) Report.*

Mackie, J., Groves, K., Hoyle, A., Garcia, C., Garcia, R., Gunson, B., and Neuberger, J. (2001). Orthotopic liver transplantation for alcoholic liver disease: A retrospective analysis of survival, recidivism, and risk factors predisposing to recidivism. *Liver Transplant* 7(5), 418–27.

Osorio, R. W., Ascher, N. L., Avery, M., Bacchetti, P., Roberts, J. P., and Lake, J. R. (1994). Predicting recidivism after orthotopic liver transplantation for alcoholic liver disease. *Hepatology* 20(1) Pt 1, 105–10.

Pereira, S. P., Howard, L. M., Muiesan, P., Rela, M., Heaton, N. and Williams, R. (2000). Quality of life after liver transplantation for alcoholic liver disease. *Liver Transplant* 6(6), 762–68.

Pirenne, J., Van Gelder, F., Coosemans, W., Aerts, R., Gunson, B., Koshiba Fourneau, I., Mirza, D., Van Steenbergen, W., Fevery, J., Nevens, F. and McMaster, P. (2001). Type of donor aortic preservation solution and not cold ischemia time is a major determination of biliary strictures after liver

transplantation. *Liver Transplant* 7(6), 540–45.

Porte, R. J., Ploeg, R. J., Hansen, B., Van Bockel, J. H., Thorogood, J., Persijn, G. G., Hermans, J. and Terpstra, O. T. (1998). Long-term graft survival after liver transplantation in the UWera: late effects of cold is chemia and primary dysfunction. *Transplant Int* 11 Suppl. 1, S164–67.

Rhodes, R. (1995). Love thy patient: Justice, caring and the doctor–patient relationship. *Cambridge Quarterly of Healthcare Ethics* 4(4),434–47.

Rhodes, R., Miller, C. and Schwartz, M. (1992). Transplant recipient selection: Peacetime vs. wartime triage. *Cambridge Quarterly of Healthcare Ethics* 4(4), 327–31.

Scanlon, T. M. (1998). *What We Owe to Each Other*. Cambridge, MA: The Belknap Press, Harvard University.

Shalala, Donna. (1998). Letter to Congress, June 1.

Showstack, J., Katz, P. P., Lake, J. R., Brown, Jr., R. S., Dudley, R. A., Belle, S., Wiesner, R. H., Zetterman, R. K., and Everhart, J. (1999). Resource utilization in liver transplantation: Effects of patient characteristics and clinical practice. *JAMA* 281(15), 1381–86.

Stratta, R. J., Wood, R. P., Langnas, A. N., Duckworth, R. M., Markin, R. S., Marujo, W., Grazi, G. L., Saito, S., Dawidson, I. and Rikkers, L. F. (1990). The impact of extended preservation on clinical liver transplantation. *Transplantation* 50(3), 438–43.

Tang, H., Boulton, R., Gunson, B., Hubscher, S., and Neuberger, J. (1998). Patterns of alcohol consumption after liver transplantation. *Gut* 43(1), 140–45.

United Network for Organ Sharing (UNOS), (2000). *1999 Annual Report to the U.S. Scientific Registry of Transplant Recipients and the Organ Procurement and Transplantation Network: Transplant Data 1989–1998*. Rockville, MD, and Richmond, VA: HHS/HRS/OSP/DOT and UNOS. [<http://www.unos.org/Data/anrpt main.htm>].

United Network for Organ Sharing. (2000). *UNOS Policy 3.6 Allocation of Livers*. [Available online at <http://www.unos.org/frame Default.asp?Category=About]

United Network for Organ Sharing. (2001a). *UNOS Critical Data* [Available online at <http://www.unos.org/data.htm>]

United Network for Organ Sharing. (2001b). *UNOS Principles and Objectives of Equitable Organ Allocation 1995–2001*. [Available online at <http://www.unos.org/

Resources/bioethics_rationale_objectives.
htm#top]

UPMC News Bureau Release (Nov. 18, 1997).
Data analysis supports idea of broad sharing
of donor livers. Available online at <http://
www.upmc.edu/NewsBureau/consad.htm>
(Dec. 4, 1998).

Veatch, R.M. (2000). *Transplantation Ethics*.
Washington, DC: Georgetown University
Press.

28

Priority to the Worse Off in Health-Care Resource Prioritization

Dan W. Brock

Resources available to the health-care system are and always will be scarce, however much many Americans would like to deny it. It is not possible, nor would it be rational or just, to provide all potentially beneficial care to everyone, no matter how small the benefits and how great the cost. As a result, use of potential resources must be given priority in a way that reflects the individual and social values at stake.

In the face of scarce resources available for health care, many will respond that such resources should be used in whatever manner will maximize the overall or aggregate health benefits for the population they serve. Cost-effectiveness analysis using measures of benefits like quality-adjusted life-years (QALYs) is the analytic tool for comparing different health interventions and programs for their aggregate health impacts (Gold et al., 1997; Brock forthcoming 2002). However, this utilitarian or consequentialist approach suffers from a familiar problem, which is that it looks only to the overall benefits to a population

without any direct concern for how those benefits are distributed to distinct individuals. It does not matter who receives how much benefit as long as resources are used to maximize overall benefits. Distributive justice and fairness, however, concern how individuals are treated relative to other individuals—which inequalities between individuals or groups are just or unjust.

Perhaps the most common feature of different theories of justice and of the thinking of ordinary people about justice is a special concern for the worse off members of society. This is seen in popular aphorisms such as "the justice of a society can be seen in how it treats its least fortunate members." Many otherwise different religious traditions also share this concern for the worse off in their teachings and work on social justice. Concern for the worse off has a long tradition in political philosophy as well, and in more recent decades has been a central focus of the work of John Rawls and the many others he has influenced (Rawls, 1971). Rawls's well known "Difference Principle" requires that the basic social and economic institutions of society be arranged so as to maximize the expectations of the worst off representative group, though the absolute priority it gives to this group is extremely controversial. However, this principle has a specific and qualified application in Rawls's work, and he did not apply it to health care. This chapter addresses how a concern for the worse off should be reflected in health-care resource prioritization. Norman Daniels (1993) has characterized this as one of several important unsolved rationing problems.

Because the U.S. health-care system is extremely heterogeneous and complex, prioritization decisions will take different forms and will be made in different ways by different parties at different places in that system. Moreover, because our health-care system often fails clearly to assign responsibility to anyone for using available resources to meet the health needs of a population, we often lack the practical institutional and policy means for making explicit and rational resource prioritization decisions. Too often resource priorities are de facto determined by myriad decisions made by many individuals acting under a variety of often perverse incentives; it should hardly be a surprise that the result is often both irrational and unjust.

However, a rational and just health-care system should be able to make explicit prioritization decisions such as these: a state mental health department must decide whether to use limited resources to expand services to severely and chronically mentally ill patients, or to expand treatment programs for less severely ill patients with mild to moderate obsessive compulsive disorder; a hospital must decide whether to use limited resources to expand its medical intensive care unit, which serves the most critically ill patients, or to expand its clinic serving teenage pregnant women and mothers; a health department must decide whether to use limited resources for a health-care outreach program for homeless persons or to expand hypertension screening programs for the general population. For each of these decisions, data are needed on the expected benefits and costs of the different programs, but they each raise as well, in different and complex ways, what priority, if any, should be given to the worse off.

If a cost-effectiveness standard for prioritizing health-care resources in decisions such as these is rejected in part in order to give priority to the worse off—that is, in favor of a "prioritarian" view—then we face three main sets of issues. First, why, for what reasons, should the worse off receive priority for health-care resources? Second, who are the worse off for the purposes of health care resource prioritization? Third, how much priority should the worse off receive? These issues are complex, controversial, and unsettled in general theories of distributive justice, and so here too in theories of just or equitable health-care resource prioritization and allocation; if anything, the problem is worse in the health-care context because the issues have received less sustained attention there and so, I believe, are less well understood. This means that it will not be possible to provide anything like a precise and definitive account of what priority the worse off should receive in health-care resource prioritization, but we can at least explore some of the issues that must be resolved to develop that account.

MORAL JUSTIFICATIONS OF PRIORITY TO THE WORSE OFF

Why does justice require some priority to the worse off in health-care resource prioritization and allocation? Perhaps the most natural reason is a concern for equality. When disadvantages are undeserved, then the moral baseline would appear to be equality, for it eliminates those undeserved disadvantages. This view has been challenged by philosophers like Robert Nozick, who has argued that, although advantages may not be morally deserved, it does not follow that individuals are not entitled to them or that others may justly take them away (Nozick, 1974). Nevertheless, many will share Larry Temkin's view that it is bad if some individuals are worse off than others through no fault of their own (Temkin, 1993). And some commitment to equality is a central feature of nearly all theories of justice, with most of the dispute being in what respects should people be equal. However, whatever the relevant arguments, strong objections exist to a fundamental commitment to equality in outcomes or conditions, both in general and as the basis of a special concern for the worse off.

First, the goal of equality in outcomes is different from the goal of improving the condition of the worse off, and so equality in outcomes will not always support improving the position of the worse off. For example, consider distributions 1 and 2 for individuals A, B, and C below:

	A	B	C
1	10	20	20
2	11	15	25

Distribution 1 is more equal, whereas distribution 2 has the better outcome for the worst off. An egalitarian view is fundamentally relational—it evaluates distributions by how equal the positions of the different parties are. A prioritarian view gives greater priority to improving individuals' positions the worse off they are, without regard to whether doing so makes the overall distribution more equal. Second, equality in outcomes or conditions is a problematic goal in its own right, even for egalitarians and even if achievable. The central difficulty is what Derek Parfit has called the "leveling down objection." If it is a morally desirable—even if not always, all things considered, decisive—feature of states of affairs that individuals are equal in some relevant respect, then to take Parfit's example

it would in one way be better if we removed the eyes of the sighted, not to give them to the

blind, but simply to make the sighted blind. That would be in one way better even if it was in *no* way better for the blind. This we may find impossible to believe. . . . [I]t is not enough to claim it would be wrong to produce equality by leveling down. . . . Our objection must be that, if we achieve equality by leveling down, there is *nothing* good about what we have done. (Parfit 1991)

Note that this objection is not just that equality is one of our moral ideals or commitments among others, as moral pluralists like Temkin acknowledge; according to Temkin, the increase in equality here is a good, but it is outweighed by our additional concern for well-being (Temkin, unpublished). However, I believe "leveling down" objections do not just show that we are moral pluralists, but rather call into question a noninstrumental commitment to equality in outcomes in general, and whether such a commitment explains our special concern for the worse off in particular.

An alternative egalitarian view looks not to whether outcomes are unequal, but rather to whether inequality is brought about by unjust treatment or action; Parfit calls these "telic" and "deontic" egalitarianism, respectively. However, whereas some of the conditions that make particular individuals or groups disadvantaged are the result of unjust treatment, such as discrimination against minorities, other conditions are not, such as suffering from genetically transmitted disease or from accidental injuries for which no one is at fault, and so deontic egalitarianism would not support giving priority to all the worse off in health-care or other contexts.

A more promising egalitarian appeal, especially in the health care context, might be to equality of opportunity. The most well-developed theory of justice in health care, that of Norman Daniels, focuses on the impact that disease has in limiting people's function and in turn opportunity (Daniels, 1985). Some principle of equality of opportunity is common to most theories of justice, and so they would require providing health care that prevents or restores loss of function so as to protect equality of opportunity. To avoid the "leveling down" objection, the requirement must be to bring people up to the normal opportunity range for their society, not strictly to *equality* of opportunity, but this is a common way of interpreting equality of opportunity principles. In general, the greater the loss of function caused by illness, the more removed people will be from enjoying the normal opportunity range, and so in that respect the worse off they will be.

How this view of equality of opportunity applies to the worse off depends on how it is interpreted. The greater the loss of function that health care can prevent or restore, the greater the increase in opportunity it will produce. If equality of opportunity is given a maximizing interpretation as requiring eliminating as much as possible the aggregate reduction in opportunity from the normal range suffered by members of society, then providing health care that prevents or restores a greater loss of function and opportunity should have priority over preventing or restoring a lesser loss. This is not equivalent to maximizing opportunity, as in a consequentialist view that focuses on opportunity instead of well-being, since raising people above the normal opportunity range does not have the same moral importance as bringing people up to it. But it does not give priority to the worse off when a greater loss of function and reduction of opportunity can be prevented or restored for better-off individuals than can be achieved for others who are worse off.

The issue of priority for the worse off, however, concerns whether and to what extent we should give priority to the needs of the worse off when we could provide greater overall improvement in function and opportunity by directing resources to better-off groups—that is, whether and how much we should depart from a maximizing cost-effectiveness applied to opportunity and accept a lower level of aggregate gain in health and opportunity in order to respond to the needs of worse-off groups.

To support this priority for the worse off, an equality of opportunity account must be interpreted as holding that the lower a person's level of opportunity is, the greater the moral importance of raising it. Most accounts of equality of opportunity are not clear on how they are to be interpreted in this regard. The general point then is that a shift in focus from well being to opportunity together with a commitment to equality of opportunity will not support priority to the worse off without an independent argument for the prioritarian instead of the maximizing interpretation of equality of opportunity; thus, let us pursue further how this prioritarian commitment for the worse off might be justified.

Whether in the context of equality of opportunity or more generally, we need an account of why the worse off should receive priority *because they are worse off*, not because we can often produce greater benefits by treating their greater needs. Here is how Derek Parfit states "The Priority View: Benefiting people matters more the worse off these people are" (Parfit, 1991). He characterizes the view as "weighted beneficence"; benefits have greater moral weight the worse off those who receive them are. This leaves open how much greater moral weight they have, and in particular does not commit a prioritarian adherent to a maximin position that gives absolute weight to improving the position of the worse off. How might one justify this prioritarian view? The issues are very complex and cannot be at all fully explored here, but I will at least mention three potentially promising responses especially relevant to the health-care context.

First, the worse off that people are, the greater the relative improvement a given size health benefit will provide them, and so the more the health benefit may matter to them; "mattering" could be given a subjective or objective interpretation in this context. To illustrate, suppose that on a scale of health-related quality of life like the Health Utilities Index (HUI), on which death equals 0 and full unimpaired function equals 1, person A is very seriously disabled and at level 0.20, whereas person B, who is less seriously ill and impaired, is at level 0.60; if we could use a given amount of health-care resources to move either of them up the HUI scale by 0.20—that is, produce the same size health gain for each, doing so would provide A with a 100% increase in his health-related quality of life but only a 33% increase for B. (Many will find precise quantification of health status problematic, but I use it only for ease of explication; it is not essential to my argument.)

This may be what people had in mind in empirical studies in which they were offered choices between using limited resources for a treatment program that would serve a group like A or a group like B, but where those same resources would produce a larger health gain for B than for A (Nord, 1993). Most people preferred to treat the worse off group A even when doing so would produce substantially less aggregate health benefits than would have been achieved by treating group B instead. The reason many people offered for this preference was that they believed it would be more important to the more seriously ill to get treatment, even though they would receive less benefit from treatment; one reason that it could be more important is because the worse off's relative health improvement, although not absolute, would be greater. Now, of course, giving priority to the greater relative improvement will afford only limited, not absolute, priority to the worse off: for example, if A can only be raised from 0.20 to 0.25, while B could be raised from 0.60 to 0.90. But if relative improvement is the morally important consideration, this may only reflect that the worse off should not get absolute priority no matter how large the sacrifice to better-off groups.

A different line of justification for the priority view focuses on the different strength claims generated by the different degrees of undeserved deprivation A and B

suffer from their substantially different degrees of undeserved poor health relative to their being in full health. Because worse-off A's undeserved deprivation is greater, he has a greater complaint and so a stronger moral claim than does B for his deprivation to be reduced or eliminated. It is morally more important or urgent to reduce A's greater deprivation than B's just because it is the greater undeserved reduction in health-related quality of life from full health. (This line of argument, of course, relies on the health disadvantage being undeserved and so will not apply in cases where individuals are at fault or responsible for their own poor health; determining which cases of health disadvantages are not undeserved is, naturally, controversial, but many people believe that a substantial portion of health problems result from behavior for which individuals are responsible.)

Some line of reasoning of this sort is common in contractualist moral theories like those of Thomas Scanlon (1998) and in Thomas Nagel's work on inequality (1979, 1991). In this view, individuals' moral complaints and, in turn, their claims are determined by how well off they are in comparison with other individuals, but not other aggregates of individuals; a group of individuals with lesser claims cannot combine together to take priority over individuals with greater complaints and claims. The idea is to minimize the complaint of those with the greatest complaint, and one interpretation (there are others) of who has the greatest complaint is those worst off; if we make the position of the worst off as good as possible, we minimize the complaint they have based on their disadvantage. A principle of minimizing complaints is a *maximin* principle that gives absolute weight to improving the position of the worst off, and so is different from weighted beneficence that allows aggregation, but weights benefits to the worse off more than benefits to the better off. If minimizing complaints is given this maximin interpretation, then minimizing complaints might be balanced against other moral concerns such as beneficence in raising average or aggregate well-being.

A similar view can be put in terms of needs, and it has a special resonance in the context of health care. Many people believe that the basic or most urgent needs of all should be met before meeting the less urgent needs or wants of any. The purpose of health care in particular should be to meet health care needs, and more urgent needs should take priority over less urgent needs. This view also requires that individual patients should confront other patients as individuals and that those with the most urgent needs should receive priority for treatment. This is a "prioritarian" view in the context of health care, though it also may be too strong in giving absolute priority to the most urgent needs.

Treating the most urgent needs first, as well as minimizing the greatest complaints, bring out the relation of the prioritarian view to the "aggregation problem"—when should greater aggregate benefits to a larger number of patients receive priority over lesser aggregate, but equal or larger individual benefits to fewer patients? (Daniels, 1993; Kamm, 1993). Consequentialists in principle accept no limits on aggregation in seeking to maximize overall benefits, and so small benefits to many individuals may in the aggregate be greater than, and so take priority over, large benefits to a few individuals. However, if we must treat the most urgent needs, or meet the strongest claims, of individuals first, we will place very strong constraints on permissible aggregation—individuals with a less urgent need or weaker claim no matter how large their number would not be treated before anyone with a more urgent need or stronger claim. This view does not rule out all aggregation, for it would not bar preferring to treat more rather than fewer patients with equally urgent needs—for example, saving more lives rather than fewer. But determining whether doing so without giving the fewer any chance to

be treated is problematic. Many non-consequentialists would also permit some aggregation when needs are not equally urgent. Again, determining when to do so is a very difficult and controversial matter (Kamm, 1993). If always giving priority to more urgent needs or stronger claims is too strong and rules out too much aggregation, we should only give some but not absolute priority to the worse off; I return to this issue later in the chapter.

WHO ARE THE WORSE OFF FOR HEALTH RESOURCE PRIORITIZATION?

Suppose that one of these or some other line of reasoning, suitably elaborated, succeeds in establishing that it is morally more important to benefit people the worse off they are, and more specifically that it is more important to improve people's health the worse off they are. We then face the second question of who is worse off for the purposes of health-care resource prioritization and allocation. There are several parts to this question. The first is whether for purposes of health-care resource prioritization, the worse off should be understood as those who are sicker, that is, those with worse health, or as those with worse overall well-being. In a general theory of distributive justice that gives some priority to the worse off, it is overall or global well-being that is important; for example, Rawls's statement of the general form of his principle of justice does not distinguish any particular aspect of well-being, although his "Difference Principle," which requires maximization of the expectations of the worst off representative group, applies to the basic institutions that determine the distribution of income and wealth (Rawls, 1971). Thomas Nagel (1979, 1991) also argues that the "units" for distributive principles are whole human lives.

We could then treat health care as one among other goods whose distribution should be arranged to give priority to improving the condition of those who are overall worse off. This fits the common idea that a disadvantage in one aspect of well-being can be compensated for by an advantage in a different area; for example, the loss of rich cultural opportunities in moving from a large city may be compensated for by new outdoor recreational opportunities in the country, or a loss of income from taking a less pressured and demanding job may be compensated for by increased time to spend with one's family. One might argue, however, that health is not like these other goods in its substitutability with other aspects of well-being. To the extent that health is an all-purpose means necessary for the pursuit of nearly all people's aims and ends, its loss may not be able to be compensated for by other goods, leaving people's overall well-being intact; however, this nonsubstitutability of health, or of specific aspects of health, seems to hold only partially at most.

Applying the "prioritarian" view to overall or global well-being would have what for many are highly counterintuitive implications for health-care prioritization. For example, we would have to give lower priority to treating the rich than the poor, even when the rich are much sicker than the poor, if the overall well-being of the rich is higher despite their much worse health. If this is unacceptable, it indicates that we think of the distribution of health care as a separate sphere, subject to its own distributive principles, not simply as one aspect of overall well-being regulated by general principles of distributive justice (Walzer, 1983; Kamm, 1993, 2002; Brock, unpublished). Thomas Scanlon has argued explicitly that priority to the worst off does not have general application within contractualist moral theory, but that "for differences in level to affect the relative strength of people's moral claims to help, these differences have to be in an aspect of welfare that the help in question will contribute to" (Scanlon, 1998, p. 227).

A "separate spheres" position, which restricts the definition of the worse off in health-care resources prioritization to those with worse health, holds that a theory of justice will apply to different spheres of goods to be distributed. Those spheres should be treated separately or independently. Thus, a concern for the worse off, for purposes of prioritizing educational resources, should look to those who are worse off with regard to education and educational opportunities, and similarly to the extent that there are other additional separate spheres. Likewise, a concern for the worse off for purposes of prioritizing health-care resources should look to those with the worse health (and perhaps as well to their capacity to benefit from treatment, but this still keeps the assessment within the health domain); this fits common practices of giving the sickest patients priority for treatment (again, typically taking some account of capacity to benefit from treatment as well) when resources are explicitly scarce; for example, who is treated first in hospital emergency rooms or who gets scarce intensive care unit beds or organs for transplantation.

A view of "separate spheres" might be justified on pragmatic policy grounds—it would be too difficult, costly, intrusive, and controversial, as well as too subject to mistake and abuse, for health professionals to evaluate people's different levels of overall well-being; health professionals are experts in the evaluation of people's health, not of their overall well-being. Alternatively, some have argued on principled grounds for the autonomy of different spheres of distribution—income and wealth, health care, votes, and so forth—with different moral principles applying to different spheres.

For example, Kamm has argued that health care is an activity or good complete unto itself and it is corrupted when other aims besides health intrude into it. Yet in many human activities we often pursue multiple aims, and it is not clear why it must be wrong to do so in the health-care system. Kamm has also argued that there is a Kantian reason for observing separate spheres in health-care resource prioritization (Kamm, 1993). If we give one group of patients lower priority for treatment than a second group solely because treating the latter will, for example, produce indirect economic benefits for their employers by reducing lost work days that will not be produced by treating the former, we violate the Kantian injunction against treating people solely as means. The first group is treated solely as a means in the sense that they and their health-care needs are given lower priority solely because treating them is not a means to the indirect nonhealth benefits from treating the second group. The arguments for separate spheres are controversial, and their force may depend both on the contexts and levels of the health-care system in which prioritization decisions are made, as well as on the roles and responsibilities of those making them (Brock, unpublished).

Even if there is good reason to restrict the concern for the worse off to those with worse health in the prioritization and allocation of health-care resources, additional issues remain. One is how to determine who has worse health. This may seem obvious and straightforward, even if there will be disagreement about close cases, but it is not. One question is whether the worse off are those with the worse overall health or those with the most serious disease now in need of treatment?

For example, suppose A has a serious disability that leaves his overall health-related quality of life as measured on the HUI at 0.5, while B's is much better at 0.9; A and B each contract the same disease, but B's case is more serious and will reduce her health-related quality of life to 0.7 without treatment, whereas A's less serious case will reduce his to 0.4 without treatment. Should a special concern or priority for the worse off favor A or B? A's overall health is worse, and will be worse than B's even if he and not B is treated, but B has the more serious illness that is now in need of treatment because her illness will have a greater adverse impact on her health-related quality of life than will A's on his;

a natural description would be that B is the sickest now, but A's overall health is worse. It is doubtful that a separate sphere's argument implies that we should ignore large background differences in current health or health-related quality of life and attend only to the seriousness of the illness for which each patient now needs treatment. A case for separate spheres seeks to restrict health-care resource prioritization to considerations of patients' health, not other factors such as their economic productivity, but patients' background health state is a health consideration. And while treating B would produce the most health benefits, it would only increase the degree to which A's health is worse than B's. This question has obvious importance for the priority that should be given to treatment of patients with serious background illnesses or disabilities besides the current condition in need of treatment.

How sick a patient is now is the consideration Nord calls "severity," and his and others' research indicates that people give more weight to it than to treatment effect or benefit, as long as patients will receive a significant benefit from treatment (Nord, 1993; Nord et al., 1995). Giving great weight to severity could be one explanation for the strong priority that people typically give to saving life over improving others' quality of life. Losing one's life is typically seen as losing everything, and in quantitative scales of health-related quality of life, death is the typical zero point (this leaves aside the problem of states worse than death). This supports the idea that patients with life-threatening conditions are the most severely ill and should receive priority over others less severely ill.

Another aspect of the question of who is worse off, again assuming the assessment is restricted to health, is whether only individuals' present health, or instead their health over time, including past and expected future health, is relevant. Suppose A was diagnosed with multiple sclerosis (MS) 20 years ago, has had numerous acute episodes, and has been on medications during this period, but has been left with a functional limitation in only one leg. Recently, B has been diagnosed with MS after an acute episode that leaves him with a functional limitation of one arm and one leg. A new treatment of the condition is developed that would restore the full use of their limbs to each patient, but we can only treat one of them, and no future treatment of the other will be possible. Who should be considered the worse off? Patient B's illness is more serious and results in a greater loss of function than A's, but A has suffered his lesser loss of function for 20 years while B has been healthy all his life and only now has suffered his more serious case of MS and loss of function. Patient A seems the worse off with regard to health because he has had the condition for so long, even though his condition now is less serious than B's. People's lives extend continuously over time, and our moral concern should be for the lives they lead, not simply for how good their lives are at a particular point in time, whether now or sometime in the past or the future. A concern for the worse off should reflect this concern for people's lives as a whole and so not ignore the duration of people's poor health. Moreover, in other areas besides health we often take what a person has had or suffered in the past to be relevant in distributing scarce benefits now; if one child has had little opportunity for travel in the past in comparison with her well-traveled sibling, fairness supports giving a travel opportunity to her now that can only go to one of them, even if the well-traveled sibling might enjoy and benefit from the trip more.

Differences in the duration of expected future health impairments seem relevant as well for who is worse off; for example, if both A and B contract a disease now at age 65, but A will suffer his lesser impairment for the rest of his life, while B will suffer his greater impairment only for a few years and then will regain normal function, A appears to be the worse off. In this case, if both diseases are fully treatable, what makes patient A worse off also makes treating her produce the greater benefit.

Who will be worse off in the future is sometimes treated as urgency, but that concept is in fact more complex. Urgency is a function at least of how great a harm a patient will suffer if not treated, how soon a patient must be treated to prevent the harm, and how soon the patient will suffer the harm without treatment; it is a major factor in selecting candidates for transplantation of scarce organs as well as for "triaging" patients under emergency conditions.

Frances Kamm (1993) distinguishes two senses of urgency to reflect its complexity: urgency$_t$ which refers to how soon the harm will be suffered; urgency$_q$, which refers to how much the patient's quality of life will be reduced without treatment. However, as there are two aspects of the temporal component of urgency—how soon it is necessary to treat the patient to prevent a harm and how soon the harm will be suffered if the patient is not treated—they may conflict. For example, it might be necessary to treat A now to prevent her suffering a harm a year from now and necessary to treat B in six months to prevent her suffering a harm at that time; B is more urgent in how soon she will suffer the harm, A in how soon she must be treated to prevent the harm. Notice that the aspect of urgency of how great a harm the patient will suffer without treatment, Kamm's urgency$_q$ is in fact a measure of expected benefit from treatment; this illustrates how potential treatment benefit determines one respect in which patients are worse off. Urgency captures the aspect of who is worse off that is future directed, but ignores how well or badly off a person has been in the past. I believe that both expected and past health states are relevant to a judgment of how badly off people are, not just how bad a person's health is now.

HOW MUCH PRIORITY SHOULD THE WORSE OFF RECEIVE IN HEALTH RESOURCE PRIORITIZATION?

The third issue in developing a moral framework for determining what priority the worse off should receive in health-care resource prioritization is how much priority they should receive. The reasons for support of priority to the worse off will affect the answer. Contractualist reasoning, which requires minimizing the complaint of the person with the greatest complaint, may support maximizing the position of the worst off, or giving the worst off absolute priority. However, giving the worst off absolute priority over others for health-care resource prioritization is not plausible because it encounters what has been called the "bottomless pit" problem (Daniels, 1985). If the worst off are understood, for example, as the very severely cognitively and physically disabled who have an extremely low health-related quality of life, health interventions in the form of health care and other supportive services may provide them with only very small benefits but at very great cost. If improving their condition is given absolute priority, there may be almost no end to what could be done to provide them with minimal marginal gains consuming near limitless resources; greatly expanded medical research on their conditions, even if very unpromising and at very great cost, could also have some very small expected benefit for them. Even if some minimal threshold of significance of benefits must be met for the claim of the worst off to receive priority, great resources would be required to go to the worst off before any needs of others could be met. If we give absolute priority to the worse off, not just the worst off, and maximize the health-related quality of life of each next most worse off group after doing everything possible for those worse off than they, few resources would remain for the important health needs of most of the population who enjoy a higher health-related quality of life.

Some balance is clearly required between giving special priority or weight to the needs of the worse off and other relevant moral considerations such as using limited resources to maximize overall health benefits and to meet the needs of those better off. Ideally, we want a principled basis or

reason(s) for how much priority to give the worse off, but it is not clear what that principled basis would be. Rather, it seems that most people have independent moral concerns for the worse off and for aggregate health benefits that must be balanced, but no precise weight for the different concerns. John Stone (2000) has suggested a "proportional benefit" principle as a way of balancing these two concerns. For example, if on a HUI a person is seriously disabled and at 0.30 and would be raised to 0.45 with treatment, his proportional benefit is 50%; he would have priority over another patient at 0.60 who would be raised to 0.80 with treatment, thereby receiving greater benefit, 0.20, but a lesser proportional benefit, 0.33. The balancing required will be more complex still, because other moral concerns that bear on overall health-care resource prioritization and allocation, but not on my focus here on the worse off, must be taken account of as well. Lacking any principled basis for how much priority to give to the worse off, we could ask people, using the person trade-off methodology with various hypothetical choice scenarios, how much benefit to others they are prepared to sacrifice in order to treat the worse off; empirical research of this sort by Eric Nord and others has begun, but the data are very limited at this point (Nord et al., 1995; Ubel et al. 1996 Nord, 1999). Alternatively, we could turn to fair procedures, either political procedures or procedures within private health plans, to make these trade-offs (Daniels and Sabin, 1997).

CONCLUSION

I hope it is abundantly clear by now that the question of what priority the worse off should receive in health-care resource prioritization raises a large agenda of normative issues that have received far too little attention to date. The full details and complexities of the three questions I have briefly discussed must be systematically explored: What is the moral justification for giving priority to the worse off for health-care resource prioritization? Who are the worse off for health-care resource prioritization? How much priority should the worse off receive in health-care resource prioritization?

Moreover, in applying a moral framework for priority to the worse off in health-care resource prioritization, it will likely be necessary to distinguish different contexts in which decisions are made—for example, funding different health programs versus selecting among patients for scarce treatment, and the various roles and responsibilities of different decision makers in those different contexts. I have raised many questions and issues without providing and defending solutions to many of them; in part, this is no doubt my own failing, but I believe it reflects as well the quite undeveloped state of serious work on the issues of health-care resource prioritization and allocation. Bioethicists and others of a normative bent should get to work.

REFERENCES

Brock, D.W. (2002). Ethical issues in the use of cost-effectiveness analysis for the prioritization of health care resources. In S. Anand and A. Sen (eds.), *Ethical Foundations of Health Equity*. Oxford: Oxford University Press (in press).

Brock, D.W. Unpublished. *Separate Spheres and Indirect Benefits*. Available online at: http://www.who.int/whosis/fairness/

Daniels, N. (1985). *Just Health Care*. Cambridge: Cambridge University Press

Daniels, N. (1993). Rationing fairly: Programmatic considerations. *Bioethics* 7(2–3), 224–33.

Daniels, N. and Sabin, J. (1997). Limits to health care: Fair procedures, democratic deliberation, and the legitimacy problem for insurers. *Philosophy and Public Affairs* 26(4), 303–50.

Gold, M.R., Siegel, J.E., Russell, L.B., and Weinstein, M.C. (1997). *Cost-Effectiveness in Health and Medicine*. New York: Oxford University Press.

Kamm, F.M. (1993). *Morality-Mortality. Vol. I: Death and Whom to Save From It*. Oxford: Oxford University Press.

Kamm, F.M. (2002). Deciding whom to help, the principle of irrelevant good and health-adjusted life-Years. In S. Anand and A. Sen (eds.), *Ethical Foundations of Health Equity*. Oxford: Oxford University Press.

Nagel, T. (1979). Equality. *Mortal Questions*. Cambridge: Cambridge University Press.

Nagel, T. (1991). *Equality and Partiality*. Oxford: Oxford University Press.

Nord, E. (1993). The trade-off between severity of illness and treatment effect in cost-value analysis of health care. *Health Policy* 24, 227–38.

Nord, E. (1999). *Cost-Value Analysis in Health Care*. Cambridge: Cambridge University Press.

Nord, E., Richardson, J., Street, A., Kuhse, H. and Singer, P. (1995). Maximizing health benefits vs. egalitarianism: An Australian survey of health issues. *Social Science and Medicine* 41, 1429–37.

Nozick, R. (1974). *Anarchy, State and Utopia*. New York: Basic Books

Parfit, D. (1991). Equality or priority? *The Lindley Lecture*. Copyright: Department of Philosophy, University of Kansas.

Rawls, J. (1971). *A Theory of Justice*. Cambridge, MA: Harvard University Press.

Scanlon, T. (1998). *What We Owe to Each Other*. Cambridge, MA: Harvard University Press.

Stone, J. (2000). *Disadvantage and the Allocation of Health Care Resources*. Unpublished doctoral dissertation, Brown University, Providence, RI.

Temkin, L. (1993). *Inequality*. New York: Oxford University Press.

Temkin, L. Unpublished. *Equality or Priority in Health Care Distribution*. Available online at: http://www.who.int/whosis/fairness/

Ubel, P., Scanlon, D., Lowenstein, G. and Kamlet, M. (1996). Individual utilities are inconsistent with rationing choices: A partial explanation of why Oregon's cost-effectiveness list failed. *Medical Decision Making* 16, 108–19.

Walzer, M. (1983). *Spheres of Justice*. New York: Basic Books.

29

Whether to Discontinue *Non*futile Use of a Scarce Resource

F.M. Kamm

In this chapter I consider some of the ethical problems presented by the desire to discontinue the *nonfutile use* of a resource because it is scarce. It might be said that doctors should not do "rationing at the bedside" with patients. Rather, rationing should result from a systemwide macropolicy that ties doctors' hands and prevents them from allocating resources as they wish. However, I shall argue that there may be an in-between case: When individuals are involved in trials for use of drugs, treatment to them might be discontinued because they do not do well enough, if and only if treating those who do better makes it possible to treat more candidates who are equally worthy. The drug clozapine, uniquely useful for treating schizophrenia, is taken as an example of such a resource made scarce because of its costliness.[1]

In the first section of the chapter I consider relevant available medical data, and I review current treatment policy involving the drug. In subsequent sections I isolate three major issues that arise in the morality of discontinuing aid: regression, doctors' commitments to patients, and the temporal gap between denying aid to one person and providing better aid to someone else; I also deal with whether differential outcome should affect who gets helped. To examine this topic, I present, in outline, some general principles for the distribution of scarce resources[2] and then begin to make clear what these principles might imply for the case of differential outcomes with clozapine. The concluding sections consider the role of differential numbers of people who might be helped and the significance of urgency relative to outcome. I attempt to provide a morally justified principle that tells us how to relate the *outcome* we expect in treating patients to the *urgency* of patients' condition and the *number* of potential recipients of treatment. The final section of the chapter considers the fate of those individuals who are only moderately ill and suggests a possible change in policy that might be of benefit in achieving just distribution to them.

BACKGROUND

Suppose that clozapine is the most effective treatment for schizophrenia, helping people who would not otherwise be helped, helping them more than alternative treatments, and causing fewer side effects. However, suppose it is more expensive than other treatments, at least in the short run. Whether it is more expensive in the long run than other treatments depends on the outcomes it produces.

In some people, clozapine treatment essentially results in a return to normality. These people can leave hospitals so hospital beds can be eliminated. Such patients must continue to take medication costing about $5,500 per year. But they can become self-supporting, returning to work and family. This implies they themselves could fund their medication. In this population, clozapine is overall less expensive than other treatments.

Other people show only moderate improvement, both in the sense that the difference between their condition with clozapine and without it is not great and in the sense that they do not return to normality. These individuals must continue the drug in order to get benefits that only clozapine can provide to them, but they cannot live independently. They may move to outpatient facilities, supported by both state and federal funds, or they may have to remain in state-run hospitals. In this population, clozapine use is overall more expensive than other treatments.

In a third group, clozapine produces no differential benefits over other drugs. However, the possibility that it produces fewer side effects, even if it is no more effective than other treatments, raises the question of whether its use is nonetheless indicated.

Suppose that there is no way to tell before treatment into which of these three groups a person will fall. For example, there is an equal distribution of big successes (normality) in severe and nonsevere patients. However, once someone is on treatment, one can tell within six months

whether that person will respond, and to what degree.

Assume that when clozapine must be provided at public expense, it is a scarce resource owing to its costliness. A significant ethical problem that arises is whether to continue treating those who cannot pay for their own treatment and who make only moderate gains that do not lift them to normality. This is one of the most expensive groups to treat, and discontinuing their treatment would allow us to help more people become normal. In other words, should the maintenance of someone on the scarce resource depend on the outcome it produces?

At present, it is said,[3] the publicly funded treatment policy being followed is essentially twofold: (1) Keep on treating all those who achieve normality on the drug (indeed, this is taken for granted). (2) Give medication in accordance with the severity of the illness and *keep on* treating even those who improve only to a subnormal level. This means that others who, at the start, are not so severely ill but who might achieve normality are not treated. For prongs (1) and (2) of this policy to be consistent, it must be assumed that most of the normals who are continued on treatment would be severely ill without treatment, even if not all the severely ill who are treated attain normality.

ISSUES SPECIFIC TO DISCONTINUING TREATMENT

The decision to stop treating those who are achieving a moderate level of well-being—the rejection of prong (2)—in order to try to increase the number who can achieve normality raises several ethical questions. The first asks: Is there a moral difference between (a) not beginning treatment that would help someone achieve only a moderate level of well-being in order to help others more, and (b) terminating such treatment once it has begun in order to help others more? All the issues (for example, concerning action versus omission) that are familiar from the discussion of discontinuing life-sustaining treatment might be thought to arise here. It could be said, however, that *not* giving yet another dose of a drug is not the same as terminating (by action) a life-support system. At most, it is like a case involving a life-support machine that needs to be reset every day. Then the issue is also whether it is permissible to omit resetting it.

Whatever the philosophically best way to treat the termination-versus-not-beginning-treatment issue may be, psychological studies might support the view that, if people form *expectations* about future treatment on the basis of past treatment, this will set a baseline from which noncontinuation of treatment, even by failure to give another dose, will be perceived as a loss.[4] For those who have not yet received treatment and have not formed expectations about getting treatment, not being treated may be perceived as a no-gain situation. Losses tend to be rated more negatively than "no-gains," even when they both leave the patient at the same absolute level of well-being. Would this be a reason not to terminate drug use, even when we may refuse to begin it? It is possible that one could prevent the development of expectations concerning further treatment by explicitly warning people that beginning treatment does not guarantee that treatment will continue. Then the expectation of treatment would not be a reason to continue, for there would be no expectation. Furthermore, ceasing treatment should then be seen as a no-gain rather than as a loss. Deliberately characterizing the first six months of use of the drug as a *trial* may succeed in stemming expectations.

However, there might be other reasons not to stop treatment. For example, if we are clear about what terminating treatment with clozapine leads to in a patient, we may see another ground for objecting to it. Theoretically, there are two possibilities for the trial: (a) treatment must be continued for up to six months in order for us to know (by some sign) whether someone will

become normal but there is no change in the patient's condition during that time period; (b) treatment must be continued for up to six months in order for us to know whether someone will become normal and there is an improvement in the patient's condition during that time period. I believe it is (b) rather than (a) that raises a moral problem for terminating treatment. In (b), terminating treatment does not merely stop a patient from achieving further progress (as it may in [a]); it allows the patient to regress, to fall back down to the level from which he was already lifted. It is not stopping treatment per se, even when we know this will prevent some future improvement, that seems morally significant relative to not starting treatment. What seems morally significant is *stopping an improvement in the patient's condition that has already occurred by stopping what was already being done to achieve it*. The latter condition is important. For suppose a regress would occur unless we increase the dosage already given. I do not believe that refusing to prevent the regress in order to help others instead would raise the same concern. Hence, it is not even the regress per se but its occurrence as a result of not continuing to do what was already being done that may be problematic. (Call this regression*.)

This concern with regression* assumes that improvement to a point below normality is still better than being in a much worse condition. Some may challenge this assumption. They might point out that individuals who are severely mentally ill live in a world of pleasant delusions. When patients recover partially, they become aware of their problems and for the first time experience misery. Several points can be made in response to this challenge. First, if severely ill schizophrenics are already very miserable, the challenge does not apply to them. Second, the challenge depends on a completely experiential conception of the good life: What you do not experience as bad is not bad for you and there are no nonexperiential goods that compensate for experiential harms. If this were a correct conception of the good life, it would imply that a good life could be had by taking drugs that give one pleasant experiences and the illusion of living a productive life. It also denies that pain experienced in coming into contact with reality can be compensated by the mere fact that one is in contact with reality. There is much to be said against the experiential conception of the good life.

Let us now consider a doctor's point of view on stopping treatment that involves regression*. A doctor who omits to continue the same treatment may view herself as fully responsible for the decline in a patient and think that "producing" this decline is worse than not aiding the patient to start with. Yet a philosopher might reasonably argue that it is as permissible (or impermissible) not to continue aid that one has been providing as it is not to start aid, even if the patient declines, as long as he or she declines to a state that is no worse than the patient would have been in had aid not begun, assuming there is no independent commitment (e.g. a promise) to continue aid once started. But is one worse off if one improves for a few months and then declines than if one had never improved at all? I do not believe so, for if all we could ever do for any patient was improve him for a few months before an inevitable decline, doing so would be better for him than not.

Admittedly, a doctor has a duty to aid (unlike an ordinary bystander), but even with this duty, a doctor may refuse to start helping one patient in order to help a greater number of other patients. Why then may she not stop the aid once started, in order to help others more, if the patient will be no worse off overall and being in the trial gave him a chance? Must the fact that the patient gets worse again through failure to continue what has already been done be definitive? I suggest not.

It is also inappropriate to apply the Hippocratic doctor's concern with not doing harm above all to the case of the patient's decline. First, the doctor would be refusing to continue aiding and this is not, strictly, harming. Furthermore, looking only at what happens if we do not continue aid relative to the patient's improved condition considers too narrow a time slice; it fails to consider the overall period from before the doctor intervened: The doctor produced the improvement and would not have been duty bound to do so if he could alternatively have helped more people. Not helping someone retain an improvement and instead helping others may be aesthetically less pleasing than not helping to start with—declines to a level may be less pleasing than maintenance of a status quo at the same level—but it is not clear that it is morally different.

This brings us to another objection to terminating treatment based on the idea that a doctor might simply become committed to a specific patient once treatment starts. I do not believe that this gives rise to an obligation to continue aid in all cases. Commitments may be overridden, for example, by the attempt to help greater numbers of people, especially if these are also one's patients. In addition, commitments might be undertaken by doctors in an explicitly conditional form, for example: "You will be provided with a drug on condition no one else needs it more." It may be part of the *responsibility of patients* to accept that their useful treatment may be stopped for morally legitimate reasons. Most importantly, the idea of a commitment to a patient suggests that a doctor would be wrong to stop treatment that had not yet had *any* effect on the patient when the doctor knows that continuing treatment will lead to some subnormal improvement in the future. But I do not believe the doctor would be wrong to drop treatment for such a patient in order to offer it to others who can reach normality. All this suggests that it is regression* that raises the moral problem, not simple failure of commitment or simple termination of treatment.

It is true, however, that playing down a doctor's commitment to individual patients makes the establishment of special bonds (comparable to the ones we form with friends or family members) impossible. Such special bonds are thought to legitimately impede meeting even the more pressing needs of other people. Should we exchange the possibility of such bonds between doctor and patient for fairer treatment? The suggestion is that we could morally afford to do so by having trials that can be ended.

Nevertheless, there are particular facts of the clozapine case that further complicate the decision not to continue aid to someone in order to help others more. Terminating aid so as to *definitely help* others more is different from terminating aid to *go searching* for others who will do better. In the latter case, we cannot be sure that we will be helping the next person more than we are helping the person already being treated, and it will take up to six months to find out. The person on whom we try our drug next may do no better, and possibly worse, than the person we dropped. If he does worse, this means that we could have been doing more good by having continued treatment for the first patient. What if he and subsequent trial subjects do only as well as the person dropped? It might be argued that this is still a better outcome, for there is a fairer distribution of temporary moderate improvements. For example, instead of n months of moderate improvement going to one patient, m patients each get n/m months of moderate improvement. If we had to distribute the good of moderate improvement to begin with, we might well divide it over several people rather than concentrate its duration in one person, as long as what we distribute is still a significant good. (Notice that this is not the same as saying that we would deny normality to someone by dividing a normality-producing dose so as to produce only moderate well-being in many.) Regression*, admittedly, poses the dominant countervailing consideration to such a fairer distribution of moderate improvement.

Still, there is at least a chance that the drug will prove *very* successful in the next person, and this is no longer true of the person we would drop. The probability of finding people who do much better is an empirical question, and we may be reluctant to stop helping one person unless there is a sufficiently high probability of helping others much more in the *near future*.

This last point makes salient the time gap that can exist between stopping aid to one person and finding another person whom we can help reach normality. At worst, it is possible that by the time we find someone who does better and help him, we may no longer be helping someone who was suffering at the same time as the person we originally dropped. If this is so, we will have put off helping someone who is suffering *now* with the consequence that we help others more who will suffer *in the future*. This raises the question of whether we should adopt an attitude of *temporal neutrality*, not distinguishing between those who need help now and those who will come with need later. (I shall return to a related issue below.)

SEVERITY, OUTCOME, AND A GENERAL THEORY OF DISTRIBUTION

Here is another ethical question raised by the decision to not continue treatment of those who are achieving moderate well-being in order to increase the number of individuals who can achieve normality: Should the attempt to achieve normality for some lead us to deprive others of their chance for moderate improvement, even if these others are more severely ill than those who would be substituted for them in drug trials? This question arises independently of the possible moral problem of stopping treatment, for theoretically it could also arise in cases where we must just decide whether to start aiding someone. This question has two subparts: (a) Should better outcomes dominate equal chances for help? (b) Should better outcomes dominate greater severity?

In this section, I shall deal with subpart (a). It will be useful to first present some general principles for distributing scarce resources. I have elsewhere attempted to describe a distribution procedure that takes account of four factors: need (N), urgency (U), outcome (O), and waiting time (WT).[5] Factors besides these four may be relevant; however, I believe one should not start by cluttering the picture. In general, the method is to begin with two factors, holding the others constant in the background, and to see what the relation is between these two factors—for example, which takes precedence over the other. Then we introduce a third factor to see whether it makes a difference to the relationship between the first two factors as well as how the third relates to each of the two others. If we follow this procedure patiently, adding additional factors in an orderly way, we have some hope of making progress.

Let me first describe three of the four factors, N, U, and O. A patient's *urgency* (U), as I use the term, is a measure of how bad his future prospects are if he is not treated; it is a function of how bad his future will be and the likelihood it will come about. (This is not quite the ordinary notion of urgency, which also focuses on how soon treatment is needed. Someone could face very bad prospects but not need treatment to avoid such prospects as soon as someone else, in which case the ordinary notion says his need is not as urgent.) *Need* for treatment (N), as I use the term, connotes how badly someone's life will have gone overall if that person is not treated. Unlike urgency, need is not merely a forward-looking concept; it takes someone's whole life into consideration. Person A could be more *urgent than B*, in that A will die in a month if he is not treated now and B will die in a year if he is not treated now, and yet B could be more in need (of life-giving treatment) because he would die at age 20 whereas A would die at age 60. This assumes that one will have had a worse life overall if one dies at 20 than if one dies at 60 (other things equal). Because need takes into account someone's past about which one can no longer do anything, it implies that how we treat someone in the future could at least compensate someone for the past, and that such compensation could be as morally important as preventions of harm in the future. (This may be a contentious assumption.)

Outcome (O) refers to the expected difference that treatment will make. In cases where life and death are at issue, I believe that the relevant measure of outcome is additional time alive independent of quality, as long as the patient would find the quality of life acceptable. This means that in life-and-death cases, we should not use QALYs (quality-adjusted life-years) in evaluating different possible outcomes. In cases where life and death are *not* at issue, outcome is appropriately measured in terms of (some types of) quality-of-life differences, such as relative freedom from the symptoms of schizophrenia.[6]

What are some of the things we can say about the relative weights of N, O, and U? First, let us consider distribution of a scarce, *lifesaving* resource between *A* and *B*, holding need, urgency, and outcome (as well as any other factor) constant. Fairness requires giving each an equal chance. It is important to understand that giving equal chances is *not* a symptom of the desire not to be responsible for making a choice. It is, rather, the fair way to choose when there is no morally relevant difference between potential recipients.

Now add a third person, *C*, whose need, urgency, and outcome are the same (and who can also be saved only if we save *B*). What I call the "Balancing Argument" claims that in such a case, justice demands that each person on one side should have her interests balanced against those of one person on the opposing side; those who are not balanced out in the larger group help determine that the larger group should be saved. Hence, the number of people saved counts morally.

Now consider conflicts when the individ-

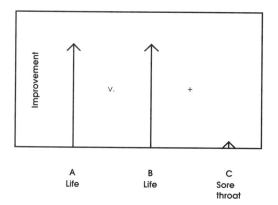

Figure 29–1. The sore throat case.

uals are not equally urgent. Figure 29–1 represents a choice between saving *A*, on the one hand, and on the other hand, saving *B and* curing *C*'s sore throat with left-over medicine. The overall outcomes will be different depending on whom we save, as more good, spread over two people, will occur if we save *B* and *C*. My claim is that we should treat the difference in outcome as morally *irrelevant*.

The reasoning behind this is as follows: From an impartial view, we should not favor *A* over *B* per se (given that they are assumed alike *in themselves* in all morally relevant respects). If they were alone (independent of *C*), we should give them equal chances. From the impartial perspective, we also see that *A* and *B* each has his own partial point of view; *A* prefers his own survival to that of *B*, and vice versa. It is important to each, therefore, that he retain his equal chance to survive. The fact that we could save *C* from a sore throat is a matter of minor importance to him, he is not very needy or urgent and, in addition, the difference in outcome achieved by helping him is small. These three points lead to the conclusion that we should not deprive *A* of his 50% chance of survival merely to also help *C*. Hence, *C*'s cure should be a morally irrelevant good in choosing between these people. (This contrasts with the view that we should *aggregate* the gains to *B* and *C* and help them because we pro-

duce a benefit that is larger than the benefit possible to *A* alone.)

This form of reasoning gives equal consideration to each individual's partial point of view from an impartial point of view, so it combines subjective and objective perspectives. Hence, I call it *sobjectivity*. It implies that certain extra goods (like the throat cure) can be morally irrelevant; I call this the "Principle of Irrelevant Goods." Whether a good is irrelevant is context-dependent. Curing a sore throat is morally irrelevant when others' lives are at stake, but not when others' earaches are. The *Sore Throat Case* shows that we must refine the claim that what we owe each person is to balance her interests against the equal interests of an opposing person and let the remainder help determine the outcome.

If small increases in good to a person are sometimes morally irrelevant, this can help provide one reason why someone who has a big and even irreplaceable effect on society *in aggregate* should not necessarily be favored in the distribution of a scarce life-saving resource over someone else. If the big effect amounts to only small effects on the lives of many people, then these effects should not, I believe, be aggregated so as to help outweigh the claim of someone else to have 50 % chance to have his life saved.

Aggregating small benefits to many people, *none* of whom are very needy or urgent, to outweigh the grave need of a single person can be even more problematic than aggregating saving a life and providing such small benefits in order to outweigh someone else's equal chance to live. Such a problematic procedure would be exemplified by public policies, that, for example, provide marriage counseling to the great number of people who will need it rather than provide care for a far fewer number of the severely schizophrenic.

Suppose (as in Fig. 29–2) that if we save *B*, we can also save *C*'s arm. This is the prevention of a large loss to *C*. I believe that when the loss to *C* becomes so significant, it is no longer an irrelevant good,

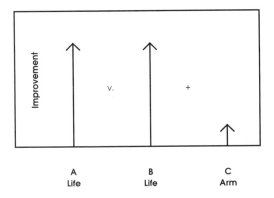

Figure 29–2. The extra arm case.

given that we can only save one life no matter what we do. This is true even though C does not stand to lose as much as A or B and so is not as needy or urgent as each of them. Explaining why this moral shift occurs is not easy, and I shall not attempt it here. This shift would mean either that we should give the treatment outright to B and C or at least that we should give them a greater proportional chance of getting the treatment.

What if the extra good is concentrated in the person whose life would be saved? For example, suppose we could save A's or B's life, but, if we save B, we could also save him from having a sore throat, which A will suffer if she is saved. Here the need and urgency of A and B are the same, but the outcome each presents is different. My claim is that the sore throat is an irrelevant difference in a decision of life and death, and we should not deprive A of her chance to live because of it, even though no more than one person can be saved.

Suppose we could save A or B, but, if we save B, we will also prevent his arm from falling off, whereas A's arm would fall off anyway. Is the saving of an arm here a morally relevant good that should incline us to save B rather than A? (See Fig. 29–3.)

I believe that B's arm is morally irrelevant. Further, I believe this is consistent with my conclusion earlier that C's arm is relevant in Figure 29–2. When the im-

provement in quality of life would occur in the very same person for whom the primary good at stake is life itself—that is, when the good is concentrated rather than distributed—I believe the additional good we can do him should not necessarily lead us to deprive A of her chance at a life that she finds acceptable. Two principles underlie this conclusion. First, *we are more concerned with helping someone avoid a very bad condition than with providing the very same person whom we help in that way with an additional improvement.* Second, *each person wants to be the one who avoids the very bad condition and come close to being normal.* (The fact that A might be willing to run a risk of death [in surgery] to be saved without the loss of an arm does not imply that he would run a greater risk of death so that B can have a greater chance at being saved with both arms).[7]

Finally, suppose we have a choice between helping one person, A, who will be very badly off and much benefited by our aid, or helping a couple of people, B and C, each of whom will be as badly off as A but not benefited as much by our aid. As long as the lesser benefit is significant, it is morally more important, I think, to distribute our efforts over more people, each of whom would be as badly off as the single person, rather than to provide a bigger benefit concentrated in one person (other

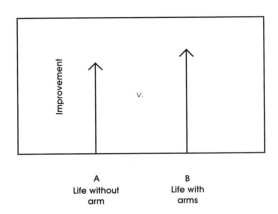

Figure 29–3. The life-with-an-extra-arm case.

things being equal). One way to analyze this situation employs what I shall call "Balancing Argument" (II): Find the part of the potential large gain to A (part 1) that is balanced by the smaller gain to B. Now we must decide how to break that tie between them. If we care about giving priority to those who are worst off, we will care more about benefiting the next person in the group, C, rather than giving an additional benefit (part 2) to A, who, having received part 1, would already have more than C. This means that instead of breaking the tie between A-with-part-1 and B by giving A a greater benefit (part 2), we break the tie by helping B and C, each to a lesser degree.

CLOZAPINE AND DIFFERENCES IN OUTCOME IN A TWO-PERSON CHOICE

In the case of clozapine, we are considering whose quality of life to improve, not whose life to save. Again, let us assume at this point that need and urgency are great and constant between people, but that outcomes will be different. Also let us assume for the time being that the only two people affected by our choices are A and B, and they can both be improved only by clozapine (Fig. 29–4).

Assume B will be improved *slightly* beyond A, to the point of normality. The view most clearly implied by my previous discussion is that in this case we should not deprive A of his equal chance to make what is a more critical change from a very bad condition to being close to normal, just in order to bring B first close to normal and then make the further less critical move slightly beyond to normality. The principles that underlie this conclusion are (1) we are more concerned with helping someone avoid a very bad condition than with providing him with an additional improvement, and (2) each person wants to be the one who avoids the very bad condition.

Here is an alternative view: Normal mental health (which need not mean perfect mental health) is a unique kind of good. It is closely associated with the characteristics that are commonly thought to account for the moral importance of being a person at all: rationality, self-control, capacity for responsible action, and so forth. The difference between normality and its absence is not just a matter of degree, like the difference between perfect pain relief and some degree of pain. Improvement to a moderate level of mental health is a good for the person who is ill, as is improvement to normality. But normality is also more than a good *for* the person; it helps account for the importance of the person. Being in normal physical condition does not have a comparable role. We might, therefore, see achieving it as an especially important goal that represents more than just an additional benefit to someone who already will have achieved the most important part of what is good for him.

Call this the "Mental-Special View." Here is a possible implication of it: Avoiding a truly horrifying mental condition could be so important that we should not deprive A of his equal chance to avoid it and improve to a substantial degree just so that B can also achieve normality. But if A and B are moderately ill, the good of B's becoming normal could override A's chance. This possible implication comes close to a guarantee that we will focus on rescuing someone from a very bad fate if

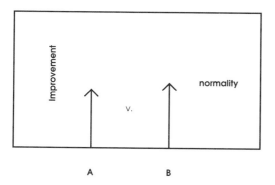

Figure 29–4. Two-person choices: the normal person case.

we can bring him up to a minimum level. Having done that, we will maximize outcome so as to produce normality where we can. Here is another implication: Suppose we could improve many moderately ill people a significant amount but not to normality by dividing a dose that would produce normality if given to one person. We should not divide the dose. (Here is an analogy with another domain—we can improve the artistic abilities of many people who are already moderately good at art to another level or we can invest in producing one great artist. We should do the latter, but not necessarily because we do a great deal of good *for* the person who becomes the great artist, but just because we produce a great artist.)

But now imagine another case. Suppose that with clozapine we can improve *B*'s condition greatly and improve *A* not very much. (We might imagine two different variations: [1] *B* is still not normal, and [2] *B* is normal. For present purposes, we need not worry about this distinction. I shall not consider the possibility that we could make someone superior to normal.) (See Fig. 29–5.)

Even someone who rejects the Mental-Special View could believe that when the difference in mental condition that we can produce becomes quite great in this way, it may be morally appropriate to favor the person in whom we can produce more good, given that need and urgency are equal in both. This means that the greater concern with helping someone avoid a very bad fate than with providing additional improvement (and the recognition that each wants to be the one helped) does not imply that avoiding the worst fate is *all* we are concerned about. At least when we are also helping someone avoid the same very bad fate, our greater concern is combined with a lesser concern to produce additional significant improvement, and this may override concern for equal chances to avoid the very bad fate. However, the worse *A*'s and *B*'s conditions are in absolute terms without the drug, the harder it is for extra good in *B* to overcome the claim that *A* has to an equal chance for significant improvement. The fact that the better *A*'s and *B*'s conditions are in absolute terms, the easier it is to override equal chances by a great good, makes this position close to a position requiring a guaranteed minimum beyond which we can maximize regardless of whether anyone achieves normality. (Notice that we can favor the person in whom we can produce much greater quality-of-life in non–life-and-death cases, even if the same sort of quality-of-life distinction does not count in life-and-death cases.)

Let us change one of our assumptions and imagine that candidate *B*, but not *A*, is susceptible to moderate improvement with a drug other than clozapine—call it "mozapine"—that is inexpensive and so not scarce. Candidate *B* will not improve on mozapine as much as on clozapine, but he will improve as much as *A* would improve on clozapine. Suppose one of our principles is that we are more concerned with helping someone avoid a very bad fate than with providing additional improvement. Does this imply that we should make *B* ineligible to receive clozapine, for we can then treat both *A* and *B*, moving each away from a very bad fate? Not necessarily, for if we treat *B* with clozapine *and he attains normality* and self-sufficiency, he will be

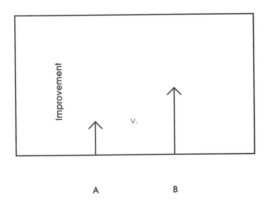

Figure 29–5. Two-person choices: the below normal case.

able to pay for his own maintenance on clozapine. We (i.e., public institutions) will then have money with which to treat *A* with clozapine as well. The trouble is that we may have to wait at least six months before we can treat *A* in this way, whereas if we keep *B* on mozapine, we can treat *A* right away. The question is whether some extra months of suffering on *A*'s part are worth the goal of producing normality in *B*. The answer may vary depending on how bad *A*'s condition is.

HELPING MORE PEOPLE

The last case reminds us of the additional crucial factor in the clozapine case that we have so far deliberately ignored: More people can be helped if some rather than others are helped. Suppose that if and only if *B* is treated rather than *A* will money be freed up from his care so that someone else can be treated as well. This is because only *B* achieves normality.

Suppose that all those who might be treated have the same need and urgency, and these are great. Then only if we treat *B* can we treat another person, *C*, who is as needy and urgent as *A* is (by hypothesis). This is a determinative reason for treating *B* rather than *A*, at least if the improvement in *C* is significant. But now suppose that we had to choose whether (*1*) to help *B* and *C* or (*2*) to help *B* and *D*, when *C* will improve to a moderate level but *D* will achieve normality. If money is freed up only if we help someone who becomes normal, and *E* (with the same need and urgency as *A* and a possibility for a significant outcome) is also waiting, then we should treat *B* and *D* rather than *B* and *C* (or *A*), for we can then treat *E* as well (see Fig. 29–6).

The principle that accounts for these judgments is that when need and urgency are constant, we ought to treat whoever allows us to treat as many people as possible, at least when the greater number of people will be helped significantly. Above, I argued that we should not always choose *B* over

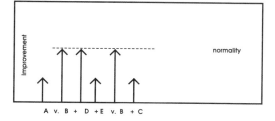

Figure 29–6. Case of multiple persons choices.

A when only these two people are in great need of help just because *B* will do better. Hence, if we should help *B* when other people's welfare is at stake, this implies we are treating *B* as a means to the good of others, though not as a mere means since he also benefits.

Several objections can be raised to this analysis. The first objection is connected to the last point: The problem, it may be said, is not that we choose to help one person in part because this is a means to helping others. The problem is that the person who is *not helped* is treated *merely* as a means. To make this clearer consider the following example: If we face a choice between saving a doctor and a teacher, the fact that the doctor will be irreplaceable in saving lives should not mean that all the lives he will save (an indirect effect of the resource he gets) are counted on his side against the teacher (Doctor Case). It might be suggested that this is true because the person who would *not* be selected for aid would be inappropriately evaluated from too instrumental a point of view, and not sufficiently as an end-in-himself. That is, it is only because he is *not* useful as a means in saving others that he is rejected for treatment. Is this not, it may be said, how the person who only improves moderately on clozapine is treated?

But now consider the following additional case: We have a scarce resource to distribute, and if we give it to *A*, he can then also carry it to another person, *C*, who needs our resource as much as A and B do. Person *B* cannot do this. In this case, it is permissible, I think, to select A over B, excluding B merely because he cannot be instrumentally useful. Doing this helps us to better serve those who directly need our resource. Hence (surprisingly), it seems it is not essentially distinguishing people on the basis of whether they have an instrumental role that determines if our behavior is objectionable, but rather whether our choice leads us to use our resource for its best *direct* (rather than indirect) effects. In the clozapine case, we select someone who will allow for the best direct use of our supply of clozapine, hence the "treating as a mere means" objection does not defeat the strategy.[8]

A second objection, it may be said, is the difference between (a) denying someone treatment (either by not starting it or terminating a trial) in order to treat a greater number of other people *here and now*, and (b) denying someone treatment in order to treat a greater number of people *later*. Suppose we should give preference to the *here and now*. But, by hypothesis, we cannot treat B, D, and E simultaneously, for we must wait for B to recover in order for money to be freed up to treat D, and for the same reason we must wait for D to recover before we treat E. Theoretically, it could be a year before we get to helping E, if it takes six months each for B and D to reach normality. Hence, here and now, it is a choice between A and B, and so, it might be said, we should toss a coin between them. However, even if we accept the correctness of giving preference to the here and now, we can answer this objection by noting that D and E do *here and now need to be treated*, even if we cannot treat them until later. Therefore, their case is different from the case of persons (statistical or even identifiable) whom we predict will need care in the future.

However, a third objection is waiting. We have assumed that we *know* that B and D will achieve normality, but in reality the problem is that we do not know who will achieve normality. So, at the time we must choose between A and B, we have no rea-

son to believe B will do better. Still, suppose we have already treated A for six months and he only improves moderately. Then there is at least a chance that B will achieve normality but none that A will. If we drop A, we would do so in order to *go searching* for someone who will achieve normality so that we may help a greater number of people.

Therefore, even if numbers of those we can help matters morally, we must decide whether it matters more than (a) dropping someone after we have started treatment, in order to (b) only possibly help someone else more, in order to (c) only eventually help a greater number. I suggest that at least *when there is as yet no positive change in the patient's condition*, the moral appropriateness of doing this depends on how long it will take to find someone who will achieve normality and whether we are doing as much good in the interval as we would have done with the person dropped. Suppose that instead of six months, it took only one day to find out who would be normal ("One Day Case"). I suggest that objections arising from (a), (b), and (c) would then not be weighty, and we could morally afford to go searching for those who will allow us to treat the greater number. This suggests that what is problematic in the real case, where we must wait six months before we know if someone will be normal, is not (a), (b), and (c). Rather, it is (in addition to regression*) the possibility of a lengthy time during which no one is being helped who will increase the numbers helped as much as or more than A can.

But notice that what happens in one day in the One Day Case could be our *knowing* that someone will achieve normality, without his achieving it for six months. So we may still have to wait six months before treating someone else. When the *payoff* of treating more people is not achieved quickly, do factors (a), (b), and (c) loom larger again? I suggest not. This implies that it is morally more important, at least when the person dropped has not yet improved, how long the gap is between dropping him and beginning treatment for someone else who will achieve normality, rather than how long the gap is between dropping him and treating a greater number of people.

What if *A* has already improved before we contemplate dropping him? Does the speed with which we can identify and begin treatment of someone who can become normal affect the permissibility of dropping *A*? If one thinks that doing what leads to a patient's regression* is impermissible, the speed with which we find others to treat more successfully will not affect the impermissibility of dropping *A*. If regression* is not a barrier to helping a greater number of other people, the speed with which we can identify a candidate who will be normal and producing sufficient good should increase the permissibility of dropping someone.

CONFLICTS OF URGENCY AND OUTCOME IN A TWO-PERSON CHOICE

We have been assuming that all candidates for clozapine have the same need and urgency, and only varying outcomes. Now we come to deal with whether outcome dominates difference in severity (subpart [b], p. 377). But degree of need and degree of urgency may themselves differ in the candidates. For example, there may be unequal need (as I have defined it), but equal urgency: Suppose *A* is 20 years old, has had 10 years of severe mental illness, and faces a bad future. Suppose *B* is 20 years old, has experienced moderate mental illness for the last year, and faces as bad a future as *A*. There is unequal need here, as *A*'s life will have gone worse overall if he is not treated than *B*'s life will have gone if he is not treated.

The type of case I wish to deal with in detail involves holding pasts equal, but varying urgency. How do we deal with differences in outcomes when some will be worse off than others if not treated (i.e.,

they are more urgent)? Let us start with two-person cases.

An easy case of this type is represented in Figure 29–7, where "U" stands for urgency, "O" for outcome, and the numbers indicate the degree of each.

Here *A* is both more urgent *and* promises a better outcome (normality) if treated. Here there is no conflict between taking care of the person who would be worse off and treating the one who will produce the best outcome, at least if the difference in urgency between the two people is significant. But, of course, in another case, a conflict could arise between helping the person who would be worse off if not treated and producing the best outcome (normality). For example, see Figure 29–8.

If U_{10} is a very bad prospect and O_5 is a significant outcome that lowers *A*'s urgency to the level at which *B* is already, then it might be argued that we should first improve the condition of the worst off person, *A*, before producing a bigger benefit that goes to someone who is already better off. This follows from *maximin*, which is based both on a principle of fairness between people and the idea that we produce a morally more valuable outcome if we give even a smaller outcome to the worst-off person. It even follows from a nonmaximin principle, such as trying to bring those very badly off in an absolute sense to a

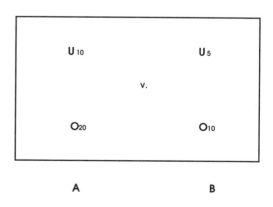

Figure 29–7. Case of greater urgency and outcome coinciding.

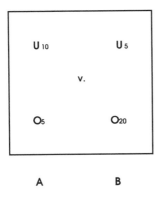

Figure 29–8. Case of urgency and outcome not coinciding.

minimal level, even if not always favoring the worst off person.

An alternative position argues that we need not always favor the worst-off, even when they are very badly off and we could make a significant improvement up to a minimal level, if we can instead produce a much greater benefit in the life of someone else. According to this position, we should show that helping the worst off counts for somewhat more than merely producing the best outcome by assigning a factor with which we can multiply the outcome score of the worst off, in accord with the absolute (and relative) badness of his or her condition. This means that we give the worst off an edge, but someone less badly off and with a better outcome could always win out. (Presumably, it would take a bigger outcome in the less urgent person to override the weight of urgency in the worst person by comparison to the outcome it takes in someone equally urgent to override the tendency to give the two equal chances.)

All these policies on how to deal with conflicts between urgency and outcome conflict with certain claims made about current clozapine policy.[9] For example, it is said that treating in accord with urgency and jeopardizing better outcomes is "against intuition." Policies I have described favoring the worst-off individuals claim that it is not against intuition to do so. (Of course, given that urgency is no in-

dication that clozapine will not lead to normality, sometimes there will be no conflict between favoring the urgent and producing the best outcome.)

It is also said that "no one argues against treatment where there is a dramatic response," that is, marked reduction of symptoms and restoration of normality. If this means that no one could reasonably argue against treating the most urgent who become normal, that should be true. But if it means that no one could reasonably argue against treating those who would *not* be the worst off without treatment but who can achieve normality, that is not true, at least in the two-person case.

HELPING MORE PEOPLE AND HELPING MORE URGENT PEOPLE

Let us expand our conclusions about conflicts between urgency and outcome to deal with the additional crucial factor in the clozapine case, namely that the number of people we can help may depend upon whom we help. Suppose A is more urgent than B but only B can achieve normality. (This assumes, hypothetically, that we could know before treatment who will become normal.) Suppose C is as urgent as A is and will produce as good an outcome. We free up money to help C only if we help B. So, should we help B and then C rather than A? (See Fig. 29–9.)

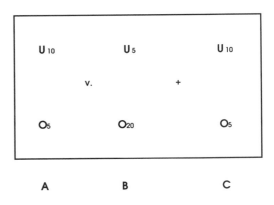

Figure 29–9. Case of helping more people.

That choice seems peculiar. For if C is already in need now, why would we not choose to help him immediately? That is, why isn't it just a contest between A and C? The only answer available is that if we treat A or C first, we will never get to treat B, for A or C will not free up money for another patient. Here we are asked to consider letting a more severe patient suffer for some months while we treat a less severe patient simply because this allows us to treat both.

Suppose we can help B and C *or* B and D but not both sets. Patient D is as urgent as C (and A), but D and not C will achieve a normal outcome. Suppose E, who is as urgent as C but cannot achieve normality, is also waiting to be treated. Only if we help D can we also help B and E, and so we should do this rather than helping B and C. We can then help two people who are as urgent as A instead of one person (see Fig. 29–10).

One way of interpreting the general principle at play here is as follows: Pay complete attention to better outcomes when doing so conflicts with taking care of the more urgent only if this makes it possible to significantly help more of those who are as urgent as those we might otherwise have helped. We do not so heavily favor those who give better outcomes per se; we favor them so heavily only when it helps us treat more who are urgent.

In the clozapine case, however, we are told that there will be no reason to think, at the time we make a choice, that someone as urgent as A will not have as good a chance of reaching normality as B and, hence, freeing up resources. It is also more important to treat the most urgent. Thus, it seems unlikely that it ever makes sense to treat the moderately ill B instead of someone more urgent. This means we should look for those who can produce normal outcomes among the urgent people only. (For one radical alternative to this, see the section titled "The Moderately Ill" below.)

Also, we are told, we cannot know that A will not produce a normal outcome until we treat for six months. On the basis of our previous discussion, we can see that two issues then arise. First, may we stop treating A after six months to test another urgent person for restored normality, or does regression* matter morally? Second, does it matter how long it is expected to take to find someone who will respond better than A and how much good we produce in the interval? On the assumption that there are now always additional urgent cases who could reach normality, and that it is not always wrong to stop or not start treating the most urgent who confront us, we should drop those who are urgent but have only moderate outcomes after six months of treatment, so as to search for those who are now urgent and who will achieve normality (as long as the probability of finding these is sufficiently high and sufficient good is done in the interval of the search).

This policy, however, gives lexical priority to helping significantly as many of the worst-off individuals as we can. As noted above, an alternative is to give only somewhat greater weight to claims of the worst off or focus on them only if they are below a minimal state. On this alternative, we would not ignore the possibility of better outcomes in the less urgent or do whatever is necessary to maximize the number of most urgent people who get treated. This

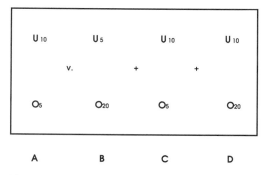

Figure 29–10. Case of producing more normal people.

might mean also taking care of moderately ill people who will achieve normality in order to increase the number of people who achieve normality.

THE MODERATELY ILL

Most importantly, if there were no more urgent cases to treat who could achieve normality, a maximin policy says that those urgent individuals who could only achieve moderate outcomes should be favored over other patients who were already only moderately ill regardless of the outcomes they would produce. Here is where the concern for treating the worst off comes into real conflict with the desire to produce good outcomes and with the desire to treat as many patients as possible. For if we treated "moderates" rather than those "urgents" whom we know cannot achieve normality, we might achieve more cases of normality (albeit in those only moderately ill). Of course, if a policy of treating moderates who become normal freed up enough money to bring more urgents up to the level of moderate well-being in a reasonable time, we would get the benefits to moderates without too great a sacrifice to urgents.

A radical alternative that opens up more possibility for treating the moderately ill suggests itself. Consider that if we continue treating only those urgents who will become normal, they will wind up *better off* than those who were moderately ill to begin with. Out of fairness, we might stop fully treating the urgents at the point where they become moderately well—assuming we could maintain them at that degree of moderate well-being if full treatment did not continue—and then decide whether to bring them or those who were already moderately ill (independent of clozapine) up to normality.

This proposal may strike many doctors as morally problematic: It would have them stop treatment although more good for a patient could be achieved. However,

it is not problematic in the way regression* is, and I have already argued that commitment to one patient is not necessarily a strong enough consideration to override concern for other patients. Of course, in this situation, it is just a concern for fairness rather than better outcome that is driving the proposal, since either patient (it is being hypothesized) could become normal.

A problem with this proposal is that we lose cost-effectiveness, for we will use some of our clozapine resources to keep some people who would be urgent at the level of only moderate well-being. Those who survive at a moderate level without clozapine are costly because they require institutionalization, but they are not as costly as those who require institutionalization *and* also require clozapine treatment to achieve moderate well-being. Furthermore, when we partially treat a patient who could become normal to *search* for a moderate who could also be normal, we give up on a sure bet for many possible failures followed by a random choice.[10]

NOTES

1. Other drugs may (or perhaps already have) come to supplant clozapine for treatment of schizophrenia. That will not affect the relevance of my discussion, because I take clozapine only as an example of a scarce resource. My discussion also applies to other scarce resources, such as places in intensive care units. However, the method I employ in this discussion may lead to different results where other scarce resources are involved because they do not share a particular characteristic assumed to be true of clozapine: the severely ill (what I call the most urgent cases) have as good a chance of attaining normality as those not already severely ill. In other situations (e.g., involving scarce organs for transplantation), severity of illness tends to be correlated with worse outcomes.

2. These are principles I have (for the most part) discussed in detail in my *Morality Mortality*, Vol. 1. New York: Oxford University Press, 1993, and in my "Nonconsequentialism" in *Guide to Ethical Theory* (Oxford: Blackwells), 1999.

3. In Hastings Center Background Document, "Mental Health Services: Ethics of Resource Utilization" (unpublished) 1994,

4. I here make use of Prospect Theory developed by Daniel Kahneman and Amos Tversky. For more on this theory see my "Moral Intuitions, Cognitive Psychology, and the Harming/Not Aiding Distinction, *Ethics*, April 1998

5. See *Morality, Mortality*, Vol. 1.

6. These claims are discussed in more detail in Morality, Mortality, vol. 1.

7. For reasons I will not go into here, I do not believe an *ex ante* perspective on this issue yields a different result.

8. I believe there is a striking similarity—indicating that the same underlying principle is at work—between what distinguishes the Doctor and Clozopine cases and what (I have elsewhere argued) distinguishes cases in which it is impermissible to favor using scarce resources on a nondisabled candidate rather than on a disabled one from cases in which doing so is permissible. There, once again (I surmise), it turns out that we may favor a candidate whose makeup allows us to use our resources to do a better job but may not favor a candidate who yields a better outcome simply by virtue of characteristics he brings to the situation. For more on this, see my "Disability, Discrimination, and Irrelevant goods" (unpublished).

9. As reported in Hastings Center Background Document, (see note 3).

10. This article was originally conceived in 1994 as part of a Hastings Center Project on Mental Health. I thank John Oberdick for his comments.

REFERENCES

Hastings Center Background document, Mental Health Services: Ethics of Resource Utilization. (unpublished) (1994)

Kamm, F.M. (1993). *Morality, Mortality, Vol. 1*. New York: Oxford University Press.

Kamm, F.M. (1999). Nonconsequentialism. In *Guide to Ethical Theory*. Oxford: Blackwell's.

Kamm, F.M. Disability, discrimination, and irrelevant goods. (unpublished, forthcoming).

30

Disability, Justice, and Health-Systems Performance Assessment

Jerome E. Bickenbach

In a bold move, the World Health Organization (WHO) has set out a framework for assessing the overall performance of health systems around the globe (WHO, 2000). The media's interest in the *World Health Report, 2000* (herein *Report*), was sparked, not so much by the complex assessment framework it uses, as by the fact that the *Report* ranks 191 countries by their performance, revealing surprises such as the first place position of France and the relatively low ranking of the United States (37th). Ministries of Health around the world either proudly displayed their unexpectedly high ranking, used their relative position as an argument for reform, dismissed the exercise as an invidious "health Olympics," or else expressed concern about the quality of the data or the methodology. On its release, WHO Director General Gro Harlan Bruntland made it clear that WHO is committed to its assessment framework and plans yearly recalculations based on more valid and reliable country-level data. At the same, when

WHO's Executive Board met in February 2001, it failed to give unalloyed support to the project, and several member countries expressed concern about the methodology employed.

MEASURING HEALTH-SYSTEM PERFORMANCE: THE *WORLD HEALTH REPORT, 2000*

Arguably, the WHO *Report* represents a dramatic change in the WHO traditional health agenda—a change that brings it closer to the Organization for Economic Co-operation and Development (OECD) and the World Bank (both of which have proposed cost-effectiveness assessment frameworks: OECD, 1998, 1999; Hsiao, 1995). Nonetheless, the direction WHO has chosen is fully consonant with recent interest, in the United States and elsewhere, with performance measurement as a first step in health-system reform.

On the face of it, the WHO framework is vulnerable to a range of criticisms readily found in the literature. As the framework adopts a standard economic efficiency analysis, it is open to the objection that it ignores considerations of justice. In addition, the framework relies on the notion of disability-adjusted life expectancy (DALE), a mathematical variant of disability-adjusted life-years, or DALYs, a notion that has attracted widespread criticism. The DALYs, many have argued, perpetuates systematic discrimination against persons with disabilities and others with health or functional limitations (e.g., Harris, 1987; Lockwood, 1988; Nord, 1993; Williams, 1987; Brock, 1989, 1992, 1995, 1997; Edgar et al., 1998; Hadorn, 1992). The essence of the critique comes to this: If health-system performance is understood as a matter of weighing health attainment against resource expenditure, then, given resource scarcity, we are driven to allocation decisions that sacrifice the lives or well-being of individuals whose present or future disabilities create poorer and more costly health outcomes. Doing so, however, is fundamentally unjust inasmuch as it sacrifices the interests of people with disabilities, the elderly, and fetuses or infants with severe disabilities in order to maximize average health attainment.

Unlike the earlier WHO-sponsored "burden of disease" study (Murray and Lopez, 1996), the recent WHO framework for health-system performance assessment addresses these objections by integrating justice considerations directly into the assessment process. To appreciate how this is accomplished, the framework needs to be spelled out in some detail.

WHO's ASSESSMENT FRAMEWORK

Rather than reviewing existing health performance indicators, or surveying variations in health-system design, the WHO *Report* more intuitively opens by enumerating the intrinsic goals of health systems to delimit the outcomes for which it is plausible to hold health systems accountable. Although the bulk of the *Report* concerns the organizational functions (service delivery, investment, financing, and stewardship) that make achievement of its goals more likely, and offers suggestions for improving their efficiency, justice issues arise in the basic building blocks of the framework.

The WHO *Report* identifies three intrinsic goals of a health system: *health, responsiveness,* and *fair financing.* Improving the health of the population it serves is the obvious goal of a health system. Still, health systems must also respond to our legitimate expectation that health-care delivery respect the dignity of the person (by way of respecting autonomy and confidentiality) while maintaining a "client orientation" (by providing prompt attention, appropriate amenities, access to social supports, and choice of provider). These responsiveness values are intrinsic to what health systems are for. We also insist that the provision of our health care is financed in a fair manner. Health expenses are unforeseeable and, potentially, catastrophically expensive. Fairness requires that health be financed by means of a regime of prepaid, risk-spreading insurance joined with cross-subsidization to ensure equal access to the poor.

Levels of the attainment of health and health-system responsiveness can be measured as a population average, and this average is a plausible metric of the quality of the health system. Equity is a different matter. The average health attainment across a population may be high, even though health attainment is unequally distributed (a characteristic feature of the situation in the United States as it happens). Similarly, a health system may score well on all the responsiveness goals because of the manner in which services are delivered to most people, while at the same time a minority is flatly denied those benefits. Attainment goals, in short, are both a matter of average and equity. (Fairness in financing, by contrast, is simply an equity issue. The question of how much of a country's overall resources are allocated to the health system, however, is a macro-allocation issue outside the scope of health-system assessment.)

The WHO framework therefore identifies five distinct goals of a health system (two of which have a total of seven subgoals): the average and equity of health attainment, the average and equity of responsiveness, and fair financing. Together, these goals capture essential considerations of both goodness and fairness, where "[g]oodness means a health system responding well to what people expect of it; fairness means it responds equally well to everyone, without discrimination" (WHO, 2000, p. xi).

The WHO *Report* describes in general terms how each goal is operationalized and measured (leaving the details to a collection of technical papers). Because the five goals cannot be measured in terms of a single scale, in order to create the composite measure the goals have to be weighted. To do this, WHO performed two international surveys, the first to yield a weighing of the individual components of responsiveness, the second to weigh the achievement of the separate goals that together form the composite score. Only the overall weighting results are relevant here (see Table 30–1).

These weights are intuitive: Health attainment is regarded as the most important (indeed, defining) goal of the health system, so it dominates the overall weight. Moreover, both the goodness and the fairness of health attainment are equally weighted, suggesting recognition of the importance of equality of distribution. Responsiveness

(also equally weighted between average and equitable achievement) and fair financing are equally important, although, as intrinsic goals, secondary to health. The WHO *Report* speculates that respondents' ranking likely reflects the fact that both responsiveness and fair financing indirectly contribute to health achievement (by increasing and facilitating the use of the health system), while acknowledging that "a well-functioning health system should do much more than simply promote the best possible level of overall health" (WHO, 2000, p. 39).

As mentioned, the WHO *Report* provides tables of attainment rankings for each goal for all 191 member countries. A table of overall or weighted goal attainment is also given (with estimates of uncertainty for each value). Some expected patterns arise from these scores: Rich countries can afford to spend more on health, and so enjoy high levels of health attainment; they can also afford amenities and attention to responsiveness and, finally, tend to have more or less universal, prepayment financing schemes in place. As a result, ranking by overall attainment is closely correlated to country wealth. The fact that equity issues are significant components of the overall score means, however, that countries that are not rich but have managed a high level of equity of distribution of health resources rank relatively high (Andorra, Cyprus, and Cuba, for example, all fall within the top 40, although their health budgets are relatively small). Because of exceptionally high life expectancy, Japan leads the list of health attainment, although falling to 6th for responsiveness and 8th for fair financing. The United States is first in responsiveness, but 34th in equality of health attainment, and 54th in financial fairness, yielding a composite ranking of 15th.

Composite attainment of the five health-system goals, though interesting in itself, is just the first step in health-system performance assessment. Performance is a matter of comparing attainment level with expenditure. Because the WHO *Report* takes this

Table 30–1. Health System Goals: Weighting

Health	
Overall or average	25%
Distribution or equality	25%
Responsiveness	
Overall or average	12.5%
Distribution or equality	12.5%
Fair financial contribution	
Distribution or equality	25%

step, it presents an economic assessment of health systems, rather than a mere ranking of goal attainment. Indeed, even if the *Report* did not turn to efficiency explicitly—but merely discussed ways health systems could improve attainment levels—it would still, implicitly, be offering an economic assessment of health systems. This is because the fair financing goal makes progressive prepayment an implicit goal (perhaps instrumental, perhaps intrinsic), not merely because such a financial scheme shelters all households from catastrophic expenses and subsidizes the poor for essential health services, but also because it is an economically efficient way of financing health care. Economic efficiency, in short, is taken to be the overriding goal of a health system. The WHO *Report*'s advice to health-system decision makers is to take performance levels seriously. Identifying factors that influence performance and articulating policies that will achieve better performance are the primary responsibilities of public officials (it forms the operational content of what the WHO *Report* calls the "stewardship" role of public officials and agencies).

But how do we know when performance is lower, or higher, than it should be? The performance of a health system is a comparison of actual composite attainment with the *best the health system could have accomplished* as measured by two variables representing resource input. The first is the country's actual financial expenditures on health (measured in the *Report* as a proportion of GNP). The second—the country's average level of educational attainment—is a measure of human capital, which serves as a proxy measure for the country's contribution to factors outside of the health system that contribute to health status, degree of responsiveness, and how the health system is financed. Together, these variables account for a country's direct and indirect input into health systems; they also establish each country's relevant "frontier" or upper limit of performance—the most that could be expected of that health system given that level of resources.

A country's actual performance is thus a proportion of this upper limit. In fact, the *Report* estimates two performance relationships. The first relates resource input only to average health-status attainment, measured in DALEs; the second relates that same input to the overall composite attainment.

Although only the second of these indicators is consistent with WHO's insistence on a composite indicator derived from the five goals of health systems, the first indicator provides interesting information as well. It clearly shows, for example, that the expected direct correlation between level of expenditure and average health attainment creates a threshold effect: No country can hope to achieve more than 75% of the life expectancy that should be possible if its health budget is below $10 a person annually. Moreover, when the two indicators are compared, it becomes clear that a significant source of some wealthy countries' high achievement score lies not so much in average health attainment as in their ability to afford responsiveness and fair financing. Whereas the United States ranks 72nd in performance on health levels, it rises dramatically to 37th when responsiveness and fair financing levels are added in.

Only time will show whether WHO's commitment to health-system performance assessment will survive the increasingly hostile reception it is receiving from some member states, or, more importantly, whether the commitment will contribute to a measurable improvement in world health. But we need not wait to debate the question of whether the WHO's assessment framework escapes the kinds of criticisms that its predecessors have attracted.

Justice Concerns About Health-System Performance Assessment

Adopting the WHO *Report*'s distinction between attainment and performance, we can say that the enterprise of measuring how well a health system performs presupposes agreement both over a measure of attainment and a standard of performance.

In theory, we could use the measure of attainment itself to set the standard—for example, by defining appropriate units of outcome and measuring performance in terms of an optimal, ideal, or a "frontier" level of outcome. But it is far more sensible to measure performance as a function of outcome in light of the costs of producing that outcome.

Financial expenditure or opportunity costs, of course, need not be our exclusive focus. We could also add (or substitute) costs understood as violation of human rights, limitation of freedom, equality, well-being, or, indeed, a limit on any other value, individual or social. For example, Amataya Sen has long argued for development "efficiency" to be measured in light of the cost in freedom (Sen, 1999). Whatever our choice, for assessment to be meaningful, this "cost" must be measurable and linked to outcome.

In recent years, summary measures of population health (SMPH) have become the tool of choice for measuring health attainment. The SMPH scales are particularly attractive to WHO because one of its longest standing mandates has been to collect and render comparable health data across countries. Valid and reliable health information is an international public good that can be used to further international health cooperation. Country-level estimates of mortality, morbidity, and functional status by age, gender, and cause are useful for a wide range of public health purposes. However, to adequately describe health patterns across WHO's 191 member states a vast array of estimates need to be generated. With this deluge of information, it is nearly impossible to isolate main findings or salient trends, or even to compare levels of population health across countries, unless the data are summarized in some way.

Theoretically, too, SMPH are valuable instruments. Mortality data about causes of death, or proxy population health data such as infant mortality rates, or even symptom-oriented measures of illness or morbidity, do not capture all that we mean by "health." In addition, the health of a population, like the health of an individual, is a matter of the level of capacity or performance of basis human functions, activities, and roles. There are nonfatal as well as fatal health outcomes. Although the boundaries between what is health and what is not are controversial, aspects of human functionality do seem to be intrinsic features of a person's or a population's health status.

Both DALY, and its variant DALE, are composite health measures that combine information about mortality (life expectancy) and nonfatal health outcomes (disability) into a single number, understood as a portion of a year of life (Murray, 1996). Assuming that a state of perfect health has a weight of 0, and death that of 1, living with a disease-related disability has a weight somewhere between these end points. In the original Global Burden of Disease study, for example, angina was assigned a weight of 0.223, major unipolar depression 0.619, and quadriplegia 0.895. Thus, a year lived in one of these health states is "discounted" by the appropriate disability weight: A year lived with angina is equivalent to 0.78 of a year, with depression 0.38 and with quadriplegia 0.1 of a year. To the degree that we have reliable data on the prevalence of these conditions, it is possible to calculate for a population the overall "burden" of each condition. Given that we have a common metric in disability-adjusted years lost, it is possible also to compare the relative burdens of different health states, in different populations.

If we had reliable data on the cost of prevention, treatment, and cure of particular diseases and disabilities, then we could give an economic value to the prevention of a unit of DALYs for each condition. Assuming this information was available, the move to cost-effectiveness analysis, even for the noneconomist, appears so natural as to be inevitable. With it we can determine, across the health system, the relative economic value of alternative therapies for the same disease, or the opportunity cost of moving resources from prevention to cure, or the relative benefit of funding treatment of one disease rather than another, and other such comparisons. Assuming full and accurate information at each stage, the DALYs measure, joined with cost-effectiveness analysis, appears to provide a sound basis for resource allocation questions at all levels.

There is, however, a missing step. Cost-effectiveness analysis is not itself a decision-making standard; it merely lays out the options, ranking them in terms of a ratio of cost and outcome. It rests on the normative claim that resources ought to be used in the most cost-effective manner possible, that is, the economic standard of efficiency. The standard of economic efficiency, stripped to its core intuitive meaning, entails that we should aim at producing an output at the lowest cost (or producing a maximal outcome for a fixed budget). Although economists are reluctant to admit it, this is plainly an ethical proposition, akin to the underlying maximization claim of utilitarianism.

In what way would the use of DALYs as a measure of health-system output, against a background of cost-effectiveness analysis, be an unjust or inequitable or discriminatory way of making policy decisions about how a health system should work? Perhaps because it is the most explicit and dramatic arena of medical decision making where cost-effectiveness would be used, situations requiring extreme medical resource allocation or rationing decisions have typically been the focus of critique. There are, to be sure, defenders of cost-effectiveness as a rationing tool in medicine (see, e.g., McKie et al., 1998; Ubel, 2000), but there are also many who object both to the theory and the practice, on grounds of justice. Four representative justice concerns are described next.

Unfair construction of summary measures of population health

Several critiques of QALYs, DALYs, and other SMPH have pointed to the fact that the weights given to nonfatal health outcomes are provided by a consensus of health professionals rather than by people who actually live their lives with the conditions being weighted. The concern is not merely that this produces inaccurate or prejudicial weighting (although that is certainly arguable), but also that it is fundamentally unfair to deny a voice to those whose lives will be more directly affected by the results of the weighting exercise (e.g., Loomes and McKenzie, 1989; Menzel et al., 1999).

Unjust use of cost-effectiveness for allocation decisions

It has been argued that as allocation of health resources involves fundamental matters of life, death, and well-being, such resources should be allocated by means of a just and participatory political process, rather than by turning the issue over to experts who rely on utilitarian calculation, disguised as neutral and objective science (e.g., Daniels, 1988, 1993, 1998).

Cost-effectiveness analysis is distributively neutral

More generally, it is argued that as a fundamentally utilitarian decision-making method, cost-effectiveness analysis ignores considerations of distributive justice. For example, a higher average health attainment might be achieved by cutting off the flow of expensive health resources to a few very ill or disabled individuals, and spreading those resources over a huge pool of individuals, each of whom will enjoy a very small improvement of health—although this total improvement is larger than the health loss of the few. This is an intuitively unjust result (e.g., Broome, 1988; Daniels, 1988; Williams, 1988, Anand and Hanson, 1997, 1998; Brock, 1997, 2001).

Allocation decisions that discriminate against specific populations

Individuals with disabilities and the elderly, it has been argued, are treated unfairly by SMPH in a cost-effectiveness analysis for allocation decisions. Because of preexisting health conditions or fewer years to live, or both, these populations will achieve lower health outcomes from interventions than will people who are younger or healthier; therefore, they will be discriminated against in allocation decisions (e.g., Harris, 1988, 1994; Lewis and Charny, 1989 Brock, 1995, 2000; Arnesen and Nord, 1999).

On the whole, these concerns rely on a priori arguments grounded in moral and political theory. Increasingly, however, critiques have appeared based on empirical work—drawn from surveys, key informant interviews, and focus groups—seeking evidence for public views about allocation decision making. In his recent book, Norwegian economist Erik Nord reviews this empirical work and concludes that the basis for QALY determination—and, by implication, DALY determination as well—ignores salient, well-documented social preferences that run directly counter to the presumptions of cost-effectiveness and disability weighting (Nord, 1999; cf. Menzel et al., 1999).

Philosophically, the link between this empirical evidence and the argumentation for or against the WHO performance assessment framework is not always obvious. There is nothing to prevent one from arguing that social preferences are invidious or prejudicial and ought not to be determinative of allocation decisions. But, if we grant that these objections have prima facie merit, there is ample reason to believe that legitimate doubts can be raised about the degree to which the WHO framework satisfactorily addresses them.

JUSTICE CONCERNS AND THE WHO FRAMEWORK

Subtle refinements notwithstanding, the WHO framework for health-system performance assessment assumes that the construction of its summary health measure, DALEs, based as it is on the DALY measure, is unproblematic. To be sure, a considerable amount of effort has gone into the technically sophisticated task of estimating—in the face of a dearth of solid evidence about prevalence of disability around the world—the DALE average scores for the 191 countries in the WHO survey (Mathers et al., 2000). Yet the fact remains that the DALE measure adopts without alteration the disability weights of DALYs. And it was precisely these weights of the "burden" of various disabilities, or rather the methodology for determining these weights, that was the object of this first justice concern.

Searching through the WHO *Report* and its background technical papers, all that one finds to address the concern is the following brief comment: "These weights do not represent the lived experience of any disability or health state, or imply any societal value of the person in a disability or health state. Rather they quantify societal preferences for health states in relation to the societal 'ideal' of good health" (Mathers et al., 2000, p. 13).

This remark begs the question for a variety of reasons. First, what needs to be shown—either empirically or by argument—is that the methodology that was used to determine the relative disability weights (a "person trade-off" exercise involving health professionals—described and critiqued in Nord, 1999) truly represents a societal value, rather than a dubious professional proxy for such a value. Second, the current methodology for assigning disability weights has moved away, using societal preferences in favor of utilities measured by individual preferences (Murray et al., 1999). Finally, neither conceptually nor in practice is there is a meaningful distinction between "quantifying societal preferences for health states" and expressing a "societal value of the person in a disability or health state"; this is because health states have no independent existence but are embodied in individuals with those states. In rationing contexts, if resources are restricted or denied by disability type, the effect is to restrict or deny resources to people with that disability. In short, the WHO *Report* fails to address or answer this first concern.

As for the second justice concern, the *Report* makes a determined effort to respond to the objection that health policy in general, and allocation issues in particular, ought to be debated and settled within the political process rather than, behind the scenes, by experts. It is, admittedly, no criticism of the WHO to observe that, as an international agency, it is estopped from making political recommendations relevant to the political process by which health policy is determined. Nonetheless, the *Report* does state that the responsibility for the performance of a country's health-care system lies with its government responsibility for efficient and sensible management of resources. However, a government's obligation of "stewardship"—the *Report*'s carefully chosen term to capture evidence-based systems management—need not include any form of direct participation by the citizenry. Perhaps it was felt that the equity goals could stand as surrogates for a more fully participatory process, on the assumption that the outcome of such a process would look seriously upon justice considerations of how health resources should be distributed.

Of course, this does not answer the basic challenge that Daniels and others make that distributive justice demands a fair and deliberative process, not only because there is no a priori mechanism for deciding difficult allocation questions, but also because there is no stable consensus about how these issues should be answered. The *Report* merely assumes what we have no clear social consensus (applicable around the globe) on rationing issues.

More to the point, all of this rests on the assumption that the framework does adequately incorporate distributive values. This assumption is precisely what the third justice concern challenges by way of insisting that, however sophisticated, cost-effectiveness analysis will always be distributively neutral. The *Report* has a clear response: Cost-effectiveness as an analysis is relevant only for achieving the best overall or average health; this is but one of five

intrinsic goals of health systems by which attainment is defined and measured. Moreover, except in the richest countries, cost-effectiveness analysis has limited practical value because it requires unavailable detailed information about intervention costs and results. To offset these obstacles, other and more technically complex versions of the cost-effectiveness analysis were used to prepare the WHO *Report* (Murray et al., 1999).

It is instructive to compare the *Report*'s reaction to cost-effectiveness analysis to two other approaches, both of which favor a role for cost-efficiency considerations in the allocation of health-care resources. One approach is to insist that the virtue of using QALYs, DALYs, or some other SMPH in a cost-effectiveness analysis is precisely that it is distributively neutral. By separating health maximization from distributional concerns, the argument goes, we can make more clear-headed allocation decisions and then adjust them to satisfy whatever considerations of distributive fairness society at large decides upon (see McKie et al., 1998). This makes more sense, not only because of the imminent rationality of cost-effectiveness in health-resource allocation, but also because health, for all its importance, remains but one component of well-being, opening up the prospect of further securing justice by means of compensation or some other redistributive technique.

The second approach begins by flatly denying that it is possible to compensate for ill health and concludes that the role of cost-effectiveness must therefore be restrained or limited by an independent array of values including distributional equity (Richardson and Nord, 1997; Menzel et al., 1999; and cf. Culver and Wagstall, 1993). These values (or "equity weights") might identify the desirability of giving priority to the severity of illness, to lifesaving, to ensuring that everyone has a fair chance at a normal life span, or to some other important consideration. Needless to say, how the precise allocation answers given by pure cost-effectiveness analysis are to be "adjusted" by these other factors poses a challenge to this approach.

The *Report* does not adopt, or even acknowledge the first approach, because its focus is entirely on the performance of health systems. On first reading, one might think the *Report* adopts the second approach; but this impression is incorrect, for no attempt is made to alter directly the cost-effectiveness analysis by means of equity weights. Instead, the equity goals of health equality, responsiveness equality, and fair financing are said to be wholly independent of cost-effectiveness analysis. And so there are, at least at the first stage. In the second stage (the performance determination) these goals are not independent of economic assessment. For although no direct form of economic analysis is used to determine the attainment levels of these equity goals, performance determination is itself nothing more than a direct application of economic productive efficiency.

Thus, unlike the compensation and equity weight approach, the approach taken in the WHO *Report* rests upon the plausibility of applying an unmodified form of efficiency analysis as the core analysis. Performance, in short, is economic efficiency by another name. This raises the suspicion that, although the *Report* insists it is taking equity and distributive justice seriously, in fact it ends up endorsing a purely economic analysis of health systems. Even though distributive concerns are explicitly incorporated into the framework is not the overall performance assessment is distributively neutral? Are not equity goals implicitly transformed into efficiency goals? Perhaps the best way to test this suspicion is to look at the last justice concern and ask whether people with disabilities and others with less than ideal health are discriminated against by the WHO framework.

One might argue that the very choice of intrinsic goals, if not discriminatory against the interests of people with chronic health conditions, is at least prejudicial to their interests. The *Report* argues that whereas health, responsiveness, and fair financing are intrinsic goals of a health system, considerations such as accessibility are merely instrumental aims. For people with disabilities, however, accessibility has always been a major concern; for them, the availability of health services and their provision in accessible physical and social surroundings are not trivial issues. They are fundamental issues of justice. Why does the *Report* view responsiveness and fair financing as intrinsic goals, but not accessibility?

The argument given is this: A goal is intrinsic when we agree that to raise the achievement of that goal, without lowering the attainment of other intrinsic goals, represents an overall improvement. Health is indisputably an intrinsic goal, so there is no issue there. But so too are financial equity and assuring that people are treated promptly, with respect for their dignity and their wishes; they are intrinsic goals because people would be generally unhappy with a system that fails in these areas, even when the health outcomes are satisfactory (WHO, 2000, p. 24). Accessibility to services is different. Accessibility to services may be an explanation of good or bad health attainment, but it is not itself an intrinsic goal as it is possible to imagine a situation where accessibility is increased without health being increased.

This argument is circular; it assumes that people would not be unhappy with decreased accessibility to the health system unless they perceived their health to be directly affected by inaccessibility. This may be true of people who are generally healthy or do not perceive themselves to be vulnerable to ongoing or episodic downward shifts in health status—such as are experienced by individuals with severe disabilities, chronic health conditions, or the elderly. For people with disabilities, securing a guarantee of accessibility to health care undoubtedly looms larger than ensuring that they have choice in health-care provider, good quality hospital food, confidentiality, or access to social services, the features of the purported intrinsic goal of responsiveness. This might seem to be a major criticism because minor adjustments in wording related to accessibility concerns might be incorporated into the responsiveness goal. Still, the next worry strikes deeper, and it replays arguments made by persons with disabilities against SMPH and cost-effectiveness as a standard of health-system performance.

Indisputably, the central message that WHO is sending to member states is that health-system performance improvement is both possible and desirable. Because performance is a matter of both goal attainment and resource expenditure, various paths are open to the responsible government agency wishing to improve performance. The agency can either hold costs constant and improve attainment, or hold attainment constant and lower costs, or optimally improve attainment and lower costs. More subtle options are always possible, such as altering the system in a manner that in fact reduces attainment as well as costs, but lowers costs proportionally more.

Generally, in the short run it is almost always easier to lower costs than to improve attainment levels. Improving overall attainment invariably incurs short- and medium-term costs in terms of shifting priorities, initiating and carrying out research into new methodologies, changing patterns of service provision, altering work force, and other systems changes that are costly and may not immediately produce better levels of health or responsiveness.

As a tool for summarizing health improvements, DALEs, like their close cousin DALYs, helpfully extend our notion of health outcomes from mere extension of life to levels of functioning. Yet these measures assume that disabilities are always a burden, both for the individual (in terms of lower health related quality of life) and society (in terms of a variety of costs and expenses). A life with disabilities, in the words of the WHO *Report*, is a "stunted"

life, expressed quite literally in DALEs, as a life year that is "shorter" than a full year. Understandably, this fact has never sat well with individuals who have disabilities.

Combining this devaluation of life with economic efficiency in a rationing context yields the concern that has been repeatedly expressed in the literature: On efficiency grounds, providing health resources to people with disabilities is an economically suspect proposition because, at least in comparison to people without disabilities, the same health expenditure will tend to yield a lower health outcome. Disabilities, in other words, are not only 'burdens' for people who live with them, they are costly and burdensome to the health system. For this reason, attempts to reduce costs will disproportionally prejudice the interests of people with disabilities and others with compromised health, including, as a matter of course, the elderly (but see justifications for such practice in Walters, 1996).

From this premise, any number of consequences have been argued to follow: People with disabilities will be more vulnerable to service cutbacks than others; when services are rationed, these individuals will be less likely to receive them, irrespective of the level of benefit they may receive; in end-of-life situations, resources should not be wasted on keeping their "burdensome" lives going when cost savings can be secured, either by letting them die, or by more active forms of euthanasia (see Koch, 2000; Rock, 2000). All of these social consequences represent examples of how a group of people can be sacrificed for the greater health benefits of others—a prima facie case of discriminatory treatment.

Arguably, the WHO framework disallows these results because health attainment is not one, but two goals: "the best attainable average level—goodness—and the smallest feasible differences among individuals and groups—fairness" (WHO, 2000, p. 26). The second of these goals is characterized as equality of distribution of health expectancy (that is, the expected number of years lived in full health) (Gakidou et al., 2000), a robust egalitarian measure of equity. So understood, equality of distribution of health expectancy ignores the effects of chance, choice, and any difference in health expectancy not currently amendable to change, each of which would dilute the aim of achieving equality of result. Because there is no likely decrease in the margin of utility of health improvements, Gakidou and colleagues are reluctant to rely on the standard measure of income inequality (the Gini coefficient) and they make tentative proposals for an alternative approach.

Although the discriminatory impact of the WHO framework will be blunted by its health-equity goal, it will not be eliminated. The health-equity goal has the same weight as the health-average goal, so improvements in either translate into potential improvements in overall performance (assuming no budget change). Each country must decide whether it is more feasible to improve average health attainment or reduce the gap between those with the lowest and those with the highest health expectancies. It is not obvious which is more efficient, nor does the WHO Report give guidance here. We are left with the fact that, at least in theory, overall improvements are possible by rigorously restricting access to health resources to those with the worst health. If these individuals were to die, both population health average and equality of distribution would improve.

This point is highly provocative, for it suggests that health planners would seriously consider restricting health resources to people for whom the prospect and amount of health improvement is less than it is for healthier individuals. If our ultimate evaluation of a health system is economic, then, as the Report clearly states, we must look not at health outcomes alone, but at the cost of achieving them: "In economic terms, performance is a measure of efficiency: an efficient health system achieves much, relative to the resources at its disposal. In contrast, an inefficient system is wasteful of resources, even if it achieves high levels of health, responsiveness and fairness. That is, it could be expected to do still better, because countries spending less do comparably well or countries spending a little more achieve much better outcomes" (WHO, 2000, p. 42). But we should add that performance improvement would also result from spending less and attaining poorer outcomes, when the savings outpace the loss in attainment.

Without data, we cannot tell whether this last option will be the most attractive to health planners, so that people with disabilities, the elderly, and other groups whose health expectancy is low will become the most cost-efficient targets of this strategy for health systems performance improvement. It is not an option that the Report rejects, regrets, or even comments upon. By being agnostic about the potential efficiency of discriminatory practices, the Report allows that a responsible government could create and implement such a policy. If justice considerations—as operationalized by the three intrinsic equity goals—are outcomes that are weighted against other outcomes, circumstances may arise in which the values they represent must give way in favor of performance improvement strategies.

ASSESSING HEALTH SYSTEMS: ANY ALTERNATIVE?

But do we have any option? If we accept the assumption that health resources are, and will always be, scarce and if it is pointless to assess the performance of a health system exclusively in terms of needs met or health goal reached, without any reference to cost, then perhaps policies that sacrifice some group of people are just inevitable. In the face of scarcity, have we reached a point where it becomes obvious that goodness and fairness are ultimately irreconcilable? Several responses are possible.

First, if we are going to factor into SMPH the "burden" of disability, we should do so in a manner that is true to the nature of disability. Although the debate over the appropriate "model" of disability has a long history involving many disciplinary perspectives (see the general discussion in Bickenbach, 1993), there is a consensus that disability is not some distinct and inherent trait that individuals possess. Rather, disability is the outcome of an interaction between features of the person (disease conditions, injuries, impairments) and physical and social environmental factors. What "disables" a person is, at least in part, a feature of the overall context in which the person wants to, or is required to, perform activities. Limitations in the major life activities a person can participate in are mediated by the environmental demands, barriers, and facilitators that create the lived experience of having a disability. In this sense, disability is a universal human experience that needs to be approached from various perspectives, some biomedical, some social and political (Imrie, 1997; Bickenbach et al., 1999).

This account has profound consequences for the underlying rationale of SMPH in general, and DALEs in particular. For the "burden" of having a disability, or what limits the quality of life of a person with a disability, is not entirely a matter of the biological or biophysical limitations that directly arise from impairments. It is also a matter of stigma and discrimination, of lack of accommodation and other facilitating resources, of denial of opportunities, respect, and of basic rights.

But the point here is not that in the weighting exercise for DALEs no account is taken of these sources of burden. The problem is that these burdens are implicitly taken into account, but mistakenly, and unfairly, associated with the health condition rather than the ambient social environment. Moreover, the social and environmental sources of the burden of disabilities are not remedied by the health system as normally conceived. The burdens associated with mobility limitations (no ramps, no elevators) or sensory impairments (lack of signing facilities for deaf individuals), or

psychiatric impairments (stigma and fear) require social interventions of one sort or another, rather than (what is usually thought to be) health interventions. Ironically, attributing these burdens to a social sector wholly unprepared to deal with them is yet another source of the burden of disability.

In other words, the problem with SMPH lies in presumptions that are made about the source and character of the burden of disability. Insofar as the lived experience of disability is burdensome both intrinsically (pain, discomfort, functional limitation) and extrinsically (stigma, prejudice, discrimination, lack of accommodation, inequality), by conflating these factors, SMPH reproduce misperceptions about what makes disability a burden, and further entrench these misperceptions by recasting them as clinical assessments, freed of cultural or other influence.

As a result, when DALEs are used to determine the performance of a health system, what might have been merely a question of validity, becomes an issue of fairness. Using a performance assessment framework that relies on DALEs in order to rationalize judgments about how to allocate health resources "more efficiently" prejudices people with disabilities by ascribing to their health condition "burdens" that are not caused by the state of their mind or body, but by social arrangements. These arrangements may be cheaper to alter—or, once altered, may have additional economic benefits that far outstrip their costs—than health interventions. The burden of disability, in short, may be relieved by means of interventions that are not health interventions at all and so, from the point of view of the health system, costless.

Finally, why should we think it desirable, or even elegant, to summarize performance information. Erik Nord, in a recent critique, has argued that the WHO's summary number is meaningless, of no real use, and potentially invidious (Nord, 2001). Great dangers exist in distilling inherently vague, multifactorial, and qualitative assessments into a single (falsely precise) quantitative expression: Information is lost and vital moral and political considerations are ignored. The single numerical expression may raise public awareness that a "problem" in the performance of their nation's health system exists, but little is gained if in the process more is hidden by the techniques we use to quantify the problem than is revealed.

Moreover, there are other ways to proceed. For example, Norman Daniels and colleagues have proposed and subjected to limited testing a scheme of possible "benchmarks of fairness" for assessing health-care reform (Daniels et al., 1996; Daniels et al., 2000). The benchmarks provide a highly detailed and nuanced policy tool for analyzing and evaluating the overall fairness of health-care reforms. They capture facets of fairness that are parallel to, but extend far beyond, the goals specified in the WHO *Report*, identifying intersectorial public health issues, financial and other barriers to equitable access, comprehensiveness of benefits, quality of care, administrative efficiency, and democratic accountability and empowerment (Daniels et al., 2000). Each benchmark is operationalized to apply to specific outcomes or processes.

The salient difference between the benchmark approach and the WHO framework is that Daniels provides a moral and political account of the value of health that justifies the relevance of each of his fairness indicators. Briefly, he argues that inasmuch as ill-health is a disvalue to the extent that it reduces the opportunities open to individuals, the principle of equal opportunity should govern the regulation of health systems. By contrast, the *Report* lacks any account of what makes health valuable (and indeed, what health is), and appears to float in midair: We are left wondering why the goals of the health systems are worth pursuing at all. This moral and political agnosticism is understandable coming from an international organization that must tread softly on such matters, but there is

little doubt that it undermines the overall plausibly and theoretical integrity of the WHO framework.

Of more practical significance, the benchmark approach comprehends health intersectorially, thereby integrating the health-care system into the myriad other organizations and social agencies with jurisdiction over social determinants of health. The first benchmark, in particular, identifies a wide range of determinants—nutrition, housing, clean air and water, sanitation, health education, public safety, and violence reduction—that need to be reviewed in order to evaluate the efficiency and fairness of proposed health reforms. By understanding health as an intersectorial outcome, the benchmark approach boldly confronts an issue that the WHO framework ambiguously gestures at—namely the role of the health system in the production of health.

Finally, Daniels's benchmark scheme does not produce a summary judgment of the fairness of health reform. The benchmarks represent indicators of fairness that are jointly relevant to an overall assessment of the fairness of a health reform. These indicators (unlike the *Report*'s assessment goals) are not always commensurable; nor is there a predetermined weighting of each benchmark. Instead, they are matters for public discussion that may yield different results in different countries. What ultimately is required for fairness in health reform, Daniels argues, is procedural fairness in the process of coming to judgment about the fairness of the reform.

No doubt the WHO framework is a technically sophisticated version of a political–economic approach to health systems assessment that is more attuned to the ideological temper of the times. As Vincente Narvarro in a recent critique argues, in the "new wisdom" embodied in the WHO *Report*, "client demand replaces patients' needs, risk is valued over security, market shares dominate over government planning, and entrepreneurship dominates over public services" (Narvarro, 2000, p. 1601).

Yet as Daniels's benchmark approach attests, there are viable alternatives to health system performance assessment. The World Health Organization could benefit from a rethinking of the value and validity of its own framework.

Acknowledgment

Although the author is a consultant to the World Health Organization on issues concerning disability epidemiology and modeling, he did not participate in the preparation of the *Report* or any of its technical papers. This chapter wholly represents the author's own views and does not reflect in any way the position of the WHO.

REFERENCES

Anand, S. and Hanson, K. (1997). Disability-adjusted life years: a critical review. *Health Economics* 16, 685–702.

Anand, S. and Hanson, K. (1998). DALYs: Efficiency versus equity. *World Development* 26, 307–10.

Arnesen, T. and Nord, E. (1999). The value of DALY life: Problems with ethics and validity of disability adjusted life years. *British Medical Journal* 319, 1423–24.

Bickenbach, J.E. (1993). *Physical Disability and Social Policy*. Toronto: University of Toronto Press.

Bickenbach, J.E., Chatterji, S., Badley, E.M. and Ustun, T.B. (1999). Models of disablement, universalism and the ICIDH. *Social Science and Medicine* 48, 1173–87.

Brock, D.M. (1989). Justice, health care, and the elderly. *Philosophy and Public Affairs* 18, 297–312.

Brock, D.M. (1992). Quality of life measures in health care and medical ethics. In A. Sen and M. Nussbaum (eds.), *The Quality of Life*. Oxford: Oxford University Press, pp. 95–132.

Brock, D.M. (1995). Justice and the ADA: Does prioritizing and rationing health care discriminate against the disabled? *Social Theory and Policy* 12, 159–84.

Brock, D.M. (1997). Considerations of equity in relation to prioritization and allocation of health care resources. In Z. Bankowski, J. Bryant, and J. Gallagher (eds.), *Ethics, Equity and Health for All*. Geneva: Council of International Organization of Medical Sciences.

Brock, D.M. (2000). Health care resource prioritization and discrimination against persons with disabilities. In L.P. Francis and A. Silvers (eds.), *Americans with Disabilities* New York: Routledge, pp. 223–35.

Brock, D.M. (2001). Ethical issues in the use of cost-effectiveness analysis for the prioritization of health care resources. Unpublished manuscript.

Broome, J. (1988). Goodness, fairness and QALYs. In J. Bell and S. Mendus (eds.), *Philosophy and Medical Welfare*. Cambridge: Cambridge University Press, pp. 57–73.

Culver, A. and Wagstall, A. (1993). Equity and equality in health and health Care. *Journal of Health Economics*. 12, 431–57.

Daniels N. (1988). Distributive justice and the use of summary measures of population health status. In *Institute of Medicine, Summarizing Population Health: Directions for the Development and Application of Population Metrics*. Washington, D.C.: National Academy Press, pp. 58–71.

Daniels, N., Bryant, J., Castano, R.A., Dantes, O.G., Khan, K.S., and Pannarunothai, S. (2000). Benchmarks of fairness for health care reform: a policy tool for developing countries. *Bulletin of the World Health Organization* 78, 740–50.

Daniels, N. (1993). Rationing fairly: Programmatic considerations. *Bioethics* 7, 224–33.

Daniels, N. (1998). Distributive justice and the use of summary measures of population health status. In M. Field, and M. Gold (eds.), *Summarizing Population Health: Directions for the Development and Application of Population Metrics*. Washington, D.C.: National Academy Press, pp 58–71.

Daniels, N., Light, D. and Caplan, R. (1996). *Benchmarks of Fairness for Health Care Reform*. New York: Oxford University Press.

Daniels, N., et al. (2000). Benchmarks of fairness for health care reform: A policy tool for developing countries. *Bulletin of the World Health Organization* 78, 740–50.

Edgar, A., Salek, S., Shickle, D. and Cohen, D. (1998). *The Ethical QALY*. Haslemere, UK: Euromed Communications.

Gakidou, E., Murray, C. and Frenk, J. (2000). Defining and measuring health inequality: An approach based on the distribution of health expectancy. *Bulletin of the World Health Organization* 78, 42–54.

Hadorn, D. (1992). The problem of discrimination in health care priority setting. *JAMA* 368, 1454–59.

Harris, J. (1987). QALYfying the value of life. *Journal of Medical Ethics* 13, 117–23.

Harris, J. (1988). More and better justice. In J. Bell and S. Mendus (eds.), *Philosophy and*

Medical Welfare. Cambridge: Cambridge University Press, pp. 75–96.

Harris, J. (1994). Does justice require that we be ageist? *Bioethics* 8, 74–83.

Hsiao, C. (1995). A framework for assessing health financing strategies and the role of health insurance. In D. Dunlop and J. Martins (eds.), *An International Assessment of Health Care Financing.* New York: The World Bank.

Imrie, R. (1997). Rethinking the relationships between disability, rehabilitation, and society. *Disability and Rehabilitation* 19, 263–71.

Koch, T. (2000). Life quality vs the "quality of life": Assumptions underlying prospective quality of life instruments in health care planning. *Social Science and Medicine* 51, 419–27.

Lewis, P. and Charny, M. (1989). Which of two individuals do you treat when only their ages are different and you can't treat both? *Journal of Medical Ethics* 15, 28–32.

Lockwood, M. (1988). Quality of life and resource allocation. In J.M. Bell, and S. Mendus (eds.), *Philosophy and Medical Welfare.* Cambridge: Cambridge University Press, pp. 33–55.

Loomes, G. and McKenzie, L. (1989). The use of QALYs in health care decision making. *Social Science and Medicine* 28, 299–308.

Mathers, C., Sadana, R., Salomon, J., Murray, C. and Lopez, A. (2000). *Estimates of DALE for 191 Countries: Methods and Results.* Global Programme on Evidence for Health Policy Working Paper Paper No. 16. Geneva: World Health Organization.

McKie, J., Richardson, J., Singer, P. and Kuhse, H. (1998). *The Allocation of Health Care Resources.* Aldershot, UK: Ashgate.

Menzel, P., Gold, M., Nord, E., Pinto-Prades, J-L., Richardson J. and Ubel, P. (1999). Toward a broader view of values in cost-effectiveness analysis of health. *Hastings Center Report* 29, 7–15.

Murray, C. (1996). Rethinking DALYs. In C. Murray, and A. Lopez (eds.), *The Global Burden of Disease: A Comprehensive Assessment of Mortality and Disability from Diseases, Injuries, and Risk Factors in 1990 and Projected to 2020.* Cambridge, MA: Harvard University Press, pp. 1–98.

Murray, C. and Lopez A. (eds.) (1996). *The Global Burden of Disease: A Comprehensive Assessment of Mortality and Disability from Diseases, Injuries, and Risk Factors in 1990 and Projected to 2020.* Cambridge, MA: Harvard University Press.

Murray, C., Evans, D., Acharya, A. and Baltussen, R. (1999). *Development of WHO Guidelines on Generalised Cost-Effectiveness Analysis.* Global Programme on Evidence for Health Policy Working Paper Paper No. 4. Geneva: World Health Organization.

Murray, C., Salomon, J., and Mathers, C. (1999). *A Critical Examination of Summary Measures of Population Health.* Global Programme on Evidence for Health Policy Working Paper Paper No. 2. Geneva: World Health Organization.

Navarro, V. (2000). Assessment of the *World Health Report 2000. Lancet* 356, 1598–1601.

Nord, E. (1993). Unjustified use of the quality of well-being scale in oregon. *Health Policy* 24, 45–53.

Nord, E. (1999). *Cost Value Analysis In Health Care.* Cambridge: Cambridge University Press.

Nord, E. (2001). *World Health Report, 2000,* a brief, critical consumer guide. *British Journal of Medicine* (in press).

OECD (1998). *Health Outcome Measurement in OECD Countries: Toward Outcome-Oriented Policy Making.* Paris: OECD DEELSA/ELSA/WP1 (98)6/ANN.

OECD, Health Policy Unit (1999). *An Assessment of Health System Performance Across OECD Countries.* Paris: OECD DEELSA/ELSA/WPI (99)3.

Richardson, J. and Nord, E. (1997). The importance of perspective in the measurement of quality-adjusted life years. *Medical Decision Making* 17, 33–41.

Rock, M. (2000). Discounted lives? Weighing disability when measuring health and ruling on "compassionate" murder. *Social Science and Medicine* 51, 407–17.

Sen, A. (1999). *Development as Freedom.* New York: Alfred A. Knopf.

Ubel, P. (2000). *Pricing Life.* Cambridge, MA.: MIT Press.

Walters, J. (ed.) (1996). *Choosing Who's to Live.* Chicago: University of Illinois Press.

Williams, A. (1987). Who is to live? A question for the economist or the doctor? *World Hospitals* 13, 34–45.

Williams, A. (1988). Ethics and efficiency in the provision of health care. In J. Bell and S. Mendus (eds.), *Philosophy and Medical Welfare.* Cambridge: Cambridge University Press.

World Health Organization (WHO). (2000). *World Health Report, 2000.* Geneva: WHO.

31

Responsibility for Health Status

Lance K. Stell

> Each is the proper guardian of his own health, whether bodily, or mental or spiritual. Mankind are greater gainers by suffering each other to live as seems good themselves, than by compelling each to live as seems good to the rest.
> John Stuart Mill, *On Liberty*

> The principle of mutual love admonishes men constantly to come nearer to each other; that of the respect which they owe each other, to keep themselves at a distance from one another.
> Immanuel Kant, *The Doctrine of Virtue: Part II of The Metaphysics of Moral*[1]

> [F]ortune is the arbiter of half the things we do, leaving the other half or so to be controlled by ourselves.
> Niccolo Machiavelli, *The Prince*

The Appellate Court's frustration was obvious. "Occasionally, a case will challenge the ability of the law and society, to cope effectively and sensitively with fundamental problems of human existence. This is such a case. . . ."

After the birth of her twins, Brenda Payton's[2] kidneys failed. She received a transplant but lost it, owing to rejection. To survive, she needed regular hemodialysis, a type of medical treatment to which she was entitled by federal law. Brenda proved to be a remarkably difficult patient for which to care. She often missed her appointments or showed up late, drunk. She abused illicit drugs. She regularly failed to keep her weight within the range prescribed by her doctor. She gained as much as 30 pounds between treatments, increasing her risk of heart failure and sudden death. She required hospitalization for emergency dialysis 30 times in 11 months. Brenda picked fights with other patients in the dialysis center, exposed her genitals to them, cursed them. She would interrupt her dialysis—by demanding that the dialysis machine be turned off or by pulling the needles from the shunt in her arm, causing blood to spew. Her repeated outbursts jeopardized the care of other patients. Brenda and they were dialyzed simultaneously by the same machine. If the machine were turned off, they would not receive needed treatment. Brenda demanded so much attention from the nurses that other patients' dialysis-associated complications might not be noticed promptly.

After more than three years of such behavior, Brenda's physician, John Weaver, notified her that he would no longer treat her at his dialysis center.[3] He provided her with the names and phone numbers of other nephrologists in town to facilitate her finding another doctor. Unfortunately, Brenda had made herself notorious in the health-care community. No other kidney specialist would accept her as a patient. This meant that, if Dr. Weaver severed his relationship with Brenda, she would lack a regular physician. She would have to get treatment for her kidney failure at hospital emergency departments.

Brenda went to court asking it to order Dr. Weaver to continue treating her. Because no other kidney doctor would accept Brenda as a patient, Dr. Weaver's abandoning her put her at risk of death. Brenda's lawyer even asked the court to impose on her an involuntary conservatorship on grounds that she was "gravely disabled as a result of mental disorder or impairment by chronic alcoholism."[4] Brenda's self-acknowledged alcoholism notwithstanding, the California court refused to find that it rendered her "gravely disabled."

The ensuing litigation resulted in the trial court's issuing of a stipulated order according to which Dr. Weaver agreed to continue treating Brenda for her kidney failure on the conditions that she would agree to follow his medical instructions, regularly attend an addiction counseling program, and cease her disruptive behavior at the dialysis center. Brenda promptly broke the agreement in every respect, whereupon the court found that her noncompliance was "knowing and intentional." The court ruled that Dr. Weaver had discharged fully his obligations to Brenda and that there was no basis in law or equity to saddle him with continuing obligation for her welfare. Brenda appealed. But the Court of Appeals could find no error. It sustained, agreeing that Brenda's behavior was of such a nature as to justify refusal of dialysis treatment on either an individual or collective basis. "Whatever collective responsibility may exist, it is not absolute, or independent of the patient's own responsibility." An appeal to the California Supreme Court was denied.

As for the legal arguments, the court felt compelled to address "what alternatives exist for assuring that Brenda does not die from lack of treatment as a result of her non-cooperative and disruptive behavior." Lamely, it suggested (because it had no power to order) that Brenda reconsider consenting to a voluntary conservatorship. Brenda was aware that were she to agree to this suggestion her conservator would probably admit her to a private, closed psychiatric facility. However, Brenda previously had rejected such an arrangement, and even were she to change her mind, by law, she would retain authority to revoke a voluntary guardianship simply by giving notice of her decision.

RESPECT VERSUS BENEFICENCE

It is axiomatic in law and ethics that an adult of mature years and sound mind has a fundamental right to determine what shall be done to her body.[5] How a person exercises her right of bodily control in determining what, when, and how much she eats, drinks, injects, associates, exercises, and whom she permits to touch her and in what manner (whether intimately with chosen reproductive consequences or therapeutically) tends to have at least as much effect as anything else on that person's health status.[6] The autonomy-regarding principle of respect requires that others keep a proper distance as a person makes such determinations. Ordinarily, consent (tacit or explicit) regulates further closing that distance.[7]

But as Immanuel Kant points out, the distancing-principle of respect, its evident importance in law and morals notwithstanding, is not the whole of ethics. On the contrary, Kant characterizes the moral duty of respect as "a negative one . . . analogous to the juridical duty of not encroaching on another's possessions." Its force must be counterbalanced by the welfare-regarding duty of beneficence. *Beneficence* requires that we consider each other as "fellowmen—that is, rational beings with needs, united by nature in one dwelling place for the purpose of helping one another."[8] Thus, the moral life, as Kant understands it, presents a continual problem for practical reason—*how properly to ration motivation between the moral law's requirements of respect and of beneficence.*[9]

Kant insists that respect and beneficence are equally imperative. Each summons motivation from an agent's rationally directed will, but each pulls in opposite directions; yet if either fails to recruit its share, moral disaster results. Excessive motivation allocated to respect results in callous indifference. Excessive motivation allocated to beneficence accelerates a slide from weak paternalism, which mildly demotes self-determination, to strong paternalism, which obliterates it altogether.[10] Mencius (Meng-tzu) captured the moral dynamics succinctly. "To feed a man without showing him love is to treat him like a pig; to love him without showing him respect is to keep him like a domestic animal."[11] So the moral agent must, somehow, do justice to both respect and beneficence.

THE JUST DISTRIBUTION OF RESPONSIBILITY

The moral agent's problem of counterbalancing respect with beneficence recurs for a theory of justice. The Kantian seeks an institutional arrangement that is consistent with the concept of a self-governing society composed of rational, free, and responsible individuals living under the rule of law. Its rules must not obliterate the responsibility presupposed by respect for human dignity, but its rules must be such that a rational, free, and responsible individual would be willing to live under them. This eliminates from consideration the beneficence-obliterating maxim, "Let each one be as happy as heaven wills or as he can make himself." It could not be chosen, because every rational person knows that "instances can often arise in which [one] would need the love and sympathy of others, . . . [and, no one would choose to rob himself of what he might need]." The just (equitable) arrangement for a particular community would be the one it actually chooses under its rules for making such choices. Which eligible option would be chosen cannot be predicted in the abstract, but we can be confident that Kantian

thinking would oppose allowing a patient to reduce her physician to a mere prop for her self-abusive behavior. Nor would it allow her extravagant preferences to hijack more than her share of health-care resources.

Rather than recognizing the equal validity of opposing ethical principles, John Stuart Mill works with only one, namely the "greatest good for the greatest number." He claims that utilitarian considerations favor a social rule assigning guardianship responsibility for health status to each (competent) individual, an arrangement that beats a rule requiring social approval for each decision regarding health effects. Also, by distinguishing physical health from mental and spiritual health, Mill alerts us to the trade-offs that must be made between them. The liberty-rule allows a "fitness nut" to maximize his physical health at the expense of his mental and spiritual health. It allows a religious fanatic to mortify his body as he promotes his spiritual health. Yet another person might strike a moderate balance among his physical, mental, and spiritual lives but fall short of remarkable achievement. Because these decisions concern the individual primarily, he must be free to reap the resulting benefits or suffer the decrements. Society must not interfere except to prevent harm to unconsenting others. It may, however, hold individuals liable when their intemperance results in their defaulting on their "distinct and assignable obligations"—for the default, not for the intemperance. Thus, it seems that Kantian and utilitarian considerations converge in assigning primary responsibility for health status to individuals.

Let us assume that a plausible conception of justice institutionalizes respect by recognizing a right to bodily integrity. As a result, it requires respect for Brenda Payton's opposition to involuntarily subordinating her to the supervision of a benevolent guardian in the dialysis case above. But let us also assume that society should institutionalize beneficence by underwriting the costs of treating patients with kidney failure. Must not Brenda, as the guardian of her own health, take responsibility for doing her part? At a minimum, shouldn't she avoid recklessly making her health worse? If she repeatedly makes herself a "medical emergency" by knowing and intentional noncompliance with the stipulated arrangement to which she consented, isn't it justified to infer that she has, in effect, rejected the reasonable terms for obtaining regular dialysis and reduced her rights to "emergency dialysis only"?

PERSONAL RESPONSIBILITY FOR HEALTH?

The idea of personal responsibility for health status is ancient and has become well entrenched in law and in morals. Robert Veatch (1980) disagrees. He claims that the ancients thought a person's health status was determined by fate or divine caprice, not by his own conduct. He alleges that holding individuals responsible for their health status is a new theme.[12] This is demonstrably wrong.

The ancients may have been mistaken about how personal choices affected health status, but they clearly believed that one's health status was subject to a degree of intentional control, by training, self-doctoring, and by judicious use of science. For examples, Plato criticized Herodicus who, by training and self-doctoring, overcame his mortal disease and in the process invented something worse, a lingering death, "and so dying hard, by the help of science he struggled onto old age."[13] Marcus Aurelius says of his father: "He took reasonable care of his body's health, not as one who was greatly attached to life, nor out of regard to personal appearance, nor yet in a careless way, but so that, through his own attention, he very seldom stood in need of the physician's art or of medicine or external applications."[14] Nor did the ancients need a knowledge of blood chemistry to appreciate that, by the order of natural justice, reckless or immoderate living tended to upset vitally balanced forces with

resulting loss of function and felt distress. It was well-known that an evening's heavy drinking could render a person unconscious, afflict him with vomiting, and a fuzzy head when he awoke.

Leaping ahead to the mid-nineteenth century, the American Medical Association's first Code (1847) provided, "The obedience of a patient to the prescriptions of his physician should be prompt and implicit. . . . A failure in one particular may render an otherwise judicious treatment dangerous, even fatal." And currently, at least one U.S. state holds that individuals who are ill or injured bear a responsibility to facilitate, or at least not to frustrate, their own recovery. For example, New Mexico law states thus: "If any patient shall persist in any injurious practice which imperils, retards or impairs his recovery or increases his injury or refuses to submit to such medical or surgical treatment as is reasonably essential to promote his recovery, the court may in its discretion reduce or suspend his medical care and related benefits until the injurious practice is discontinued."[15] Its workers' compensation statute similarly provides that a worker who suffers job-related injuries must avoid "injurious practices" that tend to imperil, retard or impair his recovery, or increase his disability.[16]

BLAMING THE SICK FOR BEING SICK?

It may be objected that it is morally retrograde to hold a person responsible for causing serious decrements in her health status. Holding the ill accountable, even in cases of self-victimization, amounts to "blaming the victim," encouraging a slide to smug, cold-heartedness.[17] Morever, holding the noncompliant patient accountable for the harm she self-inflicts, especially when she likely suffers from *focal incompetence, secondary to her various substance-addictions*, tends to obscure important social and economic determinants of health,[18] thereby diverting attention away from social responsibility. For example, John Stuart Mill claimed that "If society lets any considerable number of its members grow up ... incapable of being acted on by rational consideration of distant motives, society has itself to blame for the consequences."

It may be argued that socially inflicted harms are so flagrant in Brenda Payton's case that her defaults are comparatively insignificant. In the United States, the Volstead Act proved that prohibiting production and commerce of a health-harmful addictive substance is within the federal government's power. Public health data from the period of Prohibition reveal a substantial decline in alcohol consumption and in alcohol related mortality and morbidity.[19] Prohibition's repeal further illustrates society's control as the popularity of Victorian temperance (abstinence) gave way to hedonism (among other reasons). It is now society's chosen policy to "allow" alcohol production and consumption, yet society has defaulted on its associated responsibility to tax alcohol sufficiently to provide adequate care for the predictable casualties of legalization.[20] Native American communities in particular have been disproportionately harmed by the legalization of alcohol, but without adequate social compensation.

Conversely, society criminalizes production, sale, or possession of cocaine and heroin despite being no more dangerous than alcohol. This policy perversely makes consumption of these drugs comparatively more risky (medically and legally) than alcohol consumption, but it has not made them sufficiently pricey to deter their use. Even society's poorest citizens can afford cocaine. Society's declaration of "war" on (people who use) drugs creates a social responsibility to allocate adequate resources to care for the war's reasonably foreseeable civilian casualties. Inner-city minority communities have been decimated by this war.[21] Building prisons to house drug-law violators consumes resources that would be better spent on addressing educational and health-care needs of the addicted-poor.

Similarly, hemodialysis was once a home-care medical treatment. Government policy decisions have made it advantageous for kidney specialists to herd patients into "centers" for treatment with decidedly disadvantageous consequences for patients like Brenda Payton. Moreover, society has followed a rigoristic "de-institutionalization" policy for 40 years. By over-emphasizing the principle of "liberty-respect" at the cost of "beneficence-care" for a mentally disabled population, society's moral vision has turned from jaundiced to blind.

Despite its (harmful) addictiveness, tobacco growing remains subsidized by some states. Federal and state governments gain more revenue from taxes on the sale of tobacco products than do tobacco growers. Excise taxes on tobacco approximately offset the social costs of smoking, yet these funds are not reserved for treating the consequences of the unhealthful behavior the state allows, nor are they wholly dedicated to efforts to prevent or deter smoking. For example, if excise taxes raised the price of a cigarette to that of a good cigar, say, $5 each, cigarette smoking would cease to be a discussed public health issue.

There is moral power in the preceding argument. But the consequence of releasing Brenda Payton from responsibility, seeing her defaults "as comparatively insignificant," reduces her to "domestic animal" status. Animal husbandry at its best is compassionate. Extending its dominion to human persons subordinates the moral empire to the rule of beneficence and compassion—precisely the ethical disaster Kant warned about. To avoid this result, our institutions must (somehow) recognize that endlessly accommodating a patient's knowing and intentional noncompliance obliterates respect, subsidizes self-contempt, encourages the patient to treat others with similar needs contemptuously, and to discount their welfare as sharply as the patient apparently discounts her own. Society's first obligation is to establish and uphold just institutions. These strike a proper balance between respect and benef-icence. Simplicity is justice's ally.[22] Tragic stories in league with perfectionism are the enemies of such patients.

RESPONSIBILITY AND CONTROL

"Responsibility" is etymologically linked with having to answer for what one has *made* to happen or what one has *allowed* to happen, including what one has *let* others do. To *be responsible* presupposes *having the ability to be responsive*—to recognize when one has been challenged to produce an accounting for one's acts or omissions, and to respond to the challenge by providing an accounting of the appropriate sort to whoever is in a position to demand answers.[23] In other words, holding people responsible for their acts/omissions presupposes their competence to respond with an appropriate accounting.

One is not responsible for everything one makes happen or fails to prevent. We are *responsible for* things over which we have (or had) some degree of control, or things over which we should have had control. A theory of agent responsibility may implicate more or less of what the agent made to happen, more or less of what the agent let (or allowed) to happen. Agents typically exercise control by coordinating "make happen" with "letting happen." This applies, even at the most basic level, namely to coordinated physical movements. For example, when one reaches for and grasps a cup of coffee, both flexors and extensors come into play. Some muscles must relax (let arm motion occur), some must contract (make arm motion occur) in the right way and at the right time to reach for and grasp a cup successfully.

We do not hold responsible a person who suffers from Parkinson's disease for the mess he makes by spilling his coffee. He lacks sufficient control over the "making–letting system" to enable a high success rate at the task: "reaching and grasping without spilling." Conversely, if he could have avoided making a mess by requesting and securing help and if he had control over

whether to make the request and was reasonably assured of assistance upon request, the issue of his responsibility for the mess recurs. "Why didn't you ask someone to help you?" It is not uncommon to hold people responsible for attempting alone what they should have secured help for. It is also common to hold responsible potential helpers who neglected to make help apparently available.

HOLDING RESPONSIBLE AND TAKING RESPONSIBILITY

Holding a person responsible for her health status presupposes that she had (and still has) ability to take responsibility for herself and to give an accounting for her health-affecting choices. This means that (*1*) she had (and/ or has) ability to exercise *control* over factors with health-status modifying effects; and (*2*) she has the cognitive capacity to believe and understand that this is so, the evaluative capacity sufficient to make her control matter to her and to give coherence to her preferences, and the volitional capacity sufficient to timely choose an option and then to follow through in light of her understanding and evaluations.

That a person is able to take responsibility for herself does not preclude that she mistakenly takes more or less responsibility for her health status than she should. One can be faulted for avoiding responsibility for what one has caused. Taking (appropriate) responsibility for the way things are presupposes neither that one is or is not responsible for having caused things to be as they are. One may act commendably in taking responsibility to care for what one did not cause. The Good Samaritan is an example.

GLOBAL COMPETENCE, DECISION-RELATIVE COMPETENCE, FOCAL INCOMPETENCE

Incompetent persons should not be held to account for their decisions. Their incompetence precludes it. The court in California found that Brenda Payton suffered from significant, chronic decisional impairments secondary to her addictions. However, she functioned effectively much of the time. She was able to give a remarkably good account of herself in court. Admittedly, Brenda was argumentative and occasionally offensive. She chronically neglected to observe the discipline required to manage her kidney failure in a manner that would keep her out of the hospital. But Brenda presented no imminent danger to others, nor was she suicidal. Her multiple medical, behavioral, and substance abuse problems notwithstanding, she was not "gravely disabled," all things considered.

Perhaps the court in the Payton case erred in its thinking about competence. Instead of thinking of competence "globally," it should have imagined it "focally." Thus, it might be argued that the court failed to appreciate that substance addiction may impair decisional capacity focally. It may even "gravely disable" a person, rendering her "focally incompetent," specifically with respect to the decision whether stop abusing drugs, to seek treatment for substance abuse, whether to remain in treatment, whether to accept voluntarily the supervision of a conservator.

Arguably, this is not overly subtle for the court to have accepted. Courts regularly adjudicate people to be incompetent with respect to their financial decisions. The inquiry is "focal," not "global." So is the remedy. A guardian appointed to make financial decisions on the (financially incompetent) person's behalf is not thereby made guardian of the person. Similarly, a person may be adjudicated (focally) incompetent to drive an automobile, or to drive at night. Again, the inquiry and resulting determinations of incompetence and the restrictions of privilege are all focal, and task-relative. How should we understand this, theoretically?

The Elements of Competence: Cognitive and Evaluative Ability

Buchanan and Brock (1989) offer a theoretical framework for analyzing this problem. Their theory makes competence a decision-relative concept fundamentally. They argue that making a decision is similar to performing a task or solving a problem. Some problems are harder than others. Having the ability to solve some problems of a particular kind does not imply having the ability to solve all problems of that kind. One may have the ability to solve a problem at a particular time and under some circumstances but not at other times and under other circumstances. Injury, illness, fatigue, fear, hunger, pain, and chemicals can impair and even render ineffective otherwise effective problem-solving skills. Even so, a resulting incompetence is presumptively "focal" not "global." For example, alcohol intoxication, of some degree, will render a person focally incompetent to drive a car, or to give valid consent to elective surgery, but a degree of intoxication sufficient to render one focally incompetent to perform those tasks does not necessarily make one incompetent to give valid consent to sexual relations or to form the intent necessary for many criminal offenses. Buchanan and Brock make the concept "focal incompetence" coherent.

According to Buchanan and Brock (1989), the capacities needed for competent decision making are primarily cognitive and evaluative, namely the ability to understand, reason, and deliberate, and the ability to apply one's values to eligible options and to communicate a resulting choice. Whether one is competent to make a specific decision will depend on one's possessing the abilities to understand, to reason, and to evaluate to a sufficient degree. When discussing mental illness, Buchanan and Brock observe that it "often attacks the same thought processes that are necessary for competent decisions about hospitalization" (1989, p. 319).

If addiction were a species of mental illness, then addiction might cause focal incompetence in the same manner as mental illness, namely when it sufficiently impairs one or more decision-making abilities. Addiction-related craving may increase impulsiveness, impairing the ability to reason or to deliberate. When a specific decision requires deliberative ability, but addiction-related craving impairs it, resulting in an impulsive, snap decision, one's addiction may have impaired a relevant ability sufficiently to render one focally incompetent to make that decision. Impulsivity does not always have a foundation in addiction, however. An impulsive temperament may well have its basis in the neurobiology of dopamine.[24] Indeed, thrill-seeking may be a brain-management strategy common among individuals with comparatively low levels of this neurotransmitter.[25]

A Lesion of the Will?

Buchanan and Brock's theory of competence lacks an adequately robust volitional component. In particular, "volitional follow-through" is an ability that should bear on a competency assessment of addicts to make certain decisions. Tacitly, Buchanan and Brock (1989) recognize the importance of self-control, pre-apparent-choice. For example, if one lacks ability to suppress distractions in order to focus sufficiently, if one lacks ability to control his emotions sufficiently to attend to the information that bears on evaluating one's options, then one will lack ability to understand, reason, deliberate, apply his values to the available options and make a choice.[26]

However, for it to be true that one has chosen, the ability to control oneself to an appropriate degree remains important for determining whether one has in fact chosen (performed the task). Sufficiently large deficits in self-control post apparent-choice will count against one's having chosen. And if self-control deficits post apparent-choice may make it false that "you chose *x*", while not altering the truth of "you reported that *x* was your choice" they should also count in an inventory of abilities relevant to assessing competence to make decision *x*. For example, a competency assessment directed at "volitional follow through" would have been directly relevant to determining whether Brenda Payton was

competent to consent to the stipulated agreement with Dr. Weaver concerning her dialysis treatment.

There are distinctions between making a decision, only to change one's mind quickly; making a decision only to forget that one has decided; reporting one's decision (deceptively) when one knows that one has not decided (similar to crossing one's fingers when promising); and reporting that one has decided despite lacking the volitional follow-through ability to have decided. Behavior patterns provide the evidence for discriminating. It will never be unambiguous. Ordinarily, we may prefer characterizing the phenomenon as "choice, but rapid change of mind" or "strategic nonchoice, but dishonest report of choice."

It is possible that decisions of a certain kind may overtax one's decision-making abilities (to follow through) and where the evidence implicating impaired self-control (rather than dishonesty) will emerge from a pattern of behavior post apparent-choice. If so, focal incompetence secondary to substance addiction requires recognition of an additional element in the assessment of competence, namely volitional follow-through. But it would seem that a finding that a person suffers from focal incompetence to make a certain kind of decision should result in her receiving limited supervision, not supervision of her person.

ADDICTION AND FREEDOM

Addict and *addiction* are old, quasi-legal terms. According to the *Oxford English Dictionary* (OED), to *addict a person* is to deliver him over formally (e.g., by sentence of a judge) to the service of another by *restraint or obligation*. To addict another presupposes one's *having a power* to impose restraints or obligations on him. In the first-person reflexive case, to *addict oneself* is to use one's own power of choice to attach or bind oneself to another's service, to a social cause or to a habit.

A theory of addiction will naturally address: How and by whom may addictions be (validly) imposed or abolished? What sorts of "service" may be imposed and for how long? Is total subordination of the one addicted permissible? When, if ever, is an addiction of indefinite duration permissible? May an addiction be total and indefinite?

Etymology links addiction with a loss of freedom—"by restraint or obligation." This is exemplified clearly when a judge, using his sentencing authority, addicts (binds over) another to the service of a third party. "Sentences" presuppose authority to "pronounce" and impose them. Sentences imposed typically presuppose a finding of wrongdoing. They commonly involve imposition of involuntary servitude, (e.g., "5 years of hard labor"; "10 to 15 years making license plates in the penitentiary." Sentences do not involve total subordination of the one addicted, but only so much as necessary to carry out the sentence. Obviously, the judge's addicting of the convict is "knowing and intentional." A political society exercises its addictive power when, by law, it requires its young men to register for the draft at age 18. Because the resulting liberty-loss (liability to be drafted) is sex-specific and not predicated on wrongdoing, the exercise of legislative authority may be challenged on Thirteenth and Fourteenth Amendment constitutional grounds.[27]

First-person reflexive cases involve "self-binding." The most obvious example of formal self-binding is legal contract, where the self-binding is knowing and intentional. Indentured servitude is an (archaic) example of a time-limited, personal services agreement resulting in "bondage" and enforceable by "specific performance." Informal self-binding may or may not be knowing and intentional. It may be inadvertent. It may not result in "bondage" as when one commits oneself to a social cause, or when one sets about to ingrain a (good) habit. But the self-binding also may be unintentional. One may find oneself "bound" and "in bondage" despite the absence of any intent to do so. One may find oneself bound more tightly that one intended or in a manner different from the one expected.

"Falling in love" bears the characteristics of addiction. One may intentionally put oneself at risk for falling in love. One may notice that it is happening. One may put up mild/strong resistance or decide to let it happen. Falling in love obviously involves a loss of freedom. One finds his thoughts and feelings "taken over" as he becomes progressively "enthralled." Thoughts of his beloved pop into his mind forcefully and unbidden at inopportune moments, distracting him, making him "lovesick." A person may find falling in love rapturously pleasant or decidedly unpleasant, or one may be ambivalent toward both "falling in love" and toward "being in love." Recall the disciplined, jealous-of-his-independence Professor Higgins' response to recognizing that he was not merely "fond" of Eliza but that had fallen in love with her—"Damn! Damn! Damn! I've grown accustomed to her face!"

Although addiction implies loss of freedom, addictions are not thereby bad. Self-acquired addictions may advance one's interests; they may be self-expressive commitments. For example, the OED gives examples where self-addiction and "devotion" are synonyms. Thus, a person may be addicted (devoted) to her work, which suggests an attachment stronger than merely liking one's work or enjoying it. Medicalized, it is called "monomania."[28] Activities to which one is devoted (addicted) are not subject to casual self-termination. Casual self-termination of an activity rules out one's devotion to it. A workaholic may be convinced that she should spend more time with her family, decide to spend more time "at home," but yet have great difficulty reducing the amount of time she devotes to her work, despite that she spends less time "at work." People who prize their independence above all else will tend to avoid devoting themselves to anyone or anything. (Monomaniacs to independence? Was Dostoevsky's underground man addicted to independence, "the most advantageous advantage"?) When coupled with self-control, their valuing independence so highly may result in their living shallow lives, albeit freer ones. Willingness to make commitments, to be devoted, increases one's susceptibility to loss of freedom. It may also put one at increased risk for the adverse health effects associated with "monomania."

Addiction logically implies a loss of freedom A theory of addiction implicates *a theory of freedom*. We are blessed with a surfeit of theories. Adequately discussing them here is impossible. According to desire-regarding theories, a person is made unfree only if she is rendered unable to satisfy her desires, especially those that matter most to her. Her freedom is reduced only if her desire-satisfying abilities or opportunities are impaired or diminished. On a desire-account, a desire for cocaine counts as addictive only if it disables her, impairs formerly effective desire-satisfaction abilities, or otherwise reduces her opportunities for desire satisfaction overall. Many theories of addiction make it a defining condition (of addiction) that there be an inability to cease consumption despite a strong desire to do so.

Nondesire regarding theories hold that a person may be rendered unfree irrespective of any loss of desire-satisfying ability or opportunity. Freedom losses can result from internal psychological disorder, conflict of desires, from unreasoned, impulsive, debased choices, however voluntary, that express servility rather than human dignity. A desire for cocaine would count as addictive (and freedom-reducing) only if the desire were servile, expressive of insufficient self-respect.[29] The servile person may act voluntarily, but yet unfreely because the desires on which she acts are unworthy, perhaps acquired in an unjust socialization.

Yet other theories of freedom claim that a person's acts are rendered unfree only if she *identifies* the etiology of those acts as *alien*—for example, as prompted by oppressive, distracting cravings and that satisfying them requires the person to act "out

of character." It follows that if a person who fully identifies with one's own personal desire for cocaine and finds nothing out of character associated with what the person does to get and consume it, then cocaine use will be self-expressive for that individual, not an addiction.

ADDICTION AND PERSONAL IDENTITY

A theory of freedom further implicates a theory of the self or of authenticity. We distinguish among: (1) when a person speaks assertively with his own voice, (2) when anger gets the better of him and takes over his voice, and (3) when his addictive craving for a substance is doing the talking. The latter two imply increasingly severe loses of self-control. This is puzzling. How do we distinguish "his" (authentic) voice, from his (less authentic) anger's voice, from his addiction's (alien-possession) voice? Each speaks from the same mouth! First and third-person characterizations may diverge. "I won't take that comment seriously; I recognize when your addiction's talking." "That wasn't 'my addiction' talking, that was me!" "No, that's not you, I know you, and that wasn't you!"

Ainslie (1999) analyzes the dynamic this way: "The 'mind' or 'self' is a population of reward-seeking operations that survive insofar as they actually obtain reward. The mental operations selected for by a particular reward of class of rewards constitutes the person's interest in that reward; interests within the person are very like interests within a community" (p. 67). Gary Becker similarly models the person as a "community," namely a family. Davidson invokes dual-agency to explain self-deception. Compound-models of the self are at least as old as Plato's tripartite soul.

None are particularly helpful in providing a causal explanation of self-formation, dissolution, reformation. What are the truth conditions for "Now you're hearing 'the real me' talking, at last." And, "Yesterday, when I said you were hearing me speak with my own voice for the first time . . . well that wasn't true." "Don't worry, I didn't believe you yesterday. Nor do I believe you today."

If the self is identified with rationality, rational acts will be free and irrational acts unfree. Irrational acts, in virtue of their etiology in the self's "periphery," will be comparatively unfree irrespective their apparent voluntariness. If emotions, for theoretical reasons, are made peripheral to the self,[30] acts with an emotional etiology will be less free or even unfree. "His anger got the better of him." "She's so emotional, just not at all herself today." Acts not expressive of the self's "core" will tend to be regarded as less free than acts motivated centrally. None of these metaphors do more than raise the problem. Any theory of addiction that fails properly to incorporate ability/disability/opportunity into its analysis of freedom/unfreedom and personal identity courts paradox, namely the phenomenon of a person's doing regularly what (the theory says) he is unfree to do.

The preceding complexities aside, addictions are person-relative. What addicts one person may not addict another, or addict him to the same degree. Addiction is linked by logic to a loss of freedom. Causal theories of action address the mechanism whereby the loss results. Some addictions are associated with greater freedom losses than are others. Some addictions are harder to break than are others. "Loss of control" is commonly associated with addiction. Loss of control is comparative between times and is a matter of degree. Some people have more trouble breaking an addiction than other people do. Addiction is not inherently bad. Some addictions may be advantageous or laudable (e.g., devotion to a worthwhile cause). Some may be risky or self-destructive.

Theories of Addiction

Rational addiction
Economists Gary Becker and Kevin Murphy (1988) note that, "People get addicted

not only to alcohol, cocaine, and cigarettes but also to work, eating, music, television, their standard of living, other people, religion, and many other activities."[31] Indeed, Ainslie has further catalogued addictive behaviors in association with gambling, caffeine, sugar, chocolate, romantic relationships, emotional dependence, promiscuity, masturbation, haste, shoplifting, self-mutilation, spending money, and competitiveness."[32]

Becker and Murphy's analysis does not beg the question of harmfulness of addiction. They argue that some addictions may be beneficial and propose a general model of rational choice within which "addictions, even strong ones, are usually rational in the sense of involving forward-looking maximization with stable preferences." They define addiction as a habit with the characteristic that greater consumption earlier stimulates greater, not lesser consumption later. Harmful addictions are marked by "tolerance," which means that higher past consumption lowers the present utility of the same level of consumption. Beneficial addictions do not have this feature.

Critics of Becker and Murphy claim that addicts violate the "stable preference" criterion of rational choice. They allege that addicts display remarkable ambivalence about their consumption of addictive substances or that they time-discount "hyperbolically."[33] If so, addiction to health-harmful substances is not rational, yet an addict's continuing consumption of a health-harmful substance may be a better guide to his true preferences than his testimony. If so, his real preferences may not violate the stability requirement.

Rational addiction theory has a desirable ethical consequence. By underwriting the duty to respect the addict's still-intact rationality, it constrains paternalism. Beneficently directed attention should focus on the contingencies affecting the addict's consumption choices. Getting her to stop must involve her having sufficiently good reasons and her perceiving them as such as she makes choices. Such reasons might include increasing substantially the price she pays for consumption, increasing the positive consequences associated with nonconsumption, and increasing the negative consequences associated with consumption. Becoming employed in a fulfilling occupation will tend to help; becoming employed in an unsatisfying or overly demanding job will not.

Addiction as Mental Illness

Disease models focus on health-harmful addictions—primarily those to nicotine, alcohol, opiates, cocaine, and the amphetamines. Adherents of disease theories tend to regard "health-harmful addiction" as a redundancy and "beneficial addiction" as paradoxical or oxymoronic. A crude disease model claims that addicts fail to limit their consumption of harmful substances because the dynamics of addiction *renders them totally unable* to control their consumption, despite their evident desire to do so. Alcoholics Anonymous claims that "Alcoholism is a disease which manifests itself chiefly by the uncontrollable drinking of the victim, who is known as an alcoholic." The key premises in the crude disease model claim that substance addiction destroys completely the addict's self-control and that the addict's *professing* a desire to quit entails that he *has a strong desire* to quit.

Alleging that the alcoholic loses self-control completely must be hyperbole. Otherwise it becomes mysterious that the alcoholic notices when his glass is empty, that he refills it from a liquor bottle rather than from the kitchen tap, or that he remembers to travel to the toilet to drain his bladder. Of course, when the individual is sufficiently intoxicated, loss of control becomes complete—the drunk topples insensate from his chair and may besmirch himself where he lands.

Sophisticated disease models claim (more modestly) that addictive substances *reduce or diminish* the addict's ability to control her consumption. Loss of ability is a matter of degree, sometimes greater, sometimes lesser. Co-factors, such as *stress, environmental cues, or one's associates*, may exert greater or lesser causal influence. It is unclear whether disease models make "addiction" a threshold concept: addictions may vary more or less continuously in their strength parallel with variability in "control loss." Might an addiction be stronger on some days, or some times during the day, than on others? Might it exert lesser influence during some times of year than in others?

Disease models tend to be substance-specific. For example, alcohol is mood-altering and tends to be constantly present in the alcoholic's thoughts; his craving for it chronically elevates it to psychological predominance, eclipsing concern for all else. This characterization fits well with addictive consumption of cocaine, the opiates and barbiturates, and with amphetamines.

Nicotine, however, is ill-fitted to this characterization.[34] It is not mood-altering. Even when craved, nicotine does not swamp the smoker's concern for all else (he can transport himself to a "smoking allowed" area), and despite nicotine's classification among the "stimulants" (along with cocaine and the amphetamines), many smokers report (paradoxically) that smoking helps them to relax, a psychological state associated with depressants (alcohol, barbiturates, and opiates).

There is little question that cigarette smoking has health-harmful effects for many smokers. The U.S. Surgeon General first reported on the harmful effects of cigarette smoking in 1964; subsequently, 26 Surgeon General reports have warned of the increased risk of mortality and morbidity associated with tobacco use of any kind. The Centers for Disease Control and Prevention (CDC) report that each year more than 430,000 deaths in the United States result from tobacco use, making tobacco use the leading *preventable cause* of death and disease in the nation. The CDC further reports that 3,000 young people join the ranks of tobacco users each day. The social costs attributed to smoking exceed $50 billion annually. Lost earnings and lost productivity, ordinarily classified as personal costs, total an additional $47 billion. Lost tax revenues secondary to lost personal earnings and productivity increase the social costs of smoking. The U.S. Department of Health and Human Services claims that preventing tobacco use is one of the nation's most important health challenges.

For fiscal 2001, the CDC has allocated $104 million to promote smoking cessation. The Syndar Amendment requires the states to adopt and enforce laws prohibiting the sale of tobacco products to anyone under the age of 18. On August 9, 2000, the Surgeon General released "Reducing Tobacco Use." Claiming that a 50% reduction in smoking rates could be achieved over the next decade, the report proposed widespread use of programs that had proven effective in substantially reducing the number of people who are *addicted to nicotine*.[35]

Many smokers die from diseases linked to smoking—principally heart disease, emphysema, and lung cancer. Yet not all smokers die earlier than average. Nor do they all die from smoking-related illnesses. It is tempting to assume that smokers would tend to live longer, healthier lives if they refrained from smoking. Not necessarily. If smokers are addiction-prone, then nicotine almost certainly plays an important role in their brain-management even though its effects on the cardiovascular system are bad. Smoking cessation (or never starting) presumably would lead an addiction-prone person to search for alternative brain-management strategies. These may be less health-harmful, but may not.

Recent research holds promise for enhanced success in extinguishing specific health-harmful chemical addictions, especially for addicts who would welcome medical assistance in quitting "cold turkey." If vaccinated voluntarily with good informed consent, the addict knowingly renders himself unable to experience the psychotropic effects of the health-harmful substance. If vaccinated nonvoluntarily, someone besides the addict renders him unable to experience the substance's psychotropic effects. The re-vaccination decision raises further interesting questions. Does being vaccinated enable the addict's true self freely to address the re-vaccination decision? Would an addict's refusal of revaccination be an informed but unfree choice?

ADDICTION AND THE PUBLIC HEALTH?

Some harmful addictions are associated with high social costs. These include recurrent hospital admissions for which the individual does not pay, transmission of infective/infectious diseases associated with injection drug use, participation in a violent, illegal market of untaxed transactions, and related factors. The "social cost" in each case refers to *social resource consumption* resulting from addictive behavior for which the individual does not pay and that might have gone to socially better uses.

Public health professionals are preventionists dedicated to reducing the social costs of unhealthful behavior. They can be reasonably expected to make a "social responsibility" argument for using the government's police power to make "throffers" (threat-offers) to proven cocaine addicts—accept vaccination ("offer") to treat your addiction or go to jail ("threat"). It is also reasonably expected that public health professionals will appeal to *parens patriae* to justify population-wide screening to facilitate early identification of addiction-susceptible individuals. Those identified could then be enrolled in a program of regular vaccinations to prevent addiction to specific stimulant or sedative chemicals. Preventing chemical addiction with a vaccine seems cost-effective compared with mitigating the harmful medical and criminal consequences of addictive behavior.

From an anti-utilitarian perspective, John Rawls (1971) has argued that an adequate theory of justice must nullify the effects of the natural lottery and the contingencies of social circumstances. If addiction-susceptibility has a genetic component, and if environmental exposure to addictive chemicals adversely affects prospects for a successful life of the genetically susceptible, then preventing addiction by some minimally invasive but effective method, such as vaccination, would be presumptively required by justice.[36] Indeed, fair equality of opportunity would give prima facie support to social screening programs and childhood vaccination. The equality-of-opportunity principle would trump parental discretion to decide whether to screen children for addiction-susceptibility.

Substantial ethical concerns arise, however. Would testing occur at birth? What degree of increased addiction-susceptibility would trigger vaccination? Would it be mandatory to vaccinate infants identified at (low/moderate/high) risk for addiction to stimulants or sedatives? Would respect for a child's "right to an open future" make it mandatory for parents to vaccinate their addiction-susceptible children? Would it count as child neglect if they fail? How would access to test results be regulated? Would employers have access to results? Would schools?

Depending on one's theory of freedom, mandatory vaccination may or may not count as a loss of freedom. Some theories of freedom find no paradox in "forcing to be free" just as some theories will underwrite "forcing to be sane."[37] Also, extinguishing one harmful addiction (whether or not by vaccine) does not preclude substitution of another addiction equally harmful or more harmful. Even if a vaccine deprives cocaine of its psychotropic effects, it will not necessarily block its cardiogenic/cardiotoxic effects. Some vaccinated cocaine addicts may continue consuming cocaine for its cardiogenic effects. Preventing harmful addictions by vaccination will almost certainly have unintended consequences.

MANAGING THE PROBLEM OF ADDICTIVE DESIRE: ULYSSES

In *The Odyssey*, Homer described a provocative solution to the problem of addiction-related loss of self-control. In the episode Ulysses and the Sirens,[38] an enchantress, Circe, tells Ulysses that his journey unavoidably will take him within earshot of an island inhabited by the Sirens. Circe warns him that the Sirens' present a fatal attraction to seafarers. Their song is beautiful, addictive, and ultimately irresistible. Listeners, initially attracted from afar by the song's faint beauty, desire to hear it more clearly. As they draw nearer, their desire to listen grows stronger and stronger as the singing grows louder and louder. Ultimately, auditors, captive to an irresistible desire to listen, are "warbled to death."

Circe instructs Ulysses how to pass by the Sirens safely. To eliminate the threat to his men, he must stop up their ears with wax. However, Circe well-knows Ulysses's character—remarkably bold and curious. She anticipates that he will desire to hear the Sirens' for himself. Thus, she further advises him how to satisfy both his first-order desire to listen to the Sirens and his second-order desire that he be spared the fatal consequences that typically result from listening to them.[39] Prior to stopping up his crews' ears with wax, Ulysses must (1) order his crew to lash him securely to the ship's mast; (2) order that they disregard as invalid any directives he might seem to give them while he is restrained; and (3) that when the danger has passed and he has regained himself, his men should untie him, restoring him fully to command.

Ulysses fears that Circe's scheme may not work. He also thinks that it would not be right to put his men at risk without their knowledge. Hence, he discloses the entire plan to them "so that whether we live or die we may do so with our eyes open." It turns out that the plan works as advertised.

ANALYZING THE HOMERIC SOLUTION TO ADDICTIVE DESIRE

Homer describes Circe as "a great and cunning goddess." She has remarkable insight into Ulysses's character and is benevolently dedicated to preparing him to face his ultimate challenge, still years away. She has supernaturally accurate prognostic ability, yet Circe knows she cannot disclose to him completely his curriculum, all at once. She must ration his lessons progressively. His vices (fearlessness and prideful overestimation of his power) superficially resembled real virtues (bravery, audacity, self-confidence). Circe's individualized curriculum teaches by experience ("test first, lesson later"). For example, Ulysses' fearlessness makes him reckless and unmindful of his limitations. He could not become brave until he felt and overcame fear in the face of real danger. Ulysses was not easily frightened. So Circe sent him into Hell—literally, where he was scared to death (figuratively).

Having been terrified in hell, Ulysses was no longer fearless. His pride had taken a blow. He was ready for his next lesson in self-knowledge—to experience loss of self-control to an addictive desire. Circe knows that Ulysses's will power, however imposing under many circumstances, is no match for the Sirens' challenge to it. In other words, she knows with certainty that Ulysses will become acutely self-destructive when exposed to the pleasure of the Sirens' addictive song. To learn a character-building lesson, Ulysses' insatiable curiosity must acquaint him with the power of a (lethal) irresistible desire. Were Circe's prescription for Ulysses solely survival-regarding, then she would have prescribed the wax prophylactic for him as well as for his men. But he would have learned nothing from "Just say no." Circe's plan enables Ulysses to feel the motivating power of that most dangerous of irresistible desires—for divine knowledge and foresight—and to survive the experience.

Ulysses's response to Circe's plan is mindful not prideful.[40] He does not take offense at Circe's implication that his will power cannot save him from the force of his own desires, yet he is not completely confident in her plan. Everything is at stake, the risk is high for him and his men, so he discloses everything to them beforehand so that all shall proceed "with their eyes open." Obviously, Ulysses trusts his men to do their part. They prove worthy of it. They do not exploit his vulnerability in any way. They accurately recognize when Ulysses has regained his capacity for self-command and they restore him to his position of command over them.

THE ULYSSES CONTRACT: A SOLUTION TO CHRONIC LOSSES OF SELF-CONTROL?

Since at least the early 1980s, commentators have discussed whether the law should recognize as valid and enforceable some version of the Homeric solution to predictable losses of self-control due to mental illness.[41] The proposals vary in detail, but all recommend an institutional arrangement whereby a competent person would authorize strangers (albeit professionally certified) to disregard his future demands for personal liberty in order that his mental illness should receive full and adequate treatment. For example, the Norwegian law of psychic health protection recognizes and enforces an individual's voluntarily irreversible decision to admit himself to a mental hospital.[42] Whether time-indefinite or time-limited, the so-called Ulysses Contract would require a revision in American moral and legal rules that currently recognize that the liberty to refuse treatment trumps benevolently directed professional care.

Epistemic and ethical disanalogies between myth and reality show why institutionalizing the Homeric solution to addictive desire would be unwise. In the Homeric myth, the trust between Ulysses and Circe is personal and merit-based, not status-based. Not all members of Circe's "profession" are trustworthy. Some are malicious or capricious. The trust Ulysses places in Circe is not transferable on the basis of professional status. That Circe was available when Ulysses needed her was just lucky. Nor did Ulysses have a "pick-up" crew. He trusted his men completely because they had proven their reliability in shared peril.

Not only is there variable trustworthiness among human professionals (some are incompetent, others are venal, many are overworked) none can claim goddess-like analytical insight into the individualized dynamics of self-development. None can claim near-perfect prognostic foresight. On the contrary, even the best human professional therapists (whether psychiatrists or psychologists) see best retrospectively. Prospectively, they see "through a glass darkly." Their diagnostic categories are imprecise, based on majority vote of human practitioners—not consultation with "a great and cunning goddess."

In short, human institutions must manage uncertainty, establish standards of proof and distribute the burden of carrying it to minimize rights violations and harm associated with human professional arrogance, venality, incompetence, and plain mistake. John Stuart Mill ([1859], 1956) provided an excellent (Kantian) reason against recognizing legally such self-binding: "The principle of freedom cannot require that he should be free not to be free" (p. 101).

CONCLUSION

In 1993, Malcom Dean, writing in *The Lancet*, reported that British surgeons at two separate medical centers refused to schedule for nonurgent coronary bypass surgery those patients who refused to stop smoking. The journal's editorial pointed out that if this principle of "self-inflicted rationing" were extended to other medical cases, the potential savings that would accrue to the British National Health Service (NHS) would be "unlimited" (p. 1525). Al-

coholics in need of a liver transplant, HIV patients who acquired their infection through injection drug use or promiscuous sex, obese heart patients, trauma victims who were injured in auto accidents while under the influence, all sports injuries, smokers with lung cancer (and, needless to say, noncompliant hemodialysis patients), all might be plausibly denied access to care underwritten by the NHS on grounds that they had brought trouble on themselves.

Isn't this an irony? Employees of the NHS, a system best rationalized under a principle of social beneficence, invokes individual irresponsibility to justify ignoring medical need in the name of social responsibility! But the irony disappears when we recall that social insurance in the context of controllable risk itself creates moral hazard. Especially at the margin, individuals tend to be less prudent and take fewer precautions to prevent insurance-covered losses when risks are controllable. Expanding insurance coverage, therefore, creates greater moral hazard.

But as the moral hazard grows, the economic pressure to ration care on some basis or other becomes irresistible. Personal irresponsibility for worsening one's health status is then invoked to justify rationing social resources. Thus, a scheme that creates moral hazard ultimately invites its doctors to ration benefits to those whose self-inflicted health care needs may well have resulted, in part, from the scheme's incentives to reduce precautions.

Predictably, the British surgeons were criticized on grounds that appointment to the NHS requires providers to care for the sick without regard to the patient's role in causing his trouble; that doctors should not withhold health-care services on punitive grounds, and so forth. But if physicians may never use personal irresponsibility, no matter how egregious, to deny access to health-care resources, then what? Should we expect courts of law or legislators to do better using other criteria? Moral hazard does not disappear by ignoring it.

In 1944, F.A. Hayek claimed that

"Where, as in the case of sickness and accident, neither the desire to avoid such calamities nor the efforts of overcome their consequences are as a rule weakened by the provision of assistance—where, in short, we deal with genuinely insurable risks—the case for the state's helping to organize a comprehensive system of social insurance is very strong" (p. 121). But where assistance is provided without regard to an individual's ability to mitigate her health-harmful behavior, it should not be surprising when she fails to take steps to do so. Perhaps in the name of beneficence, the disease version of addiction-theory denies the addict's ability to control her behavior. But it does so at a heavy moral price—reducing her to a domestic animal.

My analysis of individual and social responsibility for health status is predicated on Kant's claim that the respect/benevolence tension must be managed, not resolved. Resolving the tension, whether in favor of respect or in favor of benevolence is not moral progress. On the contrary, it is moral disaster. And the problem recurs for a theory of justice: how to institutionalize an appropriate balance between respect for autonomy and rights and beneficent regard for people's welfare interests. Libertarians favor massive weighting on the respect side because of all the well-known problems of state-parentalism (in law, *parens patriae*). Libertarians prefer that social institutions not reduce people to domestic animal status.

Welfare liberals, in contrast, favor shifting the balance toward the beneficence side. They believe that libertarians overemphasize respect, with a result that is practically indistinguishable from an uncaring, inhumane social order. As I see it (and I think Kant would agree), this argument is essentially irresolvable. In political morality, the tension between respect and beneficence can only be managed by difficult trade-offs at the institutional level. Significant risks are inescapable no matter where one places the emphasis. If Kant was right, as I have assumed he is, politics must be both important and inherently frustrating. No one can claim justification in seeking total victory for his or her favorite value, yet there should be more than a little comfort in recognizing that Mencius (Meng-tzu), writing much earlier than Kant and in a markedly different culture, appreciated the same basic dynamic in ethics.

Acknowledgment

The author gratefully acknowledges that comments from the following individuals improved this chapter: Mary Anderlik, Michael Corrado, Roasmond Rhodes, Steve Miles, and Gladys White.

NOTES

1. Kant claims that the principles of mutual love and of respect are among the "laws of duty," which function in the moral world analogously to the the laws of attraction and repulsion in the natural world. He goes on to say, "And should one of these great moral forces fail, then nothingness (immorality), with gaping throat, would drink the whole kingdom of (moral) beings like a drop of water."

2. *Payton v. Weaver*, 131 Cal.App.3d 38, 181 Cal. Rptr. 225 (1982).

3. The physician–patient relationship is modeled on contract ("offer and acceptance"). Because the relationship is voluntary, either party may break it. However, while the patient may terminate the relationship at any time and for any reason, the physician must formally notify the patient that he intends to cease providing care and must allow the patient a reasonable opportunity to secure the services of another physician. Despite having the power to discontinue a relationship with a patient, the physician must not "abandon" the patient. Abandonment, an ethical and civil wrong, consists of harming one's patient by negligently failing to attend to the patient's medical needs when he or she is in need of care.

4. California's Lanterman-Petris Act, section 5350 (since renumbered), provided that a conservator may be appointed for a person who is "gravely disabled as a result of mental disorder or impairment by chronic alcoholism."

5. *Schloendorff v. Society of New York Hospital*, 211 N.Y. 125; 105 N.E. 92 (1914). The right to determine what shall be done with one's own body is one of the oldest personal rights recognized in common law. Its recognition is

Case for Voluntary Commitement?" in *Contemporary Issues in Bioethics*, Tom L. Beauchamp and Leroy Walters (eds.) 2d ed. 1982, p. 163; Rebecca S. Dresser, "Bound to Treatment: The Ulysses Contract," *Hastings Center Report*, June 1984, p. 13; Rebecca S. Dresser, "Ulysses and the Psychiatrists: A Legal and Policy Analysis of the Voluntary Commitment Contract," 16 *Harvard Civil Rights–Civil Liberties L.Rev.* 777 (1982); Roberto Cuca, "Ulysses in Minnesota: First Steps Toward a Self-Binding Psychiatric Advance Directive Statute," 78 *Cornell L. Rev.* 1152 (1993); Bruce J. Winick, "Advance Directive Instruments for Those with Mental Illness," 51 *U. Miami L. Rev.* 57 (1996); Paul F. Stavis, "The Nexum: A Modest Proposal for Self-Guardianship by Contract, a System of Advance Directives and Surrogate Committees-at-Large for the Intermittently Mentally Ill," 16 *J. Contemp H.L. & Policy* 1 (1999).

42. Elster, J. (1979). *Ulysses and the Sirens: Studies in Rationality and Irrationality.* Cambridge: Cambridge University Press, p. 38.

REFERENCES

Ainslie, G. (1992). *Picoeconomics.* Cambridge: Cambridge University Press, pp. 3–4.

Ainslie, G. (1999). The dangers of willpower. In J. Elster and O.J. Skog (eds.), *Getting Hooked.* Cambridge: Cambridge University Press, p. 65–92.

Becker, G.S. and Murphy, K.M. (1988). A theory of rational addiction. *Journal of Political Economy*, 96(4), pp. 675–700.

Buchanan, A.E. and Brock D.W. (1989). *Deciding for Others: The Ethics of Surrogate Decision Making.* New York: Cambridge University Press, chapter 1.

California's Lanterman-Petris Act, section 5350.

Can a subject consent to a 'Ulysses contract'? *Hastings Center Report*, August 1982, p. 26.

Cuca, R. (1993). Ulysses in Minnesota: first steps toward a self-binding psychiatric advance directive statute, *Cornell L. Rev.* 78 1152.

Damasio, A. (1994). *Descartes' Error: Emotion, Reason and the Human Brain.* New York: Avon Books, pp. 10–14.

Dean, M. (1993). Self-inflected rationing, *The Lancet* 341, 1525.

Dresser, R.S. (1984). Bound to treatment: the ulysses contract, *Hastings Center Report*, p. 13.

Dresser, R.S. (1982). Ullysses and the psychiatrists: a legal and policy analysis of the voluntary commitment contract, 16 *Harvard Civil Rights—Civil Liberties L. Rev.* 777.

Eigen, J.P. (1995). *Witnessing Insanity: Madness and mad-Doctors in the English Court.* New Haven, CT: Yale University Press, p. 59.

Elster, J., (1979). *Ulysses and the Sirens: Studies in Rationality and Irrationality.* Cambridge: Cambridge University Press, p. 38.

Elster, J. and Skog, O.J. (1999). *On Getting Hooked.* Cambridge: Cambridge University Press, p. 5.

Epstein, R. (1995). *Simple Rules for a Complex World.* Cambridge, MA: Harvard University Press. p. 22.

Frankfurt, H. (1971). Freedom of the will and the concept of a person. *Journal of Philosophy* 68, 5–20.

Hamilton, E. (1963). *Mythology: Timeless Tales of Gods and Heroes.* New York: Mentor Books, p. 214.

Hammer, D. and Copeland, P. (1998). *Living with Our Genes.* New York: Doubleday.

Hayek, F.A. (1944). *The Road to Serfdom.* Chicago: University of Chicago Press.

Hill, T.E., Jr. (1991). *Autonomy and Self-Respect.* New York: Cambridge University Press, p. 12.

Howell, T. et al. (1982). Is there a case of voluntary commitments? In *Contemporary Issues in Bioethics*, Tom L. Beauchamp and Leroy Walters (eds.), 2d ed., p. 163.

Kagan, J. (1994). *Galen's Prophecy: Temperament in Human Nature.* New York: Basic Books.

Kant, I. (1750–1964). *The Doctrine of Virtue: Part II of the Matephysics of Morals* (M.J. Gregor, trans.).

Lucas, J.R. (1995). *Responsibility.* Oxford: Oxford University Press, chapter 1.

Mill, J.S. (1859–1956). *On Liberty* (C.V. Shields, ed.). New York: Bobbs-Merrill.

Machiavelli, N. (1513–1981). *The Prince* (G. Bull, trans.). New York: Penguin Classics, p. 130.

Manning, W.G., Keeler, E.B., Newhouse, J.P., Sloss, E.M., and Wasserman, J. (1991). *The Cost of Poor Health Habits.* Cambridge, MA: Harvard University Press.

Martinez v. Zia Company, 99 N.M. 80; 653 P.2d 1226; 1982 N.M. App. LEXIS 968.

Mencius ([third century, B.C.], 1983). D.C. Lau (trans.). New York: Penguin Books, P. 190.

Morreim, E.H., (1991). *Balancing Act: The New Medical Ethics of Medicine's New Economics.* Dordrecht: Bluwer Acaemic Publishers, pp. 136–140.

N.M. Stat. Ann Sec 41-5-10-(2000).

Oates, W.J. (1940). *The Stoic and Epicurean Philosophers.* New York: The Modern Library, p. 494.

Payton v. Weaver, 131 Cal.App.3d 38, 181 Cal. Rptr. 225 (1982).

Plato, *The Republic, Book III*, The *Dialogues of Plato* translated into English w/Analyses & Introduction in Five Volumes. B. Jowett (trans). 2d edition. Vol. III "The Republic" Book III, p. 281 ff. Oxford: The Clarendon Press, 1875.

Rawls, J. (1971). *A Theory of Justice*. Cambridge, MA: Harvard University Press.

Rosker v. Goldberg, 453 U.S. 57 (1981).

Ridley, M. (1999). *Genome*. New York: HarperCollins, p. 163.

Selective Draft Law Cases, 245 U.S. 366 (1918).

Schloendorff v. Society of New York Hospital, 211 N.Y. 235; 105 N.E. 92 (1914).

Schmoke, K. (1994). Side Effects, *Rolling Stone*, May 5, pp. 38–9.

Smith, A. (1984). *Theory of Moral Sentiments*, Raphael, D.D. and Macfie, A.L. (eds.), Indianapolis, IN: Liberty Fund, pp. 254ff.

Stavis, P.R. (1999). The nexum: a modest proposal for self-guardianship by contract, a system of advance directives and surrogate committees-at-large for the intermittently mentally ill. 16 *J. Contem H.L. & Policy* 1.

Veatch, R.M. (1980). Voluntary risks to health: the ethical issues. *JAMA* 243, 50–55.

Waal, H. (1999). To legalize or not to legalize: Is that the question? In J. Elster and O.J. Skog (eds.), *Getting Hooked*, Cambridge: Cambridge University Press, pp. 137–172.

Washington v. Harper, 494 U.S. 210 (1990).

Wikler, D. (1987). Who should be blamed for being sick?' *Health Education Quarterly* 14, 11–25.

Winick, B.J., (1996). Advance directive instruments for those with mental illness, 51 *U. Miami L. Rev.* 57.

32

Does Distributive Justice Require Universal Access to Assisted Reproduction?

Mary Anne Warren

The growth of reproductive medicine has created new issues about who should have access to medical techniques that can enable infertile individuals or couples to have children. These techniques include artificial insemination, in vitro fertilization (IVF) and its many variants, and contract pregnancy, or surrogate motherhood. Some bioethicists hold that the right to reproductive freedom requires only that the use of these reproductive methods be legal (Robertson, 1994, p. 116). Others argue that distributive justice requires universal access to these medical services, within the limits of the available medical resources and other social needs (Andrews, 1989, pp. 387–88; Burley, 1998). I will argue that the second view is correct, with some important qualifications.

I begin with a brief examination of the reasons for regarding reproductive freedom as a basic human right. I argue that the importance which most people place upon having and rearing children supports the claim that a just distribution of medical re-sources would provide funding for medically assisted reproduction. Next, I consider some frequent objections to this claim: the objection from overpopulation; the objection from adoption; and the feminist concern that the new reproductive technologies are harmful to women. None of these objections are sound. Nevertheless, distributive justice does not require universal access to all reproductive technologies, without regard for the expense. The high cost of IVF and contract pregnancy makes it difficult, especially for poorer nations, to provide access to everyone who might benefit. Moreover, enough uncertainty exists about the long-term consequences of contract pregnancy to recommend a cautious approach to public subsidies, even if cost were not an issue.

Although distributive justice does not require universal access to all forms of assisted reproduction, it is a violation of the right to reproductive freedom to deny access on grounds that are unjustly discriminatory. Access should not be denied to individuals or couples unless there are valid medical counterindications, and/or valid grounds for believing that they are incapable of responsible parenting. I argue that this principle precludes discrimination against single women or men, female or male couples, or persons with mental or physical disabilities. Finally, I consider the use of IVF by post-menopausal women, and I argue that age is not in itself a legitimate basis for denying access to assisted reproduction.

REPRODUCTIVE FREEDOM AS A BASIC HUMAN RIGHT

Reproductive rights have been recognized as basic human rights by the international community. The Programme of Action adopted by participants in the International Conference on Population and Development, which was held in Cairo in 1994, calls for all nations to respect and protect the reproductive rights of all individuals. These include "the basic right of all couples and individuals to decide freely and responsibly on the number and spacing of their children, and to have access to the information, education and means to enable them to exercise these rights" (Shalev, 2000, p. 42).

The right to reproductive freedom includes both the right to have children and the right to avoid having them. Some moral theorists distinguish between negative rights and positive rights. *Negative rights* are entitlements to protection from some specific harm, such as physical assault. *Positive rights* are entitlements to specific benefits, such as health care. As negative rights, the right to have children and the right not to have them are equally basic. Coercively denying individuals the means of limiting their fertility, and coercively taking their fertility from them (e.g., through involuntary sterilization), are both serious violations of basic human rights.

But are these reproductive rights also positive rights? The case for a positive right not to reproduce is fairly clear. Those who

do not object to contraception or abortion on moral or religious grounds are likely to agree that universal access to the means of preventing unwanted births is a goal that cannot justly be postponed. The costs of unwanted pregnancies and births are too great for women, families, and nations struggling to escape poverty.[1] Universal access to safe contraception and abortion is economically within the reach of most nations, especially with the international assistance that could be made available. These facts provide a basis for the claim that access to contraception and abortion ought to be both legal and universally available, without economic or other barriers. Few well-informed people would prefer a system for distributing medical resources that results in women being forced to have children against their will. Such a system neither maximizes liberty nor benefits society as a whole; and it is particularly harmful to poor people, who are least able to purchase medical services independently.

A similar argument can be made in defense of a positive right to assisted reproduction. Justine Burley draws upon Ronald Dworkin's *theory of liberal equality* to argue that "justice demands that individuals be compensated for all or part of the assisted conception techniques that they undergo" (Burley, 1998, p. 129; Dworkin, 1995). The core of the argument is a Rawlsian "thought experiment," wherein rational choosers meet behind a veil of ignorance that prevents their knowing (among other things) what undeserved misfortunes or disabilities they will someday suffer. They are well informed, however, about the potential impact of each possible misfortune upon their chances of living a good life. In the light of this knowledge, they discuss and vote on the misfortunes for which individuals will be compensated at public expense. Burley's claim is that because the majority of people want to have children and raise them, and because this desire is likely to be a central part of their life plans, rational choosers would vote to make infertility one of the misfortunes for which compensation will be provided. How much compensation is appropriate will depend upon "aggregate decisions concerning the value accorded to having a genetically related child relative to the treatment of other medical conditions, and also the provision of other non-health-related public goods and services" (Burley, 1998, p. 142).

This argument provides a plausible basis for the conclusion that medically assisted reproduction should be socially subsidized. However, a number of objections exist to assisted reproduction that might persuade rational choosers not to invest public resources in it. Perhaps they would conclude that it is unwise to contribute to population growth and vote instead to encourage infertile individuals to adopt children who have been orphaned or abandoned. Or perhaps they would be persuaded by those feminist critics who argue that it is not in the interests of women to employ new reproductive technologies.

THE OBJECTION FROM POPULATION GROWTH

It is sometimes said that social resources should not be spent on assisted reproduction because there are already too many people on Earth for the biosphere reliably to sustain. To be sure, it is the total consumption of natural resources, rather than the size of the human population as such, that is damaging Earth's ecosystems. The citizens of wealthy industrialized nations consume far more resources per capita than do those of poorer nations. Unless this pattern of excessive consumption is altered, population stabilization may not be enough to prevent planetary ecosystemic disaster. However, it is equally true that poorer nations legitimately wish to improve their standards of living, and that as they do the resulting increase in consumption may be devastating to the planet if population growth is not halted or re-

versed. Thus, despite the encouraging decline in the growth rate of the global population since the 1960s, there is cause for continued concern. To the extent that assisted reproduction contributes to population growth, it may be viewed as contrary to the interests of humanity as a whole.

The problem with this argument is that it is difficult to justify policies designed to limit the reproductive options of infertile persons, while the options of fertile persons are not comparably limited. It is unjustly discriminatory to permit fertile couples to have as many children as they wish—children whose education and medical care will be substantially subsidized—while denying infertile persons even a modest subsidy for assisted reproduction.

Furthermore, withholding support for medically assisted reproduction is unlikely to have a significant impact on birth rates, which depend primarily upon the behavior of the fertile majority. Most of the declines in birth rates that have occurred in the past two centuries have been the result of social and economic changes that have facilitated the voluntary limitation of family size. The major exception is China, where the one-child policy has been in effect for over two decades and has been enforced coercively (Nie, 1998). Birth rates generally decline in proportion to improved social and economic conditions—including better educational and economic opportunities, especially for women, and declines in infant and child mortality. These changes are independently desirable, and they are usually sufficient to bring birth rates to sustainable levels.

THE OBJECTION FROM ADOPTION

It is sometimes argued that infertile individuals or couples ought to adopt children rather than to use medical technology to have children of their own. Assisted reproduction may enable them to have a "biological" child—that is, one who is genetically related to them, or at least conceived and born at their instigation. However, adoption may appear to be a morally better option, for it benefits an existing child and does not contribute to population growth (Mahoney, 1995, p. 51). International adoption has created new opportunities for infertile people who would find it difficult to adopt domestically. Why, then, should public resources be invested in enabling the infertile to have biological children?

This argument presupposes that most infertile persons have the option of adopting a child, and that most of them would find that option satisfactory. Both assumptions are questionable. Adopting a child can be both very difficult and very expensive. The increased availability of contraception and abortion has greatly reduced the number of infants available for adoption in most of the industrialized world. Many private adoption agencies charge fees that are prohibitively high for many potential adoptive parents. Charitable and state-funded agencies are likely to exclude many applicants on the basis of economic considerations, marital status, age, health, or sexual preference. Some agencies seek to match children and applicants for ethnicity, which can lengthen the waiting periods.

It is equally doubtful that most people who want to have children would find adoption a satisfactory option. As Barbara Berg points out, the great majority of people who wish to raise children strongly prefer to raise biological children, and they consider adoption only when that option is foreclosed (Berg, 1995, p. 81). Furthermore, Berg notes, "This nearly universal preference . . . reveals not only a value placed on the genetic linkage but on other aspects of the experience of parenting a biological child (e.g., the experience of pregnancy and childbirth)."

The rationality of the preference for biological children is questionable, as the bonds between adoptive parents and children can be just as strong and mutually rewarding as those between biological parents and children. But, rational or not, it is

often very resistant to change. Many people consider having and rearing biological children to be an essential part of a good life. This goal can usually be pursued without harming others, or taking more than a fair share of society's resources. That is why rational choosers, voting in ignorance of their individual circumstances, would vote to insure themselves against the risk of infertility by subsidizing assisted reproduction (Burley, 1998, p. 142). They would also vote to facilitate adoption. But rather than promoting adoption by limiting access to assisted reproduction, they would seek better ways of bringing together children who need to be adopted and potential adoptive parents.

FEMINIST OBJECTIONS TO IVF

Access to medically assisted reproduction cannot be a positive right unless it is a genuine benefit. However, some feminists have questioned whether new reproductive technologies provide net benefits to women. Most of their objections are directed not against artificial insemination, but against IVF and contract pregnancy. If these objections are valid, then the case for universal access to the latter forms of assisted reproduction will be weakened. This section focuses on the feminist objections to IVF; the objections to contract pregnancy will be considered in the next section.

Many feminists have expressed the concern that IVF is excessively dangerous to women, and possibly to their children (Rowland, 1992, pp. 49–73; Raymond, 1993, pp. 11–4). Various studies have shown that pregnancies begun after the use of drugs such as clomiphene (which is used to induce superovulation) are more likely to be ectopic, or to be spontaneously aborted (Rowland, 1992, p. 51). Others have found that infants conceived through IVF are more likely to die in the perinatal period, or to suffer from serious abnormalities such as anencephaly, Down syndrome, and congenital heart lesions (Kurachi et al., 1983, p. 187; Lancaster, 1987, pp. 1392–93); and still others have linked the use of clomiphene with an increased incidence of ovarian cancer (Rowland, 1992, pp. 54–5, Raymond, 1993, p. 13).

Some feminists also argue that even if IVF were not medically dangerous, it would not be beneficial to women because they do not freely choose it. Instead, they are subtly coerced by social pressures, and by pronatalist ideologies that depict childbearing as women's primary function (Raymond, 1993, pp. ix–xii, 103–107; Brazier, 1998, p. 76). Coercion need not be overt to be effective. If social pressures prevent women from making voluntary decisions about IVF treatment, then the appearance of voluntary consent is an illusion.

A third feminist objection is that women ought not to use IVF, because in supporting this technology they are contributing to a process that is depriving women of control over their own reproduction. In Robyn Rowland's words,

[W]e are changing the nature of being human and eroding the control which women have had over procreation. In its place, male-controlled technological intervention is beginning to determine how children will be conceived, [and] what kind of children will be born. (Rowland, 1992, p. 3)

The medical risks of IVF are not as well understood as they ought to be 23 years after the birth of the first IVF baby. It is also true that social pressures on women to have children sometimes amount to coercion. And it is possible that, in the future, IVF will be used to pursue inappropriate eugenic goals, with results that cannot be predicted. However, none of these facts refute the presumption that access to IVF provides a net benefit to infertile women (and men[2]) who wish to have biological children.

Although the medical risks associated with IVF are serious, their magnitude should not be exaggerated. The great majority of infants born after IVF are healthy. Moreover, it is difficult to establish that statistical differences in outcomes between IVF and non-IVF pregnancies are the result of IVF treatment, rather than of genetic or physiological problems associated with infertility. Thus, a well-informed woman who wants to have a biological child might reasonably conclude that the risks are worth taking. Women have always had to face risks to their lives and health in order to bear children, with no guarantee of success.

It is equally unclear that the majority of women who undergo IVF have not given voluntary and informed consent. As Barbara Berg points out, feminist discussions of the dangers of IVF frequently pay too little attention to the perspective of infertile women. In her experience, women who seek IVF are typically well educated and have often reflected at length on their reasons for wanting biological children. Berg argues that it is unfair to depict their desire for motherhood as merely a reflection of pronatalist socialization, when the same desire on the part of fertile women is not depicted in the same way (Berg, 1995, p. 85). All decisions about childbearing are influenced by social and economic realities, but it does not follow that they are always coerced, or influenced, in ways that make responsible decision making impossible (Warren, 1995, pp. 448–50).

There are also reasons to doubt that women who use IVF are acting against the interests of other women. Any medical technology can be used in ways that are harmful to patients, or disrespectful of their autonomy, and IVF is no exception. The physiological risks of IVF have often been underplayed, especially in media reports about "medical miracles." Some clinics have routinely exaggerated their success rates (Raymond, 1993, pp. 9–11). In the United States, the lack of federal and state funding for research involving human embryos has contributed to a dearth of public oversight and regulation. However, asking infertile women to boycott IVF is not the best way to combat these abuses. A better option is to advocate for improved oversight and regulation, to ensure that IVF patients are aware of the risks, and to eliminate clinical practices that increase the dangers to which such patients are exposed. Here, too, the opponents of IVF may be suspected of unjust discrimination against the infertile (Berg, 1995, pp. 94–95). The experience of motherhood is everywhere shaped by oppressive social institutions; but it is rarely argued that fertile women are are morally obliged to resist oppression by forgoing motherhood.

THE CASE AGAINST PUBLIC FINANCING OF CONTRACT PREGNANCY

The arguments thus far considered do not refute the claim that a just distribution of resources would provide economic support for medically assisted reproduction. However, this claim does not entail that all forms of assisted reproduction are equally worth funding. Some are apt to be prohibitively expensive, while others may prove to be medically unsafe, or to have other seriously harmful consequences that could not readily be avoided by better oversight and regulation.

Contract pregnancy is an arrangement whereby a couple or individual hires a woman (usually through a commercial broker) to bear a child and surrender it to them. The surrogate mother may either be inseminated with the sperm of the contracting father, or implanted with an embryo derived from the gametes of the contracting couple. In the first case, the surrogate mother is the infant's genetic mother; in the second case, the contracting mother is. There are three major objections to contract pregnancy of either sort. None are sufficient to establish that it is always morally objectionable, or that it ought to be prohibited by law. However, the third objection may provide a reasonable basis for withholding large public subsidies for it.

The first objection is that contract pregnancy is difficult to distinguish from the selling of an infant, which is generally

agreed to be morally wrong. The surrogate mother is evidently paid not merely for her labor, but for giving birth to a live infant and surrendering it; she is usually not paid (or not paid in full) unless both these conditions are met. If she is not literally selling the infant, then she is evidently selling her parental rights and responsibilities toward it—a transaction that is also morally problematic.

This argument is unpersuasive without proof that the sale of an infant is morally wrong in every instance. The widespread conviction that selling infants is always seriously immoral may be based upon reaction to a quite different range of cases—for example, cases in which desperately poor parents are forced to sell some of their children in order to keep others alive, or in which heartless parents sell their children because they find them tiresome and are indifferent to their welfare. Contract pregnancy is different from these distressing scenarios in that the child is conceived and born at the instigation of the contracting parent(s), rather than purchased from parents who are abandoning their initial commitment to the child. This difference is significant, because it is the difference between separating members of an existing family and forming a new family, albeit with assistance. It also provides a basis for doubting that contract pregnancy is best understood as the sale of the infant. If it is mutually understood from the start that the infant will be born a member of the family of the contracting parents (or parent), then it may reasonably be maintained that—despite appearances—what the contracting parents have purchased is not the infant itself but rather the surrogate's time and labor in bringing it to birth.

A second objection to contract pregnancy is that it will be psychologically harmful to children to learn that they were born as the result of a pregnancy contract, even if the contracting parents care for them in an exemplary fashion. Adopted children may also suffer from the knowledge that their birth parents chose not to keep them; but they can take comfort from the thought that their parents may have wanted to keep them but were unable to care for them adequately. The knowledge that one was born as the result of a commercial arrangement may be more disturbing.

This argument is unpersuasive, because the claim that children born of contract pregnancies will be psychologically harmed is highly speculative. It is at least as likely that most children born of contract pregnancies will take the knowledge of their origin in stride, especially if being born in this way is not socially stigmatized. The initial fears that children born from IVF would be stigmatized have proved unfounded. New ways of reproducing that at first seem strange and even perverse may later be accepted as routine.

The third major objection to contract pregnancy is that it is a wrongful exploitation of surrogate mothers, even when they participate voluntarily. A contract can be exploitative even though it is accepted by all parties. For example, purchasing the kidneys or other important and irreplaceable parts of living persons is widely viewed as immoral, even when the "owners" are willing to sell, because the removal of such body parts is often severely harmful. If contract pregnancy causes serious harm to surrogate mothers, then perhaps it should also be regarded as a wrongful form of exploitation.

One response to this argument is that on this criterion a great deal of wage labor would be wrongfully exploitative. People who work on keyboards are vulnerable to repetitive stress injuries, but few argue for banning that form of labor. This response is inadequate, because much wage labor is indeed exploitative, in that workers are exposed to avoidable risks for the sake of increased profits. Furthermore, the commercial exploitation of childbearing may be harmful in a special way. Margaret Jane Radin argues that sex, pregnancy, and parenthood are such central parts of the self that their commodification is inherently degrading (Radin, 1996, p. 127). This is one

reason, she says, why sex work is often regarded as more degrading than most forms of wage labor. Contract pregnancy may be degrading in an analogous way.

A stronger response to the objection from exploitation is that there is little evidence that women who freely choose to be surrogates are likely to be severely harmed or degraded by the experience. There is evidence that some women who relinquish children for adoption experience severe and long-lasting grief, which may resurface years or decades later (Winkler and van Keppel, 1984). Thus, it is reasonable to speculate that some surrogate mothers might also experience lasting grief because they cannot rear the child to whom they have given birth. However, the analogy between adoption and contract pregnancy is inexact. Unlike most relinquishing mothers, surrogates agree in advance of conception to give birth to a child they will not raise, and they may therefore be less likely to experience lasting grief. A more typical response might be pride and pleasure in providing a service of great value. Thus, direct evidence of serious harm to surrogates would be needed to prove that contract pregnancy is inherently exploitative; and such evidence is lacking.

Another telling response to this objection is that it is objectionably paternalistic to prohibit well-informed women from voluntarily entering forms of employment that involve significant risks. Contract pregnancy is surely no more physically or psychologically dangerous than being in the military, and few still argue that women need to be protected by exclusion from military service. What needs to be shown to prove that contract pregnancy (or military service) is wrongfully exploitative is not just that it entails significant risks, but that these are such that no well-informed person would endure them in return for the compensation offered, unless she were compelled by dire economic need, or some other form of duress. The risks associated with contract pregnancy have not been shown to be of this magnitude.

These objections to contract pregnancy

fail to prove that it is immoral, or that it ought to be prohibited. However, it does not follow that it ought to be publicly funded. Distributive justice supports only subsidies that are likely to produce net benefits great enough to outweigh those that could be achieved through alternative investments of public resources. Although there is little evidence that contract pregnancy is often seriously harmful, neither is there much evidence that it is not. The analogy with surrendering a child for adoption, though inexact, may prove to be important. Future research might show that contract pregnancy often causes severe psychological harm to surrogate mothers and/or members of their families, and that it is impossible to determine in advance who would harmed by it. Such evidence would not automatically justify banning contract pregnancy, for competent adults are entitled to enter some quite dangerous professions. However, it could substantially alter the cost-benefit picture for the public funding of contract pregnancy. The current inadequate understanding of the long-term consequences of contract pregnancy, together with its high cost, provides a reasonable basis for provisional opposition to large public subsidies.

ECONOMIC OBSTACLES TO UNIVERSAL ACCESS

Artificial insemination is the oldest, safest, and least expensive form of assisted reproduction. It is a valuable option not only for heterosexual couples in which the male is infertile, but also for single and lesbian women, who are enabled to have children without the personal danger and legal complexities attendant upon conceiving through heterosexual intercourse. For these reasons, it is the form of assisted reproduction that is most immediately eligible for public subsidy.

In contrast, the high cost of IVF makes universal access difficult to achieve in all but the wealthiest nations. While the cost varies between nations, it is in each case high. In the United States, IVF has been es-

timated to cost on the average $8,000 per treatment cycle (Neuman et al., 1994). Because only 10% to 15% of treatment cycles result in a live birth, the average total cost is much higher. Funding contract pregnancy would also be very expensive. Pregnancy contracts typically cost prospective parents from $25,000 to $30,000, even without the additional expense of using IVF to enable the contracting mother also to be the genetic mother. Universal access is a goal that must be evaluated against other possible uses of medical resources, as well as the society's nonmedical needs. Now and for the foreseeable future, cost considerations preclude the assertion of a universal positive right to have children through IVF or contract pregnancy.

Although there is no universal positive right to the most expensive forms of assisted reproduction, access ought not to be denied on the basis of arbitrary and unjustified criteria. Unfortunately, unjust obstacles to access to medically assisted reproduction are common.

SINGLE WOMEN AND FEMALE COUPLES

In the United States, few legal restrictions exist on who may use IVF or artificial insemination. Nevertheless, many infertility clinics and sperm banks still prefer to provide services only to married women. In Europe, where general insurance plans often cover most infertility treatments, access is often limited by law. Norway prohibits artificial insemination or IVF for unmarried women, and Denmark, Sweden, and France permit access only to women with male domestic partners (Sandor, 2000, p. 201). These exclusionary provisions are motivated by the belief that children do best in heterosexual two-parent families. But are there any good reasons to believe this? Patriarchal law and religion typically classify children born to single women as illegitimate, and often severely penalize their mothers, yet there is no sound evidence that children cannot be well reared and provided for in the absence of an involved male parent—as long as law and cultural tradition do not unjustly magnify the difficulties faced by female-headed families.

One response to this argument is that women who lack male partners are generally poorer than married women; this is because men still tend to earn more than women with comparable education and experience. Consequently, female-headed families will be apt to have fewer material benefits to offer children and will be more likely to need public assistance. Are these not legitimate reasons for refusing to facilitate the formation of such families?

This argument fails, because it is unjust to deny important benefits to individuals on the basis of statistical properties of a group to which they belong, rather than attending to their individual traits. Many single women and female couples have the resources to undertake childrearing, and they should not be denied the opportunity on oversimplified economic grounds. Even if all female-headed families were poor, the argument would fail, because the poor have the same reproductive rights as the rich even though their children are likely to lead more difficult lives.

Another argument against the public funding of assisted reproduction for single women or female couples is that their children will face social prejudice. While this will often be true, it is not a just basis for denying access. The right to reproduce does not disappear whenever socially created obstacles to a happy family life exist. If it did, then laws against marriage between persons of different races or religions would often be justified. Society's obligation is to oppose unwarranted prejudices, not to use them as a rationale for further discrimination.

SINGLE MEN AND MALE COUPLES

Single men and male couples may also wish to have biological children, and contract pregnancy can provide a means of fulfilling this desire. However, we know very little about the long-term human consequences of contract pregnancy. Consequently, it is by no means clear that the right to have children includes a positive right to free or subsidized access to it. Nevertheless, justice forbids invidious discrimination against single persons or same-sex couples (of either gender) who wish to have a child through contract pregnancy.

Given the high cost of contract pregnancy, many single men and male couples will prefer to adopt a child. Applicants for adoption should not be excluded because they lack an opposite-sex partner. The standards of eligibility to which prospective adoptive parents are subjected are inevitably somewhat stricter than could appropriately be used to limit access to assisted reproduction. Those who are entrusted with finding adoptive parents for orphaned, abandoned, or abused children are obliged to seek the best homes from among those available. Thus, an applicant's economic viability, and the availability of a second person to share childrearing responsibilities, can be legitimate considerations. However, because there is no evidence that all men who lack female partners are incapable of rearing children responsibly, it is unjust to exclude all members of this group.

PEOPLE WITH DISABILITIES

Access to assisted reproduction should not be denied on the basis of mental or physical disabilities that are not demonstrably and irremediably incompatible with responsible parenthood. Granted, some severely mentally disabled individuals are permanently incapable of undertaking the responsibilities of parenthood. For them, the assertion of a right to reproduce would be all but meaningless. In some cases their own interests demand that they be protected from becoming pregnant, or causing a pregnancy. However, when a disabled but mentally competent adult's access to assisted reproduction is at issue, the right to reproduce becomes highly relevant.

Infertility specialists may reasonably

consider themselves obliged to ascertain that those who will become parents through their assistance are capable of responsible parenthood. Guido de Wert observes that, "A doctor assisting in reproduction shares the responsibility for creating a new human being. . . . For this reason, judging the suitability for parenthood of infertile prospective parents is part of the professional responsibility of the physician" (de Wert, 1998, p. 231). Yet great caution must be used in making such judgments about the capacity for responsible parenthood. High intelligence is not a valid criterion, and neither is freedom from serious mental or physical disability. Justice requires that judgments be made on an individual basis, and that adequate account be taken of the forms of social support that are available.

POST-MENOPAUSAL WOMEN

Women who have completed the menopause no longer produce viable oocytes. Nevertheless, some post-menopausal women have given birth by using donated ova or embryos. One Italian infertility specialist is reported to have helped 70 post-menopausal women to become pregnant in this way (Andrews, 1999, p. 100). A 1991 study (Edwards et al.) found that the success rate per treatment cycle for post-menopausal women using donated oocytes is better than for premenopausal women using their own ova. Several women in their sixties are said to have given birth to healthy infants; however, the majority of post-menopausal births have been to women in their forties or early fifties.

The American Society of Reproductive Medicine states in its guidelines concerning egg donation that, "Just as oocyte donation to prepubertal girls is unacceptable, so should it be unacceptable for post-menopausal woman to bear children" (Andrews, 1999, p. 101). In Canada, the Royal Commission on New Reproductive Technologies recommends that "women who have experienced menopause at the usual

age should not be candidates to receive donated eggs" (de Wert, 1998, p. 222). This judgment would be justified were there definitive evidence that pregnancy is unacceptably dangerous for all post-menopausal women or for their children. However, there have thus far been too few post-menopausal births, and too few outcome studies, to permit a definitive assessment of the medical risks (Fisher and Sommerville, 1998, p. 212).

The comparison between post-menopausal women and prepubertal girls is inappropriate, since it is already known that pregnancy is more dangerous for very young women, and it is highly probable that the risks for prepubertal girls would be even greater. In the absence of valid evidence that pregnancy is unacceptably dangerous for all post-menopausal women, the exclusion of all members of this group from IVF treatment is unjustified.

There is also a potential for injustice in the use of inflexible upper age limits for women's access to IVF. Though there may be an upper age limit for safe childbearing, no one knows what it is. Age is rarely a good reason for denying a potentially beneficial treatment. Although the age of a patient is often correlated with greater risks and a lower probability of successful treatment, each patient's prognosis is determined not by her age but by her physical and mental condition, which may differ substantially from the statistical average. For this reason, upper age limits for access to IVF are best treated as guidelines rather than as absolute barriers.

Another argument against permitting older women access to IVF is that an older mother is likely to have fewer years to spend with the child. Many bioethicists have noted that this concern is rarely expressed when it is the male partner who is over age 50. This disparity is difficult to justify, especially as women in most parts of the world live several years longer than men. A healthy woman of 50 or 55 is likely to have 20 or more active years left— presumably enough to give a child a good start in life. At 60 or 65, however, the odds are less favorable. As Laura Purdy points out, having children who are apt to be orphaned at an early age is morally dubious (Purdy, 1996, pp. 37–38). Nevertheless, the age of the would-be parent is not so strongly predictive of a bleak future for the child that it can justly be used as an absolutely disqualifying condition. As always, individual cases need to be considered individually.

SUMMARY AND CONCLUSION

The importance that the majority of people place upon the goal of having and rearing "biological" children supports the claim that a just system of distributing medical resources would provide funding for medically assisted reproduction. Neither the problem of human population growth nor the fact that (some) infertile persons could adopt a child justifies withholding such funding. Moreover, the feminist objections to IVF fail to show that women derive no net benefit from access to this technology.

Because having children is a basic human right, access to assisted reproduction may not justly be denied on the basis of any personal trait—such as disability, marital status, sexual orientation, or age—that is not demonstrably incompatible with the capacity for responsible childrearing. At the same time, the high cost of IVF precludes that it be made available immediately to every infertile woman or couple in the world. Universal access to contract pregnancy is also likely to remain a low priority, both because of the enormous expense it would entail, and because there is still too little understanding of the long-term consequences for surrogate mothers and their families.

NOTES

1. Worldwide, at least 120 million women who want to limit or space their pregnancies have no access to contraception (UNFPA, 1999). About 20 million women risk their lives annually through illegal abortion, and about 80,000 of them die (WHO, 1998, pp. 1–15).

2. Although initially developed as a treatment for female infertility, IVF is also used in some cases of male infertility or subfertility. For instance, a single sperm can be injected into the in vitro ovum, permitting some men with very low sperm counts to conceive.

REFERENCES

Andrews, L.B. (1989). Alternative Modes of Reproduction. In S. Cohen and N. Taub (eds.), *Reproductive Laws for the 1990s*. Clifton, NJ: Humana Press, pp. 361–404.

Andrews, L. (1999). *The Clone Age: Adventures in the New World of Reproductive Technologies*, New York: Henry Holt.

Berg, B.J. (1995). Listening to the voices of the infertile. In J.C. Callahan (ed.), *Reproductive Ethics and the Law*. Bloomington and Indianapolis: Indiana University Press, pp. 80–108.

Brazier, M. (1998). Reproductive rights: Feminism or patriarchy? In J.Harris and S. Holm (eds.), *The Future of Human Reproduction*. Oxford and New York: Oxford University Press, pp. 66–76.

Burley, J.C. (1998). The price of eggs: Who should bear the cost of fertility treatments? In J. Harris and S. Holm (eds.), *The Future of Human Reproduction*. Oxford and New York: Oxford University Press, pp. 127–49.

Cohen, C.B. (1996). *New Ways of Making Babies: The Case of Egg Donation*. Bloomington and Indianapolis: Indiana University Press.

Delhanty, J.D., Wells, D., and Harper, J.C. (1997). Genetic diagnosis before implantation. *British Medical Journal* 315, 828–29.

de Wert, G. (1998). The post-menopause: Playground for reproductive technology? Some ethical questions. In J. Harris and S. Holm (eds.), *The Future of Human Reproduction*. Oxford and New York: Oxford University Press, pp. 221–37.

Dworkin, R. (1995). The foundations of liberal equality. In S. Darwall (ed.), *Equal Freedom*. Ann Arbor: University of Michigan Press, pp. 190–306.

Edwards, R.G., Morcos, S., Macnamee, M., Balmaceda, J.P., Walters, D.E., and Asch, R. (1991). High fecundity of amenorrhoeic women in embryo transfer programs. *Lancet* 338, 292–94.

Fisher, F. and Sommerville, A. (1998). To everything is a season? Are there moral grounds for refusing fertility treatment to older women? In J. Harris and S. Holm (eds.), *The Future of Human Reproduction*. Oxford and New York: Oxford University Press, pp. 203–20.

Kurachi, K., Ano, T., Minagawa, J. and Miyake, A. (1983). Congenital malformations of newborn infants after clomiphene-induced ovulation. *Fertility and Sterility* 40, 187–89.

Lancaster, P.A.L. (1987). Congenital malformations after in vitro fertilization. *Lancet* 8275, 1392–93.

Mahoney, J. (1995). Adoption as a feminist alternative to reproductive technology. In J.C. Callahan (ed.), *Reproductive Ethics and the Law*. Bloomington and Indianapolis: Indiana University Press, pp. 35–54.

Neumann, P.J., Gharib, S.D., Weinstein, M.C. (1994). The cost of a successful delivery with in vitro fertilization. *New England Journal of Medicine* 331 (4), 239–43.

Nie, J.B. (1998). The problem of coerced abortion in China and related ethical issues. *Cambridge Quarterly of Health Care Ethics* 8, 463–74.

Purdy, L. (1996). *Reproducing Persons: Issues in Feminist Bioethics*. Ithaca, NY: Cornell University Press.

Raymond, J. (1993). *Women as Wombs: Reproductive Technologies and the Battle Over Women's Freedom*. New York: HarperCollins.

Radin M.J. (1996). *Contested Commodities: The Trouble with Trade in Sex, Children, Body Parts, and Other Things*. Cambridge, MA: Harvard University Press.

Robertson, J. (1994). *Children of Choice: Freedom and the New Reproductive Technolo-*gies. Princeton, NJ: Princeton University Press.

Rowland, (1992). *Living Laboratories: women and Reproductive Technologies*. Bloomington and Indianapolis: Indiana University Press.

Sandor, J. (2000). Reproductive rights in Hungary: a new right to assisted procreation? *Health and Human Rights* 4, 196–218.

Shalev, C. (2000). Rights to sexual and reproductive health: The ICPD and the convention on the elimination of all forms of discrimination against women. *Health and Human Rights* 4, 38–67.

Turmen, T. (2000). Reproductive rights: How to move forward? *Health and Human Rights* 4, 31–37.

UNFPA. (1999). *The State of World Population 1999: Six Billion: A Time for Choices*. New York: United Nations Fund for Population Activities.

Warren, M.A. (1995). IVF and women's interests: An analysis of feminist concern. In J.D. Arras and B. Steinbock (eds.), *Ethical Issues in Modern Medicine*. Mountain View, CA: Mayfield, pp. 447–59.

Winkler, R. and M. van Keppel. (1984). *Relinquishing Mothers in Adoption: Their Long-Term Adjustment*. Melbourne: Institute of Family Studies.

World Health Organization (WHO) (1998). Unsafe abortion. In *Global and Regional Estimates of Incidence and Mortality Due to Unsafe Abortion, with a Listing of Available Country Data*. Geneva: WHO.

33

Premature and Compromised Neonates

Ian R. Holzman

The world of neonatal intensive care strikes most people as foreign and somewhat unreal. Not unlike other intensive care units it is filled with monitors, alarms, flashing lights, and frenetic movement, but it also has rows of doll-like patients enclosed in plastic cocoons or splayed out on warming trays. The patients are often barely visible below the tubes, tape, and eye patches. It is in this setting that we confront the complex issues of resource allocation to infants with a wide array of problems—infants who are in no way responsible for their own decisions and may never reach a point of being held responsible.

In this chapter I present an overview of the technical information necessary to understand the health care allocation issues relating to newborns and then discuss the complexity of ethical problems surrounding both personal and societal decisions for this unique population. For convenience, I have subdivided the salient problems into three separate areas: management at the lower limits of viability (the "tiny baby" problem), discontinuing intensive care support for a neonate, and the problems associated with infants having multiple congenital anomalies.

BACKGROUND

The field of neonatal medicine has witnessed enormous changes during the last two decades (Avery, 1998). Technological advances in respiratory care, effective prenatal treatments to mature lungs, surfactant replacement therapy and better nutritional supplements have all led to markedly improved survival of babies as small as 1.5 pounds and as much as 16 weeks early (Lorenz, 2000). The success of assisted reproductive technologies has also led to an increasing number of multiple gestation premature births (Warner et al., 2000). For infants with complex congenital anomalies, the range of therapeutic options, including fetal surgery, extra corporeal membrane oxygenation, and transplantation, has greatly expanded, promising, at the least, improved survival.

As in all of medicine, these changes have not come without enormous economic consequences—neonatal ICUs, equipped and staffed to manage the smallest and sickest infants, are present in the majority of hospitals, and an increasing array of services are available for graduates of intensive care (Cavalier et al., 1996). Within pediatrics, the largest percentage of physicians who choose a subspecialty decide to train as neonatologists. Despite this trend having persisted for decades, employment opportunities continue to be widely advertised, suggesting a continued market for neonatal care.

It has been estimated that the total neonatal intensive care resources expended annually in the United States are between $2 billion and $4 billion (Stolz and McCormick, 1998) and there are various analyses of how these dollars are spent (Rogowski, 1998, 1999; St. John et al., 2000). At least 18,000 higher-acuity neonatal beds (levels 2 and 3) are available in the United States (Martin et al., 1998), but we also know that infants <25 weeks of gestation account for only 5.4% of the costs involved (Stolz and McCormick, 1998). Although the majority of the costs are not for the smallest infants at the limits of technology, overall neonatal-care expenditures do constitute a significant portion of child health-care costs (Stolz & McCormick, 1998). Furthermore, costs of neonatal care for tiny infants pale when compared to those for many adults with serious illnesses (Tyson et al., 1996; Lantos et al., 1997).

Nevertheless, the costs of neonatal care are probably disproportionately distributed to the public sector because the risk of premature births affects the inner-city African-American population two to three times more than the rest of the nation (Guyer et al., 1999). It has also been shown that hospitals with a higher proportion of insured patients have better neonatal resources than do similarly situated hospitals (with similar teaching status and ownership) that have fewer privately insured patients (Glied and Gnanasekaran, 1996). Economic analyses are also available for the cost of high technology care for one of the more serious congenital anomalies, diaphragmatic hernia. The hospital cost for each survivor of surgery who requires extra corporeal membrane oxygenation treatment (ECMO) is $365,000, and professional fees account for approximately 23% of the total costs (Metkus et al., 1995).

THE LOWER LIMITS OF VIABILITY

The last quarter of the twentieth century has seen a dramatic decline in the weight of newborns considered "appropriate" for delivery room resuscitation—from about 1000 grams (2lb 3oz) (or 12 to 13 weeks early) to 500 grams (1lb 2oz) (or 16 to 17 weeks early). The causes for this change are a complex mixture of advances in medicine and philosophical changes in the "mind-set" of the obstetricians and neonatologists who care for the mothers and babies. A discussion of how this change occurred is beyond the scope of this chapter, but suffice it to say that a similar analysis could have been applied in 1975 to decisions for babies a month more mature at birth than for those today. Saving 1000-gram babies was then considered a miracle.

The purely technical limit to our ability to resuscitate a tiny premature infant falls below our present operational limit—that is, the medical equipment (endotracheal tubes, intravenous lines, monitors) can be used for infants as small as ~400 grams (14 ounces) at birth or 18 weeks early. If it could be agreed that there is some weight or gestation below which it is not technically possible to provide care, should we *never* try? Should there be an attempt to develop equipment for even smaller babies? The argument to continue to try to push the limits of our abilities is based upon the success of such a philosophy during this quarter century. It could be paraphrased as "no pain, no gain." Few practitioners view resuscitation of the tiniest infants as experimental; rather, they see it as giving the babies and their families a best effort to produce a living child. Some neonatologists genuinely believe that affording every baby, no matter how small or young, a chance at survival is what doctors are required to do—any less would be playing God and deciding who should live and who should die.

The reality is, though, that the overwhelming majority of infants who are less than 500 grams at birth (excluding those who are small and poorly grown but of more advanced gestational age, as such infants are more likely to survive) will not survive. Attempts at keeping such tiny infants alive are experimentation (the physician knows survival is unlikely but believes that employing an innovative approach might allow this particular infant to survive and generate new knowledge and should be presented as such) (Peabody and Martin, 1996; Paris et al., 2000).

If all such attempts are experiments, what is their proper place within a just scheme for allocating medical resources? In a climate of unbridled autonomy where patients demand any and all treatments (Paris and Schreiber, 1996b) it might seem simplest to acquiesce to either the parental or physician demand to try to keep the smallest of infants alive. If, as argued by Tooley (1983) and Englehardt (1978), newborns have no independent interests or rights, then the wish of the parents to try to save a 400-gram infant should be honored. However, if we accept that such treatment is experimental, can we really hold every neonatologist required to "experiment" on every small baby when the parents demand it? Regardless of how one views the moral status of such tiny infants, when considered as research subjects their vulnerability seems unquestionable. Decisions to employ active intervention for infants who will not survive should only happen in a setting where protocols for acquisition of knowl-

edge and protection of subjects are in place and after informed consent is obtained (Paris and Schreiber, 1996a).

This discussion of the limits of viability has focused, to this point, on whether a mandate exists to resuscitate the very tiniest of infants. We have not addressed either distributive justice or economics, yet the incidence of prematurity falls disproportionately on the urban poor (and especially the urban African-American poor). The reasons for this higher incidence among urban African-American women are complex and only partly understood. Certainly inadequate early prenatal care, poor nutrition, smoking, and unwanted conceptions are part of the story. However, there is some greater cultural-social explanation that has evaded researchers as attempts to correct the more obvious causes have not met with great success (Hogue and Hargraves, 1995). Any decision to limit care for infants at the margins of viability would fall most heavily on that population.

Surprisingly, the reality is that decisions to be aggressive in the resuscitation of tiny infants have never been linked to experimentation on the poor. Possibly, the tiny newborns of our poorest families are not resuscitated as aggressively as newborns from other social strata, but it seems equally probable that requests for aggressive care (and physician fears of "not doing everything") are more likely to be voiced by some, but not all, sectors of our population.

Family religious beliefs may also play a role in parental requests for aggressive care, and the myriad of cultural differences, expectations for the future of a given child, and trust in the "words" of a physician contribute to the aggressiveness of resuscitation at the limits. The state of Oregon considered the concept of setting a lower limit of birth weight below which care would not be reimbursable (Bodenheimer, 1997). Because the Oregon plan was devised to redistribute *public* monies for health care in a more equitable manner, the poor would be the group not offered resuscitation for their tiny neonates. Though an economic justification might exist for such a policy, it is harder to see it as just. The idea that neonates from poor families, as a distinct group of American citizens, should be denied access to medical treatment requires careful examination.

DISCONTINUING INTENSIVE-CARE SUPPORT

Issues concerning the lower limits of neonatal viability often resemble decisions concerning "turning off respirators." Many neonatologists have adopted a policy of aggressively resuscitating small infants (although not necessarily at the lowest limits of viability) and then discontinuing support, if parents agree, when medical factors indicate a poor prognosis (Kinlaw, 1996). These factors might include severe lung disease, massive bleeding into the brain, overwhelming infections, or bowel necrosis.

On the surface, this approach seems to offer a reasonable compromise among many competing interests—that of the infant, the parents, health care workers, and the investment by society in health care. But there are problems. Parents confronted with the birth of a tiny premature are rarely well informed or unemotional. Physicians tend to be either overly optimistic or pessimistic early in the care of a sick infant, and they must counsel families at a time when physicians have limited information; meaningful outcome data must take into account the totality of the neonatal intensive-care course. It is not always obvious what the underlying justification for discontinuing support might be. If it is clear that the infant will die soon (but not soon enough) then the decision seems to involve consideration of compassion and respect for the infant and family. The arguments are not different from those marshaled by adults who choose to die without the intrusiveness of respirators and feeding tubes. Though the neonate cannot express such wishes, both parents and health-care workers together would seem

to be appropriate surrogates. When death is likely, a decision to withdraw support must be based upon considerations of the burdens of living.

Justifyng the discontinuation of treatment by the potential for a future life of misery will apply only to very few infants. For those who will develop into minimally sentient beings—blind, deaf, unable to make contact with other humans, loss of cortical function—it is hard to imagine that living per se is unpleasant. Adults who have been in prolonged coma and then awaken do not announce that being fed, bathed, clothed, and cared for by others was a horror. For those infants who are likely to be aware of their surroundings but will have years of painful procedures, incomprehensible to them, with no likelihood of an end to their pain and suffering, an argument could be made that death is not an irrational choice.

In many cases, decisions to discontinue support arise from the perceived burden to the family (and in the public policy arena, to society) rather than to the infant. It is easy to construct arguments in support of the parents' critical role in decision making (Peabody and Martin, 1996)—they are responsible for their child. It is less clear why parents are allowed to choose death rather than a complicated future in the case of neonates, while a similar choice is not acceptable for their older children who might be stricken with complicated illnesses. If society were more supportive of the severely disabled and provided the requisite financial and social assistance necessary to cope with a medically devastated neonate, would it be less acceptable to cede "quality of life" a preeminent position?

Once the burdens to the family and society of rearing a profoundly damaged neonate are brought to bear, issues of healthcare allocation come to the forefront (Emanuel, 2000). The long-term costs of caring for a handicapped infant are obviously large, and decisions about allocation in a democracy are not easy to make (Goold, 1996). In any specific case, physicians rightly feel uncomfortable about factoring in the cost of present and future care when a decision to end a life is before them. Parents are similarly uncomfortable but must consciously or unconsciously add financial burdens to their calculus. Without equal access to support (in the broadest sense) for their handicapped children, it seems dangerous to give much weight to considerations of family burden when deciding to discontinue care for a neonate.

THE INFANT WITH COMPLEX CONGENITAL ANOMALIES

Though decisions about the appropriateness of intervention or continued support for extremely premature infants have been in the forefront of public debate, neonatologists (and other pediatric subspecialists) are also often faced with decisions concerning infants with multiple anomalies. The increasing availability of organ transplantation services (although not organs) is forcing neonatologists to reconsider what conditions are truly fatal. The possibility of heart transplants for infants born with incomplete development of the left side of their heart (hypoplastic left heart syndrome) created concerns for the availability and appropriateness of heart donors (Robertson, 1999). Of more immediacy to neonatologists both then and now is whether parents have the right to refuse either palliative surgery (Norwood et al., 1980) or a transplant for their infant. The surgical treatment requires multiple visits to the operating room over the first few years of life, and both survival and intact survival rates have not been high. Outcomes have improved, although long-term outcome remains a question. The argument for respecting a family's wish not to have their infant's heart treated surgically turns on the reality of a low surgical success coupled with multiple major operations and an unknown future survival—surgery seemed like an option many would not choose for themselves and, therefore, not opting for

that course for their sick infant seemed reasonable. With the improvement in surgical technique the choice of "no treatment" is probably now only infrequently offered to families. True parental authority to decide on their child's future has given way to the imposition of the medical establishment's imperative that surgery is the norm. Transplant, though, remains an optional neonatal therapy. Because the availability of hearts is so low, to do otherwise is unreasonable.

The transplantation of other solid organs (liver, lung, kidney, intestine) is similar to that of hearts. The lack of organ availability "allows" physicians the comfort of leaving the choice to families. Were there an instant and magical increase in organ availability would physicians consider such treatment optional for infants? If the success rate were reasonably high (40%? 50%?) what would the justification be for allowing infants to die when half could live? If life with a transplanted organ was sufficiently bearable (no need for repeated surgery, no unrelenting pain, no constant danger of serious infections, no bouts of organ rejection) and there was a reasonable chance of many years of life, such treatment would be considered an infant's right. If the prospects for success were good, any other option could only be justified by society's determination that such expensive therapy was not in its best interests, that its health-care dollars could be better spent.

The above discussion has focused on infants with a single need, namely a heart or liver not properly functioning. Some children, though, are born with a complex group of defects—a syndrome that may or may not be well described. Many include mental retardation but others involve primarily cosmetic issues as well as multiple partially functional organs. There may be shortened, deformed legs, abnormal kidneys, and a deformed and bent spine. No single anomaly is necessarily fatal, but the group of defects could herald enormous health issues in childhood and adulthood.

When the group of abnormalities fits a well-described syndrome with a known prognosis, the considerations usually focus on the likelihood of a life span beyond the first year or two. For some well-defined genetic syndromes such as trisomy 13 the underlying disruption of normal cellular function seems to preclude any hope of growth and development. Though there are always single cases of long-term survivors, albeit severely damaged, this is distinctly uncommon. This should be clearly differentiated from a trisomy 21 or Down syndrome patient where prognosis for a long and happy life is much better. Few, if any, physicians would advocate multiple surgical attempts to repair heart or other organ defects in a child with trisomy 13. These "treatments" would have no coherent purpose and should be considered harmful interventions. The range of conditions in which surgeons have felt operative intervention is not indicated is fairly wide and has included various abdominal wall and urogenital defects, diaphragmatic herniae, and significant intestinal track anomalies (Hazebroek et al., 1993; Caniano et al., 1995).

The more difficult decisions involve those infants whose prognosis and syndrome are unknown or, at least, not clear. Often the concerns about an infant's potential for mental development become paramount and drive the decisions about interventions. Such discussions often begin with the invocation of "quality of life" as a reason to discontinue care. Wouldn't it be unfair to keep such a child alive? For a child who is likely to be aware of its surroundings and experience a painful future, never being able to understand the purpose, there is much to be said for a nonaggressive approach.

Conversely, mental disability, per se, does not equate with a poor quality of life. In reality, the main burden of raising a child with a mental disability is on the family and society. Decisions that impact enormously on both must be carefully examined to assure they are being decided justly

(Emanuel, 2000) and that the decisions reflect our respect for life and the fabric of society, particularly in this era of managed care.

When there are extremely complex decisions about whether to begin a prolonged course of treatments for multiple anomalies, any one of which could be repaired, it would seem that a course of action should be undertaken that weighs the desires of the family (either for or against aggressive treatment) and the imagined desires of any child to have a life with some moments of pleasure and value. If the totality of defects makes such a future unlikely or if the mortality from repeated attempts to "fix things" is extremely high, then a decision not to proceed should be acceptable.

CONCLUSION

The ethical problems faced both by healthcare workers in neonatal ICUs and the families of small and sick neonates are a microcosm of those in the rest of medicine in the twenty-first century. Technological advances such as the temporary use of an artificial lung (ECMO) and organ transplants have allowed medicine to offer life where only a few short years ago none was possible or expected. The patients in this drama are truly incompetent with no past on which to base future wishes. Their families must struggle with a desire to have a child and, at the same time, a wish not to have or give a future of misery. Caught between these wishes are physicians and nurses who want to save lives but without causing pain and who are also fully aware that the ultimate responsibility to care for the child after discharge will be borne by the family.

For the tiniest babies, at the limits of viability, society and physicians will have to draw some lines (Botkin, 1990). It is possible to make decisions that are just, fiscally sound, and respectful of infants and families, when we approach this area with the realization that intervention is experimental and must only be performed with full disclosure and with the real support of society.

For those infants who are not at the lower limits of viability but who reach the point at which discontinuation of support is proposed, there must be a careful weighing of the competing interests—the child's future, the parents' concerns and the potential burdens, the goals of medical treatment, and the need for a just distribution of health care. The latter will be an issue during the child's acute neonatal illness and for the remainder of his or her life.

Infants born with complex birth defects and failing organs bring to the forefront the cutting edge of medical science at a time when the economics of health care are in flux. For some infants, decisions to proceed are unquestionably experimental and should be treated as such. For others, physicians and families must decide whether aggressive and complicated treatment serves the child, the family, and society well. Such discussions can only occur with full and open disclosure of all the facts (as unclear as they may be) and an examination of what the future for that child might be. Such decisions, in the abstract, must also be opened to the general public where a debate on our society's commitment to its youngest members can occur. Though none of these decisions are ever easy, attempting to make them with compassion, justice, and knowledge is probably the most we can expect.

REFERENCES

Avery, G.B. (1998). Futility considerations in the neonatal intensive care unit. *Seminars in Perinatology.* 22, 216–22.

Bodenheimer, T. (1997). The Oregon health plan—lessons for the nation. *New England Journal of Medicine* 337, 651–55,720–23.

Botkin, J.R. (1990). Delivery room decisions for tiny infants: An ethical analysis. *Journal of Clinical of Ethics* 1, 306–11.

Caniano, D.A., Hazebroek, F.W.J., DenBesten, K.E. and Tibboel, D. (1995). End-of-life decisions for surgical neonates: Experience in The Netherlands and United States. *Journal of Pediatric Surgery* 30, 1420–24.

Cavalier, S., Escobar, G.J. Fernbach, S. Quesenberry, C.P. Jr., and Chellino, M. (1996). Postdischarge utilization of medical services by high-risk infants: Experience in a large managed care organization. *Pediatrics* 97, 693–99.

Emanuel, E.J. (2000). Justice and managed care—Four principles for the just allocation of health care resources. *Hastings Center Report* 30, 8–16.

Englehardt, H.T. (1978). Ethical issues in aiding the death of young children. In M. Kohl (ed), *Beneficient Euthanasia.* New York Prometheus Books, p. 78.

Glied, S.A. and Gnanasekaran, S. (1996). Hospital financing and neonatal intensive care. *Health Services Research* 31, 593–607.

Goold, S.D. (1996). Allocating health care: Cost-utility analysis, informed democratic decision making, or the veil of ignorance? *Health Politics, Policy and Law* 21, 69–98.

Guyer, B., Hoyert, D.L., Martin, J.A., Ventura, S.J., MacDorman, M.F. and Strobino, D.M. (1999). Annual summary of Vital statistics— 1998. *Pediatrics* 104, 1229–46.

Hazebroek, F.W.J., Tibboel, D., Mourik, M., Bos, A.P. and Molenaar, J.C. (1993). Withholding and withdrawal of life support from surgical neonates with life-threatening congenital anomalies. *Journal of Pediatric Surgery* 28, 1093–97.

Hogue, C.J.R. and Hargraves, M.A. (1995). Preterm birth in the African-American community. *Seminars in Perinatology* 19, 255–262.

Kinlaw, K. (1996). The changing nature of neonatal ethics in practice. *Clinics in Perinatology* 23, 417–28.

Lantos, J.D., Mokalla, M. and Meadow, W. (1997). Resource allocation in neonatal and medical ICUs, epidemiology and rationing at the extremes of life. *American Journal of Respiratory and Critical Care Medicine* 156, 185–89.

Lorenz, J.M. (2000). Survival of the extremely preterm infant in North America in the 1990s. *Clinics in Perinatology* 27, 255–62.

Martin, G.J., Gattshall, K., MacPherson, F. and Tiffany, S. (1998). Future financial neonatal shock. *Pediatric Clinics of North America* 45, 619–34.

Meadow, W., Lantos, J.D., Mokalla, M. and Reimshisel, T. (1996). Distributive justice across generations. *Clinics in Perinatology* 23, 597–608.

Metkus, A.P., Esserman, L., Sola, A., Harrison, M.R. and Adzick, S.N. (1995). Cost per anomaly: What does a diaphragmatic hernia cost? *Journal of Pediatric Surgery* 30, 226–30.

Norwood, W.I., Kirklin, J.K. and Sanders, S.P. (1980). Hypoplastic left heart syndrome: Experience with palliative surgery. *American Journal of Cardiology* 45, 87–91.

Paris, J.J., DeLisser, H.M. and Savani, R.C. (2000). Ending innovative therapy for infants at the margins of viability: Case of twins. *H. Journal of Perinatology* 4, 251–56.

Paris, J.J. and Schreiber, M.D. (1996a). Parental discretion in refusal of treatment for newborns a real but limited right. *Clinics in Perinatology* 23, 573–81.

Paris, J.J. and Schreiber, M.D. (1996b). Physicians' refusal to provide life-prolonging medical interventions. *Clinics in Perinatology* 23, 563–71.

Peabody, J.L. and Martin, G.I. (1996). From how small is too small to how much is too much. *Clinics in Perinatology* 23, 473–89.

Robertson, J.A. (1999). The dead donor rule. *Hastings Center* Report 29, 6–14.

Rogowski, J. (1998). Cost-effectiveness of care for very low birth weight infants. *Pediatrics* 102, 35–43.

Rogowski, J. (1999). Measuring the cost of neonatal and perinatal care. *Pediatrics* 103, 329–35.

Stolz, J.W. and McCormick, M.C. (1998). Restricting access to neonatal intensive care: Effect on mortality and economic savings. *Pediatics* 101, 344–48.

St. John, E.B., Nelson, K.G., Cliver, S.P., Bishnoi, R.R. and Goldenberg, R.L. (2000). Cost of neonatal care according to gestational age at birth and survival status. *American Journal of Obstetrics and Gynecology* 182, 170–75.

Tooley, M. (1983). *Abortion and Infanticide.* New York: Oxford University Press.

Tyson, J.E., Younes, N., and Wright, L.L. (1996). Viability, morbidity, and resource use among newborns of 501- to 800-g birth weight. *JAMA* 276, 1645–51.

Warner, B.B., Kiely, J.L. and Donovan, E.F. (2000). Multiple births and outcome. *Clinics in Perinatology* 27, 347–61.

34

Just Caring: Do Future Possible Children Have a Just Claim to a Sufficiently Healthy Genome?

Leonard M. Fleck

The defining theme of Philip Kitcher's book *The Lives to Come* (1996) is that we are beyond the age of genetic innocence and that we have entered irrevocably the age of genetic responsibility (p. 204). Kitcher wants us to avoid the excesses and moral wrongs associated with the eugenics movement in the early twentieth century, advocating for what he terms "utopian eugenics." He writes, "Utopian eugenics would use reliable genetic information in prenatal tests that would be available equally to all citizens. Although there would be widespread public discussion of values and of the social consequences of individual decisions, there would be no societally imposed restrictions on reproductive choices—citizens would be educated but not coerced" (Kitcher, 1996, p. 202). Three key ideas comprise the core of Kitcher's utopian eugenics: (*1*) respect for the procreative liberty of all, (*2*) equal access (no financial barriers) to the genetic technologies necessary for *effective* procreative liberty, and

(*3*) a responsible social commitment to preventing "deep human suffering" (p. 192) associated with one's genetic endowment to the extent that medicine provides us with the tools needed to achieve that objective.

The primary question in this chapter springs from the second and third of those key ideas. If we take Norman Daniels's fair equality of opportunity account of health-care justice (1985) as providing us with an essential principle of health-care justice (as opposed to a full account), then what does health-care justice require of us, as a society, when it comes to determining the genetic endowment of future possible children? Buchanan, Brock, Daniels, and Wikler (2000) address this question from the perspective of a future possible capacity to do germline genetic engineering of eight-cell embryos, either repairing or enhancing that genetic endowment through the replacement of some genes in those embryos with either normal or enhanced versions of those genes. However, I put aside that set of issues as too futuristic. Current capacities of medicine raise serious issues of health-care justice, such as our capacity to do preimplantation genetic diagnosis (PGD) of eight-cell embryos.

For couples who know they are at risk of having a child with a serious genetic disorder, such as cystic fibrosis, which will very adversely affect both the length of life and quality of life of a child, PGD is a godsend. It means that they can avoid two choices that they might find morally and psychologically unpalatable: (1) aborting an affected fetus at 16 weeks identified through prenatal testing, and (2) taking a 25% chance that a child will be born with cystic fibrosis. With PGD a woman would be given drugs that would cause her to hyperovulate. Multiple conceptions would occur in vitro, perhaps 12 to 15, grown to the eight-cell stage, and a cell would be removed from each for genetic analysis. Embryos that had no copies of the gene associated with cystic fibrosis (or only one copy of the gene) would be candidates for implantation. The cost of achieving a successful pregnancy via PGD is about $40,000, a sum those not securely in the middle class could not afford. Consequently, if nothing is done to equalize access to this technology (and associated forms of genetic testing needed to identify at-risk potential parents) for members of all socioeconomic classes, disproportionate numbers of children with serious genetic disorders will be born to parents relatively less well off in our society.

From a moral point of view how should we judge either the disproportionate aspect of that outcome, or that a substantial number of children were born with these life-diminishing genetic disorders whose births could have been avoided with access to PGD? Can we confidently judge that it would merely be an "unfortunate" outcome (certainly a correct judgment in a world without PGD)? Is this the sort of bad outcome for which no one is morally blameworthy? Or is this presumptively un-

just? Does this represent a moral wrong that citizens of a society aspiring to be both just and caring are morally obligated to remedy?

FRAMING THE ISSUE

We must next frame more precisely the moral issues comprising this subject. Our preliminary suggestion would be that PGD should be an option for any couple that knows from prior genetic testing (triggered by family history) that they are at risk for having a child with a serious genetic disorder that would adversely affect either the length of life or quality of life of that child from the early stages of life on. This would include cystic fibrosis, Duchenne's muscular dystrophy, Canavan's disease, fragile X syndrome (most common form of mental retardation), hemophilia (and other such X-linked disorders), juvenile diabetes, Tay-Sachs, disease, autism (assuming a solid genetic link), neurofibromatosis, Lesch-Nyhan syndrome, and others. Many other medical disorders with strong genetic links emerge in midlife or later that also very adversely affect length of life or quality of life, including breast cancer linked to the BRCA1 gene, or earlier-onset forms of Alzheimer's disease linked to APOE, or Huntington's disease, or various forms of cancer or heart disease to cite a few. However, for our discussion, we will stipulate there are no just claims for access to PGD for these later-in-life disorders to which potential parents may know their future possible children might be vulnerable. This implies that financially well off potential parents could access at their own expense PGD for these later-in-life disorders for future at-risk children. Further, if some of these parents chose not to purchase PGD, their children could not justifiably claim that they had been treated unjustly, either by their parents or by the larger society. Strictly speaking, they were merely unfortunate.

Several morally relevant considerations

justify our making the moral distinction we propose regarding PGD. First, the causal connections for the children are "tight" and the consequences seriously harmful to their welfare and opportunities. In contrast, the causal connections for the later-in-life disorders are much looser and less certain. With the exception of the Huntington's disease example, all the other disorders listed require for their manifestation as actual disease poorly understood complex environmental co-factors.

Second, appealing to Norman Daniels's fair equality of opportunity account of health care justice, children born with the disorders we have listed are largely deprived of the opportunity to experience anything approaching a normal human life. Their lives are severely compromised for the most part. But with later-onset disorders, individuals will have been able to take advantage of most opportunities that define a human life. Also, given a 40-year period of time and given rapid developments in medicine, there may well be either cures or very effective life-prolonging therapies for many of these disorders. There are no such realistic hopes for children born with the disorders we listed.

Third, aggregate costs are a morally relevant consideration when we have only limited resources to meet virtually unlimited health-care needs for all in our society. If we restrict socially funded PGD for the limited range of disorders we listed (or implicitly included by analogy), approximately 200,000 American children might be born each year through the use of PGD. The direct cost of that would be about $8 billion annually. But 4 million American children are born each year, virtually all of whom will carry a gene for a serious medical disorder that will diminish life expectancy and/or compromise their quality of life. If all those births were through PGD, costs would be $160 billion annually. Costs of that magnitude (or even half) cannot be justified on either moral or economic grounds, even given total health spending in the United States for 2000 of $1.2 trillion.

This argument can be fleshed out further. The dollars spent to make PGD available for the parents of future possible children at risk for childhood genetic disorders would be more than offset by the savings achieved by not having to provide very expensive medical and social interventions for children afflicted with these disorders. The children who would be born without these disorders would have a normal life expectancy, and they would be vulnerable to the whole range of other medical problems to which everyone else is vulnerable. But before many of these vulnerabilities would be actualized, most of these individuals would have enjoyed many healthy decades. However, if we used PGD to eliminate various forms of earlier onset Alzheimer's, or cancers with a strong genetic association, etc., the result would be very high front-end social costs with very little in offsetting health-care savings.

For the sake of argument we will assume that this expansive use of PGD is maximally successful, that we do eliminate thereby what would otherwise be a cause of premature death and disability for some individuals. However, we are mostly speaking of causes of premature death in the later part of life, and we assume that none of these disorders can be properly characterized as "the" cause of the future death of an individual. Instead, it would be more correct to say that we eliminated what might otherwise have been the "first" cause of death and/or significant disability. Keep in mind also that the rejection of one or another eight-cell embryo with the targeted gene might result in choosing an embryo with an unrecognized predisposition to a medical problem that would bring about an even earlier death or serious disability.

Again, given later-in-life medical disorders, we may assume that a second potential cause of death or significant disability could be lurking in the not-very-distant future for each of those individuals. Thus, relative to the decades of life gained per embryo for our first use of PGD, the gain for our second use of PGD is only "marginally beneficial." From the perspective of health-care justice, these additional years of life do not have significant moral weight. Further, though the health-care system as a whole would initially achieve savings by eliminating these potential "first causes" of death or disability, the savings would prove to be ephemeral, because similar health costs would be incurred by these individuals for the "second causes" of their death or disability. As the costs would only have been postponed a few years, our society would not be unjust to refuse to fund publicly this expansive use of PGD.

As a liberal society we would have to permit the wealthy to purchase PGD for more expansive uses. No one is made worse off by permitting this purchase, nor are any of the less well off treated unjustly. Using only their own resources, the wealthy are purchasing what at best is a very marginal and very uncertain benefit for their future possible children. Further, those who are less well off would likely rationally and autonomously reject wanting to access this expansive use of PGD for themselves and their future possible children, given other currently unmet health needs for themselves or their future possible children deserving higher priority for public funding than this expansive use of PGD. The prescription drug benefit for the Medicare elderly is one clear example of such a higher priority health need, with an estimated price tag of $310 billion over the next 10 years (which represents about 65% public funding for those costs). Even if we follow Norman Daniels's Prudential Lifespan Account (1988, chap. 4), which is aimed at showing why it would be both rational and just for each of us to allocate resources away from the latest stages in life to earlier stages in order to maximize the likelihood that each of us would reach old age, that argument would not justify allocating resources for an expansive use of PGD.

Finally, it would be disingenuous to claim that this expansive use of PGD was aimed at meeting either the best interests or the just interests of children as children. The interests that would be met would be the interests of the older adults that these future possible children would become. By way of contrast, the more limited use of PGD we recommend would obviously be aimed at improving the health prospects of children as children as the medical disorders we would seek to eliminate would be disorders that directly affected children. Still, we need to provide more argument to support the claim that justice requires such social support for this intervention.

PREIMPLANTATION GENETIC DIAGNOSIS: AN HISTORICAL SIDE NOTE

For the past five years I have been the co-principal investigator of an NIH funded project through the ELSI program (Ethical, Legal, and Social Implications of the Human Genome Project). The title of this project for its first three years (1995 to 1998) was "Genome Technology and Reproduction: Values and Public Policy." This project has sought to test a certain model of rational democratic deliberation, a more constructive approach to shaping public policy on deeply controversial moral and social issues than we have seen exhibited in the so-called abortion debates. There was a total of 13 two-hour sessions in each of seven Michigan communities with 30 to 50 individuals in each dialogue group. One session involved discussing preimplantation genetic diagnosis.

At the beginning of each cluster of six dialogues we surveyed moral and policy judgment. Responses were on a 5-point Likert scale from "strongly agree" to "strongly disagree." The survey was repeated at the end of each cluster to determine whether or not views had changed significantly over the course of the six dialogues. One item said that government should mandate that 80% of the costs of accessing PGD should be paid either by private insurance or state Medicaid programs (Fleck, 1996a, 1997).

The aggregate response from the seven communities was 21% agreement with the statement and 70% disagreement. This was at the end of the dialogue process and reflected a slight increase in the level of disagreement from the beginning (Fleck, 1997, pp. 32–33). I found this result remarkable, for I would have predicted a 50% to 60% level of agreement initially, which would increase as a result of sustained discussion. Our dialogue groups were broadly representative of each of their communities, at least as far as diversity of viewpoint was concerned. In other respects they were not so representative (e.g., 80% of our participants had college degrees or better). I have used this same item in several dozen other audiences of varying sizes, and I will rarely elicit more than 25% agreement. This suggests considerable social prevalence in this judgment, at least at present.

What I have done is not rigorous survey research. My primary objective was to elicit both policy and moral judgments relating to emerging genetic technologies that would engage participants, spark discussion, and give the discussion focus. My primary reason for believing that this proposal would elicit a fairly high level of initial agreement was that it was aimed at saving babies from considerable suffering and very abbreviated lives. I believed that these facts would connect with very strong intuitions of justice and strong feelings of compassion. This was generally true for the 21% who agreed with this proposal, but as I learned from the discussion there was considerable diversity among reasons for disagreement.

I had expected Right to Life supporters to disagree because PGD necessarily involves discarding excess embryos. I expected advocates for disability groups to disagree because the embryos that would be discarded would be those that would otherwise be born with serious disabilities. I expected political conservatives to disa-

gree because this was a government "mandated" program, and the mandate would be directed at private insurance companies. I was surprised that a number of social liberals disagreed. The most common reason for their disagreement was that stronger just claims associated with other unmet health needs in our society would have to be satisfied before this PGD proposal could be justly funded. Most often they cited the 43 million people without health insurance whose health needs are undiagnosed and often unmet.

I was also surprised by the "appeal to personal freedom" argument, which came from both political liberals and political conservatives. I had taken procreative liberty to be a background condition that had little moral salience for this argument. However, critics attributed considerable salience to this assumption of procreative liberty for thinking through the justice issues.

One version of their argument went like this: A health-care justice argument must start with health-care needs, but no needs are involved in this situation. Potential parents *wish* to have a child. They know there is either a 25% or a 50% chance that they will have a child with a serious genetic disorder. They do not *wish* to have a child with that disorder. They *wish* instead that their child will be born with at least a normal degree of health. Such wishes are quite understandable, but such wishes do not generate health needs, much less any just claims to access PGD at public expense. These parents have options. They do not need to have children; they can have a very satisfying life without children, or they can adopt. They also have the less expensive alternate reproductive option of using sperm or ova from donors whose gametes are very unlikely to result in the conception of a child who will be born with a serious genetic disorder. They may want to have a child that is genetically their own. But again, this is a want, not a need. Further, we are talking about couples who have the capacity to have children of their own. They have effective freedom in this regard.

But there are the 15% of couples in the United States who are infertile, who do not have the capacity to have children of their own without some form of outside assistance. It would seem that if anyone has a moral right to have satisfied the desire to have children, those infertile couples would have a stronger prior right than the couples seeking publicly funded access to PGD. Prima facie, this is a persuasive line of argument against the claim that anyone has a just claim to PGD.

DOES JUSTICE REQUIRE PUBLIC FUNDING FOR LIMITED PGD?

Before responding to the above objections, we need to frame our issue a bit more. In the item used with the dialogue groups, we referred to private insurance companies being "mandated" to cover access to limited PGD. Some considerations of justice make that proposal problematic. Specifically, if this increases the cost of employer-sponsored insurance enough for small marginal firms, they may drop health insurance for their employees, thereby increasing the pool of uninsured. So we can imagine two alternate ways of asking our question. (1) Can a justice-based argument be made for saying that limited access to PGD ought to be considered part of a comprehensive package of health benefits that a just and caring society ought to guarantee to all its citizens? (2) Given the highly fragmented way in which we currently finance health care, and given the unlikelihood of a system of national health insurance in the United States in the foreseeable future, does justice require creating a separate federal program for funding a limited PGD benefit, something akin to the End-Stage Renal Disease Program, which will pay for kidney dialysis or kidney transplant for all who are in renal failure, no matter what their financial, employment, age, or insurance status might be?

Next, there is a metaphysically odd feature to this alleged problem of health-care justice. Ordinarily we have a person who is suffering, or at risk of suffering, a very serious health problem, which can only be addressed by a very expensive or experimental or uncertain health intervention. We want to know whether *that person*, and others similarly situated, have a just claim to that health intervention. But in the case of PGD the object of our inquiry is a *future possible person*, not an actual person with unequivocal moral standing. Moreover, the real issue is not whether we will provide to that future possible person some lifesaving or quality-of-life protecting intervention. Rather, the real issue is whether one future possible person who is at risk of being afflicted with a serious genetic disorder will be replaced by a different future possible person whom we know to be free of that disorder. (This issue does not arise with germline genetic engineering.)

A critic might reasonably ask what the justice-relevant issue is. A strong critic might argue that there is a justice issue, but not what we originally suggested. The problem instead is that we are proposing using social resources to bring one possible person into existence instead of another who is disfavored because of the disabilities with which he or she will be afflicted. The argument continues that we might have to accept reluctantly the right of potential parents to make such a choice as part of procreative liberty, but it would be clearly unjust for social resources to be used to favor existence for one person rather than another when all members of a society are entitled to equal treatment. Respect for parental procreative liberty does not require that sort of social support.

This objection rests upon one very flawed premise. It implicitly assumes that "future possible persons," as represented by some number of embryos in a petri dish, have some sort of strong moral or political right to become actual persons. However, no persuasive argument can sustain that claim. Future possible persons have no actual interests; hence, they have no actual rights. Scenarios can be imagined that might cause us to qualify this last claim, but we may ignore those scenarios for now. If multiple embryos have been brought into existence for a morally permissible purpose, such as avoiding the actual birth of children with serious genetic disorders that would adversely affect both the length and quality of their lives, then both the parents and the larger society are morally free to choose which of those embryos will have an opportunity to become actual persons. Embryos as embryos in this situation can be neither harmed nor discriminated against; this should be regarded as both a conceptual claim and a moral claim. This also implies that it is presumptively morally permissible to use social resources to assist potential parents in achieving their objective of having children born with normal health. It is *not unjust* to use social resources for this goal, unless additional arguments can be adduced to demonstrate an injustice. But we have not yet shown that justice *requires* providing social support for this purpose. In other words, a society such as our own could not be rightly judged to have acted unjustly by failing to provide social resources to support parents in these circumstances.

Advocates for the rights of individuals with disabilities have attempted to adduce arguments aimed at showing that injustices would result from social funding of our limited PGD proposal. One such objection is what is often referred to as the "expressivist objection." In brief, it is the claim that genetic interventions aimed at eliminating disabilities represent a profound devaluing of the lives of people with those disabilities. The social message expressed by such interventions is that we do not want people "like that" in our society. Buchanan (1995) and Buchanan et al. (2000) have provided an effective response to this line of argument. Here is another. As many argue, it is the disabilities themselves that are disfavored, not the people who live with those disabilities. Our society clearly has strong obligations of justice with respect to meeting the needs of individuals with a broad range of disabilities.

Most often the moral basis for this obligation is in something like Daniels's fair equality of opportunity account of health-care justice. For individuals with spinal cord injuries, a just and caring society must provide the wheelchair assistance they need to move about. And buildings must be modified for accessibility. For the blind, there are now computers that can give them effective access to an extremely broad range of informational sources necessary for their accessing the range of opportunities the sighted take for granted. That too represents a requirement of justice.

Still, these interventions are nothing more than "second best" interventions. They provide partial restoration of function but not full and effective function. However, new and extremely promising medical strategies are on the horizon. There is the hope associated with human embryonic stem cells to create any of 200 other types of cells, including nerve cells that could restore nearly full functioning to severed spinal cords or to the nerve tissue associated with sight. If such technologies were maximally successful in their therapeutic intent, then justice would require us to provide such technologies at social expense for individuals with those disabilities.

Some individuals with these disabilities might reject these interventions, but it is easy to imagine that most would embrace them. The net result would be that those with these types of disabilities would become ennabled as a result of their own free choice. Such a result undercuts the force of the expressivist objection, for it is a clear embodiment of the claim that it is the disability itself that is disfavored, not the person with the disability. That is, a real distinction exists between the person with the disability and the disability itself (see also Silvers and Satz, 2000; Silvers, 2001).

Are there considerations of health-care justice that would either warrant or require public funding for access to PGD in the limited circumstances we identified? To be clear, we will defend the view that such funding would be *warranted* by considerations of justice, but not required. In brief, the deep theoretical reason for this conclusion is that the moral terrain of justice is exceptionally complex. There is no single principle of justice that provides us with clear criteria for concluding in all, or even most, instances of need that a particular medical intervention must be provided as a matter of justice.

The moral reality is that our socially shared conception of justice is pluralistic to its core. There are times when the fair equality of opportunity strand of justice provides the surest guide to what is morally required. But, on occasion, the utilitarian strand provides that guidance, or the strong egalitarian strand does, or the libertarian strand, or urgency of need considerations, or considerations of personal responsibility, and so on. Further, when we globally view the entire expanding universe of medical needs with all the heterogeneity of that universe (protease inhibitors for HIV, prescription drugs for the elderly, left ventricular assist devices for congestive heart failure, renal dialysis, neonatal intensive care units for extremely premature infants, rehabilitation for victims of devastating disease or accidents, etc.) we realize that there are some considerations of justice that would provide moral support for meeting any one of these needs, but rarely will that support be decisive and uncontroversial.

We cannot escape the need for medical-care rationing. We have only limited resources for reasonably meeting health needs. Priorities must be established. But our various strands of justice will not yield a list of justice-authorized health-care priorities. Especially in the very broad middle range of any such list, reasonable people will be able to reasonably disagree. But justice as fair treatment will require that we not just accede to random and arbitrary judgments in this middle range. Instead, as we have argued elsewhere (Fleck, 1992, 1994, 1996b, 1998, 1999; see also Daniels and Sabin, 1997, 1998), we appeal to processes of rational democratic deliberation

to achieve a reasonable ordering among our health-care priorities, an ordering that can only be "just enough," given that we must make such judgments in nonideal circumstances under what Rawls (1993) refers to as "the burdens of judgment." It is for these reasons that funding PGD for the circumstances we identified may be *warranted* by considerations of justice but may not be required. If, for example, a fair deliberative process results in the judgment that there are many other health-care needs of higher priority for the resources available, then we may not be able to provide social resources for PGD even though there are some considerations that would support so doing.

What are the considerations of health-care justice that would warrant social funding for at least limited access to PGD? First, there are fair equality of opportunity considerations. Strong considerations of justice require that we provide access to effective rehabilitative services for individuals who have become disabled. We might think that this same response should be required for children born with serious genetic disabilities instead of providing funds for PGD. However, several morally relevant considerations distinguish the situations of the respective groups.

Individuals who acquire disabilities later in life as a result of disease or accident, or individuals who have these disabilities from near birth on as a result of disease or accident beyond our ability to predict or control, are individuals whose initial circumstances are unfortunate, but not unjust. No one could effectively alter their fate. However, given the existence of PGD, we cannot make that same claim for children who might be born with predictable genetic disorders. We cannot be morally indifferent with respect to their fate. Today, as Kitcher contends, we cannot escape responsibility for their fate.

Next, we emphasize that we are speaking of children whose lives will be seriously impaired and dramatically shortened. For many of these children no rehabilitative efforts can make more than the merest marginal difference to either the quality or the length of their lives. This will certainly be true for disorders such as Tay-Sachs or Canavan's or Lesch-Nyhan or muscular dystrophy. Adults who become disabled may have the psychological resources needed to cope with their radically altered life circumstances, but these youngsters, especially those afflicted with both mental and physical disabilities, have no such internal resources available to them because the very roots of those coping capacities are irrevocably damaged. The potential for restoring for them even a small portion of what Daniels calls the "normal opportunity range" is just not there. Hence, for the sake of making possible more lives (different lives, to be sure) in that normal opportunity range, we ought to provide the resources needed for PGD in the circumstances we identified.

We emphasize again that this discussion is based upon respect for the procreative liberty of potential parents. Recognizing this provides an important second step in our argument. Potential parents may know they are at risk for having a child with cystic fibrosis or fragile X syndrome. They may also know that PGD is a socially available option. We will even say that there is a socially funded program in place that makes this option accessible. But they may nevertheless reject that option for, perhaps, deeply religious reasons. They may believe they are religiously obligated to accept whatever children God provides to them, including children born with serious genetic disabilities. They may also have prepared themselves for this possibility, knowing that the demands of parenting were going to be much more rigorous for them than for other parents. If this is the case, then these parents are not open to the charge of having acted irresponsibly (see Andre et al., 2000). Further, they might not be morally culpable for what many would regard as harm to their future possible children.

More importantly, in a liberal pluralistic society the choices of such parents ought to be respected, at least to the extent that there can be reasonable disagreement regarding what should count as culpable harm to children. This means both that social resources should support their efforts to care for their child, and that no social policy should legally require them to use PGD or to refrain from having children. This liberal commitment is an important part of our justice argument, for one of the implications of society extending respect and support to these individuals is that such individuals should extend a similar degree of support and respect to those potential parents who would choose to avail themselves of PGD to avoid having a child with a serious genetic disorder. This is a reasonable practical construal of what fair terms of cooperation might mean in these circumstances. In other words, social resources ought to be available to sustain the choices of couples who would either use or refuse PGD. This is not a choice that emerges from political bargaining. Rather, it is a choice that emerges from a political society in which mutual respect exists for diverse reasonable conceptions of what it means to lead a good life.

The above line of reasoning provides us with resources for responding to the objection raised in the community dialogues, namely that access to PGD is about parental wishes and wants regarding possible children, not needs that would generate just claims. It also opens the question of whether social funding for PGD requires a comparable degree of social funding for infertile couples as a matter of social justice.

There is a more general justice argument for our proposal. Buchanan et al. (2000, pp. 81–82) suggest that in the future a just and caring society ought to do what is in its power to assure each child that is born a "genetic decent minimum." The context for that suggestion is a world in which we have the capacity to do germline genetic engineering, including genetic enhancement. Buchanan and colleagues reject the idea of pursuing genetic equality. The general idea behind a genetic decent minimum is that all children ought to have the capacities to access the normal opportunity range of their society; and, to the extent that those capacities require a sufficiently intact genome, society is obligated to assure that to the extent its medical capacities permitted. We do not have the capacity to do germline genetic engineering; but we do have the capacity to offer PGD for couples at risk of having children with serious genetic disorders. We cannot give a perfectly precise account of what is or is not included in the genetic decent minimum, but we do not need that level of precision for our purposes. All of the genetic disorders we have identified (or implicitly have in mind) would clearly involve serious genetic deficiencies that would deprive the bearers of effective access to large portions of the opportunity range with no compensating advantages. Hence, this consideration would support our proposal.

There remains the morally troubling objection that it seems unjust to fund access to PGD while permitting about 44 million individuals to remain without secure access to needed health care. However, it will not necessarily follow that justice would obligate us to meet those needs before funding the limited PGD program we propose. Here empirical facts, whatever they might turn out to be, will be morally relevant, perhaps determinative. For example, the approximate cost of funding access to PGD for 200,000 children would be $8 billion. These costs should be more than offset by the savings achieved from not providing to children, who would otherwise be born, very substantial health care and social support services. *If that is true*, then no social resources will have been taken away from meeting other health-care needs. No one will have been made worse off as a result of this transfer of resources; no individuals will find themselves denied health resources to which they had a stronger just claim. Our system might fall short of moral approval from the perspective of some "ideally just" health-care system, but the world

we inhabit is a world in which nonideal justice is the most we can reasonably expect to achieve (Fleck, 1987). The outcome we portray here can be fairly characterized as being "just enough."

In concluding, we return to the point made earlier, namely that providing public funding for limited access to PGD is justice-warranted for multiple reasons but may not necessarily be justice-demanded. The practical moral challenge will be to determine, through a fair process of rational democratic deliberation, how high a moral priority such a program ought to be given relative to all the other health needs. Though our major conclusion is modest, it is not without moral force and significance. It says that for the relevant population of potential parents who may be at risk of having a child with a serious genetic disorder they have a *justice-warranted* claim to access PGD at social expense. A society would not be morally justified in treating the issue of such access as merely a matter of social beneficence, something that can be given or withheld as a matter of social charity without being open to moral criticism. Instead, if our conclusion is correct, a society would be morally justified in withholding socially funded access to PGD only if that society could show, given limited resources, that there was a considerable number of other higher priority health needs that justly commanded those resources. It would not be sufficient simply to assert that there were these higher priority health needs; the reasons and arguments would have to be given in accordance with the publicity condition of health-care justice (Gutmann and Thompson, 1996 Daniels and Sabin, 1997, 1998).

A skeptic might be inclined to believe that, in this sort of situation, reasons could never be given that were persuasive and forceful enough to compel most members of a society to accept some particular ordering of health-care priorities. We have already conceded that in many circumstances the burdens of judgment will make it difficult to achieve a consensus. This motivates and justifies an appeal to fair democratic deliberative processes when we need a socially legitimated result. However, in many circumstances a consensus on a specific ordering of health-care priorities could easily be achieved. For example, consider the prioritization of Medicare funding for the left ventricular assist device for patients in end-stage congestive heart failure over funding access to the limited PGD program we have proposed. It would be exceedingly difficult to imagine justice-relevant considerations that could yield this ordering of priorities. Each left ventricular assist devices costs about $150,000. There would be about 200,000 patients each year in the United States who would potentially need that device, a device that would afford them no more than an extra year or two of life for an annual aggregate cost of $30 billion. Neither a utilitarian strand of health care justice, nor a strong egalitarian strand, nor a libertarian strand, nor a fair equality of opportunity strand, nor cost-effectiveness considerations would provide moral support for such an ordering of health priorities. The resources of public reason in this regard are much richer and stronger than philosophic skeptics recognize.

Finally, we need to address what Daniel Callahan (1990) refers to as the "ragged edge" problem with respect to our limited PGD program. In brief, it is that there is no bright line that sharply distinguishes why some individuals with a specific health need have a just claim to health-care resources while other individuals who have very nearly the same need are denied access to those resources.

Earlier in this chapter I allowed, for the sake of argument, that a sharp distinction existed between those later-in-life genetic disorders that children could be born with, and those genetic disorders that children would be born with that would manifest themselves near birth. This distinction suggested that considerations of justice warranted funding the latter but not the for-

mer. The biological and medical realities are that there is a continuum here. Some genetic disorders manifest themselves in the late part of the first decade of life, others in the second or third decade. What would justify our denying potential parents access to PGD at public expense so that they too could choose to have children not at risk for the disorders they fear? The short answer, especially as we get closer to the first decade of life, is that there are no morally compelling considerations that unequivocally justify drawing the line in one place rather than another. The best we can do is seek to achieve democratic deliberative agreement about such matters, taking into account a broad range of factors including predicted cost data for a more expansive benefit, judgments about how much is gained in length or quality of life, medical alternatives on the horizon (such as gene therapy), competing health-care needs, and so forth. The result will necessarily be non-ideal, but it will be "just enough" and "rational enough," and it will have sufficient legitimacy that it ought to be respected by reasonable people in a liberal, morally pluralistic society.

REFERENCES

Andre, J., Fleck, L. and Tomlinson, T. (2000). On being genetically "irresponsible." *Kennedy Institute of Ethics Journal* 10, 129–46.

Buchanan, A. (1995). Equal opportunity and genetic intervention. *Social Philosophy and Policy* 12, 105–35.

Buchanan, A., Brock, D. Daniels, N. and Wikler, D. (2000). *From Chance to Choice: Genetics and Justice.* New York: Cambridge University Press.

Callahan, D. (1990). *What Kind of Life: The Limits of Medical Progress.* New York: Simon & Schuster.

Daniels, N. (1985). *Just Health Care.* New York: Cambridge University Press.

Daniels, N. (1988). *Am I My Parents' Keeper? An Essay on Justice Between the Old and the Young.* New York: Oxford University Press.

Daniels, N. (1993). Rationing fairly: Programmatic considerations. *Bioethics* 7, 224–33.

Daniels, N. and Sabin J. (1997). Limits to health care: Fair procedures, democratic deliberation, and the legitimacy problem for insurers. *Philosophy and Public Affairs* 26, 303–50.

Daniels, N. and Sabin J. (1998). Last chance therapies and managed care: Pluralism, fair procedures and legitimacy. *Hastings Center Report* 28, 27–41.

Fleck, L. (1987). DRGs: Justice and the invisible rationing of health care resources. *Journal of Medicine and Philosophy* 12, 165–96.

Fleck, L. (1992). Just health care rationing: A democratic decisionmaking approach. *University of Pennsylvania Law Review* 140 (May), 1597–1636.

Fleck, L. (1994). Just caring: Oregon, health care rationing, and informed democratic deliberation. *Journal of Medicine and Philosophy* 19, 367–88.

Fleck, L. (1996a). *Genome Technology and Reproduction: Values and Public Policy. A Report on the Fall Community Dialogues.* East Lansing: Michigan State University.

Fleck, L. (1996b). *Just Caring: Rational Democratic Deliberation, Health Care Rationing, and Managed Care.* Paper presented at the American Association of Bioethics Meeting, San Francisco, November.

Fleck, L. (1997). *Genome Technology and Reproduction: Values and Public Policy. A Report on the Spring Community Dialogues.* East Lansing: Michigan State University.

Fleck, L. (1998). Justice, rights and Alzheimer disease genetics. In S. Post and P. Whitehouse (eds.), *Genetic Testing for Alzheimer Disease: Ethical and Clinical Issues.* Baltimore: Johns Hopkins University Press, pp. 190–208.

Fleck, L. (1999). Just caring: Managed care and protease inhibitors. In J. Arras and B. Steinbock (eds.), *Ethical Issues in Modern Medicine,* 5th ed. Mountain View, CA: Mayfield, pp. 679–86.

Gutmann, A. and Thompson, D. (1996). *Democracy and Disagreement.* Cambridge, MA: Harvard University Press.

Kitcher, P. (1996). *The Lives to Come: The Genetic Revolution and Human Possibilities.* New York: Simon & Schuster.

Rawls, J. (1993). *Political Liberalism.* New York: Columbia University Press.

Silvers, A. and Satz, A. (2000). Disability and biotechnology. In M. Mehlman and T. Murray (eds.), *The Encyclopedia of Biotechnology: Ethical, Legal and Policy Issues.* New York: John Wiley.

Silvers, A. (2001). Normality and functionality. In M. Mahowald, V. McKusick, A. Scheurle, and T. Aspinwall (eds.), *Genetics in the Clinic: Clinical, Ethical, and Social Implications for Primary Care.* St. Louis: Mosby.

Index

Abortion, 427
Access, 426
   free, 134
   to health care, 398–399
      universal, 178–180, 433
   to mental health care, 249
      stigma and, 255–256
"Accountability for reasonableness," 7, 15, 19,
   145
Activity-specific principles of justice, 201
Acupuncture, 322
Acute care/illness, 81, 210, 241, 242
Addiction, 411–412. *See also* Drug abuse
   defined, 412
   and freedom, 412–414
   as mental illness, 416–417
   and personal identity, 414–417
   and public health, 417–418
   rational, 415
   theories of, 415–416
Addictive desire
   analyzing the Homeric solution to, 419
   managing the problem of, 418
Addictive substances, 409. *See also* Drug abuse
Adherence, 351
Adoption, 428–429
Advocacy, 292–293
Affirmative action, 273. *See also* Fair equality of
   opportunity

African Americans. *See also* Distrust; Race
   mortality among, 173–174
Age. *See also* Elderly
   and priority of treatments, 148
   and QALY approach, 57
   and in vitro fertilization, 435–436
Age rationing, 270–271
   claims of partial compliance theory and, 272–
   276
Age standardized burden of injury and disease, 172,
   173
Agency, 123–125
   three-dimensional theory of, 126–130
Aggregation, 16, 19, 66, 69–70, 366–367, 379
   defined, 66
Aging population, 193
Aid to Families with Dependent Children (AFDC),
   112, 113
Aid-in-dying, 273–274
AIDS/HIV, 101, 219, 256
Alcoholism, 416. *See also* Addiction; Drug abuse
Alternative medicine, 319, 320
   how health plans should respond to, 326–331
      costs, coverage, and, 328–330
      promoting good care within prudent limits,
      330–331
      risks, benefits, and, 327–328
   measuring up to science, 322–325
      implications, 325–326

Alternative medicine (*continued*)
  radically different perspectives, 320–322
  research findings, 328–329
American Medical Association (AMA), 228, 408
Americans with Disabilities Act (ADA), 21n.2, 294, 296
Amundson, Ron, 240
Anderson, Elizabeth, 239
Antidiscrimination, 48
Anti-Free-Riding Principle (AFRP), 25–29, 35, 36n.5
APOE, 447
Appeals condition, 16–17, 19
Appleby, Joyce, 100, 122, 131n.2
Applied ethics, 20, 212
Archer, Margaret, 131n.4
Aristotle, v, 3, 121, 216
Arneson, Richard, 238
Assisted suicide. *See* Physician aid-in-dying
Associated Provincial Picture Houses Ltd v. Wesnesbury Corp., 160
Atomistic philosophies, 176
Audi alteram partem, 159
Aurelius, Marcus, 408
Australia, 99, 170, 172, 173
Australian health system, 170
  aboriginal health programs, 180
  evolution of, 178
  responding to the social reality of health, 177
  universal access to services, 178–180
Australians, indigenous and nonindigenous
  death rates by age, 174
Autonomy, 122, 125–129, 153, 273–274, 348
  justice and, 60–61

"Backlash attitudes," 273
Balanced Budget Act of 1997, 107
"Balancing Argument" claims, 378, 381
Barry, Michael, 162–164
Basic human interests, 91
Basic need(s), 88, 306. *See also* Need(s)
  health care as, 88–89
Becker, Gary, 415
Bedside justice, 235–237, 245
  clear-sighted, 246
Benchmarks of fairness, 402–403
Beneficence, 406
  respect *vs.*, 406–407, 421
  "weighted," 365–367
Benevolence, 261, 298
Bentham, Jeremy, 56
Berg, Barbara, 430
Berkeley, George, 56
Best-interest standard, 265–266
  as an ideal, 266
Beta-interferon, 150
Bingham, Thomas, 166
Birth defects, 243
Blame and blamelessness, 238
Blaming the sick for being sick, 408–410

Bobbitt, Philip, 67
Bone marrow transplant, 325
"Bottomless pit" problem, 371
Bourdieu, Pierre, 132n.14
BRCA1 gene, 447
Bridge, Lord, 162
British National Health Service. *See* National Health Service
Brock, Dan W., 411, 412
Buchanan, Allen E., 411, 412
Bunch, Charlotte, 229
Burdens of disease, 148, 177, 274, 401
Burdens of judgment, 453
Burley, Justine, 427

Calabressi, Guido, 67
Callahan, Daniel, 21n.4, 270, 456
Canada, 144
Canavan's disease, 454
Canavan's Lesch Nyhan, 454
Cancer treatments
  alternative, 321
  bone marrow transplant, 325
Capabilities, 8, 10, 48
  "basic," 175
Capabilities view/approach, 14, 132n.20, 169, 175
Caplan, Arthur, 241, 349
Care, 291. *See also* Advocacy
Caregivers, 210, 232, 278–279, 283–285, 293, 294
Caring, 347–348
"Case law," 17
Cassell, Eric J., 235, 240
Chapman, Audrey, 95n.1
Charity, 87, 112, 211, 310
Child health care, 259–261
  efficiency and social utility, 264–265
  empathy and sympathy for children and, 261–262
    need for more, 262–263
Childrearing, 262
Children, 282
  and equality of opportunity, 263–264
Children's Health Insurance Program (CHIP), 111, 114, 116, 262
Children's rights
  empathy and sympathy as basis for, 262
Child-Turcotte-Pugh (CTP) scoring system, 350, 351
Choice, 10, 67–68, 153–154
  freedom of, 124. *See also* Liberty(ies)
Chronic care, 150–151, 162
Chronic illness, 150–151, 162
Chronically Sick and Disabled Persons Act 1970, 162
Civil Rights Act of 1964, 104
Claim rights, 5
Clinical trials, 101, 197–198. *See also* Randomized controlled trials
  coercive offers, 201–202
  exploitation of subjects, 202–204
Clinton, Bill, 106

Clozapine, 374, 375, 381–383, 386
Coercion, 26–27, 201–202
Cognitive ability. *See also* Mental incapacity; Mentally retarded persons
　and competence, 411
Common good, 18
Common law, 305
Communitarian approach, 62
Communitarianism, liberal, 45
Community rating (of premiums), 274
Compassion, 211, 256
Compensatory justice, vi
Competence, 209, 412. *See also* Incompetence
　elements of, 347, 411
　focal *vs.* global, 411
Complaint account, 71–74
　limits of, 74–75
　model, 71–72
Congenital anomalies, 243
Consent, 27, 31
　informed, 202, 267
　prior, 25, 30
Consequentialism, 66, 165, 367. *See also* Utilitarianism
　semi-consequentialist position, 296
Consequentialist view, full, 296
Constitutional theory, 103
Constructed-environment, 293, 296
Context in health-care decision making, 66–68
Context-sensitive morality, 67–69
Contraception. *See* Reproductive freedom
Contractarianism, 297
Contractualist theory/reasoning, 368, 371
Correlative thesis, 79
Cost containment
　strategies for, 195
Cost-effectiveness
　combining it with other values, 146–147
　ethical issues and, 147–151
　unfair use of, for allocation decisions, 395
Cost-effectiveness analysis, 55, 362, 363, 395, 397–398
Cost-efficiency, 3, 29
Cost-worthiness, 36n.7
Council of International Organizations of Medical Societies (CIOMS), 202–203
Counterfactual endorsement of disadvantaged person, 72
Cranston, Maurice, 86–88
Cultural diversity, 38, 39
Culture, 210
Cystic fibrosis, 447, 454

DALE (disability-adjusted life expectancy), 317, 391, 401. *See also* QALY and DALY
DALY (disability-adjusted life year[s]), 148, 394–395. *See also* QALY and DALE
Daniels, Norman, vi, 3, 21n.2, 46–48, 95n.8, 144, 239–240, 270, 402, 448, 449
de Wert, Guido, 435
Decent minimum, 13

Decision-making abilities, 412
Deinstitutionalization, 250–251, 409
Democracy/democratic society regimes, 10, 39, 40, 49, 94, 123
　justice and, 61
Democratic deliberation, rational, 453
Denmark. *See* Scandinavia
Dental care/treatment/disease, 81, 151, 210, 257–258
　compassion, urgency, and, 256–257
Deontological rights, 165
Dependency, 224, 253, 298–299
　"inevitable," 291
　justice and, 296–298
Dependency consequentialism, 298
Dependency relation, 293
Dependency relationships, moral importance of, 294–296
"Dependency" work(ers), 232, 294, 295
Descartes, René, 126–127
Descriptive ethics, 212
Deserts, 53, 55, 126
Deserving, 209
Desire accounts, 136
Developing nations, 198
　coercive offers, 201–202
　exploitation of subjects, 202–204
　justice of using placebo control group, 198–201
DeVille, Kenneth, 223
Diagnosis, 309
Difference principle, 13, 263, 362–363, 367
Dignity, human, 78
　health care and, 89–90
Disability-adjusted life expectancy (DALE), 317, 391, 401. *See also* DALY; QALY
Disability-adjusted life year(s) (DALY), 148, 394–395. *See also* DALE; QALY
Disability(ies), 453. *See also* Preimplantation genetic diagnosis
　"burden of, 400–401
　drug addiction and, 411
Disabled persons, 99, 162, 210, 239
　assisted reproduction and, 434–435, 452
Discontinuing nonfutile use of a scarce resource, 373–374, 388n.1. *See also* Urgency
Discontinuing treatment, issues specific to, 374–377
Discrimination, 8, 48
　allocation decisions that discriminate against specific populations, 395–396
Distributive justice, v–vi, 122–124, 302
　and health care, 7–8, 213–214, 307, 426
Distrust, 213
　among African Americans, 209, 215–218
　problem of, 218–219
　ways to overcome, 219–222
Donnelly, Jack, 90
Double effect, 59
Double jeopardy, 150–151
Doulia, 296, 297, 299n.12

Down syndrome, 236, 237, 299n.6, 429
Dresser, Rebecca, 226
Driver, Julia, 217
Drug abuse, 352, 406, 407, 409. *See also* Addiction
Drugs
  prescription, 111, 146, 156, 178, 195, 197
    research on, 324, 325
  "war" on (people who use), 409
Duchenne's muscular dystrophy, 447
Duration of poor health, 370. *See also* Chronic
    illness
Duties, 79, 406, 421n.1
  negative and positive, 80
  to protect best interest of incompetent people, 265
    threshold for intervention and reasonable
      judgment, 265–266
Dworkin, Ronald, 100, 123–126, 131, 427
Dying persons, 149–150
Dystrophy, 454

Early and Periodic Screening, Diagnosis and
    Treatment program (EPSDT), 112–113
Education, 13
  "suitable," 163
Education Act 1993, 163
Effectiveness
  defined, 152
  evidence of, 152–153
Efficacy, 350–351. *See also* Utility
Efficiency, 393, 394
  justice and, 309–310
Egalitarianism, 35, 39, 364
  medical, 32, 33
Egoism, 58
Egoism, rational, 58
Elderly, 193, 210, 275–276
  indigent, 111
  vulnerability of the frail, 275
Emanuel, Ezekiel, 40, 44–46, 49
Embryonic stem cells, human, 446, 452
Embryos, 451, 452
Emergency care, 408
Emergency Medical Treatment and Active Labor
    Act (EMTLA), 28
Emergency room (ER), 4, 65, 71, 73–74
Emergency departments, 102
Empathy, as grounding for justice, 261–262
Enforcement condition, 17, 19
Engelhardt, H.T., Jr., 40–45
England. *See* United Kingdom
Epidemics, 81
Epstein, Richard, 305, 307–310
Equal Importance Principle, 124, 126
Equal Opportunity for Welfare (EOW), principle of,
    25, 32–35
Equality
  of opportunity, 18, 263–264, 364–365, 446
  theory of liberal, 427
Equity, 3, 316, 349–350
  principle of, 153

Ethics, 20
  branches of, 212
Eugenics, 446
European Convention of Human Rights, 157, 161
Evaluative ability, and competence, 411
"Evidence-based" medicine, 324–326, 328–329
Expressivist objection, 452
Extra arm case, 379–380

Fair equal opportunity, 184, 188
Fair equality of opportunity, 8–9, 48, 49, 263, 446,
    448, 452
Fair financing, 391–392
Fair process, 7
Fair terms of cooperation, 14, 16, 18, 19, 47
Fair-mindedness, 18
Fairness, 11, 47, 137, 399–400
  benchmarks of, 402–403
  justice as, 7, 8, 11, 16, 47
  of limits to health care, 14–20
Faith, 321, 327–328
Families, 210, 280. *See also* Caregivers
  embodying patterns of injustice, 282
  and individualism, 280
  injustices to, 279–281, 287
  practical identities, 281–282, 286–287
  threats to, 281–282
    propensity for exploitation, 281
"Family care," right to, 285–288
Faulkner, William, 271
Fault, 10
Federal Insurance Contributions Act (FICA), 274,
    277n.8
Feminists, 224, 227–228
  difference, 226–227
  diversity, 225, 229
  dominance, 225, 227, 229
  sameness, 225–227
Fertility. *See* In vitro fertilization
FICA (Federal Insurance Contributions Act), 274,
    277n.8
Financing, fair. *See* Fair financing
Finland. *See* Scandinavia
Food and Drug Administration (FDA), 324, 325
Fragile X syndrome, 454
Freedom. *See also* Liberty(ies)
  addiction and, 412–414
Free-market systems, 3, 42
Free-riders/free-riding, 25–27
  and compulsory universal insurance, 27–29
Fried, Charles, 72
Functionings, 175
Future possible persons, 451

Gay couples, and contract pregnancy, 434
Gender, 9
Gender justice in health care
  dependency approach to achieving, 230–232
  difference approach to achieving, 224, 226–227
  diversity approach to achieving, 224, 229–230

dominance approach to achieving, 224, 225, 227–229
sameness approach to achieving, 224–226
Genetic counseling, 230
Genetic decent minimum, 454–455
Genetic disorders, 230, 447, 451–452
Genetic responsibility, 446
Genetic technologies, 230, 446, 447, 454
German health-care system, 28, 195
Global (principles of) justice, 201
Godwin, William, 56
Goffman, Irving, 294, 295
Good, the, 399. *See also* Public good(s)
conceptions of, 39, 40, 245
giving some sway to patients' view of, 244–246
Goodness, universality of, 58
Gornick, Marian E., 220
GP (general practitioner) system, 187
Grimes, 266–268
Gross domestic product (GDP), 11–13, 130, 170, 191
Gross national product (GNP), 185, 262
Group homes, 294
Growth-hormone deficiency and treatment, 10, 18
Guide cost, 147–151

Hacker, Andrew, 218
Handicap. *See* Disability(ies)
Happiness, 8, 54. *See also* Utilitarianism
Harris, John, 57–59, 150
Harrison, Michelle, 227
Hart, H.L.A., 156
Hastings Center Report, 242, 244–245
Hayek, F.A., 420–421
Health. *See also specific topics*
defined, vi, 78
factors influencing societal, 12–13
Health care. *See also specific topics*
as basic necessity, 308–309
as special, 6
special moral importance of, 7–10
Health Care Financing Administration (HCFA), 107, 109, 115
Health-care systems. *See specific topics*
Health Maintenance Organizations (HMOs), 108, 109, 125
Health outcomes (measures), 100
persistent inequality in, 12–13, 171
income inequality and, 172–173
income level, social class, and, 170–172
position of disadvantaged groups, 173–174
Health Utilities Index (HUI), 365–366, 369
Health-care delivery systems, 104
Health-care enigma, the, 121–123
Health-system performance assessment
alternatives in, 400–403
vs. health attainment, 391–394
justice concerns about, 393–396
Hedonism, 136
Hegel, Georg Wilhelm Friedrich, 161

Hemophilia, 447
Hidden dependencies, 293
Hippocratic Oath, 80
Hippocratic physician, 82, 376
HIV, 101, 174. *See also* AIDS/HIV
HIVNET 012, 197, 199
Hobbes, Thomas, 126–127
Holdout(s), honest, 26, 27, 34–35
Holmes, Oliver Wendell, 292
Home-based care, 157, 285
Homeopathy, 322, 332n.14
Homer. *See The Odyssey*
Hospitalization for mental illness, 250–251
Human rights, 84–85, 87. *See also* Right(s)
defined, 84
secular, 157–159, 161–163
Human Rights Act 1998, 161, 162, 164
Human Rights Committee, 87
Hume, David, 261
Huntington's disease, 448
Hutcheson, Francis, 53

Ideal justice (theory), 99, 210, 270, 272–274
Identifiability of claimants, 68, 71–74
and limits of complaint account, 74–75
Identifiable patients, favored over nonidentifiable patients, 148–149
Identities
personal, 414–417
practical, 281–282, 286–287
Immigration, 38
Imminence of harm, 66, 68–70
Impact, 152
Impartiality, 56, 58
In vitro fertilization (IVF), 230, 426, 429–431. *See also* Reproduction, medically assisted
dangers, 429–430
and post-menopausal women, 435–436
single women and female couples, 433–434
Incentives, 351
Income inequality(ies), 12–13, 170, 172–173
Incompetence, 265, 410–411. *See also* Competence
Independence, 252. *See also* Dependency; Self-sufficiency
Indigent elderly, 111
Indirect benefits, 369
Individualism, 122, 176, 252–253
ethical, 124–126
families and, 280
Individuality, 137
Inequalities in health, as unjust, 10–14
Inequities in health care, 105
Infants, 260. *See also* Neonates
Informed consent, 202, 267
Institute of Medicine (IOM), 353
Insurance, health
compulsory universal, 27–29
discriminatory practices, 252
disparities, 253–254
giving special status to, 9

Insurance, health (*continued*)
   national, 103–107
   private, 251
   reimbursement for mental health care, 249–251,
      254
   single-payer, 131
   state-administered, 110–111, 115–117
   universal, 100, 102, 116
Integrity, principle of personal, 25, 29–30
Intelligence, and moral status, 293–294
Intensive care units (ICUs), 438. *See also* Neonatal
   medicine
Interests, collective
   vs. rights, 164–165
International Covenant on Civil and Political Rights
   (ICCPR), 89, 93
Italian health-care system, 191–196
   National Health Care Plan, 191–192, 194
Italy, 99, 101. *See also* National Health Service

Johnson, Karen, 227
Judicial review, 100, 156, 159, 160, 163
Just Sharing, principle of, 25, 34–35
Just society, defined, 175
Justice, 32. *See also specific topics*
   defined, v, 3
   global, 201
   health care and, 304–309
   is good for health, 237–238
      equalizing opportunity, 239–240
      equalizing welfare, 238–239
   nonideal, 455. *See also* Ideal justice (theory);
      Partial compliance (theory)
   and the social reality of health, 174–177
   three questions of (a theory of), 6–7
   types of, vi
Justice Laws, 157, 158

Kamm, Francis M., 16, 21n.6, 67–69, 73, 76nn.4–
   7, 317, 368, 370
Kant, Immanuel, 216, 405–407, 421, 421n.1,
   422n.9
Kennedy-Krieger Institute, 266–267
Kerr-Mills program, 106, 111, 112
Kidney disease. *See* Renal disease
Kidney transplantation, 359n.1, 451
Kind, P., 55
Kitcher, Philip, 446
Kittay, Eva, 224, 231–232, 295–296
Korsgaard, Christine, 281

Lead poisoning, 266–268
Learning disabilities, 151
Legal positivism, 158–161, 163
Legitimate expectations, 275
Lesbian couples, and in vitro fertilization, 433–
   434
Leveling down (objection), 136, 364, 365
Levine, Carol, 282–284

Liberal communitarianism, 45
Liberalism, 41, 116, 125–126
   "neutralist," 44
Liberals, welfare, 421
Libertarian response to pluralism, a, 41–44
Libertarianism, 25, 31, 34, 42, 53, 189, 421
Liberty rights, 5
Liberty(ies), 3, 24, 53, 60, 407. *See also* Choice;
   Freedom
   vs. responsibility, 25
Life expectancy, 101, 150
Life span
   increasing average, 193
   normal, 8
"Life span" approach to justice in health care, 193
Life-extending *vs.* quality-enhancing treatment, 151
Life-maintaining care, 89
Life-sustaining treatment, discontinuing. *See*
   Discontinuing treatment
Life-with-an-extra-arm case, 380
Limbs, persons lacking, 243, 245–246
Limb-threatening disease, 73–75, 76n.5–6, 77n.11
Literacy, adult, 13
Liver allocation (transplants). *See also*
   Transplantation
   advances in the justice of, 356–358
   UNOS policy, 345–346. *See also* United Network
      for Organ Sharing
Lottery theory, 146
Luck, 10

Madison, James, 103, 118
Managed care, 250
Market competition, 304, 310
Martin, D.K., 144
Maximin principle, 15, 138, 366, 386, 388
Mazimize position, 15
Means-tested health coverage, 111–115, 276
Medibank, 179
Medicaid, 82, 229, 231
   state-run and means-tested, 111–115
   structure of, 111
Medical decisions, depersonalizing, 236–237
Medical savings accounts (MSAs), 110
Medicare, 230, 273
   in Australia, 179–180
   and mental health care, 249
   political economy of, 106–107
      distributive politics, 109
      redistributive politics, 109–110
      special-interest politics, 107–109
      the year 1965 reconsidered, 110
   privatization, 110
"Medicare Buy-In" program (QMB/SLMB), 111,
   114, 115, 119n.6
Medicare Catastrophic Coverage Act (MCCA), 114
MELD/PELD Scoring Systems, 356–358
Men, single
   and contract pregnancy, 434

Mental Health: A Report of the Surgeon General (MHR), 248–250, 252, 255
Mental health care, 248–249
  deinstitutionalization and insurance reimbursement disparities, 250–251
  insurance reimbursement and disparities for medical *vs.*, 249–251, 254
  outpatient, 251
  stigma, compassion, and, 255–258
Mental Health Parity Act, 250, 255
Mental illness, 210, 248–249
Mental incapacity, 267, 293–294
Mentally retarded persons, 290–299, 443
  advocacy for, 292–293
  intelligence and moral status, 293–294
  justice and inevitable dependency, 296–298
Mental-Special View, 381–382
Meta-ethics, 212
Midwives, 228
Mill, James, 61
Mill, John Stuart, 60, 405, 420
Minimal security, 88–89
Model for End Stage Liver Disease (MELD) Scoring System, 356–358
Modus vivendi, 40
Moral catastrophe, 165
Moss, A., 237
Multiculturalism, 38, 50, 210
  justice, pluralism, and, 38–41
Multifunctionalism, 236
Multiple person clinics, case of, 383
Multiple sclerosis (MS), 150, 369–370
Mummery, Lord, 160
Murphy, Kevin, 415
Murray-Wagner-Dingell health insurance proposal, 105

Nagel, Thomas, 137–138, 366, 367
Najman, J.M., 170
Narvarro, Vincent, 402
National health insurance and the Madisonian design, 103–107
National Health Interview Survey, 261
National Health Service (NHS)
  British, 10–11, 100, 134–135, 151, 156, 420
  Plan of 2000, 140–142
  and treatment according to need, 140–143
  Italian, 191, 192
National Institute of Clinical Excellence (NICE), 151
National Institute of Health (NIH), 65
Natural law, 158, 159
Natural rights, 79–81
Need(s), 306. *See also* Basic need(s)
  constant. *See* Basic need(s)
  for health care, 135–136, 378
  nature of, 135
  vs. preferences, 8
  treatment according to, 136–140
Needs theory, 146

Need-satisfaction, 135, 137–139
Nemo judex in rem suam, 159
Neonatal medicine, 438–439
Neonates/newborns, 260–261
  with complex congenital anomalies, 442–443
  premature and compromised, 438–439, 443–444
    discontinuing intensive care support, 441–442
    lower limits of viability, 439–441
Netherlands health care system, 28, 195
Neurofibromatosis, 447
"Neutralist liberalism," 44
Neutrality, temporal, 377
Neutrality constraint, 44
Newachecket, Paul, 261
Nicotine, 416
Non-consequentialists, 66, 67, 73
Nord, Erik, 16, 75n.2, 369, 396
Nordic countries. *See* Scandinavia
Normal functioning/normalcy, 7, 21n.1, 240–241, 245, 252, 377, 381–382. *See also* Rehabilitative care
  enhancing, 10
Normal opportunity range, 7, 33, 286, 287, 454
Normal people, case of producing more, 387
Normal species function, vi
Normative ethics, 212
Norway. *See* Scandinavia
Nozick, Robert, 363–364
Nussbaum, Martha, 175
Nutrition, 81. *See also* Alternative medicine

Odyssey, The, 418–419, 423n.38
"One Day Case," 384–385
Opportunity costs, 394
Opportunity-based view, 14
Opportunity(ies), vi, 3, 33
  protecting, 10
Oral Health: A Report of the Surgeon General (OHR), 256–257
Organ Procurement and Transplant Network (OPTN), 345, 353
Organ Procurement Organizations (OPOs), 345, 349, 353, 359
Organ transplantation. *See* Transplantation
Organization for Economic Co-operation and Development (OECD), 390
Oscar effect, 422n.18
"Ought implies can," 79–80
Outcome, 377–388
Overlapping consensus, 40
Oxfordshire Health Authority, 145, 147, 149, 151, 152
Oxfordshire Priorities Forum, 148, 151–152
  ethical framework, 152–154
  types of decisions, 154
Ozar, David, 88–89, 96n.11

Palliative care, 149–150
Parfit, Derek, 364, 365

Partial compliance (theory), 99, 210, 270, 271–
   272
   claims of, 272–276
Paternalism, 9, 187, 188, 221, 226, 422n.10
Patient's rights. *See* Right(s)
Payton, Brenda, 405–411
Pediatric End Stage Liver Disease (PELD) Scoring
   System, 356, 357
Peffer, Rodney, 124
Personal identities, 414–417
Personal integrity, principle of, 25, 29–30
Personal Responsibility and Work Opportunity Act
   of 1997 (PROWRA), 277n.10
Personhood, 293
PETRA trial, 198
Physician aid-in-dying, 273–274
Physician–patient relationship, 194–195
Physicians, beliefs and attitudes of, 220–222. *See*
   also Alternative medicine
Placebo control groups, 198–201, 267, 323–324
Placebo effect, 323, 326
Placebos, 333n.20
Plato, 408
Pluralism, 39, 40, 50
   legal, 161
   a liberal communitarian response to, 44–46
   a libertarian response to, 41–44
   and Rawlsian political liberalism, 46–49
Pluralistic market system, 24–25, 32, 35
Pluralistic society, 39
Pogge, Thomas, 296
Political conception of justice, 40
Political liberalism. *See also* Liberalism
   Rawlsian, 46–49. *See also* Rawls
Political parties, 118
Poor law model, 185
Poor persons, 99. *See also* Poverty
Population growth, 93, 428
Positivism, legal, 158–161, 163
Poverty, 111, 211, 301–304. *See also* Poor persons
Practical identities, 281–282, 286–287
Pregnancy, contract, 431
   public financing of, 431–433
Preimplantation genetic diagnosis (PGD), 447
   costs, 448
   framing the issue, 447–449
   historical side note, 449–451
   public funding for limited, 451–456
Presumed Prior Consent, principle of, 25, 30
Prevention, 10, 241
Primary institutions, 156
Prior consent, 25, 30
Prioritarianism, 363–365, 367, 368
Priorities Forum. *See* Oxfordshire Priorities Forum
Prioritization. *See also specific topics*
   absolute priority view, 137
   how much priority for the worse off, 370–371
   priorities and, 362
   "priorities problem," 15
   who are the worse off for, 367–370

Prisoner's dilemma, 354
Private goods, 129–130
Private health-care sector, 187, 189–190, 251
Privatization of Medicare, 110
Procedural justice, 16
Procreative liberty, 446
Professional roles, 70–71
Proportional benefit principle, 371
Prospective payment system (PPS), 107–108
Prudential grounds, 40
Prudential Lifespan Account, 449
Psychiatric illness. *See* Mental illness
Public good(s), 18, 25, 129–130
Public health care. *See also specific topics*
   categories of, 95n.2
Public law, 156–158
Public reason, 20, 47
Publicity condition, 16, 17

QALY. *See* Quality-adjusted life-year(s). *See also*
   DALE and DALY.
QMB/SLMB. *See* "Medicare Buy-In" program
Qualified Individuals (QI), 115
Quality of life (QL), 54, 323
Quality-adjusted life-year(s) (QALY) approach/
   model, 57, 58, 61, 146, 147–151, 153, 164,
   265. *See also* DALE; DALY; Utilitarian
   critiques of QALY model
   essence of, 146
   guide cost and, 147–151
   as utilitarian approach to justice in health care,
   54–55

Race, 9, 130
   and mortality, 173–174
Racism, health care and, 214–215
"Ragged edge" problem, 456
Randomized controlled trials (RCTs), 322–324,
   328, 329. *See also* Clinical trials
Rational agency, 127
Rational democratic deliberation, 453
Rationing, 30, 31, 453
   to a core service, 142–143
Rationing decisions, 15–16
   cost-effectiveness as starting point for, 146
Rawls, John, 8, 39–40, 49, 121, 280
   "detached" conception of democracy, 123
   on stability, 217–218
   theory and principles of justice, vi, 3, 8, 11, 13–
   14, 20, 123–124, 175, 213, 417–418. *See*
   also Difference Principle
   justice as fairness, 7, 8, 11, 16, 47
Rawlsian framework, 48, 123, 124
Rawlsian liberalism, 39–41
Reasonable conceptions, 40
Reasonable effort, 71
Reasonable pluralism, 41. *See also* Pluralism
Reasonableness, 16, 18, 145
   accountability for, 7, 15, 19, 145

Reciprocation, 296
Reflective equilibrium, 212
Regression, 375, 376, 384, 385
Rehabilitative care, allocating, 244–246
    pursuing the goal of normal functioning, 240–241
    referring to patients' personal traits and values, 242–244
Relationships, special, 70–71
Relative-income hypothesis, 12
Relevance condition, 16–19, 144, 145
Relevant personal features, 174
Religion and religiosity, 56–57, 159, 454
Renal disease, end-stage, 273
Reproduction, 228
    intervening in, 93
    medically assisted, 426, 428. *See also* In vitro fertilization
Reproductive freedom, as basic human right, 127, 228, 427–428
    objections to
        from adoption, 428–429
        feminist, 429–430
        from population growth, 428
Rescue, rule of, 148–149
Research, 324–325
Research standards, 199, 200
Resource(s). *See also specific topics*
    allocation, 7, 72, 77n.11, 145, 151, 192
    allocation decisions, 156
    limited, 156
Respect, 318, 406
    vs. beneficence, 406–407, 421
Responsibility(ies), 10, 25, 129. *See also* Blame
    attitudes toward individual and social, 122
    collective, 305–307
    and control, 410
    genetic, 446
    just distribution of, 407–408
    personal
        for health, 405–406, 408
        holding responsible and taking, 410
    shared, 195
Responsiveness, 391, 392, 398
Restorative justice, vi
Retributive justice, vi
"Ribicoff children," 112
Right(s), 83n.1. *See also* Human rights; *specific topics*
    abandoning the concept of, 165
    and cans, 79–83
    to health, vi, 5, 82, 85–86
    to health care, 5, 48, 81, 85–86, 130, 185
        arguments against, 78–83
        as basic right, 90–91
        content of, in international law, 92–95
        justifying, 88–92
    infringement of, 165
    of man, 87. *See also* Human rights
    negative *vs.* positive, 5, 427

    as shield, 166
    social and economic, 87
    violation of, 90, 165
Rights-based judicial reasoning, 157–159, 161–163, 166
Right-to-choose principle, 188
Risk-budgets, 72, 74
Rosser, R.M., 55
Ruddick, Sara, 291
Rule of rescue, 148–149
Rule utilitarianism, 58, 165
Rule-based reasoning, 157, 166

Sabin, J., 144
Saltman, R.B., 184
Sanctity-of-life doctrine, 57
Sandel, Michael, 125, 169, 176
Scandinavia, 99, 183, 184
    future challenges, 187–188
    problems in 1980s and 1990s, 183, 184
    Scandinavian approach, 183–185
    welfare states in the twenty-first century, 189–190
Scanlon, T.M., 71, 138
Scarcity, 4, 72, 102, 163
Schauer, Frederick, 166
Schizophrenia, 249, 317, 374, 375
Science
    and alternatives, 322
    in medicine, 322
        metaphysics of, 332n.11
        philosophical obstacles to, 322–324
        practical obstacles to, 324–325
Secular rights-based judicial reasoning, 157–159, 161–163, 166
Self, conceptions of, 176, 177. *See also* Identities, personal
Self-control, chronic losses of. *See also* Addiction
    solution to, 419–420
Self-sufficiency, 122, 123, 126, 128, 131, 252
Sen, Amartya, 14, 121, 122, 126, 131n.1, 132n.15, 169, 175, 238
Separate spheres, 368
Severity of illness, 369
    severity, outcome, and a general theory of distribution, 377–381
Shalala, Donna, 346
Shared responsibility, 195
Short children, 10
Shue, Henry, 90–91
Sidgwick, Henry, 58
Siegler, Mark, 237
Silvers, Anita, 296–297
Singer, P., 144
Single persons, and contract pregnancy, 434–435
Single-payer insurance, 131
Smith, G. Davey, 170, 171
Smith, Tom, 240
Smoking, 416–417. *See also* Tobacco
Sobjectivity, 76n.4, 379

Social determinants of health, 5
impact of social structures, 46
inequalities and health, 12–13
social class and health outcomes, 170
and mortality rates, 170–172
social reality of health, 170, 177
socioeconomic gradient, 12, 14
Social justice, vi. *See also specific topics*
defined, vi
Social resource consumption, 417
Social Security, 109, 110, 116
Social unmooring, 126
Solidarity, 101, 184
Sore throat case, 379
Special Responsibility Principle, 124, 126
Specified Low-Income Beneficiary (SLMB), 115
Stability, 217–218
Stages of life, 9
"Stewardship," 393, 397
Stigma/stigmatization, 210
and access to health care, 255–256
and ethical validation of insurance disparities, 251–253
Substance abuse. *See* Drug abuse
Suffering, 446
Sufficiency, 140
Suicide, assisted. *See* Physician aid-in-dying
Summary measures of population health (SMPH), 394, 395, 399–401
unfair construction of, 395
Surgeon General. *See Mental Health*
Surrogate mothers. *See* Pregnancy, contract
Survival lottery, 58–59
Sweden. *See* Scandinavia
Sympathy, as grounding for justice, 261–262

Tandy, Beth, 162–164
Tay-Sachs, 454
Temkin, Larry, 364
Temporal neutrality, 377
Terminally ill, 149–150
Termination of treatment. *See* Discontinuing treatment
Thomas, Laurence, 218
Thomasma, David, 93
Threshold effect, 393
Threshold principle (TP), 139–140
Tobacco, 409. *See also* Smoking
Toebes, Brigit, 92–93
Tolerance, 318
Tooley, M., 440
Total dependence, 292
Total institutions, 294, 295
Trade-offs, 4, 68, 71–73
Tragic choices, 4, 65
Translation barriers, 31, 36n.9
Transplant centers, organ
small *vs.* larger, 355
expertise, 355
fairness, 356

research, 355–356
trust among, 353–355
Transplant organs, 4, 58–59, 89, 237, 345
Transplantation, organ. *See also* Liver allocation
goals for, 349
appropriate, 348–349
efficacy, 350–351
equity, 349–350
unsupported distinctions, 351–353
trust and, 347
caring and, 347–348
professional competence and, 347
respect for autonomy and, 348
Transplantation Ethics (Veatch), 353
Truman, Harry, 105
Trust, 194–195, 209, 347, 353–355. *See also* Distrust; Transplantation
Tuskegee Syphilis Study, 209, 216–217, 219
Two-person choice(s), 381–383
conflicts of urgency and outcome in, 385–386

Ultra vires, doctrine of, 159–160
Ulysses, 418–419, 423n.38
Ulysses Contract, 419–420
Uncertainty, 58–59
taking it seriously, 59–60
Unitary health-care system, 25, 31, 32, 35
United Kingdom, 82, 99. *See also* National Health Service
mortality by social class, 172
United Nations, 81
United Nations Charter, 89
United Network for Organ Sharing (UNOS), 316, 345, 346, 350–354, 357–359
United States, 102. *See also specific topics*
Universal access to services
in Australian health system, 178–180
economic obstacles to, 433
Universal Declaration of Human Rights, 84–85
Universal health insurance, 100, 102, 116
Universality, 134
of goodness, 58
Urgency/urgent, 8, 345, 350, 357, 370, 378
conflicts of outcome and, 385, 386
in a two-person choice, 385–386
and helping more people, 383–388
and the moderately ill, 388
two types of, 370
Urgent people, helping more, 386–388
Utilitarian approach to justice in health care, 53–54
QALYs as, 54–55
Utilitarian critiques of QALY model
liberal, 57–58
theological, 56–57
Utilitarian defense of QALY model, 55–56
Utilitarian framework, "liberal," 60
Utilitarian ideal, 4
Utilitarianism, 395, 407
act, 165
defined, 53

vs. egoism, 58
  problems with, 54
  theological, 56–57
"Utilitarianism of lives," 59
Utilitarians, 61–62
  and nonutilitarians, 62
  "skeptical," 62
Utility, 8, 53, 165. *See also* Efficacy
  social, 264–265
Utopian eugenics, 446

Vaccinations, mandatory, 418
Value, defined, 152
Veatch, Robert, 296, 297, 353
Veil of ignorance, 270
Virtue, 94
Volitional follow-through, 412
Voting Rights Act of 1965, 104
Vouchers, 43
Vulnerable persons and populations, 209, 211, 268,
  273–276. *See also* Mentally retarded persons

Waiting time (WT), 378
Wales, mortality by social class in, 172
Walzer, Michael, 188
Wednesbury, 160
Weighted beneficence, 365–367
Weighted-need principle, 138
Welfare, 48, 99. *See also* Equal Opportunity for
  Welfare
  equalizing, 238–239

Welfare legislation, 122–123
Welfare liberals, 421
Welfare model, intrinsic tensions in, 188–189
Welfare programs, 115, 123
Welfare right to health, 43
Welfare state, 185
Welfare theory, 144, 145
Welfarist health-care system, 213
Well-being, 92, 135
Whitlam, Gough, 179
Will, 412
Williams, Alan, 55
Willowbrook, 294, 299n.8
Women, 130, 209, 225, 229, 282, 430. *See also*
  Gender justice in health care; Reproductive
  freedom
  changing roles of, 127, 128
  empowerment of, 128, 232. *See also* Feminists
World Bank, 95n.2
World Health Organization (WHO), 78, 101, 390,
  399, 403. *See also* World Health Report
  2000
  assessment framework, 391–393, 399–400
    justice concerns about health-system
    performance assessment, 393–396
  justice concerns and the, 396–400
World Health Report 2000 (Report), 185–186, 192,
  317, 390–393, 396–398, 402
Worse off, 362, 365
  moral justifications of priority to the, 363–367
Worst off, 13, 368, 386–388